Management of Gender Dysphoria

Carlo Trombetta • Giovanni Liguori
Michele Bertolotto
Editors

Management of Gender Dysphoria

A Multidisciplinary Approach

Springer

Editors
Carlo Trombetta
Department of Urology
University of Trieste, Cattinara Hospital
Trieste
Italy

Michele Bertolotto
Department of Radiology
University of Trieste, Cattinara Hospital
Trieste
Italy

Giovanni Liguori
Department of Urology
University of Trieste, Cattinara Hospital
Trieste
Italy

ISBN 978-88-470-3939-1 ISBN 978-88-470-5696-1 (eBook)
DOI 10.1007/978-88-470-5696-1
Springer Milan Heidelberg New York Dordrecht London

Printed on acid-free paper

Springer is part of Springer Science+Business Media (www.springer.com)

To all those in the medical field whom have taken time to learn, to study, and to help and to all the patients, this book is dedicated to you

Contents

Part IV Legislative, Ethical and Health Policy Aspects

Abbreviations

2P-IPP	2 pieces inflatable penile prostheses
3P-IPP	3 pieces inflatable prostheses
ACMI	Arlington Community Media
AD or A.D.	Anno domini
AGIO	Atypical Gender Identity Organisation
aHR	Adjusted hazard ratios
AID	Artificial insemination by donor
AIDS	Acquired immunodeficiency syndrome
ALT	Anterolateral thigh flap
AMH	Anti-Mullerian hormone
AMS	American Medical Systems
APA	American Psychiatric Association
AQ	Autism Spectrum Quotient
ARs	Androgen receptors
ART	Antiretroviral therapy
ARTs	Assisted reproductive technologies
ASD	Autism spectrum disorders
BC	Before Christ
BCE	Bell Canada Enterprises
BDNF	Brain-derived neurotrophic factors
BMG	Buccal mucosa graft
BMI	Body mass index
BOO	Bladder outlet obstruction
BPH	Benign prostatic hyperplasia
BSPED	British Society of Paediatric Endocrinology and Diabetes
BSRI	Bem Sex Role Inventory
BSTc	Bed nucleus of the stria terminalis
CAMHS	Child and Adolescent Mental Health Service
CAPE-V	Consensus Auditory-Perceptual Evaluation of Voice
CDC	Centers for Disease Control and Prevention
Ch	Charrière
CHT	Cross-sex hormonal treatment
CI	Confidence interval
CPA	Cyproterone acetate
CPATH	Canadian Professional Association for Transgender Health
CT	Computed tomography
CVD	Cardiovascular diseases

CYP17	Cytochrome P450 17
DEXA	Dual-energy X-ray absorptiometry
DHEA	Dehydroepiandrosterone
DHHS	US Department of Health and Human Services
DNVB	Dorsal neurovascular bundle
DSD	Disorder of sex development
DSM	Diagnostic and Statistical Manual of Mental Disorders
DSM IV-TR	Diagnostic and Statistical Manual of Mental Disorders, 4th Edition, Text Rev.
DUS	Distal urethral sphincter
EBRT	External beam radiation therapy
ECG	Electrocardiography
EEG	Electroencephalography
ENIGI	European Network for the Investigation of Gender Incongruence
ERbeta	Estrogen receptor beta
ERs	Estrogen receptors
ESEMeD	European Study of the Epidemiology of Mental Disorders
F0	Fundamental frequency
FDA	Food and Drug Administration
Fig	Figure
fMRI	Functional magnetic resonance imaging
FTM	Female-to-male
FTMT	Female-to-male transsexuals
GCI	Gender-confirming interventions
GD	Gender dysphoria
GEI	Global Educational Initiative
GH	Growth hormone
GID	Gender identity disorder
GIDC	Gender identity disorder of childhood
GIDNOS	Gender identity disorder not otherwise specified
GIDS	Gender identity development service
GIRBAS	Grade, instability, roughness, breathiness, asthenia, and strain
GnRH	Gonadotropin-releasing hormone
GnRHa	Gonadotropin-releasing hormone analogue
GP	General practitioner
GRS	Gender/genital reassignment surgery
HAV	Hepatitis A virus
HBIGDA	Harry Benjamin International Gender Dysphoria Association
HBV	Hepatitis B virus
HCV	Hepatitis C virus
HCW	Heath-care workers
HDL	High-density lipoprotein cholesterol
HERS	Heart and Estrogen Replacement Study
HPV	Human papillomavirus
HRT	Hormonal therapy
HSV	Herpes simplex virus
ICD	International Classification of Diseases

ICSI	Intracytoplasmic sperm injection
IM or i.m.	Intramuscular
INAH3	Interstitial nucleus of the anterior hypothalamus
INF	Infundibular nucleus
IUI	Intrauterine inseminations
IVF	In vitro fertilisation
LCFA	Lateral circumflex femoral artery
LDL	Low-density lipoprotein cholesterol
LH	Luteinizing hormone
LM	Labia minora flap
LUT	Lower urinary tract
MDCT	Multidetector computed tomography
MINI-Plus	Mini International Neuropsychiatric Interview – Plus
MIP	Maximum intensity projection
MR	Magnetic resonance
MRI	magnetic resonance imaging
MSM	Men who have sex with men
MtF	Male-to-female
NAC	Nipple areola complex
NHS	National Health Service
NHSLS	National Health and Social Life Survey
NKB	Neurokinin B
nPEP	Non-occupational postexposure antiretroviral prophylaxis
NY	New York
OAB	Overactive bladder
OC	Osteocutaneous
OHSS	Ovarian hyperstimulation syndrome
PAHO	Pan American Health Organization
PCOS	Polycystic ovarian syndrome
PCP	Primary care providers
PDD	Pervasive developmental disorders
PDD-NOS	Pervasive developmental disorders–not otherwise specified
PET	Positron emission tomography
PGE	Prostaglandin
PH	Pubic hair
PrEP	Pre-exposure prophylaxis
PUS	Proximal urethral sphincter
QoL	Quality of life
RAFFF	Radial artery based forearm free flap
RAP	Radial artery phalloplasty
RFF	Radial forearm flap
RR	Relative risk
RV fistula	Recto-vaginal fistula
SCID-II	Structured Clinical Interview for DSM-IV Axis II Personality Disorders
SCIP	Superficial circumflex iliac perforator
SEP	Sensory evoked potentials
SICPRE	Società Italiana di Chirurgia Plastica Ricostruttiva ed Estetica

SMR	Standardized mortality ratio
SOC	Standards of care
SOM	Number of somatostatin
SRS	Sex reassignment surgery
SRY	Sex-determining region Y protein
SSI	Surgical site infection
STD	Sexually transmitted diseases
STSG	Split-thickness skin graft
SUI	Stress urinary incontinence
TDF	Testis-determining factor
TFL	Tensor fasciae latae
TRUS	Transrectal ultrasonography
TSE	Turbo spin echo
TSEQ	Transgender Self-Evaluation Questionnaire
UF	Ulnar forearm
UGDS	Utrecht Gender Dysphoria Scale
UI	Urge incontinence
UK	United Kingdom
UN	United Nations
UNAIDS	Joint United Nations Programme on HIV/AIDS
UPF	Urethral plate
US	United States
USA	United States of America
UTI(s)	Urinary tract infection (s)
V	Version
VAS	Visual analogue scale
VHI	Voice handicap index
VR	Volume rendering
VTE	Venous thromboembolism
WHO	World Health Organization
WPATH	World Professional Association for Transgender Health

Introduction: My Personal Experience Through the Years

1

Carlo Trombetta

Not often does it happen that once one decides to edit a book, the DSM changes the name of the matter of interest. The initial title of this book was *Management of Gender Disease* that was then changed to *Management of Gender Dysphoria* according to the new DSM V definition.

In this brief introduction, I will try to explain how I have arrived to this moment.

My initial knowledge of the 'problem' started in 1990 when I encountered my first patient, who at that time we called 'transsexual'. In that period at the Department of Urology of the University of Sassari, we had experience in operating children affected by 'male pseudohermaphroditism'. Surgery often consisted in creating a neo-vagina in little patients who presented external female aspect but in the complete absence of a vagina. As one can easily understand, it is very difficult to operate in such little space as there is the rectal-prostatic area especially in such small patients.

So I was very happy when 1 day, my teacher and chief, *Emanuele Belgrano*, told me we had to operate on a … 22-year-old patient. The surgical treatment was very similar, but in this case, he/she was a healthy biological male who wished to become a female. The surgery was easier, the result was satisfactory, but that day my life changed a lot.

C. Trombetta
Department of Urology, University of Trieste,
Cattinara Hospital, Trieste, Italy
e-mail: trombcar@units.it

I followed her medical history with particular care and interest, and I hope I am correct in stating that both changed each other's lives and careers for the better.

At the beginning, I thought I was enough to handle all that came along with these patients alone; I tried to follow the psychiatric-psychological part, the hormone therapy, and the follow-up (rehabilitation and physical therapy), but soon I realised that this was not the case.

My initial mistake was due to the fact that at that time, competent medical staff on this specific area of interest was scarce and scattered across Italy.

In 1994 when I arrived in Trieste, I organised myself better because I had the good fortune to meet doctors who accepted to become involved in my project:

- *Giovanni Liguori*, a young urologist who from the very beginning showed enthusiasm to partake in this field of surgery
- *Michele Bertolotto*, a curious and ambitious radiologist, incredibly competent in all areas of his specialty

In these years, I founded CeDIG (Centro per la diagnosi e la terapia dei Disturbi d'Identità e di Genere) the first Italian centre who wanted to deal with all the medical aspects and problems that are part of the lives of these patients.

The psycho-sexologists are the fulcrum of this venture: *Laura Scati* has followed more than 1,500 patients and starting from Trieste has created two other centres, in Pordenone and Genoa,

C. Trombetta et al. (eds.), *Management of Gender Dysphoria: A Multidisciplinary Approach*,
DOI 10.1007/978-88-470-5696-1_1, © Springer-Verlag Italia 2015

in order to help them all. When necessary, the help of *Elisabetta Pascolo Fabrici*, psychiatrist, is requested.

Bruno Fabris, an internal medicine specialist, developed a great experience in hormone treatment and took part in writing with us our first book in Italian, *Il Transessualismo: identificazione di un percorso diagnostico e terapeutico* (Kurtis ed., Milan, pgs: 1–374) in 1999.

Michele Pascone was a great plastic surgeon who operated with me on the first female-to-male patient with the cooperation of his young co-workers *Giovanni Papa* and *Vittorio Ramella*, who actively continue to cooperate with us, under the direction of *Zoran Arnez* actual head of the plastic surgery department of the University of Trieste.

Secondo Guaschino, gynaecologist, followed many female-to-male patients who underwent ovariectomy and hysterectomy, which sometimes took place at the same time of mastectomy and/or penile reconstruction.

Maria Assunta Cova, head of the radiology department of the University of Trieste, headed the world's first radiological evaluation of neo-vaginal width and depth in male-to-female patients by the use of the MR imaging.

Marina Bortul, general surgeon, applied with me for some laparoscopic techniques in those cases in which male-to-female patients needed to undergo re-surgery after partial atrophy of their initial neo-vagina.

CeDIG was officially presented in 2001 at our medical faculty meeting, and subsequently, the cooperation between all of us increased and widened to include other specialties.

On example, we learned the importance of having an infectious disease specialist: since 2010, *Roberto Luzzati*, and his co-workers, started to work with us, especially in the cases of HIV-positive patients.

Everybody knows that this topic, the management of GID, is particularly difficult and is an issue that can become overwhelming, and I have found in all of these people a great resource for reciprocal help; in particular in the operating room, we experimented this feeling when urologist, plastic surgeons and gynaecologists must work together for a common final result.

The anaesthesiology team has always actively participated in these surgeries; in particular, *Simonetta Fasiolo* has identified the importance of keeping liquids very low in male-to-female reassignment surgeries in order to prevent excessive swelling of the neo-labia in the immediate post-operative period. This precaution has avoided many post-op complications.

Throughout the years, starting in 2003, our nursing staff as well as the OR staff has organised several courses in order to better comprehend and therefore teach important aspects of how to interact with these patients, from how to greet them to how to teach them the physical rehabilitation.

Starting from the beginning of our experience, my co-worker and I contacted various important persons who have dealt with different aspects of the management of gender dysphoria:

- *Iole Baldaro-Verde* and her younger colleague *Alessandra Graziottin* (gynaecologist and sexologist) who wrote the first Italian book on transsexualism
- *Marten Perolino* who operated on the first Italian transsexual, in Turin
- *Sava Perovic* who came to Italy twice from Beograd (Serbia) and operated two female-to-male patients, who underwent clitoroplasty, with me

Another important international contact was established when I went to Ghent (Belgium) for a congress organised by the World Professional Association for Transgender Health (WPATH), formerly known as the Harry Benjamin International Gender Dysphoria Association (HBIGDA). WPATH is a well-known professional organisation devoted to transgender health.

Thanks to WPATH and ONIG (Osservatorio Nazionale di Identità e di Genere), the Italian national reference point, I was able to apply the international standards of care in all the procedures of CeDIG.

Every time I organise a 'little' congress or meeting on this topic, I find how important it is to speak about these issues. At the end of these meetings, my colleagues often tell me they have learned a great deal of things. Moreover, every time we have involved in this organisation the patient and their associations (such as the LGBT community), the final result has been even greater.

I know that it is difficult to organise new initiatives because the costs are not covered by pharmaceutical industries, who have little interest in this field; for this reason, this particular aspect of medicine needs to be properly inserted in the more important congresses of the scientific society.

Since my effort during the last 15 years, EAU, ESGURS, SIU and SIA have dedicated congressional sessions and work groups to this topic.

Unfortunately, this area of medicine is not given scientific importance due to the fact that nowadays it is still a relatively small reality and thus the research on it has not given much scientific weight. Every time I tell one of my young co-workers to publish a paper on this topic, I perfectly know that if he spent the same amount of time and energy publishing something on prostate or urological cancer, surely his impact factor would be much higher. We are still far from being able to change this way of thinking, but it is a change that needs to happen because the more attention we bring to this field of interest, the better it will be for these patients.

A great part of my life in the last 20 years has been dedicated to:

- These persons that often I continue to call 'patients'… sometimes friends
- Connecting patients with the correct medical doctors who can help him/her
- Informing patients of the existence of self-help groups
- Informing different colleagues on this topic and the correct way of dealing with our patients
- Coordinating the work of lawyers, medical doctors and psychologists

I graduated from medical school in 1981 with full grades, and some time ago, I was curious to see what I had done in school with regard to gender dysphoria. I went back and looked through my books and unfortunately was not surprised in seeing that little to no information was given on what at that time was called 'transsexualism'.

Starting from this observation, I decided to change this and nowadays:

- Our medical students at the University of Trieste learn different aspects of the management of gender dysphoria during psychiatry, urology, andrology, plastic surgery and endocrinology lessons.
- Our residents in Urology, during their 5-year formation period, follow more than 80 patients after different sex reassignment surgeries (MtoF and FtoM). Residents are directly involved in at least 35 operations and often perform as first surgeon a part of the male-to-female surgeries.
- As of 2008, I have organised a postgraduate surgical master's programme available to both residents and specialists, dedicated to gender dysphoria. Every year, three to four doctors learn in depth how to deal with male-to-female and female-to-male patients and often decide to continue this interest in their hospitals.

To all those in the medical field whom have taken time to learn, to study, and to help and to all the patients, this book is dedicated to you.

To those who are interested in the scientific work on gender dysphoria by Prof. Trombetta and co-workers, a list of readings and congress lectures follows.

Pseudoermafroditismo maschile con persistenza delle strutture mulleriane: descrizione di un caso.

E. Belgrano, C. Trombetta, U. Repetto, P. Pittaluga, A.F.De Rose, L. Giuliani.

Atti 58° Congr. S.I.U.- Roma, 25–28 settembre 1985.

Acta Urol. Ital. 1986; 429–433

Persistenza delle strutture mulleriane: descrizione di un caso.

E. Belgrano, U. Repetto, C. Trombetta, S. Siracusano, W. Bozzo, P. Pittaluga.

Rassegna Italiana di Chirurgia Pediatrica – 1986: Vol. XXVIII, 2;120–123

Hernia uteri inguinalis : un caso particolare di pseudoermafroditismo maschile.

C. Trombetta, S. Siracusano, M. Gabriele, E. Belgrano.

Atti 5° Corso Agg. Androl. di interesse chir.- Fiuggi Terme, 27–28 giugno 1988.

"Andrologia Chirurgica in Età Pediatrica" Acta Medica 1989; 77–82

Creazione di neovagina in due casi di pseudoermafroditismo.

E. Belgrano, C. Trombetta, S. Siracusano, S.Desole.

63° Congr. S.I.U. (Società Italiana di Urologia) – Ancona, 9–12 settembre 1990

Creazione di una neovagina in caso di pseudoermafroditismo: presentazione di due soluzioni tecniche.

C. Trombetta, S. Siracusano, S. Desole, G. Foddis, V. Usai, E. Belgrano.

Atti 40° Convegno S.U.I.C.M.I.- Alghero, 23–25 maggio 1991.

Acta Urol. Ital. 1992; (suppl. 5); 231–234.

La minilaparoscopia nella chirurgia del transessualismo.

E. Belgrano, S. De Stefani, C. Trombetta, M. Raber, G. Savoca, U. Moro.

68° Congr. S.I.U. (Società Italiana di Urologia) - Roma, 2–5 luglio 1995.

9° Congr. S.I.A. (Società Italiana di Andrologia) Ancona, 14–16 settembre 1995.

44° Conv. S.U.N.I. (Società degli Urologi del Nord Italia) Loano (SV), 5–7 ottobre 1995.

Conv.Naz. "Gender Identity Disorder" – Roma, 16–18 novembre 1995.

Creazione di neovagina: presentazione di due soluzioni tecniche.

G. Savoca, C. Trombetta, S. De Stefani, M. Raber, S. Siracusano, E. Belgrano.

Atti 9° Congr. S.I.A. - Ancona, 14–16 settembre 1995.

"Andrologia '95" Monduzzi Ed.; 321–324.

Stati intersessuali.

C. Trombetta, E. Belgrano.

in Trattato di Urologia a cura di M. Pavone Macaluso. UTET - Firenze 1995; 914–929

Applicazioni intraoperatorie degli ultrasuoni in urologia.

C. Trombetta.

IPSEN Ed. 1995; 1–132

Microlaparoscopy In Sex Reassignment Surgery.

S. De Stefani, C. Trombetta, M. Raber, G. Savoca, U. Moro, E. Belgrano.

Digital Urology Journal; 1996 (http://www.duj.com/Article/DeStefani.html).

Microlaparoscopy in sex reassignment male to female surgery.

E. Belgrano, C. Trombetta, S. De Stefani, G. Savoca, M. Raber, G. Liguori.

15th World Congress of Endourology and SWL,. 13th Basic Research Symposium; Edinburgh (UK). August 31-September 3, 1997. J. Endourol., vol. 11 (suppl. 1), 1997; pag. 80

Falloplastica in tempo unico in caso di transessualismo gino-androide: caso clinico e revisione della letteratura.

C. Trombetta, G. Liguori, G. Savoca, L. Buttazzi, M. Pascone, A. Ortensi, E. Belgrano.

71° Congresso Nazionale S.I.U – Torino, 21–24 giugno 1998.

Sex reassignment surgery: Female-to-Male transsexual operation.

C. Trombetta, G. Liguori, L. Buttazzi, E. Belgrano.

eUROtraining. International Symposium on Update on Pelvic Surgery Genova, 5–7 novembre 1998

Sex reassignment surgery: Male-to-Female transsexual operation.

C. Trombetta, L. Buttazzi, G. Liguori, E. Belgrano.

eUROtraining. International Symposium on Update on Pelvic Surgery Genova, 5–7 novembre 1998.

One-stage sex reassignment surgery in female-to-male transsexuals.

E. Belgrano, C.Trombetta, G. Liguori, G. Savoca, M. Raber, M. Pascone, A. Ortensi.

2nd Meeting of the European Society for Impotence Research (ESIR).

October 1–4, 1998, Madrid (Spain). Abstract Book, pag. 56, 1998

Utilizzo della mucosa buccale in caso di stenosi della neo-uretra dopo falloplastica sec. Chang.

G. Liguori, G. De Giorgi, G. Savoca, S. Ciampalini, S. Siracusano, C. Trombetta, E. Belgrano.

XII Congresso Nazionale S.I.A. – Copanello (CZ), 9–12 giugno 1999.

Ripresa dell'attività sessuale dopo intervento di conversione andro-ginoide: valutazione mediante questionario.

L. Buttazzi, F. Plaino, G. Liguori, G. Savoca, G. Silvestre, B. Fabris, M. F. Cavallino, C. Trombetta, E. Belgrano.
XII Congresso Nazionale S.I.A. – Copanello (CZ), 9–12 giugno 1999

Il Transessualismo: identificazione di un percorso diagnostico e terapeutico.
E. Belgrano, B. Fabris, C.Trombetta.
Kurtis Editrice, Milano 1999; pag. 1–374.

L'attività' sessuale dopo intervento di conversione andro-ginoide: nostra esperienza e revisione della letteratura
L. Buttazzi, F. Plaino, G. Liguori, G. Savoca, B. Fabris, M.F. Cavallino, C. Trombetta
Atti del 72° Congresso della Società Italiana di Urologia (S.I.U.); Roma, 20–23 giugno 1999;
Acta Urol. Ital., Vol. XIII (2), Suppl., 1999; p. 147–148.

Complicanze dopo intervento di conversione andro-ginoide e loro prevenzione: come trattarle e
come prevenirle
C. Trombetta, G. Liguori, L. Buttazzi, S. Siracusano, E. Belgrano
Atti del 72° Congresso della Società Italiana di Urologia (S.I.U.); Roma, 20–23 giugno 1999;
Acta Urol. Ital., Vol. XIII (2), Suppl., 1999; p. 148–149.

Surgical treatment of male-to-female transsexual patients: our experience.
C. Trombetta, G. Liguori, L. Buttazzi, E. Belgrano.
9° Congresso A.I.U.G. (Associazione Italiana di Urologia Ginecologica e del Piano Pelvico). Milano, 25–27 novembre 1999. Supplemento a: Urogynaecologia International Journal 1998, Vol. 12bis n°3, pag 182–85.

La riconfigurazione dei caratteri sessuali (RCS) nel transessualismo andro-ginoide: 2 tecniche a confronto
G. Liguori, L. Buttazzi, C. Trombetta, I. Gattuccio, S. Siracusano, E. Belgrano
Atti del 72° Congresso della Società Italiana di Urologia (S.I.U.); Roma, 20–23 giugno 1999;
Acta Urol. Ital., Vol. XIII (2), Suppl., 1999; p. 148

Nostra esperienza nella riconfigurazione dei caratteri sessuali (RCS) in caso di transessualismo androginoide
G. Liguori, L. Buttazzi, C. Trombetta, I. Gattuccio, S. Siracusano, G. Silvestre, E. Belgrano
Atti del XII Congresso Nazionale della Società Italiana di Andrologia (S.I.A.); Copanello (Cz), 9–12 giugno 1999. Giornale Italiano di Andrologia, vol. 6, (no 1) 1999, pag. 89

Transessualismo e sindrome di Klinefelter: considerazioni su un caso clinico.
G. Liguori, F. Gattuccio, C. Trombetta, V. Pelice, A. Amoroso, E. Belgrano.
XII Congresso Nazionale S.I.A. – Copanello (CZ), 9–12 giugno 1999.

Uretroplastica con lembo della mucosa buccale in caso di stenosi neo-uretra dopo falloplastica sec. Chang.
G. Liguori, G. De Giorgi, G. Savoca, S. Ciampalini, S. Siracusano, C. Trombetta, E. Belgrano.
72° Congresso Nazionale S.I.A – Roma, 20–23 giugno 1999.

Condilomatosi uretrale e vaginale in un transessuale maschio HIV positivo sottoposto ad intervento di riconfigurazione dei caratteri sessuali: caso clinico e revisione della letteratura
G. Liguori, C. Trombetta, L. Buttazzi, S. Bucci, E. Belgrano
Atti del 73° Congresso della Società Italiana di Urologia (S.I.U.); Bologna, 28–31 maggio 2000;
Abstract Book; p. 116.
Atti V Giornate Andrologiche Italiane; Firenze, 15–17 ottobre 2000.
Giornale Italiano di Andrologia vol. 7, (no 1) 2000, pag. 37

Peritonite acuta da perforazione di abnorme neovagina stenotizzata in un maschio transessuale
G. Liguori, C. Trombetta, S. Bucci, L. Buttazzi, D. Ricci, E. Belgrano
Atti del 73° Congresso della Società Italiana di Urologia (S.I.U.); Bologna, 28–31 maggio 2000;
Abstract Book; p. 116

Creazione del cappuccio neoclitorideo nei transessuali androginoidi: note di tecnica
G. Liguori, C. Trombetta, S. Bucci, L. Buttazzi, D. Ricci, E. Belgrano

Atti del 49° Congresso della Società Italiana degli Urologi del Nord Italia (S.U.N.I.); Brescia, 21–23 settembre 2000,
Urologia (Abstract Book), p18.

Valutazione mediante questionario e biotesiometria dopo intervento di conversione androginoide
L. Buttazzi, F. Plaino, G. Liguori, S. Bucci, D. Paolinelli, C. Trombetta, E. Belgrano
Atti V Giornate Andrologiche Italiane; Firenze, 15–17 ottobre 2000.
Giornale Italiano di Andrologia vol. 7, (n° 1) 2000, pag. 70.

Dettagli tecnici nella terapia chirurgica dei disturbi dell'identita' di genere mediante riconfigurazione dei caratteri sessuali
G. Liguori, C. Trombetta, S. Bucci, L. Buttazzi, D. Ricci, E. Belgrano
Atti V Giornate Andrologiche Italiane; Firenze, 15–17 ottobre 2000.
Giornale Italiano di Andrologia vol. 7, (no 1) 2000, pag. 71.

Creazione di neoclitoride sensibile in corso di intervento di conversione androginoide: nostra esperienza
L. Buttazzi, F. Plaino, G. Liguori, S. Bucci, G. Savoca, C. Trombetta
Atti del 73° Congresso della Società Italiana di Urologia (S.I.U.); Bologna, 28–31 maggio 2000;
Abstract Book; p. 117.

Treatment of strictures of the neo-urethra after phalloplasty according to chang technique.
C. Trombetta, G. Liguori, G. De Giorgi, L. Buttazzi, M. Pascone, E. Belgrano.
XXV World Congress of the Societe Internationale d'Urologie; Singapore
British Journal of Urology Int. 2000; 86 (suppl. 3): 197–8

Our technique for treatment of male-to-female transsexual patients.
C. Trombetta, G. Liguori, L. Buttazzi, S. Bucci, E. Belgrano.
XXV World Congress of the Societe Internationale d'Urologie; Singapore
British Journal of Urology Int. 2000; 86 (suppl. 3): 202

Il lembo fasciocutaneo radiale dell'avambraccio ed il lembo miocutaneo di muscolo gracile in chirurgia urologica: cenni di anatomia chirurgica e modalità di prelievo
S. de Stefani, G. Liguori, S. Ciampalini, C. Trombetta, M. Pascone, M. Bertolotto, E. Belgrano
Archivio Italiano di Urologia Andrologia; 72 (2): 37–43, 2000 (Milano; Italia).

L'importanza dell'accuratezza dei tempi demolitivi negli interventi di conversione andro-ginoide
G. Liguori, C. Trombetta, L. Buttazzi, S. Bucci, D. Ricci, D. Paolinelli, E. Belgrano
Atti del 74° Congresso della Società Italiana di Urologia (S.I.U.); Cagliari, 9–12 maggio 2001;
Abstract Book; p. 180

Riconfigurazione chirurgica dei caratteri sessuali (RCS) in senso gino-androide in tempo unico:
tecnica e follow up a tre anni
G. Liguori, C. Trombetta, L. Buttazzi, S. Bucci, D. Ricci, D. Paolinelli, M. Pascone, E. Belgrano
Atti del 74° Congresso della Società Italiana di Urologia (S.I.U.); Cagliari, 9–12 maggio 2001;
Abstract Book; p. 179

Aspetti chirurgici nella conversione andro-ginoide
C. Trombetta, L. Buttazzi, G. Liguori, S. Bucci, E. Belgrano
25° Congresso Nazionale del Centro Italiano di Sessuologia (CIS), San donà di Piave 28–29
ottobre 2000.
Rivista di Sessuologia, 25 (2): 130–137, 2001.

Valutazione della sensibilità del neoclitoride in seguito ad intervento di conversione androginoide
L. Buttazzi, C. Trombetta, G. Liguori, S. Bucci, E. Belgrano
Atti del 74° Congresso della Società Italiana di Urologia (S.I.U.); Cagliari, 9–12 maggio 2001;
Abstract Book; pag. 40–41.

Acute peritonitis due to introital stenosis and perforation of a bowel neovagina in a transsexual.
G. Liguori, C. Trombetta, L. Buttazzi, E. Belgrano
Obstetrics & Gynecology, 97 (5): 828–829, 2001 (USA).

Trattamento chirurgico dei D.I.G. riconfigurazione chirurgica dei caratteri sessuali (RCS) in senso gino-androide in tempo unico
G. Liguori, C. Trombetta, L. Buttazzi, S. Bucci, D. Ricci, S. Ciciliato, M. Pascone, G. Papa, E. Belgrano
Atti del XVII Congresso Nazionale della Società Italiana di Andrologia (S.I.A.); Venezia, 5–8 Dicembre 2001.
Giornale Italiano di Andrologia, vol. 8, (no 3) 2001, pag. 60.

Trattamento chirurgico dei D.I.G. androginoidi: utilita' della resezione completa dell'apice dei corpi cavernosi
G. Liguori, C. Trombetta, L. Buttazzi, S. Bucci, D. Ricci, S. Ciciliato, E. Belgrano
Atti del XVII Congresso Nazionale della Società Italiana di Andrologia (S.I.A.); Venezia, 5–8 dicembre 2001.
Giornale Italiano di Andrologia, vol. 8, (no 3) 2001, pag. 60.

Ottimizzazione dei tempi operatori della conversione androginoide
L. Buttazzi, G. Liguori, S. Bucci, S. Ciciliato, C. Trombetta
Atti del XVII Congresso Nazionale della Società Italiana di Andrologia (S.I.A.); Venezia, 5–8 Dicembre 2001.
Giornale Italiano di Andrologia, vol. 8, (no 3) 2001, pag. 61.
International Journal of Impotence Research, vol. 13 (suppl. 4), pag. 23, 2001.

Risonanza magnetica dopo riconfigurazione androginoide dei caratteri sessuali
C. Trombetta, G. Liguori, L. Buttazzi, S. Bucci, M. Cova, R. Pozzi-Mucelli, E. Belgrano
Atti del XVII Congresso Nazionale della Società Italiana di Andrologia (S.I.A.); Venezia, 5–8 dicembre 2001.
Giornale Italiano di Andrologia, vol. 8, (no 3) 2001, pag. 61

Male-to-female sex reassignment surgery (SRS): technique and functional outcome
C. Trombetta, G. Liguori, L. Buttazzi, S. Bucci, E. Belgrano
4th Biennal Congress of the European Society for Sexual and Impotence Research (ESSIR); 30th September – 3rd October, 2001; Rome, (Italy).

One stage sex reassignment surgery in female-to-male transsexuals
C. Trombetta, G. Liguori, L. Buttazzi, S. Bucci, M. Pascone, E. Belgrano
4th Biennal Congress of the European Society for Sexual and Impotence Research (ESSIR); 30th September - 3rd October, 2001; Rome, (Italy).

Trattamento chirurgico del transessualismo androginoide: note di tecnica, risultati e follow-up.
C. Trombetta, G. Liguori, L. Buttazzi, S. Bucci, S. Ciciliato, R. Rinaldi, B. Fabris, E. Belgrano.
G.I.A. – Giornale Italiano di Andrologia; Vol. 8 (1–2): 24–30, 2001

Aspetti chirurgici nella conversione andro-ginoide
C. Trombetta, L. Buttazzi, G. Liguori, S. Bucci, E. Belgrano
Rivista di Sessuologia, 25 (2): 130–137, 2001

Correzione chirurgica secondaria dopo vaginoplastica nel transessualismo andro-ginoide
(G. Liguori, S. Bucci, L. Buttazzi, S. Ciciliato, M. Pascone, ed E. Belgrano).
Atti del 75° Congresso Nazionale della società italiana di Urologia (S.I.U.), Bologna 15–19 Maggio 2002

Total sex reassignment surgery in female-to-male transsexuals: a one stage technique
C. Trombetta, G. Liguori, M. Pascone, S. Bucci, S. Guaschino, G. Papa, E. Belgrano
Br. J. Urol, 90 (07), 754–7 2002

Male-to-female sex reassignment surgery (SRS): urological technique
C. Trombetta, G. Liguori, L. Buttazzi, S. Bucci, E. Belgrano
100th AUA Orlando 25–30 Maggio 2002 – J. Urol. 167, 4 (suppl): 149 (abstract no 597)

Value of magnetic resonance imaging (MRI) in the valuation of sex reassignment surgery in male-to-female transsexuals
M. Cova, E. Mosconi, G. Liguori, C. Trombetta, E. Belgrano, R. Pozzi-Mucelli
XI European Symposium Urogenital Radiology e XXVIII Scientific Assembly of the Society of

Uroradiology (ESUR); Genova 15–20 Giugno. (Italy). European Radiology, vol 12: D14, 2002 (I premio Poster)

La femminilizzazione dei genitali esterni e la creazione della neovagina

C. Trombetta, G. Liguori, L. Buttazzi, S. Bucci, S. Ciciliato, E. Belgrano

In: D. Nadalin e P. Stella, Transiti: percorsi e significati dell'identità di genere

Servizio Stampa e Informazione della Giunta Regionale Regione Emilia Romagna; Bologna,

Giugno 2002; pag. 111–118

Male-to-female sex reassignment surgery: urological techniques

C. Trombetta, G. Liguori, L. Buttazzi, S. Bucci, E. Belgrano

97° Annual Meeting of the American Urological Association (AUA), Orlando (Florida-USA),

May 25–30, 2002. Journal of Urology, vol 167 (n. 4), pag. 149, 2002

Le complicanze: il parere dell'urologo

C. Trombetta, G. Liguori, L. Buttazzi, S. Bucci, S. Ciciliato, E. Belgrano

In: D. Nadalin e P. Stella, Transiti: percorsi e significati dell'identità di genere

Servizio Stampa e Informazione della Giunta Regionale Regione Emilia Romagna; Bologna,

Giugno 2002; pag. 130–134

Riassegnazione chirurgica dei caratteri sessuali in senso andro-ginoide

G. Liguori, C. Trombetta, S. Bucci, L. Salamè, E. Belgrano

76° Congresso nazionale della Società Italiana di Urologia (SIU); Firenze, 14–18 Giugno 2003

Il trattamento chirurgico del disturbo di identità di genere andro-ginoide: note di tecnica

G. Liguori, C. Trombetta, S. Bucci, L. Salamè, E. Belgrano

20° Congresso Nazionale della Società Italiana di Andrologia (SIA); Capri, 25–28 Ottobre 2003

Value of magnetic resonance imaging (MRI) in the evaluation of sex reassignment surgery In male-to-female transsexuals

M. Cova, E. Mosconi, G. Liguori, E. Belgrano, R. Pozzi-Mucelli

Abdom Imaging. 2003 Sep-Oct;28(5): 782–32

Surgical therapy in transsexual patient: a multidisciplinary approach

C. Trombetta, G. Liguori, S. Bucci, E. Belgrano

18° Congress of the European Association of Urology; Madrid (Spagna) March 12–15, 2003.

European Urology, vol. 2, no 1, pag. 97, 2003

Imaging in sexual and gender disorders

C. Trombetta, G. Liguori, S. Bucci, L. Salamè, M. Cova, E. Belgrano

V Congress on therapy in Andrology; Pisa; 24–27 Marzo 2003

Le complicanze degli interventi di conversione andro-ginoide

Trombetta C.

Scripta Medica vol 6 n 8, 2003

Riassegnazione chirurgica dei caratteri sessuali in transessuale sottopostosi ad emasculazione: tecnica originale

G. Liguori, C. Trombetta, S. Bucci, L. Salamè, E. Belgrano

20° Congresso Nazionale della Società Italiana di Andrologia (SIA); Capri, 25–28 Ottobre 2003

77° Congresso nazionale della Società Italiana di Urologia (SIU); Milano, 19–23 Giugno 2004

Tecniche di falloplastica: nostra esperienza

C. Trombetta, G. Liguori, S. Bucci, L. Salamè, G. Garaffa, S. Guaschino, M. Pascone, S. Perovic, E. Belgrano

21° Congresso Nazionale della Società Italiana di Andrologia (SIA); Trieste, 23–26 Settembre 2004

Trattamento laparoscopico delle complicanze tardive dopo vaginoplastica

E. Belgrano, G. Liguori, C. Trombetta, S. Bucci, L. Salamè, G. Garaffa, M. Bortul

Atti del 77° Congresso dlla Società Italiana di Urologia (S.I.U.); Milano, 19–23 Luglio 2004

Condylomata acuminata of the neovagina in a HIV seropositive male-to-female transsexual

G. Liguori, C. Trombetta, S. Bucci, F. De Seta, D. De Santo, S. Siracusano, E. Belgrano

Urol Int. 2004;73(1):87–8

Radiological evaluation of vaginal width and depth in male-to-female transsexuals by the use of magnetic resonance imaging

C. Trombetta, G. Liguori, S. Bucci, L. Salame, G. Garaffa, M. Cova, E. Belgrano
World J Urol. 2004 Aug 18

Male-To-Female surgery for transsexual individuals
C. Trombetta, E. Belgrano
ANIR 6(4) 190–192, 2004

La falloplastica nel disturbo di identità di genere andro-ginoide
C. Trombetta, G. Liguori, S. Bucci, L. Salamè, A. Amodeo, M. Favero, E. Belgrano
22° Congresso Nazionale della Società Italiana di Andrologia (SIA); Sassari, 1–4 Ottobre 2005

Transverse retubularized ileal Vaginoplasty: a new application of the Monti principle –
Preliminary report
C. Trombetta, G. Liguori, S. Siracusano, M. Bortul, E. Belgrano
Eu Urol 48 (2005) 1018–1024

Neo urethral reconstruction in Pryor phalloplasty for sex reassignment surgery: notes of techniques
G. Garaffa, G. Liguori, S. Bucci, E. Belgrano, C. Trombetta
8th Congress of the European Society for Sexual Medicine; London 2005

Laparoscopic mobilization of neovagina to assist secondary ileal vaginoplasty in male-to-female
Transsexuals
G. Liguori, C. Trombetta, S. Bucci, L. Salame, M. Bortul, M. Cova, S. Siracusano, E. Belgrano
Urology. 2005 Aug; 66(2):293–8; discussion 298

La riconfigurazione chirurgica dei caratteri sessuali in senso andro-ginoide
C. Trombetta, G. Liguori, S. Bucci, E. Belgrano
In D. Dettore Disturbo di identità di genere, diagnosi, eziologia, trattamento
Ed. McGraw-Hill. 309–319, 2005

Segnalazione di due casi di tumore del testicolo e di due linfomi in pazienti con disturbi di identità di genere
S. Bucci, G. Liguori, F. Favero, E. Belgrano, C. Meriggiola, A. Godano, C. Trombetta
79th Congresso della Società Italiana di Urologia (S.I.U.); Bologna, 17–21 giugno 2006

Valutazione della qualità della vita prima e dopo l'intervento di riconversione chirurgica nei pazienti affetti da disturbi d'identità di genere (DIG)
Trombetta C., Scati L.
Urologia Vol 73 N4 n2 2007, 6–10

Terapia chirurgica del transessualismo femmina-maschio
E. Belgrano, S. Bucci, G. Liguori, C. Trombetta
In: Sessuologia Medica a cura di Jannini E, Lenzi A, Maggi M
Ed. Elsevier Masson 2007
Male to Female sex reassignment surgery
C. Trombetta
9TH Congress of the European Federation of Sexology, 13–17 Aprile 2008, Roma

Disturbi del basso tratto urinario dopo riassegnazione chirurgica dei caratteri sessuali nel disturbo di genere androginoide
G. Liguori, C. Trombetta, M.D. Perrone, L. Scati, E. Belgrano
58° Congresso della Società Urologica del Nord Italia (SUNI); 28-29-30 Maggio 2009, Udine

Violenza, discriminazione e salute mentale in un campione di pazienti transessuali
G. Gerini, F. Giaretton, C. Trombetta, P. Romito
Riv. Sessuol. – Vol. 33 n. 4; Ottobre/Dicembre 2009

Evoluzione della tecnica di adeguamento dei caratteri sessuali in senso andro-ginoide: contributi originali
C. Trombetta
XXVI Congresso Nazionale della Società Italiana di Andrologia, 25–27 Novembre 2010

Riassegnazione chirurgica dei caratteri sessuali in senso androginoide. Note di tecnica: la neouretroclitoroplastica (video)
C. Trombetta, M. Petrovic, G. Liguori, S. Bucci, S. Benvenuto, G. Mazzon, G. Ollandini, R. Napoli, B. De Concilio, E. Belgrano
XXVII Congresso Nazionale SIA, Fiuggi, 2–5 Novembre 2011

Update in male to female surgery
E. Belgrano
Consiglio Nazionale delle Ricerche; Pisa, Ottobre 11–12 2012

Round table: What's in and what's new in 7 Italian centers
C. Trombetta

Consiglio Nazionale delle Ricerche; Pisa, Ottobre 11–12 2012

Neourethroclitoroplasty in male to female transsexual patients

C. Trombetta

Mediterranean Andrological Board, 15–16 Giugno 2012, Catania

Psychological, medical and surgical management in gender identity disorder. An international highlight

C. Trombetta

First Transsexualism European Meeting, 17–18 Maggio 2012, Torino

Urinary tract symptoms after MtoF sexual reassignment surgery (poster)

G. Ollandini, G. Mazzon, G. Liguori, S. Benvenuto, S. Bucci, B. De Concilio, G. Morelli, R. Pagni, C. Mariani, R. Napoli, E. Belgrano, N. Pavan, A. Morelli, P. Umari, M. Rizzo, C.Trombetta

36° Congresso Nazionale SIUD, 24-25-26 Maggio, Firenze 2012

La valutazione dell'outcome chirurgico

C. Trombetta

Master universitario di II° livello in Sessuologia Clinica, 20 Aprile 2013, Pisa

Personality profile assessment in patients with gender identity disorder

F. Sandri, F. Fiorindo, E. Pascolo Fabrici, S. Nastasich, C. Trombetta

Convegno ONIG, Lisbona 2013

Penile Prosthesis Implantation In Female To Male Transsexual

G. Liguori, N. Pavan, P. Umari, M. Bertolotto, S. Bucci, E. Belgrano, C. Trombetta

Presented video at AUA – San Diego, CA, May 4–8, 2013.

A New Technique For Sex Gender Reassignment Surgery: The Neourethroclitoroplasty

Trombetta C., Liguori G., Benvenuto S., Napoli R., Umari P., Rizzo M., Petrovic M., Pavan N.

J. Urol., Vol. 189, Issue 4, e685 poster presentation at AUA – San Diego, CA, May 4–8, 2013.

Use Of Bowel For Vaginoplasty In Male To Female Transsexual

Trombetta C., Imbimbo C., Liguori G., Verze P., Pavan N., Mirone V.

AUA – Orlando (FL) May 16–21, 2014 (presented videotape)

Neovaginal Prolapse in Male-to-Female Transsexuals: An 18-Year-Long Experience.

Bucci S, Mazzon G, Liguori G, Napoli R, Pavan N, Bormioli S, Ollandini G, De Concilio B, Trombetta C.

Biomed Res Int. 2014;2014:240761. doi: 10.1155/2014/240761. Epub 2014 May 7. PMID: 24895556

Part I

General Aspects

Sexual Ambiguity: Development of Judgement and Evaluation Criteria over the Centuries

2

Domenico Rosselli

Sexual ambiguity has always interested human beings and has taken on very different meanings over different periods according to cultural changes, moral principles and religious ethics. It has inspired beliefs, tales of mythology, exquisite works of art and impassioned verses. Later, the topic was mulled over by philosophers, naturalists and legal experts followed, in modern times, by endocrinologists, sexologists, psychologists and surgeons, although the concept of hermaphroditism, pseudohermaphroditism and homosexuality long remained confused. The literature on the subject is therefore characterised by substantial shifts.

In ancient times, fascinating legends and myths were offset by the realistic views and medicolegal principles set forth in Talmudic and Roman law texts and the thoughts of Greek philosophers. The ethical, religious and legal issues raised at a later stage, though often contradictory and confusing in their interpretation, nevertheless revealed an attempt at scientific investigation. As research progressed and scientific concepts were rationalised, the subject was mainly dealt with from a medical angle, opening the door to our present-day judgement and evaluation criteria. The outcome has been the emergence of an intersexual being, with normal opposing male and female traits and a gender identity that is no longer forced to suffocate and conceal itself.

This chapter has been translated with permission from Kurtis Editore srl. Original publication: L'ambiguità sessuale: evoluzione nei secoli dei criteri di giudizio e valutazione, in "Il Transessualismo", 1999, E. Belgrano, B. Fabris, C. Trombetta, ISBN 978-88-85030-33-5

D. Rosselli
Plastic Surgery, Bordighera-Milan IT,
Bordighera, Italy

2.1 Summary of Historical Research

2.1.1 Ancient Period

Sexual ambiguity has been the subject of religious beliefs since the most remote times: one clear example is Astarte, the hermaphrodite moon goddess, worshipped by the Neo-Babylonian and Egyptian peoples, as well as the bearded Venus of the ancient Cypriots. This concept spread to Greece towards the end of the tenth century BC, with grotesque figures transformed into classically accepted male and female forms of beauty, such as the hermaphrodite of Polykleitos (fourth century BC), the "Mirecourt" hermaphrodite (second century BC), the sleeping hermaphrodite (second century BC) and the bathing hermaphrodite, kept in the Museum of Naples (Kylices of the fifth century BC).

Mythology includes a wealth of references to the subject and inspired the poets Hesiod, Horace, Martial and Lucretius, who all wrote passages referring to such legends. Ausonius (epigraph LXIX, C and CI) provided the most comprehensive descriptions of this disorder. Ovid wrote impassioned verses referring to the fable of Salmacis, who was madly in love with Hermaphroditus, son

C. Trombetta et al. (eds.), *Management of Gender Dysphoria: A Multidisciplinary Approach*,
DOI 10.1007/978-88-470-5696-1_2, © Springer-Verlag Italia 2015

of Hermes and Aphrodite and, due to her inability to seduce him, successfully appealed to the gods to join them eternally to form a single male and female body (*Metamorphosis*, book IV).

Among the philosophers, naturalists and historians, mention must be made of Aristotle (*De generatione animalium* – Latin translation) who observed the anomaly in sheep, while Plato, who referred to a case of hermaphroditism in humans, considered that this must have been the condition of the first living beings. In his *Histories*, Herodotus harks back to the "female sickness" of the Scythians, of which Hippocrates provides a scientific explanation in his work *On Airs, Waters and Places*. Strabone in *Geography* and Pliny in *Historia mundi* also provide explanations of the origin of the term. The interest of legal experts was present from ancient times: the topic was dealt with on a legal level in Talmudic writings, when it was strictly related to religious ethics, considering four types of androgyny: male, female, male–female and neither man nor woman. Rules of living were laid down for each one, with severe penalties for transgressors.

In the *Roman Digest*, sexual ambiguity crops up repeatedly and the chapter "De statu hominum" establishes that hermaphrodites should be attributed the gender of which they demonstrate the most evident traits (Fig. 2.1).

Customs and moral principles gradually changed with the rise of Christianity. By the time he wrote his "Letters to the Romans", St. Paul was already condemning homosexuality and obviously any inklings of sexual ambiguity. St. Augustine mentioned it in his *De Civitate Dei*, while in the scientific field, Galen's effective and conscientious description specified the anatomical and clinical traits, suggesting criteria of surgical treatment for the androgyne.

2.1.2 Mediaeval and Renaissance Period

Mediaeval literature on sexual ambiguity was inspired to a large extent by the works of Paul of Aegina (seventh century AD), who leaves us an anatomoclinical classification distinguishing three different forms of male hermaphrodite and two forms of female hermaphrodite. The suggested treatment is brutal removal of the "excess parts" because they are superfluous or harmful (Fig. 2.2). One exception was the most severe male form, which he considered to be incurable.

After Paul, we may remember the Arabs Albucasis (tenth century AD), his contemporary Avicenna and Sharaf al-Din, who came not long after him and left works that were very valuable, mainly due to their exquisitely worked coloured plates; neither must we overlook Bruno da Longoburgo with his valuable manuscript and the Frenchman Chauliac. The views of these authors hardly differed from those of Paul of Aegina, and they followed his therapeutic tenets, albeit with a few changes of minimal importance.

During the Renaissance period, significant matters such as etiopathogenesis and the evaluation of hermaphroditism from an ethical, religious and legal viewpoint are widely covered; but the fundamental anatomoclinical and etiopathogenic criteria were far too influenced by works of fantasy and superstitions, with only slight progress in the scientific field. Even cases of sex changes, which were reported in antiquity, were given serious consideration and believed to come about as a result of great physical effort. Thus, Ambroise Paré and Fabrizio d'Aquapendente, who were very great surgeons of the age, devoted much space to descriptions of cases that they had personally examined and above all the uncontrolled accounts of others, not holding back in their criticisms of Paul of Aegina. Despite this, the changes proposed to his treatment are not very significant. This late Mediaeval author thus remained an extremely important pillar who was used as a benchmark by later academics. Of these, we may remember Duval, with his *Des hermafroditis*; Uffembachius, known above all for his interesting drawings of pseudohermaphrodites and true hermaphrodites; and Jacobus Möller, who considered all matters associated with these malformations. Last but not least, Thevenin, Van Horne and Bauhin deemed hermaphrodites to be an abomination against nature and therefore doomed to die.

A proportion of these authors and other later authors followed the medicolegal teachings of Paolo Zacchia, who indicated the four elements

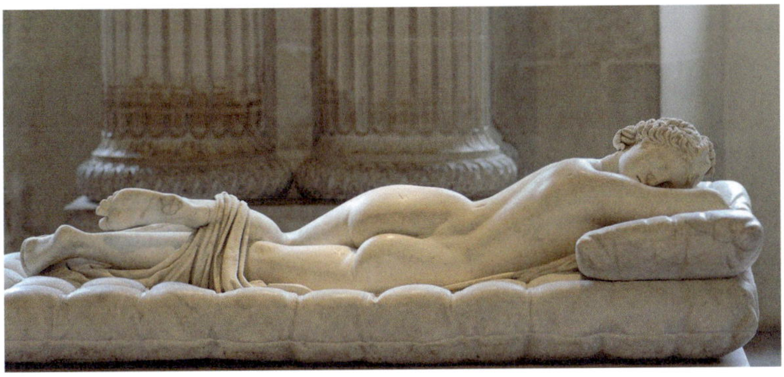

Fig. 2.1 Sleeping Hermaphroditus. Hermaphroditus: Greek marble, Roman copy of the second century CE after a Hellenistic original of the second century BC, restored in 1619 by David Larique; mattress: Carrara marble, made by Gian Lorenzo Bernini in 1619 on Cardinal Borghese's request

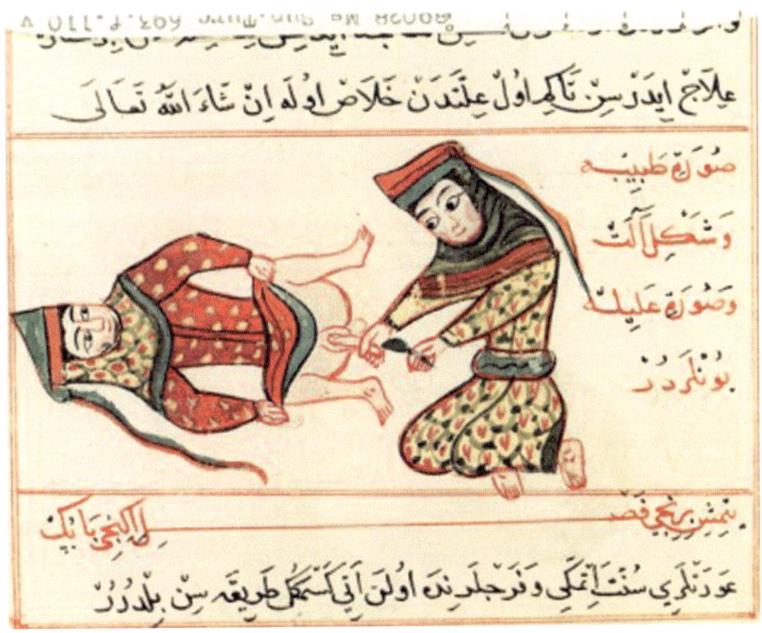

Fig. 2.2 A medical illustration by Charaf-ed-Din depicting a midwife operating on a hermaphrodite

on which an examination of androgyny should be based: the shape of the genitals, their position, *potentia coeundi*, and *generandi* (ability to perform the sexual act and generate). In the meantime, legal experts decided that individuals with ambiguous sexuality should declare the gender to which they felt most inclined and adopt that gender. Inability to keep to a difficult decision imposed too early brought very severe penalties.

2.1.3 From the Eighteenth Century to the Beginning of the Twentieth Century

Midway through the eighteenth century, we see the first signs of understanding and mercy. Albrecht von Haller touched on the essential points of the problem in a learned and wide-ranging disquisition written in 1751, concluding that it is unjust to make inferences against someone who has been mistreated by nature. In 1765, Anna Grandjean was accused of having married a woman even though she had been brought up as female, but after a long period of detention and much torture, she was more humanely judged in an appeal to the Court of Paris. In the meantime, some cases were described with more rational criteria, including that of Maret at the end of the eighteenth century.

During the next century, an attempt was made to rationalise the study of the problem based on visible genital malformations, distinguishing pseudohermaphroditism from true hermaphroditism, which many authors claimed did not really exist. One work worthy of mention is a very thorough monograph by Gaimari (1817) that accepts the existence of true hermaphroditism, even though it is very rare. Other very interesting works include ten cases described by Meyer, studies on reptiles by Geoffrey Saint-Hilaire, a case that was incompletely studied by Ricco and Sorrentino (1832) and another minutely described by Buillaud (1832). These studies started a discussion with the anatomist Manec; the former suggesting a diagnosis of true hermaphroditism and the latter referring to a diagnosis of female pseudohermaphroditism. One famous case was that of Jacqueline Foroni, presented to the Academy of Mantua and published in the Milanese Franco–Italian press, and another was that of Marie Christine Zaneboni, which was documented by detailed drawings of her external genitals. Despite the scepticism of many, the possibility of very rare true hermaphroditism was accepted and various essentially concordant definitions were formulated (Vogel 1847; Tourdes 1888).

At the beginning of the twentieth century, progress in teratology and genetics led to more modern concepts that paved the way for present-day thinking, based on criteria of endocrinology, psychology, embryopathology and surgery.

Conclusions

According to Ombredanne, the idea of sexual ambiguity in the most ancient civilisations is correlated with a pure creation of the spirit in an attempt to explain the genesis of the human species. Conversely, during an earlier age, Laugier asserted that since the dawn of time, hermaphroditism could be considered an allegory for that great vice of ancient civilisations: the unnatural use of both sexes. These apparently very conflicting hypotheses can be explained and adapted through an analysis of historical facts in such a way that one does not rule out the other. While the very ancient concept of a divinity that is neither man nor woman such as the goddess Astarte of the Neo-Babylonians and Plato's theories tend to suggest an attempt to explain the genesis of the human species; many other concepts relate to homosexuality. This idea is clear in the figures of sophisticated male and female beauty depicted by Greek artists and from descriptions of naturalists and historians of the period. We may remember, for example, the verses of Hesiod, Ausonius and, in particular, the impassioned verses of Ovid "nulla dies a me nec me diducat ab illos". On this subject, neither should we forget the descriptions of Pliny, which also suggest licentious ideas "androgynos nunc in deliciis habitos" or the "female sickness" of the Scythians described by Herodotus and Hippocrates. To sum up, in classical antiquity and above all during the Greek and Roman period, there was a close emblematic bond between visible malformation and homosexuality, but even in remote times, the phenomenon was sometimes measured using rational anatomoclinical criteria: in Talmudic writings, the various types of hermaphroditism are verified and classified; rules of life, limits of rights and duties and the protection of personal dignity are established. At other times, according to a viewpoint very far from the poetic imagination and in contrast with the interpretations we have discussed so far, the idea of the monstrous nature of the androgyne began to gain currency, seeing such beings as bringers of misfortune and therefore deserving of death. The long lists of executions, mainly determined by omens, that arose during Greek and Roman periods revealed the superstitious fear sometimes aroused by malformations, which began to abate during the period of Pliny.

During the subsequent centuries, with the advent of Christianity, a certain hostility towards hermaphroditism began to be seen again due to the belief that it might be related with homosexuality, which was harshly condemned. There were nevertheless some anatomical descriptions and a tendency to see the problem as purely scientific, albeit on the basis of very limited knowledge that was often based on fantasy and utopian views. Thus, medical and scientific tenets prevailed from the time of Galen to Paul of Aegina, the famous Arabian physicians, the Renaissance and the Age of Enlightenment. Contemporary legal practices were nevertheless closely linked to religious and ethical principles that were often poorly understood and steeped in superstition.

Establishing that malformed people had to choose the gender they felt the greatest inclination for and then strictly observe the functions of that gender led to severe penalties for infringements that in our belief were linked to the idea of homosexuality and, if marriage took place, of offence to the holy sacrament. In this case, too, we see the re-emergence of confusion with the unnatural use of both sexes. Certain heresies (Pope Gregory) founded on an interpretation of Genesis lead us towards a hypothesis of a pure creation of the spirit in order to explain the genesis of the human species. According to this theory, Adam must have been asexual or a hermaphrodite, "masculum et foeminam creavit eos". These malformed beings at last found the first glimmer of understanding and more enlightened judgements in the second half of the eighteenth century through the work of Haller (1751) and the humane appeal judgement of 1765.

During the nineteenth century, ideas were clearer, at least from an ethical, legal and religious viewpoint. Hermaphrodites were no longer seen as monsters and abominations against nature and morality but as unfortunate victims of an anomaly (Fig. 2.3).

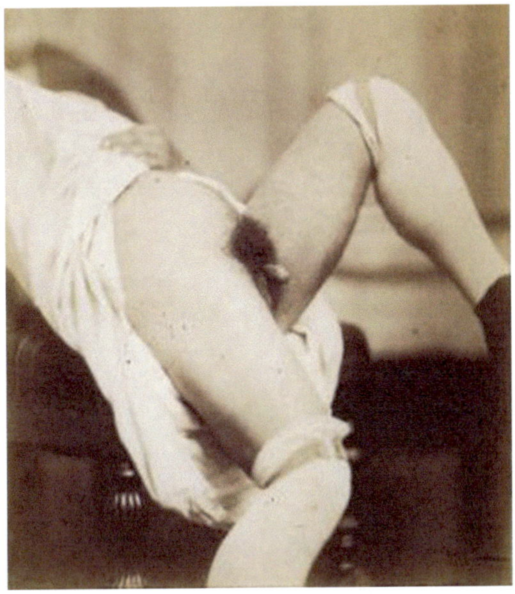

Fig. 2.3 Photograph of a hermaphrodite showing genitalia

The subject became better studied scientifically, albeit within the limits imposed by the unsatisfactory nature of the means of investigation. This approach helped pave the way towards current thinking inspired by the very latest findings in the fields of embryopathology, sexology, psychology and surgery.

Suggested Reading

1. Aristotele: De generatione animalium, in "Omnia Grecee et Latine", vol 4, ch. IV, Parisiis, 1654
2. Ausonio: Epigr. LXIX, C e CI
3. Cicerone: De diviniatione, vol 1
4. Digesto Romano: ch. De statu hominum, cit. Garcon, Toourdes et al
5. Esiodo: cit. Tourdes
6. Herodoto: Historiae, cit. Pedote
7. Ippocrate: Sulle arie, sulle acque, sui Luoghi, cit. Pedote
8. Lucrezio: De rerum natura, vol 5, cit. Tourdes, Pedote et al
9. Ovidio: Metamorphosis, vol 4, p.288
10. Platone: Symposium, cit. Mollerus, da Fabrizio d'Acquapendente et al
11. Plinio: Naturae Historia, vol 7, ch 3, cit. Zacchia P
12. Virgilio: Eneide, canto VI, 640

Gender Dysphoria: Definition and Evolution Through the Years

3

Lin Fraser

3.1 Definition

3.1.1 Gender Dysphoria

The dictionary defines gender as the state of being male or female (typically used with reference to social and cultural differences rather than biological ones) [1] and dysphoria as the state of unease or generalized dissatisfaction with life, the opposite of euphoria [2]. The term dysphoria is from the Greek word *dysphoros* meaning "hard to bear" [3].

Below are two medical definitions of gender dysphoria, both from the World Professional Association for Transgender Health (WPATH) Standards of Care (SOC), the first from the earliest (1979) [4] version, Standards of Care, The hormonal and surgical sex reassignment of gender dysphoric persons, and the second from the current and seventh version (2011) [5] Standards of Care for the Health of Transsexual, Transgender, and Gender-Nonconforming People. Both documents and their intervening versions are written and distributed by WPATH, formerly known as the Harry Benjamin International Gender Dysphoria Association (HBIGDA).

L. Fraser, EdD
World Professional Association for Transgender Health (WPATH), Minneapolis, MN, USA

Private Practice,
2538 California Street, San Francisco, CA, USA
e-mail: linfraser@gmail.com

3.1.2 1st SOC (1979)

Gender dysphoria herein refers to that psychological state whereby a person demonstrates dissatisfaction with their sex of birth and their sex role, as socially defined, which applies to that sex, and who requests hormonal and surgical sex reassignment. Gender dysphoria, herein, does not refer to cases of infant sex reassignment or re-announcement nor does it refer to those persons who, although dissatisfied with their genetically and socially defined sex status (i.e., transvestites and transgenderists), usually do not request sex reassignment. Gender dysphoria, therefore, is the primary working diagnosis applied to any and all persons requesting surgical and hormonal sex reassignment [6].

3.1.3 SOC 7 (2011)

Gender dysphoria – Distress that is caused by a discrepancy between a person's gender identity and that person's sex assigned at birth (and the associated gender role and/or primary and secondary sex characteristics) [7].

These two dcfinitions, separated by 32 years between the first and the seventh guidelines, reflect the overarching change in the evolution of the professional approach to gender dysphoria.

Using the SOC as a mirror of the evolution, the original professional approach was a medicalized one, and these guidelines of care described

C. Trombetta et al. (eds.), *Management of Gender Dysphoria: A Multidisciplinary Approach*,
DOI 10.1007/978-88-470-5696-1_3, © Springer-Verlag Italia 2015

the medical management of gender dysphoria and presumed a full transition from one sex to another (the sex-change model).

The title, as noted above, of the 1st SOC was "Standards of Care, The hormonal and surgical sex reassignment of gender dysphoric persons."

In the most recent SOC, the medical part of the definition (about requesting sex reassignment) has been intentionally omitted. The current professional approach has been to broaden the focus of transgender health [8], with an emphasis on health and not only on treatment. Individuals with gender dysphoria requesting medical care receive individualized health care, which may or may not include hormonal and/or sex reassignment. These SOC include other aspects of health care, for example, reproductive health, voice and communication therapy, lifelong preventive and primary care, and care in institutional environments [9]. Psychological care has been included from the beginning.

Thus, the title of the 7th SOC is "The Standards of Care for the Health of Transsexual, Transgender, and Gender-Nonconforming People," unlike the early ones that specifically mention sex reassignment.

Another major change from the original SOC, consistent with the above change from treatment to health, is a shift in gender paradigms.

Initially, a binary system of gender (man, woman, boy, girl) was the predominant paradigm. Now, the view is that gender falls on a spectrum and multiple gender identities and expressions are possible.

In addition, although not clear from these definitions, professional consensus has moved away from seeing gender dysphoria as a disorder and now sees it as part of an overall pattern of gender diversity [10].

The approach for providers in providing health care more broadly has, as its basis, an underlying emphasis and recognition of human rights. Health care is a human right. And trans rights are part of human rights.

The evolution of the name and approach is due to an interplay of several factors such as advancing knowledge and better clinical treatments, the aforementioned changing gender paradigms, input and participation from trans people themselves including human rights and the right to self-define, the rise of the Internet, more global participation, and evolving shifts in how transgender people are seen by the culture. Expansion of knowledge beyond Western approaches is also part of the evolution. These changes have accelerated in recent years and are exponential rather than linear.

Other names used frequently in the literature include "*gender identity disorder* [11], the formal diagnosis set forth by the Diagnostic and Statistical Manual of Mental Disorders, 4th Edition, Text Rev. (DSM IV-TR) (American Psychiatric Association 1987) which is characterized by a strong and persistent cross-gender identification and a persistent discomfort with one's sex or sense of inappropriateness in the gender role of that sex, causing clinically significant distress or impairment in social, occupational, or other important areas of functioning)", "*transsexualism* (transsexual: an adjective (often applied by the medical profession) to describe individuals who seek to change or who have changed their primary and/or secondary sex characteristics through feminizing or masculinizing medical interventions (hormones and/or surgery) typically accompanied by a permanent change in gender role) [12]", and "*transgender* (an adjective to describe a diverse group of individuals who cross or transcend culturally defined categories of gender). The gender identity of transgender people differs to varying degrees from the sex they were assigned at birth [12]".

Although gender dysphoria, an essentially neutral label, is the term most commonly used in the current medical literature, that neutrality was not always so. Until recently, the value-laden gender identity disorder, which by definition implied a "disordered condition," was the most commonly used term. Although the name gender dysphoria has come full circle, approaches to care have evolved.

These names cannot be separated from the evolution of professional understanding.

3.2 Evolution and SOC

This chapter describes the evolution of the name and professional approaches to the condition starting with the 1st international symposium on gender identity, in London, in 1969, and the beginnings of HBIGDA, in 1979, followed by the seven versions of the SOC that document the evolution of the nomenclature and the prevailing approaches to care, and then ends with the 23rd 2014 WPATH Symposium, Transgender Health from Global Perspectives, held in Bangkok, Thailand.

3.2.1 WPATH and SOC

WPATH (formerly HBIGDA) writes and disseminates the SOC.

It is the oldest and only international multidisciplinary professional organization devoted solely to the health of trans people with the mission to promote evidence-based care, education, research, advocacy, public policy, and respect in transsexual and transgender health.

Hence, the organization is in a good position to publish guidelines that reflect the state of the art and science and evolution of care.

The SOC document the evolution of the nomenclature and prevailing medical standards and are based on the best available science and expert professional consensus.

Revisions to the 1979 Standards of Care (1980, 1981, 1990, 1998, 2001, 2011) have occurred concurrent with the advancement of knowledge.

Other classification systems naming this phenomenon are the Diagnostic and Statistical Manual of Mental Disorders (DSM) put out by the American Psychiatric Association (APA) and the International Classifications of Diseases (ICD) put out by the World Health organization (WHO). These manuals have also evolved, often along parallel lines to the SOC. Although the last publication of ICD, ICD-10, was in 1990 [13], ICD-11 has a planned publication in 2017. As both the DSM and ICD have contributed to and reflect evolving notions of health care, their nomenclature will also be described.

WPATH has worked with APA and the WHO during the period of writing of SOC7 (the SOC7 process) and beyond. WPATH has had formal consensus processes advising the workgroups for APA and the WHO regarding the nomenclature for both DSM 5 and ICD-11.

This chapter will not describe the terminology and health care of children.

By necessity, broad-brush strokes will be used to provide an overview of the evolution.

Information on the background and beginnings of approaches is followed by briefer descriptions of middle periods where the interplay of factors brings us to the dramatic shifts in recent years.

Some things have not changed such as the complexity of the condition, ethical concerns, the interdisciplinary nature of the field, and the need for social understanding and education.

Major changes include the growing number of people involved in the field including more transgender people themselves. The addition of transsexual, transgender, and gender-nonconforming people joining with providers in the evolution of approaches has had a major impact. Mainstream growing acceptance is also a factor.

3.3 Pre-SOC to 1979

3.3.1 1950s and 1960s

The possibility of medical treatment for gender dysphoria entered the popular imagination in the early 1950s when Christine Jorgensen, an American GI, had a sex-change operation in 1951 in Denmark and then returned to the United States. Although not the first to have a "sex change," Dr. Harry Benjamin, an early pioneer in the field [14], remarked that Jorgensen's "sex conversion" and the worldwide publicity it created was perhaps the most important milestone in the history of transsexualism. Her surgeon Christian Hamburger in his 1953 report [14] urged the medical and legal professions to help the plight "of these unfortunate people for whom psychotherapy proved useless."

The aforementioned Benjamin, a NY endocrinologist, saw many patients and wrote the first article about the condition in 1953 [15] in the no longer existing International Journal of Sexology.

In 1966 [16], he published his magnum opus, *The Transsexual Phenomenon*. In it, he interpreted transsexualism as a form of psychic intersexuality, the intensity of which varies. He suggested that the condition was due to complex factors, most likely had more than one causation, and was primarily a neuroendocrine disorder. He argued that since there was no cure, it was in the best interest of both transsexuals and greater society to alleviate this intense suffering of transsexuals by sex reassignment, in selected cases [17].

Also in 1966, the Gender Clinic, championed by renowned medical psychologist Dr. John Money, opened at Johns Hopkins. The clinic lasted until 1979 when it was forced to close by pressure from psychiatry, asserting that it was treating a mental disorder by doing surgery [18].

Hopkins served as a model for gender clinics scattered throughout the United States.

The oldest and largest gender identity clinic in the world began operations in the mid 1960s and is still in operation located in Hammersmith in London and is sometimes known as Charing Cross Gender Identity Clinic [19].

Don Laub, M.D., Chief of Plastic Surgery at Stanford and also founder of Interplast, which was the forerunner of medical humanitarian ventures worldwide, founded another gender clinic, known as "the Stanford Program." Laub led medical teams on humanitarian surgical trips to the developing world and at the same time developed new surgical techniques for sex-reassignment surgery. Eventually, he moved to private practice but was never forced to close. Laub was instrumental in the foundation of the organization that was later to become WPATH, serving as President from 1981 to 1983 [20].

Psychiatrist and lawyer Richard Green and medical psychologist John Money (eds) published a multidisciplinary volume *Transsexualism and Sex Reassignment* in 1969, which, along with instructions on hormonal and genital sex reassignment, included sections on social and clinical aspects of transsexualism. Topics included such as psychological aspects, somatic aspects, treatment aspects, and medicolegal aspects, are themes that continue to be major topics today.

The editors dedicated the volume to Harry Benjamin, M.D., the pioneer of transsexual research, stating: His compassion and courage in treatment of the transsexual patient opened a new frontier in the knowledge of human nature [21].

Hence, foundational themes and key points from the earliest years included the following:

Gender dysphoria cannot be cured via psychotherapy.

A medical necessity for surgical sex reassignment exists in some cases.

The field is interdisciplinary.

Compassion and courage are foundational.

3.3.2 1970s

Early pioneers and early conferences

Prior to the 1st SOC, a small group of interdisciplinary professionals supported by wealthy transsexual Reed Erickson via his foundation, the Erickson Educational Foundation, assembled at six conferences in Europe and the United States to discuss the new medical condition known then as either gender disorientation, transsexualism, or gender dysphoria, starting in July 1969 with the 1st International Symposium on Gender identity: Aims, Functions, Clinical Problems of a Gender Identity Unit, London. These international symposia continue to this day, with the 23rd just held in February 2014 in Bangkok, Thailand. The next will be held in Amsterdam, the Netherlands, in 2016.

The people involved were pioneers and highly respected in their fields.

Some of the concerns of the early conferences are equally compelling today.

In the opening address of the first conference in 1969, Professor C. J. Dewhurst from Queen Charlotte's Hospital, London, states, "I actually regard this to be one of the most difficult conditions I have ever come across in clinical medicine. If we consider the condition as an anomaly that would be cured by getting the patient to accept their true anatomic sex, can we say that is ever possible?" To paraphrase Dr. Dewhurst, "What do we know of its origin? Under what circumstances does it arise? If we medically intervene, what are criteria and at what age? What is their legal sex? Can they marry?" [22].

The cover of the brochure states the following: *In addition to the medical and research aspects of the problem, there is urgent need for greater academic and professional understanding and for education*, the latter of which could be said to be the most pressing need today.

At the 1971 2nd International Gender Identity Symposium in Denmark, there was a recognition that *this is an interdisciplinary, complex condition and area of human rights*. The brochure stated that the field calls attention on the problem of gender identity and "gender disorientation, not only as a psychiatric entity but also as an area of specialized medical study and treatment and social understanding" [23].

The 1973 3rd Symposium on Gender Identity in Dubrovnik included families along with surgery and etiology as topics of discussion [24].

The 4th conference on Gender Identity in Palo Alto in 1975 was the first to use the Harry Benjamin name in the title. It also focused on the interdisciplinary exchange of scientific information and how to achieve greater acceptance. In a first-person recollection, Roy Mackenzie stated that the "first step was to make it professionally respectable to even study such material" [25].

At the 1977 5th International Gender Dysphoria Symposium in Norfolk, VA, a founding committee for an interdisciplinary international organization named after Harry Benjamin, the Harry Benjamin International Gender Dysphoria Association (HBIGDA), was founded and charged with developing Standards of Care guidelines based on knowledge and ethics at that time. Paul Walker, Ph.D., a protégé of John Money, was named as chair [26].

3.3.2.1 Literature

Aside from the literature coming from the above pioneers, most of the literature was psychodynamic and pathologizing, positing dysfunctional family, mostly mother–child dynamics, as the cause of the condition and recommended reparative psychotherapy and psychoanalysis. Examples of literature in that vein include Stoller's [27]) *Perversion* among other books [28–30] and a series of articles by psychoanalysts Ovesey and Person [31, 32] and Person and Ovesey [33, 34, 35].

Other psychological treatments were behavioral, for example, Rekers and Lovaas [36], designed to extinguish cross-sex gender expressions and reinforce gender normative behaviors.

3.3.3 Nomenclature Pre-1st SOC

SOC – The SOC did not exist.
DSM 1 (1952) – There was no nomenclature for the condition.
DSM II (1968) – (Parent) sexual deviations; (diagnosis) transvestism.
ICD-6 (1948) and ICD-7 (1955) – There was no nomenclature for the condition.
ICD-8 (1965) – (Parent) sexual deviations; (diagnosis) transvestism.
ICD-9 (1975) – (Parent) sexual deviation; (diagnosis) transvestism and transsexualism.

3.3.4 Summary

This period marked the beginning of gender clinics, the first surgeries, and the beginning of psychopathologization as a sexual deviation in the nomenclature. The paradigm was clearly binary.

The two strands of literature and approaches still continue today, but one (reparative) is now considered unethical and is not part of mainstream care. The early specialized conferences draw surprising parallels to today.

3.4 1979–1981

SOC v1. 1979 Standards of Care
The hormonal and surgical sex reassignment of gender dysphoric persons
SOC v2. 1980 Standards of Care
The hormonal and surgical sex reassignment of gender dysphoric persons
SOC v3. 1981 Standards of Care
The hormonal and surgical sex reassignment of gender dysphoric persons

The 1st 3 SOC had the same name. The healthcare approach for all was comprised of the triadic sequence, the three required steps to medically transition from one sex to another. These three included living in the preferred gender for 1 year termed the life test, hormonal, and finally genital sex reassignment. The first SOC used the name gender dysphoria.

The paradigm about gender was binary.

HBIGDA was incorporated, and the first Standards of Care were approved by the membership of the fledgling society in 1979 at the seventh conference in San Diego. From the beginning, it was made up of interdisciplinary international providers, most from Western Europe and North America, primarily from the United States. Much of the hard science came out of Europe.

One purpose of having guidelines was to gain respectability. The purpose of the new organization and the SOC was to gain academic acceptance among professional peers, to provide a place for professionals to share knowledge, to move the field forward, and to protect trans people from disreputable surgeons.

The term gender dysphoria was adopted as a descriptive and accurate label [37]. Dysphoria was about the subjective distress of the mind/body mismatch. Later, the word was extolled as being value-free compared to other labels that included the designation disorder.

The first Standards were only eight pages long, and although contributed to via professional consensus, they were actually written by Psychologist Paul Walker from the University of Texas at Galveston. Dr. Walker was the first President of HBIGDA, who later started a private practice in San Francisco, before his untimely death in 1991.

These first SOC covered such items as definitions, principles, description of the triadic sequence, and recognition of the interdisciplinary nature of the field. Strict eligibility requirements for medical treatments, including two evaluations by mental health professionals for surgery and one for hormones, were also described. Psychotherapy was compulsory.

Meanwhile, providers were excoriated on multiple fronts.

McHugh [18], pointing to studies showing that operated patients were no better off than they had been before treatment, shut down the Hopkins gender clinic in 2006. He neglected, however, to take into account that most were subjectively happy about their surgeries and few had regrets [38].

Also in 1979 radical feminist Janice Raymond, in her book *The Transsexual Empire*, proposed that male-to-female transsexuals transitioned as a way to invade female space. She also accused providers of creating a medical treatment "empire" as a means to make money [39].

The term gender identity disorder (GID) as a subset of psychosexual disorders was first introduced in DSM III (1980) [40] (for children), which initiated the language of disorder. GID would become the language for adults in DSM II-R (1987) [41]. The term suggested that one was at core disordered, this supposition becoming the basis of future protests from trans people and professionals alike. The mental disorder designation became the default position. Although no concrete evidence existed for a psychological or a physical basis for the condition, DSM III suggested that a predisposing factor was a disturbed parent–child relationship [40] consistent with Stoller [42]. One also wonders if the stigma of cross-gender behavior may have played a role in the decision regarding this placement in the nomenclature [43].

3.4.1 Nomenclature

SOC 1979, 1980, 1981 – Gender dysphoria.

DSM III (1980) – (Parent) psychosexual disorders, (diagnosis) transsexualism. Gender identity of childhood was introduced.

ICD-9 (1975) – (Parent) sexual deviations, (diagnosis) transvestism and transsexualism.

3.4.2 Summary

Today's preferred term gender dysphoria was used in the first SOC whereas the term gender identity disorder was first used elsewhere, in DSM III.

3.5 1981–1990

SOC v4 (1990) Standards of Care – The hormonal and surgical sex reassignment of gender dysphoric persons

SOC v4 had the same name as the first three versions; the health-care approach concerned medical transition from one sex to another, the triadic sequence, and used the name gender dysphoria.

The paradigm about gender was binary and the condition was still considered primarily a mental disorder.

During this period, competing theories abounded, suggesting how little was actually known.

Blanchard developed a new typology based on sexual orientation. In his view, there were two types of male to female transsexuals, one early onset and attracted only to men and the other a later onset type recognizable by a sexual orientation directed toward an inner image of oneself as a woman, which Blanchard labeled autogynephilia [44]. This eroticism of identity has created much dissension particularly among the trans community and remains a point of contention even today.

Also in 1987 Green published the influential *Sissy Boy Syndrome and the Development of Homosexuality*, which continues to have influence although the title remains controversial. In a study still cited, Green found that most children with GID grow up to be gay, not trans, and that one cannot predict adult outcomes based on childhood behavior [45]. Although this chapter is not about children, a big question regarding children has to do with who will benefit from early medical transitions and who will not? How do we predict outcomes?

Another example, presented at the HBIGDA 1989 conference in Cleveland and in his writings, Leslie Lothstein, a psychoanalytic clinician, described the etiology and treatment of FTM transsexualism. He posited that FTMs suffered from severe impaired object relations and borderline psychopathology requiring long term psychodynamic psychotherapy rather than medical intervention [46, 47].

3.5.1 Nomenclature

The SOC were still using the term gender dysphoria while others started or continued using the term GID.

DSM III-R (1987) – (Parent) disorders usually first evident in infancy, childhood, or adolescence; (diagnosis) transsexualism, gender identity disorder of adolescence and adulthood – nontranssexual type.

ICD-10 (1990) – (Parent) gender identity disorders; (diagnosis) transsexualism, dual-role transvestism, other gender identity disorders, gender identity disorder, unspecified. This ICD is still in use. ICD-11 will not be out until 2017 [48].

3.6 1991–1998

SOC Version 5 (1998) – The Standards of Care for Gender Identity Disorders

The 1998 SOC, to be consistent with DSM III, for the first time called the condition GID, rather than gender dysphoria.

Nevertheless, despite the shift in terminology, a beginning of change in approach was evident.

Although the triadic sequence was prioritized, the standards suggested that other approaches (described in the psychotherapy section) might be helpful for some people in adapting to the condition. For the first time, psychotherapy, although highly recommended, was not a prerequisite for treatment.

As a precursor to the current emphasis on human rights, the SOC stated that although GID was still considered a mental disorder, a disorder designation was not a license for stigma.

SOC v5 stated that the overarching treatment goal was "lasting personal comfort with the gendered self in order to maximize overall psychological well-being and self-fulfillment" [49]. This goal remains in place today.

Although difficult to break down how things changed exactly, a pattern emerged via an interplay of forces. The issue of labeling the condition a disorder was becoming more controversial. The literature marked a shift away from the binary into a spectrum paradigm. Biological differences were also noted. Moreover, the community started to have a larger voice.

For example, in 1994, Gil Herdt's 614-page series of articles entitled "Third Sex Third Gender, Beyond Sexual Dimorphism in Culture and History, Recognizing Global Diversity Outside the Binary" was published, describing many variations on the trans spectrum. On the biological side [50, 51], reported differences in the size of brain structures among homosexual and heterosexual men and transsexual women, in the part of the brain that regulates circadian rhythm, with the nuclei of the transsexual women being the largest [51].

3.6.1 Community

The community was beginning to have more authority among themselves and providers began to listen. The role and importance of the trans community started to grow. People started defining themselves.

The term transgender came from the community and this increasingly vocal community started to reject medical models.

For example, transgender activist and writer Dallas Denny, at a recent conference on transgender history (2014), described the impact of Holly Boswell's article (1991) "The Transgender Alternative" where she described the term transgender as a middle ground between transsexual and transvestite [52]. According to Denny, "The impact of "The Transgender Alternative" was immediate and dramatic. By 1994, the term transgender had become the consensual umbrella term for all of us. That does not mean everyone liked it. Essentialist transsexuals in particular felt they had little in common with crossdressers and transgenderists." As an aside, these differences continue to this day, hence the inclusive and respectful use of language in current terminology such as the title of SOC7. Regarding the community's relationship to the provider community, Denny noted, "It's a community in which we look to professionals for help, but not for direction. It's a community that rejects medical models of transsexualism and cross-dressing and the harmful labels that accompany them. And it's a community that has demolished all-or-nothing binary notions of gender and embraced our diversity and wholeness" [53].

Press for Change, an influential activist group (and one of the many to come), was founded in the United Kingdom in 1992. According to its welcome page on the website, Press for Change has been a key lobbying and legal support organization for trans people in the United Kingdom since its formation (http://www.pfc.org.uk) [54].

Bornstein [55] in her iconic book *Gender Outlaw* continued the theme of describing the trans perspective from outside the gender binary.

Google Search was initiated in 1997. The impact of the Internet on the rise of the trans community cannot be overestimated. Originally isolated, members were able to communicate and discuss common concerns and issues, including discussions about nomenclature. Members of the community questioned the terms used and, more tellingly, posed the question, who decides on the name of this condition? Who gives providers this right?

3.6.2 Nomenclature

SOC 5 (1998) – Gender identity disorder
DSM IV (1994) – (Parent) sexual and gender identity disorders, (diagnosis) gender identity disorder in adolescents or adults
ICD-10 (1990) – No change

3.6.3 Summary

This period was the beginning of change toward a more varied approach, marking the use of the term transgender as an umbrella term and the rise of a more vocal trans community.

3.7 1999–2001

Version 6 (2001) – The Standards of Care for Gender Identity Disorders

The SOC continued to use the name gender identity disorder.

3.7.1 Evolution and Literature

The SOC v6 offered more flexibility and more individualized treatment. Given that there was no name change and for other factors that remain unclear, an increasingly unhappy client population did not recognize these changes.

The popularized term transgender was mentioned in this SOC, not as a formal diagnosis but as a term that does not connote psychopathology [56] indicating recognition for providers to shift away from stigmatizing language and the binary paradigm.

3.7.2 Community

An example of the growing voice of the trans community was the 1999 *Reclaiming Genders* by legal scholar and Professor Stephen Whittle BCE who was later to become the first transgender President of WPATH [57].

The increasing vocal community became more critical to providers, using the common complaint that they were required to "jump through hoops" to receive medically necessary services. A growing tension developed between providers and service end users.

Trans academics groups began to form. Movies such as Boys Don't Cry (1999) and Southern Comfort (2001) portrayed trans people as recipients of horrific treatment: murder by his peers in the former when his identity as a trans man was discovered and murder by neglect from medical professionals in the second, who refused to provide treatment to a trans man with ovarian cancer [58, 59]. These sympathetic portrayals began to bear witness to trans people's plight in the popular imagination.

3.7.3 Nomenclature

SOC – No change
DSM – No change
ICD – No change

3.7.4 Summary

This period was marked by continued flexibility in the SOC, more support in the popular imagination, and continued growth of the community without change in the nomenclature.

3.8 2001–2011

3.8.1 SOC7 (2011)

Standards of Care for the Health of Transsexual, Transgender, and Gender-Nonconforming People

This 10-year period marks a major shift in the approach to health care in the SOC and among providers in general, summarized by a change from a focus on treatment to one of overall health and individualized care. In SOC7, the name has been quite consciously changed back to gender dysphoria and the condition is no longer considered a disorder.

The paradigm shifted from a binary to a spectrum.

The rate of evolution moved from linear to exponential concurrent with the continued massive growth of the Internet.

The exponential rate of change can be seen in the following chronology, which is marked by more of an emphasis on human rights. Other concrete examples include the newly named WPATH and the vastly different seventh version of the Standards of Care.

The literature began normalizing the condition with books such as the award winning and compassionate 2004 *Transgender Emergence* by Arlene Lev and the 2004 autobiographical *Becoming a Visible Man* by trans man Jamison Green, who later became WPATH President in 2014 [60, 61]. Although some literature remained focused on disorder such as Bailey's 2003 *Man who would be Queen*, supportive of Blanchard's typology emphasizing the sexual nature of the condition [62], the book was met by a tremendous outcry from the community and other professionals. Although discussion of the latter theory is outside the scope of this chapter, the degree of dissent highlights the power of the voices demanding normalcy as well as the growing power of the transgender movement.

In 2006, the Harry Benjamin International Gender Dysphoria Association's (HBIGDA) name was changed to the World Professional Association for Transgender Health (WPATH). This change was a major milestone reflecting broader changes in the field. For example, the inclusive and umbrella term transgender in the title marks an emphasis on multiple trans identities and gender diversity, accentuating the change from a binary to a spectrum paradigm. The term health, as in SOC7, underscores that the field now emphasizes health rather than treatment.

Moreover, while the Standards were being developed, the field was growing internationally.

For example, a group of experts in human rights met in Indonesia and wrote the Yogyakarta Principles (2007) on the Application of International Human Rights Law in relation to Sexual Orientation and Gender Identity [63]. Although not legally binding, these set of principles were and are intended to apply international human rights law to Sexual Orientation and Gender Identity.

In 2007, Dr. Gail Knudson, current WPATH President-Elect, founded the Canadian Professional Association for Transgender Health (CPATH), modeled after WPATH, but at the national level.

At the 2009 WPATH Oslo Conference, then President Dr. Walter Bockting announced that WPATH's primary goal would be to broaden the focus of transgender health [64].

In 2009, the Council of Europe Commissioner for Human Rights recommended that anything related to gender identity should not be classified as a mental disorder in ICD-11 [65].

In 2010, the WPATH Board of Directors issued a press release and policy statement depathologizing gender variance worldwide. This statement, now known now colloquially as the "depath statement" says the following: "The WPATH Board of Directors strongly urges the depsychopathologisation of gender variance worldwide. The expression of gender characteristics, including identities that are not stereotypically associated with one's assigned sex at birth is a common and culturally diverse human phenomenon, which should not be judged as inherently pathological or negative" [66].

This statement was shortly followed by the Identity Recognition Statement (2010), emphasizing the human right to self-define. The statement reads as follows: "No person should have to undergo surgery or accept sterilization as a condition of identity recognition. If a sex marker is required on an identity document, that marker could recognize the person's lived gender, regardless of reproductive capacity. The WPATH Board of Directors urges governments and other authoritative bodies to move to eliminate requirements for identity recognition that require surgical procedures" [67].

Consistent with self-definition, medical clinics with an informed consent model such as Fenway Health in Boston and Callen–Lorde Community Health Center in NYC flourished.

Major changes in SOC7 paralleled and underscored these changes in the field.

For example, the names used in the title are inclusive and respectful of names used by trans people themselves and include transsexual, transgender, and gender-nonconforming people rather than using the term gender identity disorder.

The title is about health, not treatment. The document is evidence based, has multiple authors, and is 115 pages long with 265 references compared to the 1st SOC, for example, that was only 8 pages long, had no references, with input from a small group of professionals, and was written by basically one author. Psychotherapy is no longer a requirement and the new SOC are compatible with informed consent models.

Finally, the 2011 SOC recognize its Western-centric nature and supports global adaptations. It calls for more partnerships outside of Western Europe and North America.

3.8.2 Community

Prior to writing SOC7, the WPATH leadership called upon an international advisory committee comprised of carefully selected leaders from the trans community. One of these, Christine Burns, commented on the improved SOC and implicit improved provider and service end user relationship with the following:

If I had to sum it up then it would be that whereas previous versions of the SOC were always perceived to be about the things that a trans person must do to satisfy clinicians, this version is much more clearly about every aspect of what clinicians ought to do in order to properly serve their clients. That is a truly radical reversal… one that serves both parties very well [68].

3.8.3 Nomenclature

SOC – Name returns to gender dysphoria.

DSM 5 workgroup is in the process of changing to gender dysphoria.

ICD-11 workgroup is in the process of selecting a name.

3.9 Post SOC7

Since 2011, a tipping point has occurred in trans health and the rate of change is clearly exponential and not linear.

SOC7 has been met with almost universal acclaim. It has been translated into eight languages, with more to come. As a living document, updates will be introduced as knowledge advances. Support for the development of companion documents for resource-poor nations exists. PAHO has developed such a document, the Blueprint for the Provision of Care for Trans Persons and Their Communities in Latin America and the Caribbean PAHO under the leadership of Rafael Mazin, M.D. [69].

Exchange of knowledge has moved from Western to global. The goal of WPATH President Lin Fraser, during this period, has been global expansion and educational exchange. WPATH 2014, the 23rd International Symposium, was held for the first time outside of Western Europe and North America. The conference, entitled Transgender Health from Global Perspectives, convened in Bangkok, Thailand, and was attended by people from 34 countries and 6 continents. Plenaries were held on the following topics, indicating new directions in the field: new research regarding transsexual brain differences; surgical centers outside the West; ICD-11 where diagnostic placement will no longer be in mental health, furthering depathologization models; uterine transplants; and reproductive and hormonal possibilities. Trans thought leaders were invited and convened a special session series on "Trans People in Asia and the Pacific."

More partnerships are developing between professionals and providers.

WPATH convened an international gathering of global thought leaders in San Francisco February 2013 to continue its ICD Consensus Process to advise the WHO on ICD-11 and invited trans activists to be part of the process. The PAHO Blueprint was a joint professional/activist process. More trans people are also professionals, who bring added richness and depth to the conversation.

The field is growing at a rapid rate and the demand for education and training is following suit. WPATH has founded a Global Educational Initiative (GEI) to address this huge need to educate providers, policy makers, and other interested parties worldwide. GEI is designed to educate from both a human rights and standard medical education models. The hope is that education will be multimodal, both face2face and via the Internet, and in collaboration with global partners.

3.9.1 Nomenclature

SOC – No change.

DSM 5 2013 – Gender dysphoria.

ICD-11 – The name is undecided but it will not include the term disorder and will not be placed in the mental disorders section.

3.9.2 Summary

This period can be summarized by the exponential growth of the field, perhaps best described by the designation "transgender beyond disorder."

Conclusion

Finally, although the field has enjoyed remarkable growth, rapid change, and new knowledge, as providers, we might still listen to the wise words of the early pioneers. We can listen to Hamburger in his 1953 report, urging the medical and legal profession to help, to the brochure at the 1969 first conference calling for the *Need for better understanding, and urgent need for education*, to heeding the topics on the program of 1971 2nd International Gender Identity Symposium in Denmark, *recognizing that this is an interdisciplinary, complex condition and area of human rights*.

The foundational themes, such as compassion and courage are as relevant today as they were 60 years ago.

The subject matter in Green and Money's 1969 epistle and the early conferences echo the plenary topics at the recent Bangkok symposium.

The call for education is as much a crying need today as it was then and needs to be responded via medical education and human rights work.

As from the beginning, much needs to be done, and as interdisciplinary health-care providers partnered with others, we have much to do. The clarion call today is for training and education as we move from transgender beyond disorder to all facets of transgender health.

We could do worse than follow in the footsteps of our forebears.

References

1. New Oxford American dictionary, definition of gender
2. New Oxford American dictionary, definition of dysphoria
3. New Oxford American dictionary, definition dysphoros
4. Walker P et al (1979) Standards of care, the hormonal and surgical sex reassignment of gender dysphoric persons. Available online http://www.wpath.org
5. WPATH (World Professional Association for Transgender Health) (2011) Standards of care for the health of transsexual, transgender and gender non-conforming people. Int J Transgenderism 13(4):165–232
6. Walker P et al (1979) Standards of care, the hormonal and surgical sex reassignment of gender dysphoric persons. p 2. Available online at http://www.wpath.org
7. WPATH (2011) SOC7. Int J Transgenderism 13(4):221
8. Bockting W (2009) XXI biennial symposium, vision of the incoming president, Oslo, June 20
9. WPATH (2011) SOC7 table of contents. Int J Transgenderism 13(4):i
10. WPATH (2011) SOC7. Int J Transgenderism 13(4): 168–171
11. WPATH (2011) SOC7. Int J Transgenderism 13(4):221. Glossary
12. WPATH (2011) SOC7. Int J Transgenderism 13(4): 222. Glossary.
13. WHO (World Health Organization) (1990) International classification of diseases and related health problems, 10th revision. World Health Organization, Geneva
14. Green R, Money J (1969) Transsexualism and sex-reassignment. Johns Hopkins University Press, Baltimore, p 3
15. Green R, Money J (1969) Transsexualism and sex-reassignment. Johns Hopkins University Press, Baltimore, p 4
16. Benjamin H (1966) The transsexual phenomenon. Julian Press, New York
17. Green R, Money J (1969) Transsexualism and sex-reassignment. Johns Hopkins University Press, Baltimore, p 9
18. McHugh P (2006) Surgical sex. In: The mind has mountains. Johns Hopkins University Press, Baltimore, p 221
19. Charing Cross Gender Identity Clinic located on internet. http://www.wlmht.nhs.uk/gi/gender-identity-clinic/
20. WPATH History of the association past leadership (1995) http://www.wpath.org/site_page.cfm?pk_association_webpage_menu=1347&pk_association_webpage=3911. Retrieved 8 June 2014
21. Green R, Money J (1969) Transsexualism and sex-reassignment. Johns Hopkins University Press, Baltimore, Dedication
22. Dewhurst CJ (1969) 1st international symposium on gender identity, London. http://www.wpath.org/site_page.cfm?pk_association_webpage_menu=1347&pk_association_webpage=4229. Retrieved 4 May 2014
23. Devor A (2013) International Symposia, the 2nd International Gender Identity Symposium (1971) Elsinore, 12–14 Sept 1971. http://www.wpath.org/site_page.cfm?pk_association_webpage_menu=1347&pk_association_webpage=4229
24. Devor A (2013) International Symposia, the 3rd international symposium on Gender Identity (1973) Dubrovnik, 8–10 Sept 1973. http://www.wpath.org/site_page.cfm?pk_association_webpage_menu=1347&pk_association_webpage=4229
25. Matte N, Devor A, Vladicka T (2009) Nomenclature in WPATH's standards of care: background and recommendations. Int J Transgenderism 11(1):45, quoting MacKensie
26. Devor A (2013) International Symposia, the 5th international Gender Dysphoria symposium (1977) Norfolk 10–13 Feb. http://www.wpath.org/site_page.cfm?pk_association_webpage_menu=1347&pk_association_webpage=4229
27. Stoller R, Vol I (1975) Perversion: the erotic form of hatred. Dell, New York
28. Stoller R (1964) A contribution to the study of gender identity. Int J Psychoanal 45:220–226

29. Stoller R (1968) Sex and gender. Science House, New York
30. Socarides CW (1969) The desire for sexual transformation: a psychiatric evaluation of transsexualism. Am J Psychiatry 125:1419–1425
31. Ovesey L, Person E (1973) Gender identity and sexual psychopathology in men: a psychodynamic analysis of homosexuality, transsexualism and transvestism. J Am Acad Psychoanal 1(1):53–72
32. Ovesey L, Person E (1976) Transvestism: a disorder of the sense of self. Int J Psychoanal Psychother 5:221–235
33. Person E, Ovesey L (1974) The transsexual syndrome in males: I. Primary transsexualism. Am J Psychother 28:4–20
34. Person E, Ovesey L (1974) The transsexual syndrome in males: II. Secondary transsexualism. Am J Psychother 28:174–193
35. Person E, Ovesey L (1978) Transvestism: new perspectives. J Am Acad Psychoanal 6:301–323
36. Rekers G, Lovaas O (1974) Behavioral treatment of deviant sex-role behaviors in a male child. J Appl Behav Anal 7:173–190
37. Fisk NM (1974) Editorial: Gender dysphoria syndrome—the conceptualization that liberalizes indications for total gender reorientation and implies a broadly based multi-dimensional rehabilitative regimen. West J Med 120(5):386–391
38. McHugh PR (1992) Psychiatric misadventures. Am Scholar 61:497–510
39. Raymond J (1979) The transsexual empire. Beacon Press, Boston
40. American Psychiatric Association (1980) Diagnostic and statistical manual of mental disorders DSM III. APA, Washington, DC, p 263
41. American Psychiatric Association (1987) Diagnostic and statistical manual of mental disorders DSM III-R. APA, Washington, DC
42. Stoller RJ (1985) Presentations of gender. Yale University Press, New Haven/London
43. Drescher J, Cohen-Kettenis P, Winter S (2012) Minding the body: situating gender identity diagnosis in the ICD-11. Int Rev Psychiatry 24(6): 568–577
44. Blanchard R (1985) Typology of male-to-female transsexualism. Arch Sex Behav 14:247–261
45. Green R (1987) The "sissy boy syndrome" and the development of homosexuality. Yale University Press, New Haven
46. Lothstein L (1989) Presentation at XI HBIGDA symposium, Cleveland
47. Lothstein L (1983) Female-to-male transsexualism, historical, clinical and theoretical issues. Routledge and Kegan Paul, Boston/London/Melbourne/Henley
48. Kismodi E et al (2014) ICD Plenary, 23rd WPATH symposium, Bangkok, 16 Feb 2014
49. HBIGDA (1998) The standards of care for gender identity disorders version 5, p 48. Available online at http://www.wpath.org
50. Herdt G (ed) (1994) Third sex third gender, beyond sexual dimorphism in culture and history. Zone Books, New York
51. Zhou JN et al (1995) A sex difference in the human brain and its relation to transsexuality. Nature 378:68–70
52. Boswell H (1991) The transgender alternative. Chrysalis Q 1(2):29–31
53. Denny D (2014) Moving trans history forward, University of Victoria Trans Archives Symposium, 21–23 Mar. Victoria, BC.
54. Press for Change Information online at http://www.pfc.org.uk
55. Bornstein K (1994) Gender outlaw: on men, women, and the rest of us. Routledge, New York
56. HBIGDA (2001) The standards of care for gender identity disorders, p 85. Available online at http://www.wpath.org
57. More K, Whittle S (eds) (1999) Reclaiming genders. Cassell, London/New York
58. Peirce K (Director) (1999) Boys don't cry (Motion picture)
59. Hill W (Director) (2001) Southern comfort (Motion picture)
60. Lev A (2004) Transgender emergence, therapeutic guidelines for working with gender-variant people and their families. Haworth, Binghamton
61. Green J (2004) Becoming a visible man. Vanderbilt University Press, Nashville
62. Bailey JM (2003) Man who would be queen. Joseph Henry Press, Washington, DC
63. Yogyakarta Principles (2007) Principles on the application of international human rights law in relation to sexual orientation and gender identity. http://www.yogyakartaprinciples.org/principles_en.htm
64. Bockting W (2009) 21st Biennial International Symposium, Vision of the incoming president, Oslo, 20 June 2009
65. Council of Europe Commissioner for Human Rights (2009). Issue Paper: Human Rights and Gender Identity. https://wcd.coe.int/ViewDoc.jsp?id=1476365. In: Drescher J, Cohen-Kettenis P, Winter S (2012) Minding the body: Situating gender identity diagnosis in the ICD-11. Int Rev Psychiatry 24(6):572
66. WPATH Board of Directors (2010) De-psychopathologisation statement released May 26, 2010. Retrieved from http://www.wpath.org/site_page.cfm?pk_association_webpage_menu=1351&pk_association_webpage=3928
67. WPATH Board of Directors (2010) Identity recognition statement released June 16, 2010. Available online http://www.wpath.org/site_page.cfm?pk_association_webpage_menu=1351&pk_association_webpage=3928
68. Coleman E (2011) XXII Biennial Symposium, Launch of version 7 of the WPATH standards of care for transgender health, Atlanta, 25 Sept
69. Mazin R (2011) Blueprint for provision of care to transgender persons in Latin America and the Caribbean, presentation at Technical Consultation PAHO meeting, Washington, DC, 19–21 Dec

The DSM-5 Diagnostic Criteria for Gender Dysphoria

4

Kenneth J. Zucker

4.1 Placement in the Nomenclature

In DSM-III [1], *gender identity disorders* were introduced into the psychiatric nomenclature, and, in the chapter on psychosexual disorders, there were three specific diagnoses: gender identity disorder of childhood (GIDC), *transsexualism* (for adolescents and adults), and atypical gender identity disorder (a residual diagnosis). In DSM-III-R [2], there were four specific diagnoses, which were moved to the chapter on disorders usually first evident in infancy, childhood, or adolescence: GIDC; transsexualism; gender identity disorder of adolescence or adulthood, nontranssexual type; and gender identity disorder not otherwise specified (GIDNOS). In DSM-IV [3], there was a reduction in diagnoses to two, now placed in the chapter Sexual and Gender Identity Disorders: Gender Identity Disorder (GID) (with distinct criteria sets for children vs. adolescents/adults) and GIDNOS. In DSM-5 [4], there is a distinct chapter called *Gender Dysphoria*, which contains three diagnoses: gender dysphoria (with distinct criteria sets for children vs. adolescents/adults), other specified gender dysphoria, and unspecified gender dysphoria. In this chapter, I will review and summarize the key changes to this diagnostic category that were made in DSM-5. A more detailed account can be found elsewhere [5].

4.2 Conceptual Issues

The DSM-5 Task Force was announced in April 2008, and the Sexual and Gender Identity Disorders Work Group (for which I was the chair) was one of 13 groups charged with the task of reviewing the DSM-IV diagnoses and to recommend the addition, deletion, or reform of diagnostic categories. The Gender Identity Disorders Sub-work Group (chaired by PT Cohen-Kettenis) published four review papers, taking stock of conceptual issues, along with empirical issues and proposals for revision to the diagnosis of GID in DSM-IV [6–9].

The most overarching conceptual issue was whether or not the GID diagnosis should be retained in *DSM-5*. Many transgendered activists and some clinicians certainly wanted the disorder to be removed, arguing that GID was not a mental disorder, and wanted its removal for reasons similar to the removal of homosexuality from DSM-II in 1973: transsexualism was nothing more than a normal variant of gender identity, that its classification as a mental disorder contributed to stigma, and that there was nothing inherently "wrong" with a gender identity that was incongruent with one's biological sex [10, 11]. For various reasons, the Gender Identity Disorders Sub-work Group recommended the

K.J. Zucker
Gender Identity Service, Child, Youth, and Family Services, Centre for Addiction and Mental Health, Intergenerational Wellness Centre,
Beamish Family Wing, 80 Workman Way,
Toronto, ON M6J 1H4, Canada
e-mail: Ken.Zucker@camh.ca

C. Trombetta et al. (eds.), *Management of Gender Dysphoria: A Multidisciplinary Approach*,
DOI 10.1007/978-88-470-5696-1_4, © Springer-Verlag Italia 2015

retention of the diagnosis in DSM-5, including the important issue of access to care [7], but with a variety of substantive changes and reforms.

4.3 Summary of Diagnostic Changes

There were ten relatively substantial changes to the DSM-IV-TR diagnosis of GID, which I summarize here (see also [5]):

1. The diagnostic label was changed to gender dysphoria (GD), which was based on two considerations: first, it was selected as a more accurate term which highlighted the aversive emotional component of the condition and was already a term that has had a long history in clinical sexology [12]. It was also consistent with the general argument that the diagnostic term should, in a more transparent manner, indicate that it pertains to "distress" (dysphoria) and not identity per se [13]. Second, there was considerable support on the website of the American Psychiatric Association during the three periods of open commentary that removal of the "disorder" label in the name of the diagnosis would be less stigmatizing (see also [11]).
2. In DSM-5, GD has its own chapter and thus has been decoupled from the sexual dysfunctions and paraphilias, which also have their own chapters. The prior placement of these three diagnostic classes in prior editions of the DSM was probably influenced by several considerations, including clinical utility. At the same time, however, it was argued that the theoretical overlap among these three broad classes of conditions was far from complete. For example, sexual dysfunctions are of little direct relevance to GD as it manifests in children. It was also argued that inclusion of GD in a section of the manual that also included the paraphilias was somewhat stigmatizing. Although GD in adolescents and adults frequently co-occurs with one paraphilia, *transvestic disorder* [14], the Gender Identity Disorders Sub-work Group recommended that the advantages of uncoupling the major diagnostic classes outweighed the disadvantages.
3. As can be seen in Table 4.1, the Point A criterion introduced a conceptual shift in how best to understand GD by describing it as "A marked *incongruence* between one's experienced/expressed gender and assigned gender, of at least 6 months durations…" The term incongruence was descriptive and reflected the core of the problem, namely, an incongruence between, on the one hand, the identity that one experiences and/or expresses and, on the other hand, how one is expected to live based on one's assigned gender (usually at birth) [8]. It was also deemed preferable to the DSM-IV-TR descriptor "cross-gender identification" in that a strictly binary gender identity concept is no longer in line with the spectrum of gender identity variations that one sees clinically [5].
4. In contrast to DSM-IV-TR, which had two sets of clinical indicators (Criteria A and B), the symptom indicators in DSM-5 were merged into a single criterion set. The distinction in DSM-IV-TR was never supported by factor analytic studies, which all pointed to one underlying dimension [9, 15, 16].
5. The GD criteria for children are potentially more conservative than they were in DSM-IV-TR because the current A1 criterion (of a total of eight symptoms) is now a necessary symptom for the diagnosis (in total, 6/8 symptoms are required for the diagnosis). The A1 criterion pertains to the child's "… strong desire to be of the other gender or an insistence that he or she is the other gender (or some alternative gender different from one's assigned gender)." The tightening of the requirement for caseness will likely sharpen the distinction between a diagnosis of GD and normative variation.

As reviewed in Zucker [9], critics of the DSM-IV-TR diagnostic criteria were concerned that some children who showed pervasive cross-gender behavior, yet who did not express a desire to be of the other gender, might be inappropriately diagnosed with GD (false-positives). Secondary data analyses

[5, 9] supported the idea that requiring the presence of a strong desire to be of the other gender, along with various surface expressions of gender incongruence, would probably raise the bar for caseness, with strong evidence for sensitivity and specificity.

6. For adolescents (and adults), the DSM-5 diagnostic criteria for GD moved to a more detailed *polythetic format* (six symptoms), replacing the somewhat sketchy criteria that were used in DSM-IV-TR. Secondary data analyses indicated that the presence of at least two indicators yielded a rate of 94.2 % sensitivity and 99.3 % specificity [5].
7. Whether or not individuals born with a physical intersex condition (now termed a *disorder of sex development*) (DSD) should be eligible for a diagnosis of GD has had a back-and-forth history since DSM-III [17]. Since the publication of DSM-IV in 1994, considerable additional evidence has accumulated that some individuals with a DSD experience GD and may wish to change their assigned gender [18, 19]. The percentage of such individuals who experience GD is syndrome dependent [20, 21]. From a phenomenological perspective, DSD individuals with GD have both similarities and differences to individuals with GD with no known DSD, and there are also similarities and differences in developmental trajectories [4, pp. 455–456]. Because the presence of a DSD is suggestive of a specific causal mechanism that may not be present in individuals without a diagnosable DSD, it was included as a specifier in DSM-5.
8. For adolescents (and adults), the DSM-IV-TR specifier for *sexual attraction* (to males, to females, to both, to neither) was eliminated in DSM-5. This decision was a highly controversial one. On the one hand, there is considerable evidence that sexual attraction (orientation), typically dichotomized as homosexual or nonhomosexual in relation to the patient's birth sex, is associated with meaningful differences among GD adolescents and adults (e.g., age of onset, birth order, degree of expression of cross-gender behavior in childhood, co-occurrence

Table 4.1 DSM-5 criteria for gender dysphoria

Children
A. A marked incongruence between one's experienced/expressed gender and assigned gender, of at least 6 months' duration, as manifested by at least six of the following (one of which must be Criterion A1):
1. A strong desire to be of the other gender or an insistence that one is the other gender (or some alternative gender different from one's assigned gender)
2. In boys (assigned gender), a strong preference for cross-dressing or simulating female attire; or in girls (assigned gender), a strong preference for wearing only typical masculine clothing and a strong resistance to the wearing of typical feminine clothing
3. A strong preference for cross-gender roles in make-believe play or fantasy play
4. A strong preference for the toys, games, or activities stereotypically used or engaged in by the other gender
5. A strong preference for playmates of the other gender
6. In boys (assigned gender), a strong rejection of typically masculine toys, games, and activities and a strong avoidance of rough-and-tumble play; or in girls (assigned gender), a strong rejection of typically feminine toys, games, and activities
7. A strong dislike of one's sexual anatomy
8. A strong desire for the primary and/or secondary sex characteristics that match one's experienced gender
B. The condition is associated with clinically significant distress or impairment in social, school, or other important areas of functioning
Specify if:
With a disorder of sex development (e.g., a congenital adrenogenital disorder such as congenital adrenal hyperplasia or androgen insensitivity syndrome)
Adolescents and adults
A. A marked incongruence between one's experienced/expressed gender and assigned gender, of at least 6 months' duration, as manifested by at least two of the following:
1. A marked incongruence between one's experienced/expressed gender and primary and/or secondary sex characteristics (or in young adolescents, the anticipated secondary sex characteristics)
2. A strong desire to be rid of one's primary and/or secondary sex characteristics because of a marked incongruence with one's experienced/expressed gender (or in young adolescents, a desire to prevent the development of the anticipated secondary sex characteristics)

(continued)

Table 4.1 (continued)

3. A strong desire for the primary and/or secondary sex characteristics of the other gender
4. A strong desire to be of the other gender (or some alternative gender different from one's assigned gender)
5. A strong desire to be treated as the other gender (or some alternative gender different from one's assigned gender)
6. A strong conviction that one has the typical feelings and reactions of the other gender (or some alternative gender different from one's assigned gender)
B. The condition is associated with clinically significant distress or impairment in social, occupational, or other important areas of functioning
Specify if:
With a disorder of sex development (e.g., a congenital adrenogenital disorder such as congenital adrenal hyperplasia or androgen insensitivity syndrome)
Specify if:
Posttransition: the individual has transitioned to full-time living in the desired gender (with or without legalization of gender change) and has undergone (or is preparing to have) at least one cross-sex medical procedure or treatment regimen – namely, regular cross-sex hormone treatment or gender reassignment surgery confirming the desired gender (e.g., penectomy, vaginoplasty in a natal male; mastectomy or phalloplasty in a natal female)

Note: Reprinted with the permission of the American Psychiatric Association

with transvestic disorder in natal males) [22]. There is also evidence that subtyping by sexual attraction (orientation) is related to differences in underlying casual mechanisms for the genesis of GD (for an exhaustive review, see [23]). On the other hand, sexual attraction per se currently plays only a minor role in contemporary treatment protocols or decisions [6]. Moreover, it has been argued that sexual attraction does not, in and of itself, reflect a difference in symptom expression of GD, which is a cornerstone of the meaning of a specifier in the DSM. Thus, the DSM-5 GID Sub-work Group recommended its deletion; however, in the DSM-5 text [4, pp. 454–456], the two sexual attraction types are described in detail with regard to *developmental trajectories* and with regard to their relevance for research that focuses on underlying casual mechanisms.

9. A lower-bound 6-month duration criterion was introduced into the GD diagnostic criteria. This decision was based on clinical consensus or expert opinion, not on formal empirical studies. The introduction of a *duration criterion* was, in part, to caution against a "hasty" diagnosis of GD (with the potential for inappropriate treatments) for cases in which the symptoms might well prove to be transitory.
10. Lastly, a *posttransition specifier* was added to the GD criteria for adolescents and adults. The addition of this specifier was prompted by the observation that many individuals, after transition, do not meet any more the criteria set for GD; however, they continue to undergo chronic hormone treatment, further gender-confirming surgery, or intermittent psychotherapy/counseling to facilitate the adaptation to life in the desired gender and the social consequences of the transition. Although the concept of "posttransition" was modeled on the concept "in [partial or full] remission" as used for mood disorders, "remission" has implications in terms of symptom reduction that do not apply directly to GD. Cross-sex hormone treatment of gonadectomized individuals could, of course, be coded as treatment of hypogonadism, but this would not apply to individuals who have not undergone gonadectomy but receive hormone treatments. In the DSM-5 text, it is noted that the course specifier of "full remission" in its original meaning does apply to many children with the diagnosis of GD and, perhaps, to a small number of adolescents and adults.

References

1. American Psychiatric Association (1980) Diagnostic and statistical manual of mental disorders, 3rd edn. American Psychiatric Association, Washington, DC
2. American Psychiatric Association (1987) Diagnostic and statistical manual of mental disorders (rev 3rd ed). American Psychiatric Association, Washington, DC
3. American Psychiatric Association (1994) Diagnostic and statistical manual of mental disorders, 4th edn. American Psychiatric Association, Washington, DC

4. American Psychiatric Association (2013) Diagnostic and statistical manual of mental disorders, 5th edn. American Psychiatric Association, Arlington
5. Zucker KJ, Cohen-Kettenis PT, Drescher J et al (2013) Memo outlining evidence for change for gender identity disorder in the DSM-5. Arch Sex Behav 42:901–914
6. Cohen-Kettenis PT, Pfäfflin F (2010) The DSM diagnostic criteria for gender identity disorder in adolescents and adults. Arch Sex Behav 39:499–513
7. Drescher J (2010) Queer diagnoses: parallels and contrasts in the history of homosexuality, gender variance, and the *Diagnostic and Statistical Manual*. Arch Sex Behav 39:427–460
8. Meyer-Bahlburg HFL (2010) From mental disorder to iatrogenic hypogonadism: dilemmas in conceptualizing gender identity variants as psychiatric conditions. Arch Sex Behav 39:461–476
9. Zucker KJ (2010) The DSM diagnostic criteria for gender identity disorder in children. Arch Sex Behav 39:477–498
10. Ault A, Brzuzy S (2009) Removing gender identity disorder from the Diagnostic and Statistical Manual of Mental Disorders: a call for action. Soc Work 54:187–189
11. Vance SR, Cohen-Kettenis PT, Drescher J et al (2010) Opinions about the *DSM* gender identity disorder diagnosis: results from an international survey administered to organizations concerned with the welfare of transgender people. Int J Transgenderism 12:1–14
12. Fisk N (1973) Gender dysphoria syndrome (the how, what, and why of a disease). In: Laub D, Gandy P (eds) Proceedings of the second interdisciplinary symposium on gender dysphoria syndrome. Stanford University Press, Palo Alto, pp 7–14
13. Knudson G, De Cuypere G, Bockting W (2010) Recommendations for revision of the *DSM* diagnosis of gender identity disorders: Consensus Statement of the World Professional Association for Transgender Health. Int J Transgenderism 12:115–118
14. Blanchard R (2010) The DSM diagnostic criteria for transvestic fetishism. Arch Sex Behav 39:363–372
15. Paap MC, Kreukels BP, Cohen-Kettenis PT et al (2011) Assessing the utility of diagnostic criteria: a multisite study on gender identity disorder. J Sex Med 8:180–190
16. Zucker KJ, Green R, Bradley SJ et al (1998) Gender identity disorder of childhood: diagnostic issues. In: Widiger TA, Frances AJ, Pincus HA et al (eds) DSM-IV sourcebook, vol 4. American Psychiatric Association, Washington, DC, pp 503–512
17. Meyer-Bahlburg HFL (1994) Intersexuality and the diagnosis of gender identity disorder. Arch Sex Behav 23:21–40
18. Pasterski V, Zucker KJ, Hindmarsh PC et al (in press) Increased cross-gender identification independent of gender role behavior in girls with congenital adrenal hyperplasia: results from a standardized assessment of 4- to 11-year-old children. Arch Sex Behav
19. Richter-Appelt H, Sandberg DE (2010) Should disorders of sex development be an exclusion criterion for gender identity disorder in DSM 5? Int J Transgenderism 12:94–99
20. Meyer-Bahlburg HFL (2005) Gender identity outcome in female-raised 46, XY persons with penile agenesis, cloacal exstrophy of the bladder, or penile ablation. Arch Sex Behav 34:423–438
21. Meyer-Bahlburg HFL (2009) Variants of gender differentiation in somatic disorders of sex development: recommendations for Version 7 of the World Professional Association for Transgendered Health's Standards of Care. Int J Transgenderism 11:226–237
22. Zucker KJ, Bradley SJ, Owen-Anderson A et al (2012) Demographics, behavior problems, and psychosexual characteristics of adolescents with gender identity disorder or transvestic fetishism. J Sex Marital Ther 38:151–189
23. Lawrence AA (2010) Sexual orientation versus age of onset as bases for typologies (subtypes) of gender identity disorder in adolescents and adults. Arch Sex Behav 39:514–545

Epidemiologic Considerations on Transsexualism

5

Fabio Barbone

5.1 Introduction

To define what key literature and source of knowledge may offer epidemiologic considerations on a human condition such as gender dysphoria and transsexualism, it might be useful to recall that etiologic epidemiology is *the scientific observation of human beings for the purpose of discovering a cause of a disease* and that clinical epidemiology is *the study of determinants and effects of clinical decisions*. In the search for both causes and effects of human conditions, the first step must be a flawless and stable definition of the condition. Once such a definition has been accepted, variants are recognized – eventually determining mutually exclusive categories – then used for a relatively long time and in many geographic populations, then epidemiologic measures can be estimated including measures of frequency, measures of association, and measures of impact [1].

The first difficulty dealing with the epidemiologic evidence accrued related to the *incongruence between a subject's experienced gender (gender identity) and assigned gender* concentrates with the apparent conundrum of what area of medicine, if any, such a condition intercepts. The difficulty of choosing a definition has been considered in other chapters of this textbook, particularly the chapter by Cohen et al. entitled *Psychological Characteristics and Sexuality of Natal Males with Gender Dysphoria* [2].

The availability of a common, consensus-based definition is essential to classify conditions that may have a common etiologic web, similar signs and symptoms, diagnostic procedures, treatments, and type and burden of care. Lack of such a background for a sufficient time period and across populations, with the obvious conclusion of possible presence of ascertainment bias, does not allow easy comparison of disease frequency estimation, much less of other more sophisticated epidemiologic measures such as associations and impacts. Therefore, such measures, if calculated, must be used with caution and, if presented, are prone to controversy.

5.2 Methodological Issues

Table 5.1 describes variations of terms by historical periods, sources of terms, and categories within the defined condition.

As listed in Table 5.1, before 1975, neither the International Classification of Diseases (ICD) by the World Health Organization (WHO) nor the Diagnostic and Statistical Manual of Mental Disorders (DSM) by the American Psychiatric Association (APA) included any terms, names, and codes that referred to the *incongruence between a subject's experienced and assigned gender*. At that time the scientific literature, as

F. Barbone
Department of Medical and Biological Sciences,
University of Udine, Italy,
Piazzale Kolbe, 2, Udine 33100, Italy
e-mail: fabio.barbone@uniud.it

C. Trombetta et al. (eds.), *Management of Gender Dysphoria: A Multidisciplinary Approach*,
DOI 10.1007/978-88-470-5696-1_5, © Springer-Verlag Italia 2015

Table 5.1 Variations of terms by historical periods, sources of terms, and categories

Term	Transsexualism, desire to change sex	Gender identity disorder, transsexualism	Gender identity disorder	Gender dysphoria	
Time period of use	<1975	1975–2013	1994–2013	2013–	
Realm in medicine	Psychiatric symptoms, within schizophrenia or borderline personality disorder diagnosis	A psychiatric condition separate from other psychiatric diseases	A psychiatric condition separate from other psychiatric diseases	A psychiatric condition separate from other psychiatric diseases with presence of clinically significant distress associated with the condition	Not a psychiatric condition? Not a disorder at all? Rather a gender variant?
Sources of term and classification	Case reports and case series (<1975)	ICD-9 (1975) [3] DSM-III (1980) [4] ICD-10 (1994) [5]	DSM-IV (1994) [6]	DSM-5 (2013) [7] ICD-11 (2017?)	Cohen et al., this book [2] Dreger in *Pacific Standard* [8]
Number of variants or level of severity within the condition	Many	2 (yes vs no)	2 (yes vs no)	Many	Many

explored by bibliographic engines developed by the US National Library of Medicine (PubMed and derivatives), depended on the clinical work conducted in the 1950s that led to Harry P. Benjamin's description of the "transsexual phenomenon" in the USA [9]. At the time the literature had already coined terms such as "androgyne," "transvestism," "transgender," and "transsexual" and symptoms such as "desire to cross-dress" and "desire to change sex" had been identified and reported mostly in case reports and case series and scientific studies [10]. In the absence of a recognized classification of these conditions, nevertheless diagnostic psychological tests (i.e., the Bem Sex Role Inventory (BSRI) were developed (1971). The BSRI characterized personality as masculine, feminine, androgynous, or undifferentiated and was based on gender stereotypes, so what it was measuring was how well the person fit into a traditional sex role. At the same time, in terms of classification and etiology, transsexualism was considered mostly just as a symptom of another psychiatric disorder, especially schizophrenia or eventually a borderline personality disorder. As a consequence, there was neither interest nor a recognized definition and unique diagnosis and coding that allowed for the measurement of disease frequency. Therefore, before 1975 its epidemiology remained vague, and there could be numerous variants and levels of severity within the condition.

As far as clinical epidemiology, i.e., the study of determinants and effects of clinical decisions based on the transgender recognition or diagnosis by the subject and or by the medical community, medical journals reported male-to-female (MtF) and female-to-male (FtM) sex reassignment even before WWII but mostly as anecdotes. In 1965, the Hopkins Hospital became the first academic institution in the USA to perform sex reassignment surgeries. Before 1975 psychoanalytic literature held the belief that beneath the desire to change sex may lie a serious psychopathology – even of a psychotic nature – and that transsexual wishes may arise from oedipal conflict, preoedipal fixation, or schizophrenic processes [11]. Only in 1977 initially the Harry Benjamin International Gender Dysphoria Association (HBIGD), later (2007) renamed as the

World Professional Association for Transgender Health (WPATH), join to provide standard of care (SOC) for transgender persons, which currently has produced its 7th edition (SOC7) [12].

In 1975 the ICD-9 of the WHO introduced specific psychiatric terms, conditions, and codes separate from other psychiatric diseases for sexual and gender identity disorders, particularly:

302: Sexual and Gender Identity Disorders, among which are:

302.5: Trans-sexualism

302.6: Gender Identity Disorder in Children

302.85: Gender Identity Disorder in Adolescents or Adults

This classification created the opportunity for any gender identity disorder and for transsexualism in particular to calculate disease frequency, associations with subject's characteristics and measures of impact.

In 1980 the DSM-III of APA confirmed the ICD-9 classification while specifying that the transsexualism diagnosis required:

A. Sense of discomfort and inappropriateness about one's anatomic sex
B. Wish to get rid of one's own genitals and to live as a member of the other sex
C. The disturbance has been continuous (not limited to periods of stress) for at least 2 years
D. Absence of physical intersex or genetic abnormality
E. Not due to another mental disorder, such as schizophrenia

Codes changed in ICD-10:

F64: Gender Identity Disorders

F64.0 Transsexualism

F64.1 Dual-Role Transvestism

F64.2 Gender Identity Disorder of Childhood

F64.8 Other Gender Identity Disorders

F64.9 Gender identity disorder, unspecified)

However, definitions remained relatively stable. Instead DSM-IV accommodated all strong and persistent cross-gender identification accompanied by persistent discomfort with one's assigned sex previously listed separately as Gender Identity Disorder of Childhood, Gender Identity Disorder of Adolescence or Adulthood, and Transsexualism at both sexes and all ages in the unique DSM-IV code 532: Gender Identity Disorder.

As a result, between 1975 and 2013, the estimate of the overall frequency of "gender identity disorder" may have been consistent between classification systems (ICD vs DSM), whereas the frequency of transsexualism could only be measured based on ICD as DSM from 1994 to 2013 collapsed all subcategories within gender identity disorders. In addition, for all epidemiologic research conducted to date in this field, we should not underestimate the chance that exists for ascertainment bias (especially underreporting) for all the individuals who did not match the five DSM-IV diagnostic criteria for transsexualism but still could fit into the "gender identity disorder." It is likely that the estimate of the frequency of such a group depended on historical period, societal pressures, sex assigned at birth, country, and especially attitudes and proficiency on the subject by the local medical communities. Differences in these nonbiological determinants may have caused biased estimates of the frequency of these conditions.

Also the future of epidemiologic estimates will depend, as for the past, primarily on case definition and attitudes toward case ascertainment. The long-lasting tendency to move gender identity questioning initially away from psychiatry and then away from the concept of "medical abnormality," as advocated by some groups of subjects and professionals, may at the end determine the elimination of gender identity disorder, as it happened for definitions of homosexuality, which was no longer listed as a category of disorder in the seventh printing of the DSM-II, in 1974, and again from the DSM-III. In fact, in DSM-5 with the new term "gender dysphoria" and its definition as "A psychiatric condition separate from other psychiatric diseases with presence of clinically significant distress associated with the condition," the clinical existence of a mental disorder in this field is restricted to the "significant distress" that may accompany gender identity issues. From the epidemiologic standpoint and to measure the frequency of this condition, it is then likely that accordingly the number of subjects meeting this definition will be reduced further, from previous, broader definitions which did not require such a "significant distress." ICD-11 (expected to be released in 2017) and SOC7 of WPATH are consistent with this approach. In conclusion, the transsexual, transgender, and gender nonconforming people are likely to be considered more and more for their health needs rather than as carriers of a pathological condition. Consequently, in the future the epidemiologic measurement of the frequency of this health characteristic is likely to identify a human variation that has no specific abnormality meaning per se but is of clinical interest because it might be associated sometimes with pathological conditions or might require clinical intervention to satisfy a need of the subject.

5.3 Epidemiologic Associations Between Gender Dysphoria and Mental Health Disorders

Reports of these associations have been relatively common. Heylens et al. investigated psychiatric problems within the European Network for the Investigation of Gender Incongruence (ENIGI) [13]. The network had study bases in Amsterdam (Netherlands), Ghent (Belgium), Hamburg (Germany), and Oslo (Norway). Participants were 305 adults seeking gender reassignment therapy and surgery at the four gender clinics and fulfilling DSM-IV-TR criteria for a diagnosis of gender identity disorder. Data were collected between January 2007 and October 2010. The Utrecht Gender Dysphoria Scale (UGDS) was used to measure the degree of experienced gender dysphoria. The Mini International Neuropsychiatric Interview – Plus version 5.0.0 (MINI-Plus) was used to measure Axis I diagnoses at the time of the interview ("current diagnosis") and disorders that have a longer history ("current and lifetime diagnosis"). The Structured Clinical Interview for DSM-IV Axis II Personality Disorders (SCID-II) was used to assess Axis II diagnoses; this is a semi-structured clinical interview. In 38 % of the individuals with gender identity disorder, a current DSM-IV-TR Axis I diagnosis was found, mainly affective disorders and anxiety disorders. Furthermore, almost 70 % had a current and lifetime diagnosis. All four countries showed a similar prevalence, except for affective and anxiety disorders, and no difference was found between individuals with early-onset and late-onset disorders. An Axis II diagnosis was found in 15 % of all individuals with gender identity disorder, which is comparable to the general population. In conclusion, people with gender identity disorder show more affective and anxiety problems than the general population [13].

Some authors found associations between GD and autism spectrum disorders. Therefore, they were cautious about irreversible treatments (sexual reassignment surgery) before autism spectrum disorders were excluded and a genuine issue of transsexualism was confirmed. In particular, John Parkinson [14] reported the incidence of Asperger's syndrome as above average in young people presenting with gender dysphoria. Patients with Asperger's syndrome, however, were prone to obsessive preoccupations and the apparent dysphoria may in some cases prove to be a transient obsession.

A recent epidemiologic survey reported that individuals with pervasive developmental disorders (PDD) often have identity crises, which sometimes include gender dysphoria [15]. It has been proposed that the rate of PDD may be almost 1 % and that many PDD cases might not be diagnosed properly in childhood. PDD are characterized by two essential symptoms: impairment in social interaction and restricted, repetitive, and stereotyped patterns of behavior, interests, and activities. PDD include autistic disorder, Asperger's disorder, and PDD-not otherwise specified (PDD-NOS). These three disorders are part of autism spectrum disorders. Among 204 children and adolescents who visited a GID clinic in the Netherlands, 7.8 % were diagnosed with autism spectrum disorders after a careful diagnostic procedure by a multidisciplinary team. Taken together, these authors considered PDD and GID still closely related to each other.

The Japanese Society of Psychiatry and Neurology published guidelines for the assessment and treatment of GID in 1997 and revised them in 2006. As a result, GID has become well known as a clinical entity in Japan, and there have been an increasing number of Japanese patients complaining of gender dysphoria. At the same time also their guidelines caution clinicians to consider an underlying diagnosis of PDD when encountering patients with gender dysphoria [15].

An association between personality disorder and gender dysphoria has been reported [16], with prevalence of personality disorder varying between 20 and 70 % in different studies. Personality disorder is defined as an enduring pattern of thinking and feeling about oneself and others that significantly and adversely affect how an individual functions in the various aspects of life (DSM-5). Personality disorder prevalence among GD cases with anxious symptoms might be even higher.

Results of positive effects of treatment were found instead in a large review of the literature conducted by Murad et al. [17]. In terms of psychological health among subjects who were treated for reassignment surgery, the authors concluded on the basis of 28 studies, with 1,833 persons with gender dysphoria (1,093 natal males and 801 natal females) and an average follow-up of 6 years, that 78 % of persons had less psychiatric problems after treatment of their GD than before. For people with GD, gender reassignment thus seemed to have positive influence on their mental health.

5.4 Suicide and Non-psychiatric Associations

A Swedish cohort study of 324 persons with transsexualism was followed after sex reassignment (also termed gender confirmation intervention) [18]. The objective of this study was to shed new light on transsexual persons' health after sex reassignment. In particular, the study investigated all-cause mortality, suicide, cardiovascular diseases, and neoplasms. Morbidity included any psychiatric disorder (gender identity disorders excluded), alcohol/drug misuse and dependence, definite/uncertain suicide attempt, and injuries. Finally, court convictions for any criminal offense and any violent offense were investigated. Gender reassignment was as follows: male-to-female (MtF), $N=191$, and female-to-male (FtM), $N=133$. For each transsexual (exposed) person, ten non-transsexual (unexposed) comparison subjects were randomly selected. Considerably higher risks for total mortality and selected causes of death were measured. Specifically, compared to unexposed subjects, overall survival of transsexual persons started to diverge from that of matched comparators after about 10 years of follow-up. The increased adjusted hazard ratios (aHR) were 2.9 (95 % CI: 1.9–4.5) for all causes of death, 2.5 (1.2–5.3) for death from cardiovascular diseases, 2.1 (1.0–4.6) for cancer death, and 19.1 (5.8–68.9) for suicide. This mortality pattern is rather consistent among both male-born and female-born subjects. Any psychiatric hospitalization, substance abuse, suicide attempts, any injury, and any crime were also significantly higher among the exposed cohort members. However, in subgroup analyses, suicide attempts were more frequent among MtF (aHR: 10.4 (4.9–22.1)) versus comparators, whereas crime was frequent only within the FtM subgroup (aHR: 4.1 (2.5–6.9)).

Another major long-term epidemiologic follow-up study of mortality was conducted in the Netherlands among 966 male-to-female (MtF) and 365 female-to-male (FtM) transsexuals receiving treatment with cross-sex hormones [19]. An increased mortality in hormone-treated MtF transsexuals (122 observed, 81 expected, SMR = 1.51; 95 % CI: 1.47–1.55) was associated with both hormone- and non-hormone-related causes. Strong associations were found with lung cancer, hematological neoplasms, ischemic heart disease, cerebrovascular accidents, AIDS, and external causes (particularly illicit drug use and suicide and unknown/ill-defined symptoms). No deaths from breast cancer were identified in this cohort. However, in previous publications from this cohort [20], breast cancer was reported in one MtF and one FtM. The former case had a 30-year exposure to estrogens. The latter occurred in a subject with bilateral mastectomy while receiving treatment with testosterone that had lasted 10 years. This occurred in residual mammary tissue and may be caused by testosterone, which is partially aromatized to estradiol. Furthermore, other results from this set of publications related to this cohort included frequent venous thrombosis (6–8 %) among ethinyl estradiol users and deleterious effects on cardiovascular risk in MtF androgen-deprived, estrogen-using transsexuals, while increased cardiovascular morbidity or mortality was not clearly demonstrated among FtM transsexuals with prolonged use of androgens.

5.5 Prevalence of GD

BMJ Best Practice (http://bestpractice.bmj.com/bestpractice/monograph/992/basics/epidemiology.html) reports the prevalence of gender dysphoria as approximately 1.67 per 100,000 born males (i.e., about 1 in every 60,000) and 1 per 100,000 born females [21]. In Northern Europe, the prevalence of transsexualism has been estimated at approximately 1:12,000 cases in males and 1:30,000 cases in females. In the USA, there seems to be no significant association between transsexualism and social class, intelligence, or ancestry. As discussed previously in this chapter, cases reported by gender identity clinics may be increasing, but this may reflect better access to diagnosis and treatment rather than increasing incidence.

In 1998, the prevalence in Scotland of gender dysphoria among patients aged over 15 years was calculated as 8.18 per 100,000, with an approximate sex ratio of 4:1 in favor of male-to-female patients. One-third of gender-dysphoric patients known to practices had registered in the preceding 12 months, suggesting that patients with this condition are increasingly likely to present for medical care. Questionnaires were sent to senior partners in all general practices in Scotland designed to elicit experience of patients with gender dysphoria: a subjective experience of incongruity between genital anatomy and gender identity. Responses were received from 73 % of practices [22].

Prevalence estimates by special interest organizations in the UK such as the Gender Identity Research and Education Society (The Number of Gender Variant People in the UK – Update 2011 http://www.gires.org.uk) [23] show much higher proportions. In terms of absolute numbers, 12,500 may have presented for treatment representing a prevalence of 20 per 100,000 (both born genders combined). The same organization suggests a strong increase also based on change of cultural climate.

According to a recent Japanese study, FtM-type GID patients are present with a point prevalence of at least 90/100,000 and an estimated lifetime prevalence of 0.001–0.002 % [24].

In Serbia, the prevalence of transsexualism according to cases seen at the only clinic performing sex reassignment has been estimated about 1/100,000. The relatively young age of those applying for sex reassignment and the sex ratio of 1:1 distinguish the population in Serbia from others reported in the literature [25].

Most previous studies of the prevalence of transsexualism have used data from individuals seeking sex reassignment surgery. New Zealand is unique in that transsexual people can apply to have an "X" for the sex on their passport if they have a name on their birth certificate that is congruent with the sex opposite to their birth assigned sex and provide a statutory declaration stating they have lived as a member of that sex. From the information provided by the New Zealand Passports Office, the authors ascertained that the prevalence of transsexualism among New Zealand passport holders was at least 16/100,000 (i.e., 1 in every 6,364). The prevalence of male-to-female transsexualism was 27/100,000 (i.e., 1 in every 3,639), and the corresponding figure for female-to-male transsexualism was 4/1,000,000 (i.e., 1 in every 1:22,714). The estimates from New Zealand were higher than most previous estimates of transsexualism prevalence. There was also a larger-than-expected ratio of male-to-female transsexual people to female-to-male transsexual people (6:1), which could in part be due to female-to-male transsexual people being relatively overrepresented among those transsexual people for whom we did not have data on the direction of sex change, or this may be indicative of the demography of transsexualism in Australasia [26].

In Belgium, the overall prevalence is 1:12,900 for male-to-female and 1:33,800 for female-to-male transsexuals. In Wallonia (the French-speaking region of Belgium), the prevalence is significantly lower than in Flanders (the Dutch-speaking region) and in Brussels (the bilingual

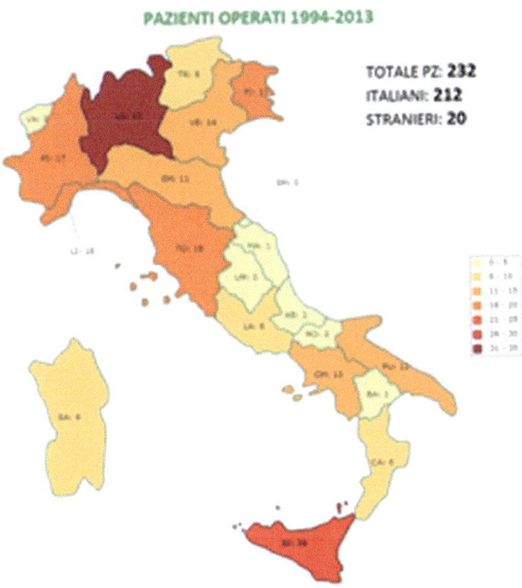

Fig. 5.1 Region of residence of subjects who underwent sex reassignment in Trieste, Italy

capital region). In the total Belgian population, the male/female sex ratio is 2.43:1, again with a substantial difference between Wallonia on the one hand and Flanders on the other. The authors suggest that transsexualism in Wallonia is socially less acceptable: persons suffering from gender dysphoria in that part of Belgium might encounter more problems accessing gender clinics and receiving treatment [27].

A much higher prevalence was calculated from a population survey in Massachusetts, USA including 28,176 respondents. 131 or 0.5 % responded yes to the question "Some people describe themselves as trans- gender when they experience a different gender identity from their sex at birth. For example, a person born into a male body, but who feels female or lives as a woman. Do you consider yourself to be transgender?" A more detailed definition of the term transgender was read to those who expressed confusion [28].

In terms of the absolute number of treated cases at the largest Italian sex reassignment clinic, Fig. 5.1 shows the geographic distribution by Italian region of residence (Trombetta C, 2014, personal communication).

5.6 Methods to Estimate Frequency in Hidden Populations and Conclusive Remarks

The validity of the evolving epidemiology of GD, inexorably dependent on its case definition and on the consistency of application of such a case definition across times and latitudes, is further at risk because it also depends on the cultural and medical acceptance of local communities. If gender-dysphoric persons or gender variants were a hidden population, because of stigma or of other reasons, it is likely that prevalence was underestimated, health services were not provided, and group was noninfluential. Subjects requiring medical attention with high probability would travel or even migrate to have their needs satisfied. On the other hand, if only the medical or surgical interventions represented a marker of the condition in time and space, this might reintroduce the abnormality to this population. To provide a correct estimate of the size of such a minority population in order to fulfill common needs associated with any human life, the surfacing of this hidden population should be pursued. It is beyond the scope of this book to present the statistical and demographic methodology necessary to reach such a goal. In brief, an ideal sampling procedure should be established that yields not only a sample independent of its starting point but also an unbiased sample of the underlying population with a known degree of consistency from which confidence intervals can be computed [29]. With some approximation, the goal might be to devise means for drawing samples that produce a good cross section or the coverage of heterogeneity in the target population. Among the many methods that may be adopted, respondent-driven sampling has been employed in subjects who might have been persecuted, who were victims of violence, who have posttraumatic stress disorder, and many others. Such a method is of special interest because it might reduce sampling bias that affects many of the current studies on this field.

References

1. Rothman K (1986) Modern epidemiology. Little Brown, Boston
2. Cohen K et al Psychological characteristics and sexuality of natal males with gender dysphoria
3. WHO Library (1975) International statistical classification of diseases and related health problems. 9th revision, Geneva
4. American Psychiatric Association (1980) Diagnostic and statistical manual of mental disorders (third edition, DSM-III). American Psychiatric Association, Washington, DC
5. WHO Library (1980) International statistical classification of diseases and related health problems. 10th revision, Geneva
6. American Psychiatric Association (1994) Diagnostic and statistical manual of mental disorders (forth edition, DSM-IV). American Psychiatric Association, Washington, DC
7. American Psychiatric Association (2013) Diagnostic and statistical manual of mental disorders (fifth edition, DSM-5). American Psychiatric Association, Washington, DC
8. Dreger A Why gender dysphoria should no longer be considered a medical disorder. In: Pacific Standard Magazine. http://www.psmag.com/navigation/health-and-behavior/take-gender-identity-disorder-dsm-68308/. 18 Oct 2013
9. Benjamin H (1966) The transsexual phenomenon. Julian Press, New York
10. Socarides CW (1978–1979) Transsexualism and psychosis. Int J Psychoanal Psychother 7:373–384
11. Rey JH, Coppen AJ (1959) Distribution of androgyny in mental patients. Br Med J 26(2):1445–1447
12. World Professional Association for Transgender Health (2011) Standards of care for the health of transsexual, transgender and gender non-conforming people, 7th Version. http://www.wpath.org
13. Heylens G, Elaut E, Kreukels BPC, Paap MSC, Cerwenka S, Richter-Appelt H, Cohen Kettenis PT, Haraldsen I, De Cuypere G (2013) Psychiatric characteristics in transsexual individuals: multicentre study in four European Countries. Br J Psychiatry. doi:10.1192/bjp.bp.112.121954
14. Parkinson J (2014) Gender dysphoria in Asperger's syndrome: a caution. Australas Psychiatry 22:84–85
15. Tateno M, Ikeda H, Saito T (2011) Gender dysphoria in pervasive developmental disorders. Seishin Shinkeigaku Zasshi 113:1173–1183
16. Lawrence A, Zucker K (2012) Gender identity disorders. In: Hersen M, Beidel D (eds) Adult psychopathology and diagnosis, 6th edn. Wiley, London, pp 601–635
17. Murad M, Elamin M, Garcia M, Mullan R, Murad A, Erwin P et al (2010) Hormonal therapy and sex reassignment: a systematic review and meta-analysis of quality of life and psychosocial outcomes. Clin Endocrinol (Oxf) 72:214–231
18. Dhejne C, Lichtenstein P, Boman M, Johansson ALV, Långström N et al (2011) Long-term follow-up of transsexual persons undergoing sex reassignment surgery: cohort study in Sweden. PLoS One 6(2):e16885. doi:10.1371/journal.pone.0016885
19. Asscheman H, Giltay EJ, Megens JA, de Ronde WP, van Trotsenburg MA, Gooren LJ (2011) A long-term follow-up study of mortality in transsexuals receiving treatment with cross-sex hormones. Eur J Endocrinol 164:635–642
20. Gooren LJ, Giltay EJ, Bunck MC (2008) Long-term treatment of transsexuals with cross-sex hormones: extensive personal experience. J Clin Endocrinol Metab 93:19–25
21. BMJ Best Practice reports. http://bestpractice.bmj.com/bestpractice/monograph/992/basics/epidemiology.html. 2014
22. Wilson P, Sharp C, Carr S (1999) The prevalence of gender dysphoria in Scotland: a primary care study. Br J Gen Pract 49:991–992
23. Gender Identity Research and Education Society. The number of gender variant people in the UK – update 2011. http://www.gires.org.uk
24. Okabe N, Sato T, Matsumoto Y, Ido Y, Terada S, Kuroda S (2008) Clinical characteristics of patients with gender identity disorder at a Japanese gender identity disorder clinic. Psychiatry Res 157:315–318
25. Vujovic S, Popovic S, Sbutega-Milosevic G, Djordjevic M, Gooren L (2009) Transsexualism in Serbia: a twenty-year follow-up study. J Sex Med 6:1018–1023
26. Veale JF (2008) Prevalence of transsexualism among New Zealand passport holders. Aust N Z J Psychiatry 42:887–889
27. De Cuypere G, Van Hemelrijck M, Michel A, Carael B, Heylens G, Rubens R, Hoebeke P, Monstrey S (2007) Prevalence and demography of transsexualism in Belgium. Eur Psychiatry 22:137–141
28. Conron KJ, Scott G, Stowell GS, Landers SJ (2012) Transgender health in Massachusetts: results from a household probability sample of adults. Am J Public Health 102:118–122
29. Heckathorn DD (1997) Respondent-driven sampling: a new approach to the study of hidden populations. Soc Probl 44:174–199

6 Etiopathogenetic Hypotheses of Transsexualism

Randi Ettner

6.1 Introduction

Ever since the beginning of time, man has tried to understand the physical world and its human occupants. Traditional, archaic societies spun stories of creation in an attempt to explain the origins of the world and its mysteries. In these myths, supernatural beings possess human motives and animation.

Cosmogonic myths, those that explain the origins of natural phenomena, also identified the origin of sickness and cure. Indeed, many religious rituals involved recitation of the creation myth to summon a sacred power. This recapitulation was necessary to make a sterile womb fertile or to cure a body or mind [1].

Both Jung and Freud provided psychological explanations for the power of myth. For Jung, the repetition of strikingly similar figures in mythology was evidence of the collective unconscious, lending support to his theory of personality development. Freud, on the other hand, focused on primordial acts, such as patricide, as symbols of repressed personal libido. This provided confirmation of *his* theory of personality development [2, 3].

The medical profession has since made great contributions toward understanding the material or "real" world, particularly in regard to the pathophysiology of disease. But human behavior does not easily capitulate to taxonomy. Not surprisingly, in the absence of observable disease, diagnostic test, or organ deficiency, one reverts to theory—the modern equivalent of myth—to explain inscrutable phenomena. Such is the case with transsexualism, surely the most misunderstood area of human behavior.

6.2 Early Theories

Recorded accounts of men and women displaying cross-gender behavior date back to biblical times. Indeed, the Old Testament expostulated against such displays [Deuteronomy 22:5], and Ovid, a first-century BC poet, referred in verse to the extract of "stuff from a mare in heat," a reference to conjugated estrogen [4]. Nevertheless, the phenomenon was unknown in the Western world prior to the middle of the twentieth century.

Although accounts of sex-reassignment surgeries were published in Germany as early as 1930, it was not until 1952 when the Danish surgeon Paul Fogh-Andersen employed an innovative surgical technique on Christine Jorgensen, a US citizen, that media reports of "sex-change surgery" captured the public's attention [5]. Harry Benjamin, an endocrinologist, is credited with identifying the condition and in 1966 published the book *The Transsexual Phenomenon*, prompting some surgeons to perform the procedure. Thus, a taboo area of human behavior became a medical specialty [6].

R. Ettner
Department of Psychology, New Health Foundation Worldwide, 1214 Lake Street, Evanston, IL 60201, USA
e-mail: rettner@aol.com

C. Trombetta et al. (eds.), *Management of Gender Dysphoria: A Multidisciplinary Approach*,
DOI 10.1007/978-88-470-5696-1_6, © Springer-Verlag Italia 2015

Opposition to surgery arose rapidly, in tandem with Ms. Jorgensen's fame. While some surgeons in Europe, Mexico, South America, and the USA were willing to perform reassignment surgery, most hospitals prohibited the procedure. The "Christine operation" generated legal controversies, religious opposition, and moral outrage. But it was the psychiatric community that was the most vociferous in challenging the legitimacy of transsexualism [6].

The debate centered on the etiology of gender dysphoria. The psychoanalytic model, which prevailed in Europe and the USA, regarded transsexualism as a psychiatric—not a biologic—disorder. The psychiatric community claimed the desire for reassignment surgery was a delusion, an obsession, or a symptom of severe psychopathology. The symptomatology arose from serious object relation disturbances: an inability to separate on the part of both mother and child giving rise to dysregulation of intrapsychic distance for the patient and an attempt to incorporate an alternate persona [7–11]. Some conceptualized this as a psychotic disorder [12]; others viewed it as a form of borderline psychopathology [13]. Lothstein opined that the transsexual was unconsciously motivated to "discard bad and aggressive features" and create in the fabric of the body "a new idealized perfection" [13].

The tenacity of the psychodynamic model, the inflammatory rhetoric of the debate, and the conflation of transsexualism, homosexuality, and transvestism left science and research trailing behind negative public perception. Many transsexual people requesting medical and surgical treatments were committed to mental institutions. The abject failure of the "talking cure" was attributed to resistance on the part of the patient, not to the failure of psychoanalysis [14]. Tragically, electroshock and aversion therapies were too often the default treatments.

Some researchers rejected the psychoanalytic explanation and continued to pursue a biological basis for the condition to "help to replace emotional controversy by rational assessment of facts" [15]. Early attempts to find an organic etiology included roentgenological examination of the skulls of transsexual patients [16], testing for anomalous hormonal milieus [17, 18], cytotoxicity assay inspection of h-y antigen status [19–22], and quantitative frequency EEG analysis. Despite the failure of these attempts to identify an organic marker of transsexualism, some investigators remained convinced that hormonal-dependent structural brain changes, although not documented, were a likely explanation [23].

Interestingly, support for a biological basis came from an unlikely source, namely, clinical psychologists [6]. By utilizing reliable and objective psychological tests, they could substantiate, or fail to substantiate, the claim that gender-dysphoric patients had rampant psychopathology. Several such studies indicated that applicants for sex reassignment showed "a notable absence of psychopathology" [24–27].

By the 1990s, significant numbers of people had sought medical interventions, and thus a "database" of historical and psychological information could be assessed. While all such persons suffered similar distress due to gender incongruity, they had no commonality in regard to biographical indices, childhood abuse, or trauma. There was no evidence to conclude that environment or parenting practices accounted for the development of the condition [28].

6.3 Later Theories

Dramatic advances in brain-imaging capacity led to more sophisticated theories of the etiology of atypical gender identity. By the late 1990s, some researchers proffered a model known as "gender transposition" as the underlying principle. Based largely on evidence from animal studies demonstrating a link between steroid hormones, brain structure, and sexual behavior [29], this theory proposed that transsexualism occurred as a result of a switch of hormone-induced cephalic differentiation at a critical gestational point [30–32]. The theory, though appealing, proved too reductionistic. It suffered from the conflation of behavior and identity, its weighty reliance on animal study extrapolation, and the erroneous assertion of a fixed critical period anchoring sexual differentiation in the fetus [33, 34].

In 1995, one study broke new ground. Zhou et al. reported differences in autopsied brains of male-to-female transsexual persons in the bed nucleus of the stria terminalis (BSTc), an area of the hypothalamus central to sexual behavior. The examined male-to-female transsexual brains had a volume of the central sulci of the stria terminalis that was comparable to those of genetic females and unlike both heterosexual and homosexual male brains, which had greater volume [35]. The study generated a great deal of publicity, as it lent support to the conviction held by many: that a structure deep within the brain might hold the answer to complex areas of identity. It also resonated with the layperson's characterization of the transsexual person as someone who insists they have a female brain in a male body [36].

But the study raised additional questions. What if the volume differences found in the BSTc were artifacts resulting from contrary hormone use? A subsequent study was designed to address this issue. Krujiver et al. quantified the number of somatostatin (SOM) neurons in the BSTc, rather than volume. Neuron numbers of heterosexual males, homosexual males, heterosexual females, male-to-female transsexuals, male and females with sex hormone disorders, a female-to-male transsexual, and an untreated individual with gender dysphoria were compared. The findings were consistent with earlier results. Regardless of sexual orientation or adult hormone usage, there was a difference in the SOM neuron number in the human BSTc. Not only did the male-to-female postmortem brain tissue have levels corresponding to that of genetic females, but the opposite pattern was displayed in the female-to-male transsexual brain tissue [37].

6.4 Current Theories

A proliferation of studies arose in the past decade, due in no small part to technological advances and the expansion of databases. Now, meta-analyses could take place, combining data from several countries. Building on the previous brain structure studies, an assemblage of studies evinced evidence in support of biological theories, none of which were necessarily mutually exclusive, each seemingly contributing a piece of a yet unsolved puzzle.

6.5 Brain Structure

The previous significant finding of a sexually dimorphic subdivision of the BSTc bolstered support for the hypothesis that gender identity develops as a result of the interaction of a developing brain and sex hormones. However, in 2002, Chung et al. made the surprising discovery that the BSTc volume did not become apparent until adulthood. The late occurrence of sexual dimorphism in the BSTc had yet to be explained. The authors suggested that perhaps long before the difference in BSTc volume became manifest, changes in fetal hormone levels, neuronal activity, or differentiation were paving the way for structural change, which would appear at a later stage of life [38].

Pol et al. used magnetic resonance brain imaging to compare total brain volume before and after hormone treatment. They found that estrogen usage decreased brain volumes in male-to-female transsexual subjects causing them to fall in the range of female proportions. Androgen treatment in female-to-male transsexual subjects increased volume, causing the brain morphology to replicate male proportions. The authors concluded that sex steroid hormones are vital in the maintenance of sexual dimorphic brain organization throughout life [39].

In 2008, a region of the brain was identified that also appeared to be related to transsexualism, namely, the interstitial nucleus of the anterior hypothalamus (INAH3) [40]. In 2012, a study of postmortem human brain tissue determined that the gene-encoding neurokinin B (NKB) in the infundibular nucleus (INF) is sexually dimorphic. In children, both sexes had equivalent levels of NKB immunoreactivity, but adulthood brought dimorphism. As with the BSTc, there was a reversal in transsexual brain tissue, indicating that gonadotropin-releasing harmone (GnRH) secretion is regulated via estrogen feedback and that a mutation in the NKB produces gonadotropin deficiencies. Clearly, the stage was set to implicate hormones, genes, and cephalic structure in the formation of gender identity [41].

6.6 Prenatal Hormonal Influences

The theory that early influences, possibly prenatal, were the precursors for later structural brain change was gaining traction. Dessens et al. reported an elevated incidence of transsexual offspring in women exposed to phenobarbital and diphenylhydantoin [42]. As phenobarbital enhances liver function, it was widely used in many countries as a prophylactic treatment of neonatal hyperbilirubinemia, prior to the use of phototherapy, and it caused a rise in postnatal testosterone. This demonstrated that certain substances could alter steroid hormone levels [43].

Simultaneously, there was rampant evidence that environmental assaults were causing endocrine disruption in wildlife. Disturbing evidence that synthetic chemicals can disrupt sex steroids and the complexity of feedback loops was mounting. Animal researchers exposed the extreme sensitivity of developing mammals to very slight shifts in hormone levels in the womb stating "hormones permanently organize or program cells, organs, the brain, and behavior before birth, in many ways setting the individual's course for an entire lifetime" [44]. Could this explain the escalating incidence of disorders of sexual development, infertility, hypospadias, cryptorchidism, double uteruses, blind vaginas, and other disorders in the human population [45]?

Diethylstilbestrol (DES), the most studied endocrine disruptor, has been implicated in numerous health problems in female offspring of exposed women [46]. Curiously, few studies have examined the impact on male offspring, the DES sons. An online forum, DES Sons International, conducted a survey of members. Of 500 respondents, 90 members indicated they were transsexual, 48 described themselves as transgender; 17 identified themselves as "gender dysphoric"; and 3 identified themselves as "intersex." By 2004, more than 130 individuals had joined a forum called "DES Trans" [44]. Clearly, the prevalence of gender dysphoria in persons exposed to DES warrants further study.

It has been well established that the ratio of the second to fourth finger (2D:4D) is smaller in human males than females. This sexually dimorphic trait was presumed to be established prenatally, due to hormones [47–49]. Galis et al. analyzed the digit ratio in deceased male and female fetuses. They determined that at 14 weeks of gestational age, there was a small but significant difference in the 2D:4D ratio among male and female fetuses and that the ratio increases during childhood. They concluded that early levels of sexual hormones have a lasting impact and that the ratio increases after birth in both males and females. Therefore, both prenatal and postnatal processes are involved in sexual dimorphism [50]. Schneider et al. compared the digit ratio between transsexual individuals and controls. They found that male-to-female transsexual subjects had a digit ratio observed in control females, a finding that clearly supports a biological etiology to the condition. No such difference was found in the female-to-male subjects or control females. The authors concluded that decreased prenatal androgen exposure is implicated in the development of male-to-female transsexualism [51].

6.7 Genetic Theories

In 2000, Green reported on familial concordance of gender dysphoria in ten sibling or parent-child dyads. He forecast that advances in technology would make the exploration of genetic variants a viable area of exploration in the quest to discover the origins of atypical gender identity [52].

Other researchers also found a co-occurrence of gender dysphoria in families. Gomez-Gil et al. looked at a sample of 995 transsexual people, both male to female and female to male, and found 12 pairs of transsexual non-twin siblings. They state, "According to our data, the probability that a sibling of a transsexual will also be a transsexual was 4.48 times higher for siblings of MF than for siblings of FM transsexual probands, and 3.88 times higher for the brothers than for the sisters of transsexual probands. This study suggests that siblings of transsexuals may have a higher risk of being transsexual than the general population" [53].

In 2005, Swedish investigators hypothesized that the sexual differentiation of brain structures is mainly due to the influence of testosterone acting on androgen receptors (ARs) and estrogen receptors (ERs) as was the case with animals. They therefore sought to examine the potential role of three particular polymorphisms for implication in the development of male-to-female transsexualism. They found one of the three, ERbeta repeat polymorphism, to differ in mean length between 29 transsexual subjects and controls. However, the small number of individuals studied demanded caution in interpreting the results [54].

Diamond reported on an investigation of transsexualism among 112 sets of twins, illuminating the relative contribution of genetics and social factors in the phenomenon. He found a 33.3 % concordance for transsexual identity among monozygotic male twins and a 22.8 % concordance among monozygotic female twins. Interestingly, among the twin probands, there were three sets of twins who were reared apart but concordant for gender transition [55].

Two landmark studies undertook to directly assess the role of specific genes. Bentz et al. found female-to-male transsexuals to differ from female controls in a gender-specific allele distribution pattern and to have an allele distribution akin to male controls. The identified gene, CYP17, is associated with female-to-male transsexualism, as is the loss of the female-specific genotype distribution [56]. Hare et al. looked at polymorphisms in genes involved in steroidogenesis. Specifically, they examined repeat length variants in the androgen receptor (AR), the estrogen receptor beta (ERbeta), and aromatase (CYP19) genes. They found a significant association between male-to- female transsexualism and the androgen receptor (AR) gene. The transsexual subjects had longer AR repeat lengths than cisgender male control subjects. The investigators concluded that male gender identity is partially mediated through the androgen receptor, as reduced androgen and androgen signaling may contribute to the formation of a female gender identity. Theirs is the largest genetic study of transsexualism, to date [57].

Conclusion

The etiology of gender identity, typical and atypical, presently remains unknown. However, the mounting evidence for a biological basis is compelling. No doubt the next decade will bring new data that elucidates the complexities of identity formation and amplifies understanding of the transsexual phenomenon.

What is clear from the existing body of knowledge is that theories that rely on consensus, rather than science, have stigmatized people by "blaming the victim." The attribution of psychopathology, deficient parenting, or childhood trauma as the "cause" of gender dysphoria must be forever relegated to the status of myth.

References

1. Eliot A (1976) Myths. McGraw Hill, New York
2. Freud S (1946) Totem and taboo. Vintage, New York
3. Jung CG, Kerenyi C (1949) Essays on a science of mythology. Princeton University Press, Princeton
4. Taylor T (1996) The prehistory of sex: four million years of human sexual culture. Bantam, New York
5. Monstrey S, Selvaggi G, Ceulemans P (2007) Surgery: male-to-female patient. In: Ettner R, Monstrey S, Eyler E (eds) Principles of transgender medicine and surgery. Haworth Press, New York
6. Ettner R (1999) Gender loving care. WW Norton, New York
7. Lothstein LM (1979) Psychodynamics and sociodynamics of gender-dysphoric states. Am J Psychother 33(2):214–238
8. Gilpin DC, Raza S, Gipin D (1979) Transsexual symptoms in a male child treated by a female therapist. Am J Psychother 3(3):453–463
9. Moberly ER (1986) Attachment and separation: the implications for gender identity and for the structuralization of the self: a theoretical model for transsexualism and homosexuality. Psychiatr J Univ Ott 11(4):205–209
10. Ovesey L, Person E (1976) Transvestism: a disorder of the sense of self. Int J Psychoanal Psychother 5: 219–236
11. Macvicar K (1978) The transsexual wish in a psychotic character. Int J Psychoanal Psychother 7:354–365
12. Socarides CW (1978) Transsexualism and psychosis. Int J Psychoanal Psychother 7:373–384

13. Lothstein LM (1984) Psychological testing with transsexuals: a 30-year review. J Pers Assess 48(5):500–507
14. Shtasel TF (1979) Behavioral treatment of transsexualism: a case report. J Sex Marital Ther 5(4):362–367
15. Vogel F (1981) Neurobiological approaches in human behavior genetics. Behav Genet 11(2):87–102
16. Lundberg PO, Sjovall A, Walinder J (1975) Sella turcica in male-to-female transsexuals. Arch Sex Behav 4(6):657–662
17. Gooren L (1986) The neuroendocrine response of luteinizing hormone to estrogen administration in heterosexual, homosexual, and transsexual subjects. J Clin Endocrinol Metab 63(3):583–588
18. Kula K, Dulko S, Pawlikowski M et al (1986) A nonspecific disturbance of the gonadostat in women with transsexualism and isolated hypergonadotropism in the male-to-female disturbance of gender identity. Exp Clin Endocrinol 87(1):8–14
19. Eicher W, Spoljar M, Richter K et al (1980) Transsexuality and X-Y antigen (abstract). Geburtshilfe Frauenheilkd 40(6):529–540
20. Spoljar M, Eicher W, Eiermann W et al (1981) H-Y antigen expression in different tissues from transsexuals. Hum Genet 57(1):52–57
21. Eicher W, Spoljar M, Murken JD et al (1981) Transsexualism and the H-Y antigen (abstract). Fortschr Med 99(1–2):9–12
22. Engel W, Pfafflin F, Wiedeking C (1980) H-Y antigen in transsexuality, and how to explain testis differentiation in H-Y antigen positive males and ovary differentiation in H-Y antigen positive females. Hum Genet 55(3):315–319
23. Gooren L (1990) The endocrinology of transsexualism: a review and commentary. Psychoneuroendocrinology 15(1):3–14
24. Greenberg RP, Laurence L (1981) A comparison of the MMPi results for psychiatric patients and male applicants for transsexual surgery. J Nerv Ment Dis 169(5):320–323
25. Tsushima WT, Wedding D (1979) MMPI results of male candidates for transsexual surgery. J Pers Assess 43(4):385–387
26. Leavitt F, Berger JC, Hoeppner JA et al (1980) Presurgical adjustment in male transsexuals with and without hormonal treatment. J Nerv Ment Dis 168(11): 693–697
27. Cole CM, O'Boyle M, Emory LE et al (1997) Comorbidity of gender dysphoria and other major psychiatric diagnoses. Arch Sex Behav 26(1):13–26
28. Buhrich N, McConaghy N (1978) Parental relationships during childhood in homosexuality, transvestism, and transsexualism. Aust N Z J Psychiatry 12(2): 103–108
29. Wu C (1995) Ancient crocodile chomped on plants. Science News August 1995, 132
30. Dorner G, Poppe I, Stahl F et al (1991) Gene and environment-dependent neuroendocrine etiogenesis of homosexuality and transsexualism. Exp Clin Endocrinol 98(2):141–150
31. Elias AN, Valenta LJ (1992) Are all males equal? Anatomic and functional basis for sexual orientation in males. Med Hypotheses 39(1):39–45
32. Giordano G, Giusti M (1995) Hormones and psychosocial differentiation. Minerva Endocrinol 20(3):165–193
33. Coleman E, Gooren L, Ross M (1989) Theories of gender transpositions: a critique and suggestions for further research. J Sex Res 26(4):525–538
34. Dumesic DA, Goldsmith PC, Jaffe RB (1987) Estradiol sensitization of cultural human fetal pituitary cells to gonadotropin-releasing hormone. J Clin Endocrinol Metab 65:1147–1153
35. Zhou JN, Hofman MA, Gooren LJ et al (1995) A sex difference in the human brain and its relation to transsexuality. Nature 378(6552):68–70
36. Angier N (1995) Size of region of brain may hold crucial clue to transsexuality, a study finds. The New York Times, November 2
37. Krujiver FPM, Zhou J, Pool CW et al (2000) Male-to-female transsexuals have female neuron numbers in a limbic nucleus. J Clin Endocrinol Metab 85:2034–2041
38. Chung W, De Vries G, Swaab D (2002) Sexual differentiation of the bed nucleus of the stria terminalis in humans may extend into adulthood. J Neurosci 22(3):1027–1033
39. Pol HE, Cohen-Kettenis P, Van Haren N et al (2006) Changing your sex changes your brain: influences of testosterone and estrogen on adult human brain structure. Eur J Endocrinol 155:S107–S111
40. Garcia-Falgueras A, Swaab DF (2008) A sex difference in the hypothalamic uncinate nucleus: relationship to gender identity. Brain 131:3132–3146
41. Taziaux M, Swaab DF, Bakker J (2012) Sex differences in the neurokinin B system in the human infundibular nucleus. J Clin Endocrininol Metab 97(12): E2210–E2220
42. Dessens AB, Cohen-Kettenis PT, Mellenbergh GJ et al (1999) Prenatal exposure to anticonvulsants and psychosexual development. Arch Sex Behav 28: 31–44
43. Swaab DF (2004) Sexual differentiation of the human brain: relevance for gender identity, transsexualism and sexual orientation. Gynecol Endocrinol 19:301–312
44. Kerlin SP (2004) The presence of gender dysphoria, transsexualism, and disorders of sex differentiation in males prenatally exposed to diethylstilbestrol: initial evidence from a 5-year study. DES Sons International Network. TransAdvocate.org
45. Colborn T, Dumanoski D, Myers JP (1996) Our stolen future. Penguin, New York
46. Langston N (2010) Toxic bodies: hormone disruptors and the legacy of DES. Yale University Press, New Haven/London
47. Phelps VR (1952) Relative index finger length as a sex-influenced trait in man. Am J Hum Genet 4:72–89
48. Garn SM, Burdi AR, Babler WJ et al (1975) Early prenatal attainment of adult metacarpal-phalangeal rankings and proportions. Am J Phys Anthropol 43: 327–332

49. Manning JT, Fink B, Neave N et al (1998) The ratio of 2nd to 4th digit length, a predictor of sperm numbers and concentrations of testosterone, leuteinizing hormone and oestrogen. Hum Reprod 13: 3000–30004
50. Galis F, Ten Broek C, Van Dongen S et al (2010) Sexual dimorphism in the prenatal digit ratio (2D:4D). Arch Sex Behav 39(1):57–62
51. Schneider HJ, Pickel J, Stalla GK (2006) Typical female 2nd-4th finger length (2D:4D) ratios in male-to-female transsexuals-possible implications for prenatal androgen exposure. Psychoneuroendocrinology 31(2):265–269
52. Green R (2000) Family co-occurrence of "gender dysphoria": ten sibling or parent-child pairs. Arch Sex Behav 29(5):499–507
53. Gomez-Gil E, Esteva I, Almaraz MC et al (2010) Familiality of gender identity disorder in non-twin siblings. Arch Sex Behav 39(2):546–552
54. Henningsson S, Westberg L, Nilsson S et al (2005) Sex steroid-related genes and male-to-female transsexualism. Psychoneuroendocrinology 30(7):657–664
55. Diamond M (2013) Transsexuality among twins: identity concordance, transition, rearing, and orientation. Int J Trans 14:24–28
56. Bentz EK, Hefler LA, Kaufmann U et al (2008) A polymorphism of the CYP17 gene related to sex steroid metabolism is associated with female-to-male but not male-to-female transsexualism. Fertil Steril 90(1):56–59
57. Hare L, Bernard P, Sanchez FJ et al (2009) Androgen receptor length polymorphism associated with male-to-female transsexualism. Biol Psychiatry 65(1):93–96

Imaging: Examination Technique

7

Michele Bertolotto, Francesca Cacciato,
Gladiola Kaso, Matilde Cazzagon, and Piero Pavlica

7.1 Introduction

Imaging has been thought to play a minor and questionable role in the evaluation of patients with gender dysphoria. However, several clinical situations require imaging investigations in these patients. Profound modifications of the natal male or female pelvic anatomy occur after sex reassignment surgery (SRS), which are best investigated using MR imaging. Moreover, perforator flap surgery has been introduced in phalloplasty procedures which often requires detailed preoperative investigation of the vessels of the donor and of the acceptor site. Multidetector-row CT (MDCT) angiography allows localization of the perforators in combination with evaluation of the pedicle course. Color Doppler ultrasonography is used to confirm the position of the perforators and is useful to assess the course of the vessels of the neopenis and of the neourethra before prosthesis insertion [1].

Concern is rising regarding breast health in the transgender population, and screening recommendations include mammography and ultrasonography [2]. Breast MR imaging is indicated for investigation of breast augmentation in male to female (MtF) SRS. Urinary fistulas and/or stenoses are the most common complications in female to male (FtM) SRS which are best investigated with voiding urethrography [3, 4].

While the majority of these imaging procedures are performed in transgender patients as in natal men and women, a dedicated MR imaging technique is necessary when looking at the complex postoperative changes after SRS and when multidetector-row CT scanning is performed to image the complex vascular anatomy of the donor and acceptor sites before phalloplasty.

7.2 MRI Investigation

The techniques used for pelvic MR imaging of transsexual patients can be implemented with virtually any MR unit. There is no significant difference in the interpretation of images obtained with any static magnetic field strength. Image quality and signal-to-noise ratio is better, however, with relatively high-field-strength MR units.

M. Bertolotto, MD (✉) • F. Cacciato • G. Kaso
M. Cazzagon
Department of Radiology,
University of Trieste Cattinara Hospital,
Strada di Fiume 447, Trieste 34149, Italy
e-mail: bertolot@units.it; francescacacciato@gmail.com; s193904@stud.units.it; matilde.cazzagon@gmail.com

P. Pavlica
Department of Radiology, Villalba Hospital,
Via di Roncrio 25, Bologna 40136, Italy
e-mail: piero.pavlica@alice.it

C. Trombetta et al. (eds.), *Management of Gender Dysphoria: A Multidisciplinary Approach*,
DOI 10.1007/978-88-470-5696-1_7, © Springer-Verlag Italia 2015

7.2.1 Coil Selection and Patient Preparation

The best results for pelvic imaging are obtained by the use of multichannel phased-array coils for parallel imaging, such as cardiac coils, which provide high-definition images with excellent signal-to-noise ratio. Appropriate patient positioning is important. In FtM transsexuals, the neopenis is dorsiflexed in the midline against the abdominal wall, if possible, and taped in position to reduce organ motion during the examination.

In MtF SRS, the neovagina is normally collapsed, and distinguishing between anterior and posterior walls can be difficult. Such distinction is important for evaluation of the neovaginal length, integrity, and vascularization of the rectal-neovaginal septum. Using gel, the neovagina and the rectum can be distended and easily evaluated.

Several different types of aqueous gels and administration techniques may be used. We use approximately 60 mL of ultrasonographic gel for both neovaginal and rectal distention. The gel is placed in a 60-mL syringe connected with a standard enema tip prepared in advance taking care to minimize the introduction of air, and stored upright with the tip facing upward.

When possible, the MR investigation is performed with a tutor in the neovagina which eases the assessment of the neovaginal dept. All metallic parts of the tutor must be removed before insertion [5–7].

7.2.2 Examination Technique

The patient is examined in at least the sagittal and axial planes. The former is ideal for imaging the neovagina, the rectovaginal septum, and the neoclitoris. In our clinical practice, optimal coverage is provided by 3-mm thin contiguous sections.

Image quality obtained without respiratory compensation can be high enough for the diagnosis if the patient is carefully instructed to breathe regularly and shallowly to minimize respiratory excursions of the abdominal wall. Administration of a spasmolytic agent (Buscopan or glucagon) is recommended to reduce artifacts due to bowel peristalsis, which would degrade image quality.

It is recommended to use turbo spin echo (TSE) pulse sequences which have the advantage of multiple contrast weightings, high-spatial resolution, and high signal-to-noise ratio. Moreover, compared to gradient echo sequences, they are less influenced by susceptibility artifacts.

T2-weighted images allow an excellent delineation of pelvic organs. Fat suppression is not routinely used. T1-weighted images can be combined with spectral fat suppression to differentiate between blood and fat. Good image quality and morphologic detail resolution are obtained with an echo time of about 10 ms and a repetition time of approximately 400–600 ms. Repeated image averaging will average out motion artifacts.

DP-weighted images may be useful in selected cases. They are obtained with an echo time of about 30 ms and repetition time of approximately 4,000 ms.

Contrast-enhanced TSE T1-weighted images with fat suppression are repeated after gadolinium contrast administration early after sex reassignment surgery in order to assess perfusion of the neoclitoris, urethral plaque, and neovaginal wall and to delineate fluid collections. Image subtraction between the non-enhanced and the contrast-enhanced images helps delineation of postoperative fluid collections containing blood when they present with high signal intensity on non-enhanced T1-weighted images.

7.2.3 Contraindications

In general, MR imaging is contraindicated for patients who have electrically, magnetically, or mechanically activated implants, such as cardiac pacemakers, implantable cardiac defibrillators, cochlear implants, neurostimulators, bone-growth stimulators, and implantable drug infusion pumps.

Ferromagnetic or metallic biomedical implants or foreign bodies are also under contraindication due to possible danger of dislodgement or movement. In addition, such objects may be subject to heating and induction of electrical currents.

7.3 MDCT Angiography

MDCT angiography is indicated in patients already scheduled for phalloplasty; it is not advised to image patients who are still uncertain about the type of surgery they will undergo for creation of the neopenis, as it could result in unnecessary radiation exposure.

Previous studies show that MDCT angiography is highly sensitive and specific in visualizing perforators with reduction in surgical time and potential postoperative complications [8]. It can visualize perforators up to 0.3 mm in diameter, provide their precise localization, and depict the course of vascular pedicle. In our institution MDCT angiography is most often performed before free septo-cutaneous anterolateral thigh (ALT) flap phallic reconstruction, which has become a valuable alternative to radial forearm flap with reduced donor site morbidity [9].

7.3.1 Patient Preparation

Patient positioning should replicate the surgical table. Underwear must be removed, as it grossly distorts and compresses the soft tissues producing inaccuracy in the coordinate system. Breath hold instruction should not be underestimated as in our experience some investigations had to be repeated for motion artifacts [10].

7.3.2 CT Scanning

A modern multislice CT scanner is a prerequisite, as is submillimetric slice acquisition. In our department, 100 mL of nonionic iodinated contrast agent (350 mg I/mL) is administered at a rate of 4.5 mL/s followed by a 45-mL saline flush. The scanning is triggered using a bolus tracking system with a ROI set on the aortic lumen at the level of L2–L3 vertebral body. The threshold and delay before starting the scan are intrinsically interconnected and should be adjusted considering the specific scanner in use.

7.3.3 Postprocessing

The volume dataset is examined on the specific workstation available, as most commercial software are adequate. The protocol can be performed by a trained operator in less than 20 min. Surgeons are usually not confident in reviewing a large number of stack images, so the aim of the workflow is to produce a limited number of very informative images.

Five-millimeter axial (Fig. 7.1a), sagittal, and coronal maximum intensity projection (MIP) reconstructions are essential to mark the perforators and depict their course.

Perforator arteries are marked with an arrow at the point where they pierce the fascia, i.e., they pass either through or in between the deep tissues (mostly muscle) to reach the skin and subcutaneous tissue. 3D rendering is then obtained to show the complete course of the pedicle from the perforator to the origin of the pedicle from the main vessels (Fig. 7.1b).

3D surface rendering of the flap is then obtained trimming the volume manually including muscles and cutaneous and subcutaneous tissue to show subcutaneous branching of the perforators (Fig. 7.1c). Manual clipping of the overlaying skin is often necessary as density is superior to subcutaneous fat. Arrows are positioned to mark the precise projection of the perforator's origin on the skin with the use of a Cartesian coordinate system centered on a reference point. In the case of the ALT flap, the system is outlined on the axis of the anterior superior iliac spine and the lateral patella (Fig. 7.1d).

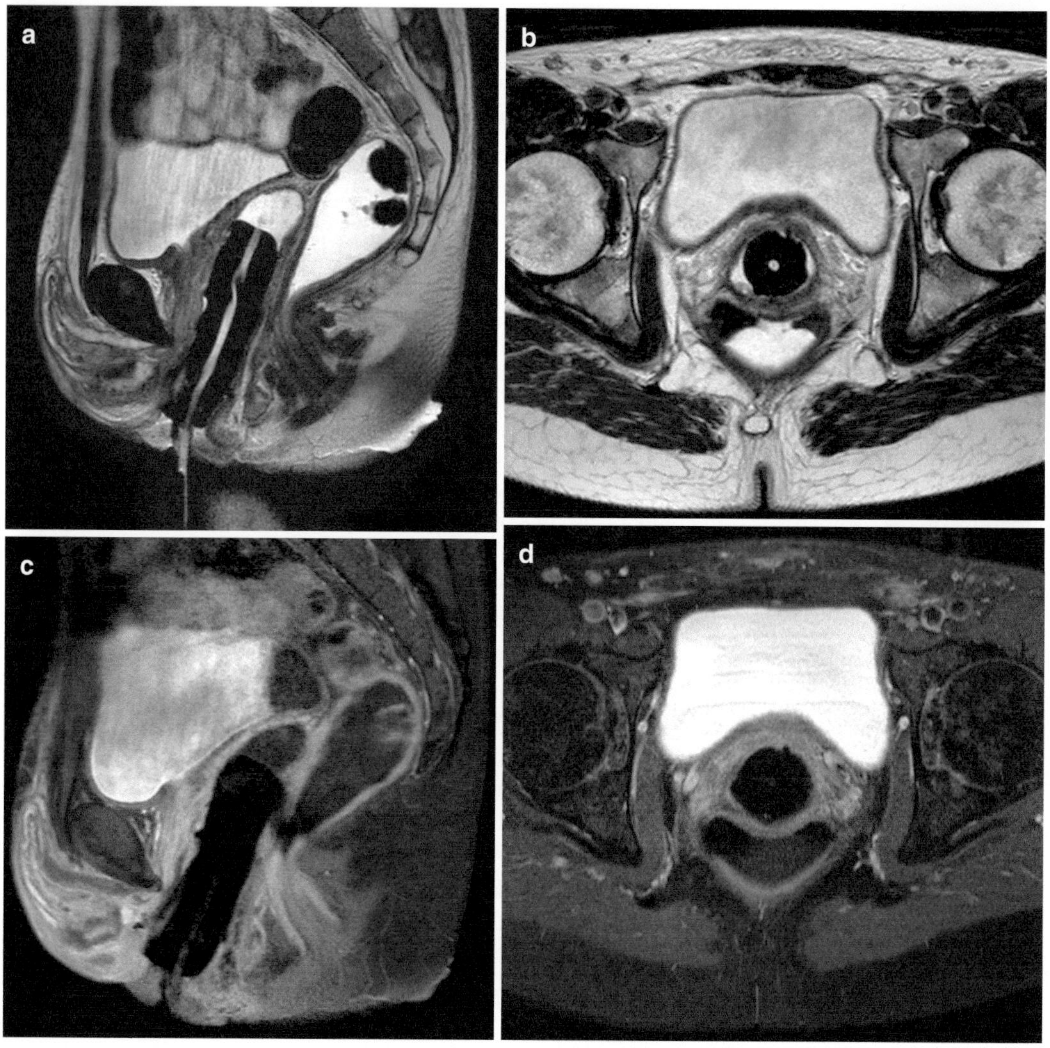

Fig. 7.1 MR imaging after MtF sex reassignment surgery. The neovagina and the rectum are distended with gel. An inflatable tutor is inserted in the neovagina. (**a**, **b**) Sagittal and axial T2-weighted images. (**c**, **d**) Sagittal and axial T1-weighted images with fat suppression obtained after gadolinium contrast administration

7.3.4 Reporting

Standard report includes description of the technique used and a qualitative judgment of the exam quality. Perforators are indexed with the Cartesian coordinate system centered on the reference point. Providing absolute diameter of perforators can be confounding, as diameter is very close to resolution limit. To visually differentiate the surgically relevant ones, perforators with caliber >1 mm can be marked with a different color. Color Doppler ultrasound is used to investigate the flow characteristics of the perforators. Besides evaluation of the vascularity, MDCT angiography allows a precise measure of the thickness of the subcutaneous fat layer, an information which is crucial to estimate the required dimensions of the flap used to manufacture the neopenis.

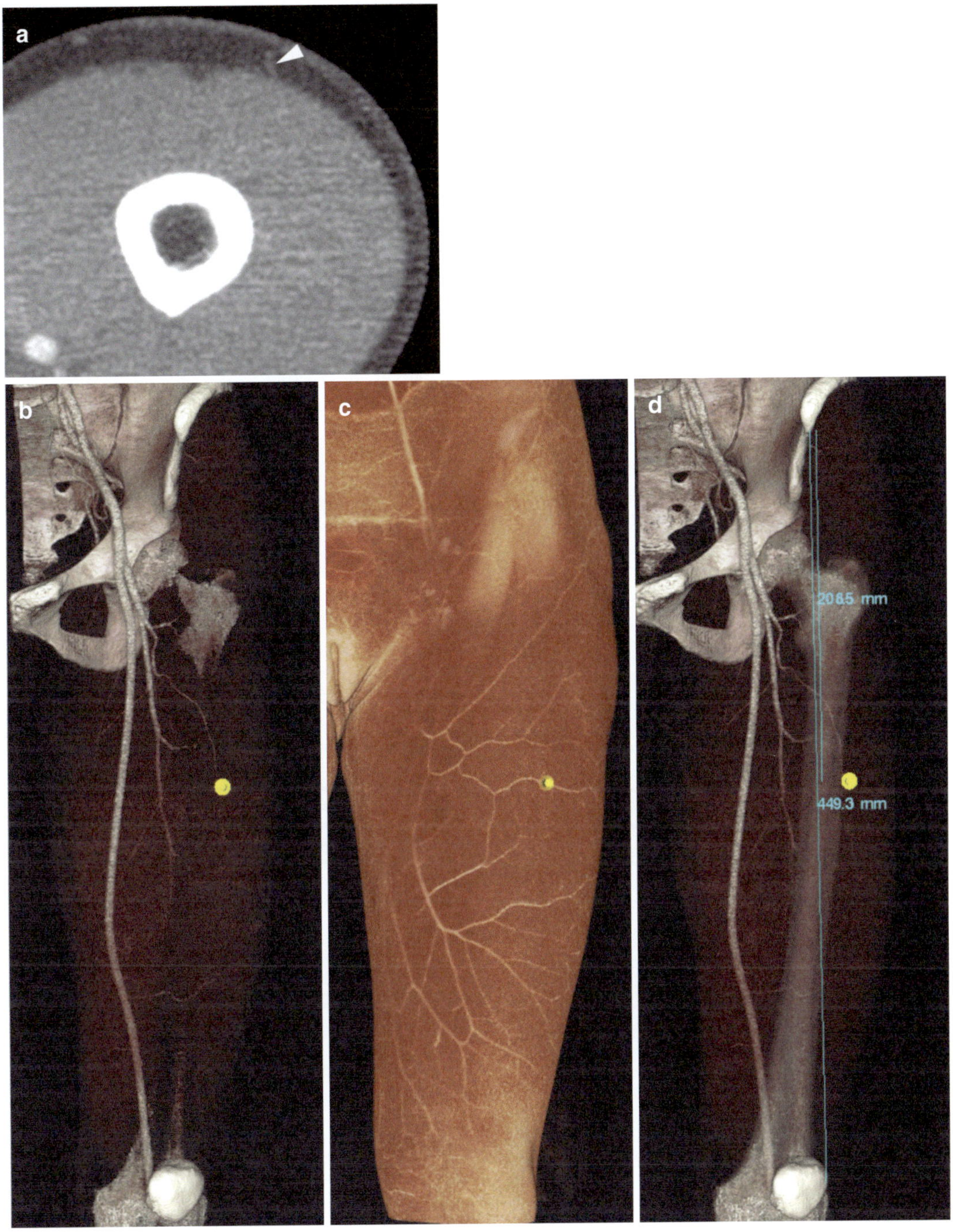

Fig. 7.2 MDCT angiography for preoperative planning of anterolateral thigh (ALT) flap for penile reconstruction. Left thigh. (**a**) Axial 5-mm MIP reconstruction shows a perforator (*arrowhead*) emerging from the vastus lateralis muscle. (**b**) 3D volume rendering (VR) reconstruction obtained to show the complete course of the pedicle. (**c**) 3D surface rendering VR showing subcutaneous branching of the perforators. (**d**) The flap is outlined on the axis of the anterior superior iliac spine and the lateral patella. The yellow mark shows the precise projection of the perforator's origin on the skin.

References

1. Bertolotto M, Serafini G, Savoca G et al (2005) Color Doppler US of the postoperative penis: anatomy and surgical complications. Radiographics 25:731–748
2. Phillips J, Fein-Zachary VJ, Mehta TS, Littlehale N, Venkataraman S, Slanetz PJ (2014) Breast imaging in the transgender patient. AJR Am J Roentgenol 202: 1149–1156
3. Babaei A, Safarinejad MR, Farrokhi F, Iran-Pour E (2010) Penile reconstruction: evaluation of the most accepted techniques. Urol J 7:71–78
4. Garaffa G, Christopher NA, Ralph DJ (2010) Total phallic reconstruction in female-to-male transsexuals. Eur Urol 57:715–722
5. Trombetta C, Liguori G, Bucci S et al (2004) Radiological evaluation of vaginal width and depth in male-to-female transsexuals by the use of magnetic resonance imaging. World J Urol 22:405–408
6. Cova M, Mosconi E, Liguori G et al (2003) Value of magnetic resonance imaging in the evaluation of sex-reassignment surgery in male-to-female transsexuals. Abdom Imaging 28:728–732
7. Brunocilla E, Soli M, Franceschelli A et al (2012) Radiological evaluation by magnetic resonance of the 'new anatomy' of transsexual patients undergoing male to female sex reassignment surgery. Int J Impot Res 24:206–209
8. Sinove Y, Kyriopoulos E, Ceulemans P, Houtmeyers P, Hoebeke P, Monstrey S (2013) Praoperative Planung der gestielten anterolateralen Oberschenkel-Lappenplastik fur Penis-Rekonstruktionen mittels Multidetektor-CT. Handchir Mikrochir Plast Chir. doi:10.1055/s-0032-1333271
9. Ali RS, Bluebond-Langner R, Rodriguez ED, Cheng MH (2009) The versatility of the anterolateral thigh flap. Plast Reconstr Surg 124: e395–e407
10. Pellegrin A, Stocca T, Belgrano M et al (2013) Preoperative vascular mapping with multislice CT of deep inferior epigastric artery perforators in planning breast reconstruction after mastectomy. Radiol Med 118:732–743

Clinical Management of Gender Dysphoria in Adolescents

8

Domenico Di Ceglie

8.1 Introduction

Before the 1960s, there was no concept of gender identity. The first definition of the term 'gender role' was given by John Money [25, 26]. Money wanted to differentiate a set of feelings, assertions and behaviours that identified a person as being a boy or a girl or a man or a woman (gender role), from the contrasting conclusion one could have reached by considering only their gonads.

The term 'gender identity' appeared in the mid-1960s in association with the establishment of a gender identity study group at the University of California. Stoller ([32]: 78) defines it as:

> A complex system of beliefs about oneself: a sense of one's masculinity and femininity. It implies nothing about the origins of that sense (e.g. whether the person is male or female). It has, then, psychological connotations only: one's subjective state.

The concept of gender identity and role having been formulated, it became possible to make sense of experiences that had until then been ill-defined and poorly understood. Incongruity between the natal gender and the psychological/behavioural manifestations of gender identity indicated the presence of a gender dysphoria. This definition opened the way to conceptualise these experiences as new identities and led to their social recognition which culminated in the UK in the passing of the Gender Recognition Act 2004. This legislation allows transgender people to change their birth certificate in accordance with their perceived gender. Similar legislation has been adopted in western countries. Together with these developments, there has been a debate on whether or not this condition should remain in the psychiatric classifications.

8.2 Classifications of Gender Dysphoria in Young People

Following the definition of Gender Identity, in 1980 the category of Gender Identity Disorder of Childhood (GIDC) and Transsexualism for Adolescents and Adults entered the *Diagnostic and Statistical Manual of Mental Disorders* (3rd edn) (DSM–III; [1]). The current diagnostic criteria for gender dysphoria in adolescents and adults are defined in DSM-V. This includes the expression of an experienced gender that is in contrast to the gender assigned at birth, the conviction that one has the typical feelings and reactions of the other gender, a strong desire to get rid of one's primary and secondary sex characteristics and acquire those of the other gender, a strong desire to be of the other gender and to be treated as the other gender (or some alternative gender different from the gender assigned at birth) [2].

D. Di Ceglie, MD, FRC, PSYCH
Gender Identity Development Service,
The Tavistock and Portman NHS Foundation Trust,
Tavistock Centre, 120 Belsize Lane,
London NW3 5BA, UK

Department of Clinical, Educational and Health Psychology, University College London, London, UK
e-mail: ddiceglie@tavi-port.nhs.uk

C. Trombetta et al. (eds.), *Management of Gender Dysphoria: A Multidisciplinary Approach*,
DOI 10.1007/978-88-470-5696-1_8, © Springer-Verlag Italia 2015

Gender identity disorder of childhood was also included in the *International Classification of Diseases, Tenth Revision* (ICD–10, F64.2; [35]). This classification is currently being reviewed.

Although there has been a shift towards the recognition of the condition as an identity, the incongruence between self-perception and body during the developmental period and beyond is a distressing condition requiring a combination of psychological, social and physical interventions during the developmental period or adulthood. This is probably the main reason for which the condition has been retained in DSM-V under the new names of 'gender dysphoria in children' and 'gender dysphoria in adults and adolescents'. The use of the word 'dysphoria' (from Greek: state of unease or mental discomfort) instead of 'disorder' emphasises the distressing nature of the condition [17] but also ensures that there is no need for the individual to retain the diagnosis of gender dysphoria once the dysphoria has disappeared through gender reassignment procedures or an evolution of the condition with the disappearance of the incongruence between self-perception and the body.

8.3 Frequency of Gender Dysphoria in Childhood and Adolescence

The incidence of childhood cross-gender dysphoria in the general population has not yet been definitively established. The studies that have been carried out have used differing criteria, such as single behaviours or identity statements. No large-scale investigation with standardised criteria, such as those of DSM–V, has yet been conducted.

Zuger and Taylor [42] interviewed the mothers of boys aged about 7 years with regard to the presence of six cross-gender behaviours: desire to be female, feminine dressing, wearing lipstick, doll play, preference for girl playmates and aversion to boys' games. The mothers were not asked how long the behaviours had been apparent nor when they started. Zuger and Taylor also showed that these behaviours were not frequently found in children (73 % never engaged in any of them).

Feinblatt and Gold [20] found that of 193 children referred to a Connecticut child guidance clinic, four boys and three girls (3.6 % of the total) were referred primarily because of 'gender-role inappropriate behaviour'.

Epidemiological data suggest that 'extreme forms of cross-gender behaviour are uncommon among boys in the general population' ([38]; see also [39]).

In recent years there has been a large increase in referrals to specialist gender identity services for children and adolescents in western countries. This is probably due to an increase in social awareness or better recognition of the conditions in these countries. The graph below (Fig. 8.1) shows the increase in referrals to the Gender Identity Development Service (GIDS) from the start of the service in 1989 to 2012.

8.4 Long-Term Follow-Up Studies

A follow-up study of children with features of gender dysphoria was conducted by Green (1987) [21]. He reported that of the 66 males in the original 'feminine boy' group, two-thirds were reinterviewed in adolescence or young adulthood, when three-quarters of them were found to be homosexual or bisexual. Only one boy in this study had a transsexual outcome.

Zucker [38] collated all the long-term follow-up studies of children with gender identity disorder (gender dysphoria) referred to mental health professionals. The study showed that a small minority of children had a transsexual outcome (5.3 %), while the majority had a homosexual or bisexual outcome (45.7 %).

More recent studies show that gender dysphoria persists into adolescence and beyond in only about ten to thirty percent of prepubertal children with gender dysphoria [19, 34]. Given the variability of outcomes, some clinicians have defined their approach to the care of children as 'watchful waiting'. Factors which may contribute to the

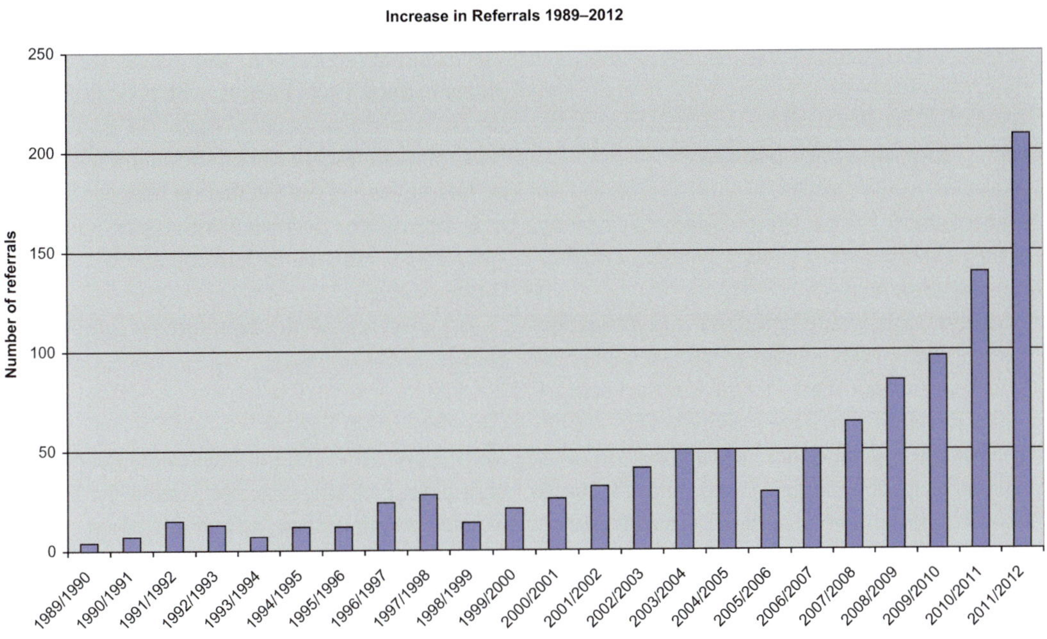

Fig. 8.1 Annual referral rates at the Gender Identity Development Service – London

persistence or desistence are unclear and the subject of current empirical research.

Gender dysphoria in adolescence tends to persist into adulthood in the vast majority of cases.

8.5 Associated Psychosocial Difficulties

Coates and Spector Person [6] have shown that children with gender identity disorders also present with separation anxiety, depression and emotional and behavioural difficulties. Suicide attempts and self-harming behaviours in adolescence are frequent, and in some cases this is how adolescents with gender identity disorders come to professional attention [29].

In a survey of the first 124 cases referred to the GIDS, we found that the most common associated features were relationship difficulties with parents or carers (57 %), relationship difficulties with peers (52 %), depression/misery (42 %), family mental health problems (38 %), family physical health problems (38 %), being the victim of harassment or persecution (33 %) and social sensitivity (31 %). This data suggest that children with gender identity problems may experience considerable isolation owing to difficulties in their relationships with significant adults and peers. They can also become the victims of persecution, which may contribute to feelings of depression and misery. In this sample, boys appear to experience more harassment than girls, and this may be due to the fact that gender nonconformity in boys is less socially acceptable than in girls. The high percentages of mental and physical health problems in the families of children and adolescents referred may indicate that factors such as parental depression or major physical illness could represent a traumatic event for the child, possibly contributing to their gender identity issues. This survey also showed that associated difficulties and case complexity increase during adolescence [16].

De Vries et al. [12] at the Gender Identity Clinic in Amsterdam reported the occurrence of autism spectrum disorders in 7.8 % in gender dysphoric children and adolescents. Jones et al. [22] reported elevated scores on the autism spectrum quotient (AQ) in female-to-male transsexual people (transmen).

For a detailed review of the associated psychosocial difficulties, see Zucker [41].

8.6 Explanatory Models

No single cause has yet been found with certainty for the development of gender dysphoria in children and adolescents.

Most authors would agree that a combination of biological, psychodynamic/psychological and social factors contributes to the development of gender dysphoria in young people. The significance of the co-occurrence in a number of cases of gender dysphoria and autistic spectrum conditions in some children is the subject of current study. Autistic spectrum features may lead to particular styles of thinking, which in some cases contributes to the persistence of gender dysphoria from childhood to adolescence and beyond.

Biological factors include differences in brain anatomy and genetic and hormonal influences during foetal development and childhood. Taziaux et al. [33] have shown that there are sex differences in the neurokinin B (NKB) system in the human infundibular nucleus. They state that these differences 'reached only significance in adulthood and that male-to-female transsexuals had a female-typical infundibular NKB system. These results suggest that: (1) in addition to the well-known perinatal period of steroid-dependent brain organisation, sex steroid hormones during puberty might also contribute to the emergence of sex differences in adulthood; and (2) the sex reversal observed in MtF transsexuals may reflect, at least in part, an atypical sexual differentiation of the hypothalamus'. These data confirm previous findings regarding the difference between sexes in some hypothalamic nuclei, in that MtF transsexual people have a configuration of these nuclei similar to those of females [23, 37]. How these differences influence self-perception remains unclear.

Psychodynamic/psychological factors contributing to the development of gender dysphoria in children and adolescents have included attachment issues [24], difficulty mourning the loss of an important attachment figure ([3], Di Ceglie 1998), consequences of traumatic experiences [8, 7], maternal depression and particular family constellations [31]. Factors which contribute to the persistence of gender dysphoria from childhood into adolescence and beyond are unclear.

On the whole, the interaction between subjective experience, hormonal influences and brain structures is not well understood and will require further studies.

For a review of the literature on aetiological factors, see [11, 40].

Case Illustration 1: Mark

Mark, aged 16 years, presented with gender dysphoria. He hated his male body intensely. Socially isolated and in despair, he had attempted suicide. Since the age of 3 or 4 years, he had felt that he was a girl. At the age of 7 years, his father sexually abused him, and this experience confirmed for him that he was a girl as, at that time, he thought that men were sexually attracted only to women. At the time of the referral, he felt that his body should be changed immediately, as he could not bear living in a contradictory situation. At this stage Mark still lived in a male role. There was also a real possibility of further suicide attempts.

A structured therapeutic programme, including individual and family sessions, and also consultation with a paediatric endocrinologist, made him feel that mind and body had been taken into consideration and helped him to tolerate a transitional phase of uncertainty by containing his feelings of despair. It also supported his hope that the incongruence between his mind and body would eventually be overcome. It was important that network meetings of the professionals involved with his care were held at regular intervals.

Exploration of the young person's expectations, gender identity and roles, body image, self-perception and other people's perception of the individual is essential preparation for the young person to begin physical (hormonal) interventions and the referral to a gender identity service for adults at the age of 18 for further treatment. Surgical intervention could be offered in the adult service. In Mark's case this exploration showed a well established – gender dysphoria.

8.7 Some Psychodynamic Considerations on the Nature of the Atypical Gender Identity Organisation: Continuity and Discontinuity

In 1964 Stoller proposed the concept of core gender identity. He saw this as:

> Produced by the infant–parent relationship, the child's perception of its external genitalia, and a biologic force, which results from the biologic variables of sex (chromosomes, gonads, hormones, internal accessory reproductive structures and external genitalia).

Stoller believed that the core gender identity is established before the fully developed phallic stage, age 3–6, although gender identity continues to develop into adolescence and beyond ([30]: 453). He further stated that the beliefs comprising the 'mental structure' of the core gender identity are the earliest part of gender identity to develop and are relatively permanent after the child reaches 4 or 5 years of age ([32]: 78).

Further research and clinical experience show that in about 10–30 % of children with gender dysphoria does the core gender identity have the enduring structural characteristics described by Stoller.

In 1998 the author proposed the concept of atypical gender identity organisation (AGIO) as a clinical entity that can be examined under a number of parameters relevant to clinical management (Box 8.1; [14]).

> **Box 8.1. Clinical Features of Atypical Gender Identity Organisation (AGIO; from [14])**
> Rigidity–flexibility
> Timing of formation of the AGIO
> Presence/absence of traumatic events in the child's life in relation to formation of the AGIO
> Position of the AGIO on continuum from the paranoid–schizoid to the depressive position

- *Rigidity–flexibility*
  This refers to the capacity of the AGIO to remain unchangeable or, alternatively, to be amenable to evolution in the course of development. Organisations which are more rigid will contribute to the persistence of the atypical gender identity development (gender dysphoria), while organisations which are more fluid will lead to shifts in gender identity development. As mentioned earlier, only in some prepubertal children (10–30 %) will it possess the unchangeable structural qualities of Stoller's core gender identity. To use a different language, one could say that there is continuity in the AGIO from childhood to adolescence/adulthood in a small proportion of children and discontinuity in the rest.
- *Timing of the AGIO formation*
  Atypical organisations that develop very early in the child's life may be more likely to become rigidly structured than organisations that develop later. The early onset of gender dysphoria is in fact one of the criteria for considering early pubertal suppression (see section on management).
- *Identifiable traumatic events in the child's life in relation to the AGIO formation*
  In some cases the AGIO is formed as a psychological coping strategy in relation to a traumatic event in childhood. The earlier the trauma occurs, the more likely it is that the organisation will acquire rigid and unchangeable qualities.
- *Where the formation of the AGIO can be located on the continuum from the paranoid–schizoid to the depressive position within Klein–Bion model of psychological development*
  The hypothesis here is that if the AGIO is formed within a mental functioning dominated by paranoid–schizoid processes in response to a traumatic event, it is more likely to become very structured, and therefore not amenable to change. Alternatively, if it is formed within a mental functioning of the depressive position, it is likely that the organisation will be amenable to evolution.

Therapeutic exploration may be able to elucidate the characteristics of the organisation and therefore guide management. The following clinical example illustrates this point.

Case Illustration 2: Jennifer

Jennifer was 17 when she presented following three suicide attempts. She was a female-to-male transgender person who presented with depressive episodes and a number of borderline features. She was still living in a female role, maintained her female name and wished to be addressed using a female pronoun. She was uncertain about physical interventions. Her mother, who had died just before Jennifer came to the clinic, suffered depression after Jennifer's birth, and her father had been physically violent towards his wife during Jennifer's childhood, until they separated. During her psychotherapy sessions, she vividly remembered episodes when her father in fits of temper had kicked her mother, even in the stomach. In one session she admitted, not without a sense of embarrassment and shame that she had identified with him, an experience that she could not explain. She loved her mother, and her main aim in life was to do something extraordinary that would have made her mother happy. There was no recollection that Jennifer herself had been physically abused by her father, but witnessing violence between her parents had been a traumatic childhood experience.

It is possible to hypothesise that the way Jennifer coped with the fear of damage to her mother and possibly to herself was to identify with a male possessing the strength of a masculine body. This belief, once established, gave her a sense of survival and also of protecting her 'damaged' mother. A female representation of herself had to be strongly avoided, as this was equated in her mind with being weak and damaged.

Another important factor also seemed to play a part. After the birth of two older sisters, her mother had miscarried a baby boy. One year later, Jennifer was born. Jennifer seemed to feel that her mother had expected her to be a boy, and in one session she alluded to her mother having 'psychic qualities', as if she had been part of a magical experience in which she and her mother could read each others' minds. She had probably received, and made her own, her mother's wish that she were a boy. This wish was probably never consciously expressed by her mother but remained unconsciously active in the relationship between them.

Two years of psychotherapeutic exploration with this young person allowed the therapist, together with Jennifer, to make this partial reconstruction of her childhood relating to her atypical gender identity development. However, any attempts to explore this understanding further with Jennifer led to continuous interruptions to the therapeutic work, which may have indicated her extreme resistance and fears of having the foundation of her gender identity revisited.

Even if she retained some of this understanding, it certainly did not alter Jennifer's gender identity development, that is to say, the sense of whom she was. Her atypical gender identity organisation was well established, and not amenable to evolution. It formed very early in her life, and traumatic events had played a large part in it. Its formation may have probably occurred under the dominance of the paranoid–schizoid position.

Towards the end of therapy, Jennifer was able to live in a male role with a male name, and his well-being improved. He did not attempt suicide again. He settled in a job, and he was more able to establish relationships with other people. One might say that therapy had helped him to cope with his well-established AGIO in a better way, to make the transition to a male role and to give him a sense of hope (an important therapeutic aim – see Box 8.3). He was eventually referred to an adult service for further treatment.

8.8 Management and Therapy: The Staged Approach

The research evidence regarding the management of gender dysphoria in young people is still poor to date. The Report of the American Psychiatric Association Task Force on Treatment of Gender Identity Disorder (gender dysphoria) states that 'the highest level of evidence available for treatment recommendations for these children can best be characterised as expert opinion' [5].

Our model of management at the Tavistock and Portman NHS Foundation Trust is based on the understanding of atypical gender identity development within a complex paradigm. It has been informed by the fact that the causation of the phenomenon of GID remains unclear, and it is probably multifactorial. It is also influenced by current cultural values and societal attitudes regarding the development of gender identity. Our therapeutic experience has shown that children are very sensitive and feel easily intruded upon by anyone attempting to change who they feel they are and by those who minimise their feelings. Therefore at the Gender Identity Development Service, we have developed a model of management in which altering an individual's perceived gender identity is not a primary therapeutic objective. Instead, emphasis is placed on the following list of therapeutic aims (Box 8.2).

Box 8.2. Primary Therapeutic Aims (From [15])

- To foster recognition and non-judgemental acceptance of gender identity issues
- To ameliorate associated behavioural, emotional and relationship difficulties [6]
- To break the cycle of secrecy
- To activate interest and curiosity by exploring the impediments to them
- To encourage exploration of the mind–body relationship by promoting close collaboration among professionals in different specialities, including a paediatric endocrinologist
- To allow mourning processes to occur [3]
- To enable symbol formation and symbolic thinking [28]
- To promote separation and differentiation
- To enable the child or adolescent and the family to tolerate uncertainty in gender identity development
- To sustain hope

It is important to add to this list the need to combat stigma which is often associated with the experience of atypical gender identity and is, at times, internalised by the individual experiencing gender dysphoria. It is also valuable to alleviate the feeling of shame that some children/adolescents and their families experience and enable people to develop skills in handling social interactions and dealing with possible hostility.

The overall aim of therapy is improving the child/adolescent's well-being. The aims outlined in Box 8.2 could be achieved through various psychotherapeutic interventions, ranging from individual to family and group therapy.

Social and educational interventions are also useful. It is important that these are well coordinated and integrated in a comprehensive management plan agreed with local services (The Network Model, [18]).

Some of these aims are more relevant in some cases than in others. The case studies above give a brief illustration of how these therapeutic objectives could be tackled in clinical work; for a more detailed account, see Di Ceglie [15].

The recognition and non-judgemental acceptance of the gender identity issue, which is not the result of the child's conscious choice, is important. Without this, the child would experience feelings of rejection and psychological splitting processes would increase to cope with this. Group work for parents of children with gender dysphoria can be very helpful in this respect, as it helps the parents to realise that their experience is not unique and that they are not isolated.

Where an inability to mourn attachment figures has interfered with gender identity development, work enabling mourning to occur may secondarily alter an atypical gender identity development.

In cases where autistic features coexist with gender dysphoria, psychological interventions aimed at increasing empathy and symbolic thinking become important (see Sect. 8.5). Although this approach has proved clinically useful, its impact is yet to be evaluated.

The general approach to the management of gender dysphoria can be best conceptualised as a process involving four stages, in line with the guidance for management originally issued by the Royal College of Psychiatrists [27] and then further developed in the Standards of Care by the World Professional Association for Transgender Health 7th version [36].

Stage 1 of the process for children and adolescents is a therapeutic exploration, as described above. In adolescents, if the AGIO persists, then physical interventions could be considered if they are requested by the adolescent and his or her family. There is often pressure for physical intervention because of the high level of distress brought about by the reality of the changing body at puberty. However, the move towards physical intervention should be carefully considered and based on a well-established process of informed consent.

Stage 2 includes wholly reversible intervention. This involves the use of hypothalamic blockers, which suppress the production of oestrogens or testosterone and produce a state of biological neutrality. In the early stage of pubertal development (Tanner stages 2–3), they induce pubertal suppression.

In order that adolescents and parents may make a properly informed decision, the Royal College of Psychiatrists' guidance recommends that young people have some experience of pubertal development. When this intervention has been properly assimilated, while continuing psychological exploration, support and physical monitoring by a paediatric endocrinologist, stage 3 can be considered.

Stage 3 includes partially reversible interventions, such as hormonal treatment that masculinises or feminises the body.

Finally, *stage 4* includes irreversible interventions, such as surgical procedures.

In the UK, since 2011, the Gender Identity Development Service can offer pubertal suppression, through the use of GNRH (stage 2/3), to children (after the age of 12) in whom the gender dysphoria persists into adolescence. This intervention is offered within a research protocol. The protocol was drafted following a wide debate involving service users, professionals and relevant professional organisations, such as the British Society of Paediatric Endocrinology and Diabetes [4]. It received ethical approval and has a well-established system of informed consent from young people and their parents/carers. It adopted the eligibility criteria similar to those of the Centre of Expertise on Gender Dysphoria in Amsterdam [9, 10]. (See Box 8.3.)

Box 8.3. Eligibility Criteria for Early Pubertal Suppression

A. Psychological criteria

Before the adolescent can be considered for inclusion in the research protocol, she/he should have been seen by the service at the Tavistock clinic site for at least 6 months and should have attended at least four interviews for assessment and therapeutic exploration of their gender identity development.

1. Standard readiness criteria relating to psychological stability sufficient to withstand the stresses of sex reassignment.
2. Fulfils the following criteria relating to GID:
   (a) Throughout childhood (defined as over 5 years), the adolescent has demonstrated an intense pattern of cross-gendered behaviours and cross-gender identity.
   (b) The adolescent has gender dysphoria that is significantly increased with the onset of puberty. Following assessment, the clinician(s) working with the young person deems that there is a high likelihood of the young person experiencing severe psychological distress consequent on experiencing full pubertal development before the blocker is implemented.
3. The young person and parents/guardians are actively requesting blockers.
4. The young person is able to give informed consent.

(Note that so called 'real-life experience' of living in a transgender role is not required, de Vries (2006, p. 91.)

B. Physical/medical criteria
  1. In established puberty:
     - For biological males, Tanner (genital and pubic hair (PH)) stage 3 and above.
     - For biological females, Tanner (Breast and PH) stage 2 and above.

     Note that these pubertal criteria match those used by the Dutch. The rationale for the sex difference is that the pubertal growth spurt which early intervention aims to avoid occurs earlier in females (Tanner 2–3) than in males (Tanner 3–4); thus, earlier intervention is required in females, but is not necessary in males to avoid unwanted growth (in males) or growth termination (in females).
  2. Normal endocrine function and karyotype consistent with biological sex.

     Note that the presence of mild elevations of androgens in biological females consistent with polycystic ovarian syndrome is not an exclusion criterion.
  3. Age 12 and above [9].

Children, particularly adolescents, and their families often find the experience of a gender dysphoria painful and unbearable, and adolescents are at high risk of suicide attempts. This sense of despair frequently leads to extreme pressure being placed on clinicians to act and to provide immediate solutions, through physical intervention. In such cases, a detailed discussion with the adolescent and the family of the treatment as a staged process may relieve the distress by creating space for thinking. This may allow time to explore the issues involved in each stage and gradually reduce the pressure for immediate solutions that have not been properly thought through.

A follow-up study of adolescents with gender dysphoria who were treated with the hypothalamic blockers shows that they had improved in their psychological functioning during the period of pubertal suppression [13].

Case Illustration 3: Laura/Rhidian

Laura was referred to the Gender Identity Development Service (GIDS) at the age of 14 by a consultant paediatrician following a series of overdoses requiring inpatient admission to a paediatric ward. Her preferred name was Rhidian, but at this stage, she wished to be addressed as a 'she'. The referrer was querying whether gender identity issues were contributing to the suicidal behaviour. Before Rhidian could be assessed by us, she had been admitted to a secure private psychiatric inpatient unit under Section 2 of the Mental Health Act as her aggressive behaviour towards others and herself had become unmanageable in the community. When we started her assessment, she was escorted by two nurses to come to our service. By this time, she was living in a secure adolescent unit.

Our assessment confirmed that she had the features of gender dysphoria associated with serious behavioural difficulties and characterised by poor impulse control and extreme sensitivity to feelings of rejection leading to explosive, violent reactions and suicidal behaviour. She was intelligent, but could not manage in any school setting.

There had been breakdowns in all her family relationships, and she could not live with her mother and stepfather. She was pressing for physical interventions to change her body as a solution to all her problems.

Our interventions involved a structured exploration of her perceptions about gender identity. We aimed to reduce her suicidal behaviour and support coping strategies. We addressed difficulties in the family relationships and within the professional network. Detailed discussion with Rhidian, her carers and professional network about the treatment as a staged process proved to be a containing and supportive framework for Rhidian's difficult feelings.

Our outreach service included meetings with the staff of the secure unit and other professionals involved. These were at Rhidian's local Child and Adolescent Mental Health Service (CAMHS) in Devon.

This gradually led to an improvement in her behaviour. She became able to live with foster parents and visited her family at weekends. Her explosive outbursts became less frequent and her suicidal behaviour stopped.

As her perception of her male gender identity had persisted for over a year and she wished to consider gender reassignment, she was assessed by our paediatric endocrinologist at 15. After further discussion, she started on gonadotropin-releasing hormone analogue (GnRHa) to suppress oestrogen production. This treatment was prescribed and monitored by our paediatrician, while Rhidian continued to be seen on a regular basis by a member of our team for further exploration of her gender identity and other associated psychological problems. By this time, Rhidian was living in a male role and wished to be addressed as 'he'.

Our regular outreach meetings continued involving social services, the local counsellor, the GP and foster parents. He was able to attend college and gained some qualifications for entry to university. He established some peer group relationships while living in a male role and gradually became able to explain his situation when appropriate. He did not require any further admission to hospital or secure accommodation. He persisted in his wish for gender reassignment. After 1 year on the GnRHa treatment, testosterone treatment was prescribed by our paediatrician. Testosterone administration could be increased in a gradual way, while the GnRHa treatment continued to suppress oestrogen production.

At 18 he was accepted at university to study nursing, and on the whole his life was more stable. He was referred to an adult gender identity service for further treatment. The member of our GID service who had been seeing him over the last 5 years attended the first appointment with the adult psychiatrist as a transitional measure.

In summary, our intervention provided a prolonged assessment of Rhidian's gender identity development, evidence of the persistence of the gender dysphoria over a long period of time and fixity of his belief of having a male identity. The treatment assisted Rhidian's development and improved his behaviour and the other psychological difficulties including his suicidality.

The outreach service supported local services and contributed to creating a stable and therapeutic environment for Rhidian, preventing the need for further expensive inpatient treatment or secure accommodation. The service initiated physical treatment at the appropriate time and paved the way for a referral to the adult services by preparing Rhidian to make informed decisions about irreversible treatment available within the adult service.

Conclusions

Gender dysphoria is a complex condition. Clinical practice and research in the past three decades have made it possible to create models of care that benefit children and adolescents. As clinical research evidence progresses, new models of care will be developed. Language and nomenclature will also change in line with new cultural and social attitudes.

The social and legal recognition in recent years of transgender experiences as new identities, protected by equality legislation, has contributed to making the assessment and diagnostic process a temporary phase which would only last as long as the experience of gender dysphoria persists and requires a multidisciplinary treatment approach.

The need remains to combat stigma and raise public awareness about gender identity issues through appropriate social interventions and policies.

For confidentiality purposes, the young peoples' names and some other details have been changed and disguised so they could not be recognised.

References

1. American Psychiatric Association (1980) Diagnostic and statistical manual of mental disorders (DSM–III), 3rd edn. American Psychiatric Association, Washington, DC
2. American Psychiatric Association (2013) Diagnostic and statistical manual of mental disorders (DSM–V), 5th edn. American Psychiatric Association, Washington, DC
3. Bleiberg E, Jackson L, Ross JL (1986) Gender identity disorder and object loss. J Am Acad Child Adolesc Psychiatry 25:58–67

4. British Society for Paediatric Endocrinology and Diabetes (2009) Statement on the management of gender identity disorder (GID) in children & adolescents. http://www.bsped.org.uk/clinical/docs/BSPEDStatementOnTheManagementOfGID.pdf
5. Byne W, Bradley SJ, Coleman E, Evan Eyler A, Green R, Menvielle EJ, Meyer-Bahlburg HFL, Pleak RR, Tompkins A (2012) Report of the American Psychiatric Association task force on treatment of gender identity disorder. Arch Sex Behav 41(4):759–796
6. Coates S, Spector Person E (1985) Extreme boyhood femininity: isolated behaviour or pervasive disorder? J Am Acad Child Adolesc Psychiatry 24:702–709
7. Coates S, Friedman R, Wolfe S (1991) The aetiology of boyhood gender identity disorder: a model for integrating temperament, development and pychodynamics. Psychoanal Dialogues 1:481–523
8. Coates S, Moore MS (1998) The complexity of early trauma: representation and transformation. In: Di Ceglie D, Freedman D (eds) A stranger in my own body: atypical gender identity development and mental health. Karnac, London, pp 39–62
9. Delemarre-van de Waal H, Cohen-Kettenis PT (2006) Clinical management of gender identity disorder in adolescents: a protocol on psychological and paediatric endocrinology aspects. Eur J Endocrinol 155:131–137
10. De Vries ALC, Cohen-Kettenis PT, Delamarre-van de Waal HA (2007) Clinical management of gender dysphoria in adolescents. J Transgenderism 9:83–94
11. De Vries ALC, Cohen-Kettenis PT (2012) Clinical management of gender dysphoria in children and adolescents: the Dutch approach. J Homosex 59:301–320
12. De Vries ALC, Noens ILJ, Cohen-Kettenis PT, van Berckelaer-Onnes IA, Doreleijers TA (2010) Autism spectrum disorders in gender dysphoric children and adolescents. J Autism Dev Disord 40:930–936
13. De Vries ALC, Steensma TD, Doreleijers TAH, Cohen-Kettenis PT (2011) Puberty suppression in adolescents with gender identity disorder: a prospective follow-up study. Int Soc Sex Med. doi:10.1111/j.1743-6109.2010.01943.x
14. Di Ceglie D (1998) Reflections on the nature of the "atypical gender identity organisation". In: Di Ceglie D, Freedman D (eds) A stranger in my own body: atypical gender identity development and mental health. Karnac, London, pp 9–25
15. Di Ceglie D (1998) Management and therapeutic aims with children and adolescents with gender identity disorders and their families. In: Di Ceglie D, Freedman D (eds) A stranger in my own body: atypical gender identity development and mental health. Karnac, London, pp 185–197
16. Di Ceglie D, Freedman D, McPherson S, Richardson P (2002) Children and adolescents referred to a specialist gender identity development service: clinical features and demographic characteristics. Int J Transgenderism 6(1). http://www.symposion.com/ijt/ijtvo06no01 01.htm
17. Di Ceglie D (2010) Gender identity and sexuality: what's in a name? Divers Health Care 7:83–86
18. Di Ceglie D (2013) The care of the gender dysphoric child. In: Kreukels BPC, Steensma TD, de Vries ALC (eds) Gender dysphoria and disorders of sex development: progress in care and knowledge (focus on sexuality research). Springer, New York, pp 151–169
19. Drummond KD, Bradley SJ, Peterson-Badali M, Zucker KJ (2008) A follow up study of girls with gender identity disorder. Dev Psychol 44:34–45
20. Feinblatt JA, Gold AR (1976) Sex roles and the psychiatric referral process. Sex Roles 2:109–122
21. Green R, Roberts CW, Williams K, et al (1987) Specific cross-gender behaviour in boyhood and later homosexual orientation. British Journal of Psychiatry, 151, 84–88.
22. Jones RM, Wheelwright S, Farrell K, Martin E, Green R, Di Ceglie D, Baron-Cohen S (2011) Brief report: female-to-male transsexual people and autistic traits. J Autism Dev Disord. doi:10.1007/s10803-011-1227-8
23. Kruijver FP, Zhou JN, Pool CW, Hofman MA, Gooren LJ, Swaab DF (2000) Mate-to-female transsexuals have female neuron numbers in a limbic nucleus. J C lin Endocrinol Metab 85:2034–2041
24. Marantz S, Coates S (1991) Mothers of boys with gender identity disorders: a comparison to normal controls. J Am Acad Child Adolesc Psychiatry 30:136–143
25. Money J (1955) Hermaphroditism, gender and precocity in hyperadrenocorticism: psychological findings. Bull Johns Hopkins Hosp 96:253–264
26. Money J (1994) The concept of gender identity disorder in childhood and adolescence after 39 years. J Sex Marital Ther 20:163–177
27. Royal College of Psychiatrists (1998) Gender identity disorders in children and adolescents – guidance for management, vol CR63, Council report. Royal College of Psychiatrists, London
28. Segal H (1957) Notes on symbol formation. Int J Psychoanal 38:391–397
29. Skagerberg E, Parkinson R, Carmichael P (2013) Self-harming thoughts and behaviours in a group of children and adolescents with gender dysphoria. Int J Transgenderism 14(2):86–92
30. Stoller R (1964) The hermaphroditic identity of hermaphrodites. J Nerv Ment Dis 139:453–457
31. Stoller RJ (1968) Male childhood transsexualism. J Am Acad Child Adolesc Psychiatry 7:193–201
32. Stoller R (1992) Gender identity development and prognosis: a summary. In: Chiland C, Young JG (eds) New approaches to mental health from birth to adolescence. Yale University Press, New Haven, pp 78–87
33. Taziaux M, Swaab DF, Bakker J (2012) Sex differences in the neurokinin B system in the human infundibular nucleus. J Clin Endocrinol Metabol 97(12): E2210–E2220
34. Wallien MSC, Cohen-Kettenis PT (2008) Psychosexual outcome of gender dysphoric children. J Am Acad Child Adolesc Psychiatry 47:1413–1423

35. World Health Organization (1992) The ICD–10 classification of mental and behavioural disorders. Clinical descriptions and diagnostic guidelines. WHO, Geneva
36. World Professional Association for Transgender Health (2011) Standards of care for the health of transsexual, transgender, and gender nonconforming people, 7th version. www.wpath.org
37. Zhou et al (1995) A sex difference in the human brain and its relation to transsexuality. Nature 378:68–70
38. Zucker KJ (1985) Cross-gender identified children. In: Steiner B (ed) Gender dysphoria. Plenum Press, New York, pp 75–174
39. Zucker KJ, Bradley SJ (1995) Gender identity disorder and psychosexual problems in children and adolescents. Plenum Press, New York
40. Zucker KJ, Wood H, Singh D, Bradley SJ (2012) A developmental, biopsychosocial model for the treatment of children with gender identity disorder. J Homosex 59(3):369–397
41. Zucker KJ (2013) Models of psychopathology in children and adolescents with gender dysphoria. In: Kreukels BPC, Steensma TD, de Vries ALC (eds) Gender dysphoria and disorders of sex development: progress in care and knowledge (focus on sexuality research). Springer, New York
42. Zuger B, Taylor P (1969) Effeminate behaviour present in boys from early childhood, in comparison with similar symptoms in non-effeminate boys. Pediatrics 44:375–380

Part II

Management of Male to Female

9 Psychological Characteristics and Sexuality of Natal Males with Gender Dysphoria

Peggy T. Cohen-Kettenis, Els Elaut, and Baudewijntje P.C. Kreukels

9.1 Introduction

The concept of gender dysphoria (GD) and its status as a mental disorder are currently strongly debated. There are several reasons why so many professionals and other stakeholders are, at this moment, involved in the debate. One reason is that the American Psychiatric Association (APA) recently published the latest version of their classification system, the fifth edition of the Diagnostic and Statistical Manual of Mental Disorders (DSM-5) [1]. Another reason is that the World Health Organization (WHO) is preparing the next version of the International Statistical Classification of Diseases and Related Health Problems, the ICD-11. Publication is expected in 2017. Finally, the World Professional Association for Transgender Health (WPATH) published the 7th version of the Standards of Care for the Health of Transsexual, Transgender, and Gender Nonconforming People (SOC7) [2]. As a consequence, professional organizations and support and advocacy groups needed to reconceptualize the diagnosis as well as the treatment of GD.

In the discussion about the concept of GD, two aspects were central. One was the very concept of GD. The other was whether it should be considered a mental disorder. Before we report on various psychological characteristics of individuals born as males (natal males) with gender dysphoria, we will address these issues shortly.

Because the diagnosis in the DSM-5 is called GD and this term is also used in the SOC7, we will use this term rather than *transsexualism*. Only when referring to specific – often older – studies, the terms *transsexualism*, *male-to-female transsexuals*, and *female-to-male transsexuals* will be used.

In the last decade, increasing numbers of individuals suffering from an incongruence between their experienced gender (gender identity) and assigned gender (usually at birth) come to gender identity clinics. The increase has been observed in gender identity clinics in many countries. An explanation for this may be that among mental health professionals, there is a growing awareness that GD [1] should be conceptualized as a multidimensional rather than a binary phenomenon. In the DSM-5, adults can receive the diagnosis of GD when they fulfill at least two out of six criteria. This implies that individuals may have forms of GD and severities of GD that are not all exactly alike. In the past, diagnostic efforts were directed toward assessing whether someone did or did not fulfill the criteria for *transsexualism*.

P.T. Cohen-Kettenis (✉) • B.P.C. Kreukels
Department of Medical Psychology,
VU University Medical Center,
Boelelaan 1117, Amsterdam 1081 HV,
The Netherlands
e-mail: pt.cohen-kettenis@vumc.nl;
b.kreukels@vumc.nl

E. Elaut
Center of Sexology and Gender Problems,
De Pintelaan 185, Ghent 9000, Belgium
e-mail: els.elaut@ugent.be

C. Trombetta et al. (eds.), *Management of Gender Dysphoria: A Multidisciplinary Approach*,
DOI 10.1007/978-88-470-5696-1_9, © Springer-Verlag Italia 2015

If they did, they could have hormones *and* surgery. If they did not, they were not eligible for any treatment but psychotherapy or other psychological interventions. By acknowledging that GD can be more than only *transsexualism*, a broader range of treatments were made available in gender identity clinics. Many persons with GD, realizing that individualized care is more widely offered, appear to pursue other forms of medical intervention than the classic hormone treatment followed by various forms of surgery [3]. For instance, natal males may just want to have estrogen treatment, whereas natal females may want breast surgery only. This may explain the increased number of referrals to gender identity clinics.

Apart from the expansion of the concept of GD, a second issue that has been a topic of intense dispute regards the question of what kind of phenomenon GD actually is. For long, GD has been considered as a symptom of another psychiatric disorder, such as schizophrenia or borderline personality disorder [4–7]. In 1975, however, the World Health Organization classified it as a distinct mental disorder in the ICD-9. For adults, the phenomenon was called *transsexualism* [8]. The APA, using the other major psychiatric classification system in the world, the DSM, introduced the diagnosis of transsexualism a few years later (DSM-III) [9]. From then on, transsexualism (later called) *gender identity disorder* [10], and even later GD [1], was considered by most clinicians as a psychiatric disorder. GD, however, is a very unusual condition. So far it is the only mental health condition that is diagnosed by mental health clinicians, but – particularly in its extreme forms – it is not treated by these clinicians, like other psychiatric conditions. In order to get rid of the symptoms, individuals with GD receive treatment from endocrinologists and/or surgeons. These clinicians do not make the diagnosis themselves, but rely on diagnoses made by mental health professionals. Over the last years, when DSM-5 and the 11th version of the ICD were prepared, the question has repeatedly been put forward whether GD indeed should be considered a psychiatric diagnosis [11]. This question seems simpler than it is. The very DSM states that psychiatry lacks a single operational definition that covers all situations. A psychiatric disorder is defined on the basis of various concepts, such as distress, loss of control, inflexibility, irrationality, a syndrome pattern, or statistical deviation from the norm [12]. Each concept is a useful indicator of a psychiatric disorder but no single concept is completely the same as the disorder. And what is called a psychiatric disorder is largely dependent on the criteria used, which are, in turn, dependent on time, Zeitgeist, and place. The APA decided in 2013 that it would still be considered a mental disorder and to retain it in the DSM-5. The WHO is still contemplating if it should be part of the ICD-11, particularly with regard to the child diagnosis, and, if so, whether it should be placed in the chapter on mental disorders or elsewhere.

An extensive discussion on the phenomenon GD is beyond the scope of this chapter. In the discussion on why GD would be a mental disorder, however, one often refers to the high rate of psychopathology (other than GD, if one would consider GD a mental disorder) among people with GD. In this chapter, we will only review the literature on psychological functioning of GD individuals who were born as males.

Besides their psychological functioning, another important characteristic of individuals with GD concerns their sexuality. In the early years, transsexuals were often portrayed as merely asexual [13–15]. This was probably because transsexualism was seen by many as a sexual perversion or aberration. By stressing the asexuality of people with GD, an attempt was made to take it out of the sexual disorder sphere. When GD became more accepted, more information became available about the sexual orientation and sexual behavior of people with GD. This made it possible to understand GD better than has long been the case. In this chapter, we will therefore also review what is known about the sexuality of natal males with GD *before* treatment.

9.2 Psychiatric Disorders: Axis I

In the DSM versions that were used until recently (III, IV, and IV-TR), a multiaxial system was followed. In this system individuals were evaluated in terms of several different domains of information that were assumed to be of clinical value. With regard to psychiatric disorders, a distinction was made between Axis I and Axis II disorders. The other axes described clinically relevant but nonpsychiatric domains. Axis I disorders referred to clinical syndromes, and Axis II primarily to personality disorders.

Studies appear to diverge largely with regard to co-occurring Axis I psychiatric problems. For example, Cole and colleagues [16] found that only 1 in 318 natal males attending their gender identity clinic had schizophrenia, whereas à Campo et al. [17] reported schizophrenia in 24 % of persons with GD (natal sex was not specified). The studies were, however, very different with regard to participants and quality of design. In an extensive recent review on psychiatric problems in individuals with GD, Lawrence and Zucker [18] concluded that Axis I psychiatric disorders in adults vary between 6 and 80 %, but the studies they discuss also cover studies on natal females. Yet, also in natal males, numbers vary. A recent and comprehensive study [19], using a structured psychiatric interview, studied coexisting psychiatric problems in a group of individuals with GD attending 4 European clinics. They observed that, at first assessment, 38 % of the natal males reported to have an Axis I diagnosis. Affective (27 %) and anxiety (17 %) disorders were most prevalent. However, if lifetime diagnoses were included, the percentage of individuals who ever had a psychiatric diagnosis increased to 68 %. When comparing the prevalence of Axis I disorders to the general population, it appeared that this lifetime prevalence was much higher than in the general population of the respective countries. This was mainly due to the high prevalence of affective and anxiety disorders in the group with GD (about 3 times higher than in the general population).

In Japan, a country with an entirely different culture, Hoshiai et al. [20] found that in a group of 230 natal males with GD, 19 % had current psychiatric Axis I problems. In their group, most common were adjustment disorders, anxiety disorders, and mood disorders. In contrast, a small Swiss study [21] found Axis I disorders in 40 % of the natal males.

Besides the study of psychiatric diagnoses, assessing the existence of psychiatric problems in an either-or way (you do have an anxiety disorder or you do not), the psychological functioning of people with GD has also been investigated by means of dimensional measures (a person may have more or less anxiety instead of fulfilling the diagnosis of an anxiety disorder or not).

A Spanish study [22] found that 75 % of their applicants for gender reassignment had no significant psychopathology, suggesting that psychopathology is not inherent to GD. Relatively low percentages of psychopathology were also found in other studies using the same instruments as were used in the spanish study and other instruments [16, 23–25]. However, in a study from Taiwan on 18 participants, it was found that natal males with GD had significantly more psychological problems than male controls [26].

If one looks at the *lifetime* prevalence of psychiatric disorders in persons with GD, the picture is that it is generally higher than in the general population. For instance, De Cuypere et al. [27] reported 45 % and Hepp et al. [21] 80 %. Heylens et al. [19] reported that 68 % of the natal males ever suffered from a psychiatric disorder as compared to 25 % that was reported in the European Study of the Epidemiology of Mental Disorders (ESEMeD) [28]. Lifetime substance abuse was found in 29 % [16], 50 % [21], and 50 % [27] of natal males. This implies that most adults with GD do struggle with psychiatric problems sooner or later in their lives. The most common problems are anxiety, depression, and substance abuse. Interestingly, Murad et al. [29] concluded on the basis of 28 studies, with 1,833 person with GD (1,093 natal males and 801 natal females) and an average follow-up of 6 years, that 78 % persons had less psychiatric problems after treatment of their GD than before. For people with GD, gender reassignment thus seems to have positive influence on their mental health.

It is notable that few studies investigated the relationship between autism spectrum disorders (ASD) and GD. Yet, this is an area that is clinically highly relevant. Making the diagnosis of GD in this group as well as making treatment decisions is usually complicated in the case of ASD. It may be hard to differentiate whether persons with

ASD "conclude" that they "must be" gender dysphoric, because of other reasons (e.g., because natal females like to be tomboyish or fall in love with girls) or whether there is a genuine GD present that only looks much like autistic preoccupations. As people with ASD are often rather rigid, it can be challenging to discuss other possible reasons for their desire to have gender reassignment while maintaining a good working relationship. The same rigidity makes it also hard for those who undergo treatment to cope with daily life situations. When transitioning and after transition, there are so many social obstacles that actually require flexibility in thinking and behavior. To date, however, few studies exist using systematic measures on this co-occurrence. The literature on the co-occurrence of ASD and gender dysphoria consists primarily of case studies on individuals with ASD and concomitant GD. Most refer to children, adolescents, or natal females; only one case study was published on an adult natal male [30]. In one study a high co-occurrence was found between GD and ADS in children and adolescents [31]. Using a questionnaire measuring autistic traits in a group of 63 natal male adults with GD, Pasterski et al. [32] found that in about 5 %, there were autistic traits consistent with a clinical diagnosis for autism.

9.3 Psychiatric Disorders: Axis II

As stated previously, GD has long been considered to be a symptom of other psychiatric disorders, borderline personality disorder in particular. This had led to a number of studies investigating the prevalence and type of Axis II disorders in persons with GD. Unfortunately some did not give separate results for natal male and natal female individuals with GD, and specific data on natal males are therefore not always available from published reports. Elevated rates of personality disorders were found by Madeddu et al. [33]. They reported 58 % personality disorders in a sample of 37 natal males. More precisely, they found that 3 % had a cluster A disorder ("odd" symptoms), 27 % had a cluster B disorder (anxious symptoms), 3 % had a cluster C disorder (dramatic symptoms), and 20 % had a personality disorder not otherwise specified. De Cuypere et al. [27] reported a prevalence of 70 % in natal males. However, there are also reports on a lower prevalence of personality disorders in persons with GD. For instance, in the previously mentioned study by Heylens et al. [19], only 12 % of the natal males had a personality disorder, which is not very much higher than the prevalence rate for personality disorders in the general population (approximately 10.5–12 %) [34]. Lawrence and Zucker [18] conclude in their review that comorbidity on Axis II in adults with gender dysphoria varies in different studies between 20 and 70 %.

9.4 Conclusions on Psychiatric Disorders

With regard to psychopathology and psychological functioning of people with GD, the most notable finding is the variation in outcome. Besides differences in design and local clinical policies, this may be caused by heterogeneity of study participants. In many studies, no distinction is made with regard to gender, sexual orientation, age, or age of onset.

Concerning gender, several [but not all; e.g., 21, 22] studies showed that natal females function psychologically better than natal males [e.g., 16, 23, 27, 35]. Sexual orientation is another neglected issue. In most studies on psychological functioning of people with GD, sexual orientation is not taken into account [e.g., 16, 21–23]. Studies that did make the distinction reported inconsistent findings. For instance, Smith et al. [36] found a difference between persons attracted to their natal or the other sex, but de Vries et al. [25] did not [for a review, see 37]. Age appears to be important with regard to psychological functioning of individuals with GD as well. Studies in small samples of adult persons with GD showed that they had a better prognosis after gender reassignment when they requested treatment before age 30 [e.g., 38]. The few studies on even younger people with GD (adolescents) showed that they had mean scores on psychological scales that were well within the normal range [25, 39, 40]. Finally, some studies [e.g., 36] found differences in psychopathology between natal males with an early and late onset GD. However, Heylens et al. [19] did not confirm these results in their study on the prevalence of Axis I, or Axis II, disorders between these subgroups. From these results it is clear that one cannot draw any firm conclusion regarding psychiatric disorders and GD from studies that do not properly describe relevant aspects of the study population.

Why individuals with GD may have more mental health problems than the general population is not entirely clear. One can think of various explanations. Lawrence and Zucker [18] mention four possibilities: (1) social stigma as a result of an atypical gender identity may lead to the development of other psychiatric disorders; (2) the presence of a psychiatric disorder contributes to the development of GD; (3) generic risk factors result in both psychiatric problems and GD; and (4) the inherent distress of GD causes other psychiatric problems.

9.5 Suicidality

Considering the high prevalence of mood disorders, one would expect that suicidality and suicidal ideation are also high. Dhejne et al. [41] indeed found that persons with GD have a much higher risk of suicide than matched controls. Suicide attempts in about one third of persons with GD (natal sex not specified) were reported in an extensive review by Haas et al. [42]. Associated factors were depression, anxiety, substance abuse, discrimination, violence, and stigma. In a large Japanese study, the rate of suicidal thoughts was, in both natal male and female persons with GD but without psychiatric problems, horrendously high: about 72 % [43]. Cultural factors likely contribute to the shame and stigma associated with GD, which in turn leads to increased suicidality in some countries.

9.6 Sexual Orientation

In the early clinical reports of GD, sexual orientation was mentioned for merely descriptive reasons [44]. Since it was assumed that applicants for treatment would show very similar histories of gender development, clinicians and researchers assumed and reported an early onset of GD and a sexual orientation directed toward one's natal sex in virtually all cases [45, 46]. During the 1960s and 1970s, as gender reassignment became more known and available, the first writings emerged on potential developmental pathways toward GD [see, e.g., 47, 48]. This increase in attention for sexual orientation in applicants for treatment was mainly driven by the attempt to identify "the true transsexual," as described in DSM-III [9], and hence select an "appropriate" candidate for gender reassignment surgery [37]. The use of sexual orientation in treatment decisions was however quite heteronormative in the sense that medicine would not support the "creation of postoperative homosexuals" [49].

The most prevalent sexual orientation-based typology pertains to the one from Blanchard [50–52]. He divided natal males into two groups with somewhat confusing names: homosexual (natal males attracted to males) and nonhomosexual (natal males attracted to females, attracted to both or neither sexes). Previous research has provided evidence for differences between these subtypes: "homosexual" natal males reported more childhood femininity, sought treatment at younger ages, reported sexual arousal during cross-dressing less often, and functioned better from a psychological and emotional point of view, leading to a lower prevalence of posttreatment regret in comparison to "nonhomosexual" natal males with GD [see, e.g., 18, 36, 37, 53–55]. Based on these results and earlier treatment practices, sexual orientation was included in the DSM as a specifier since the first introduction of the diagnosis.

As more research on posttreatment outcome became available, it was shown that sexual orientation among natal males with GD showed more heterogeneity [see, e.g., 56] and was not necessarily associated with subjective outcome [57]. In contemporary treatment protocols and decisions, sexual orientation hence started to play a minor role [49]. This continuing distinction between the concepts of sexual orientation and GD was also reflected in the most recent version of the Standards of Care (SOC7) [2], where sexual orientation is no longer mentioned. Based on the recommendations of the subworkgroup Gender Identity Disorders for DSM-5, the latest version of the psychiatric manual does no longer contain a sexual orientation specifier. It was stressed that the deletion of the specifier should however not decrease research interests in this area [49].

9.7 Sexual Behavior Before Gender-Confirming Interventions

Related to the abovementioned ideas on sexual orientation, the assumption existed on GD as a "hyposexual condition" [13–15, 58]. While this assumption was not bizarre (considering a likely causation between strong genital distress and the potential conflict this might generate when having sexual contact), very little research directed attention toward sexual health except for the general capacity to reach orgasm after gender-confirming interventions (GCI) [59–61]. Klein and Gorzalka [62] have recently provided an exhaustive overview of sexual functioning *after* GCI. During recent years, attention for the sexual health *before* treatment has increased, focusing on partnerships and frequency of sexual behavior.

9.8 Intimate Partnerships

A first indicator that GD does not represent a "hyposexual condition" is found in the reported number of sexual partners before GCI. Lawrence [63] has shown that – irrespective of sexual orientation – the number of sexual partners before genital surgery in natal males with GD was roughly comparable to the reported lifetime number of sexual partners by adult male respondents (aged 18–59) in an American population survey (NHSLS) [64]. Overall, 87 % of participants reported having had one or more female partners before surgery, 47 % reported one or more male partners, and 41 % reported both male and female partners [63].

Looking further into the (in)compatibility of the applicant's sexual orientation and the partnership constellation before treatment, Cerwenka et al. [56] observed that half of partnered natal males with GD reported partnership constellations *incomplementary* with their sexual orientation: 72 % of natal male, partnered applicants were attracted to women, while all those female partners were exclusively attracted to men. Natal males with GD who were in *complementary* partnership constellations were predominantly attracted to men (67 %) and had mostly female-oriented male partners (67 %). One must consider, however, that self-report of sexual orientation might still be somewhat biased, due to the long-standing tradition of the use of the sexual orientation specifier in the decision whether or not to provide GCI.

9.9 Frequency of Sexual Behavior

Involvement in a stable partnership however does not completely exclude a "hyposexual existence," as long-term intimate partnerships do not always include sexual activity. Therefore, with data from the same group, Cerwenka et al. [65] also looked at the partner-related sexual experiences and found a relationship between partnership constellation and the involvement of genitals during sexual contact. It was shown that higher percentages of natal males in incomplementary partner constellations reported to involve their genitals in the sexual contact with their partner (88 %), in comparison to those in complementary constellations (25 %). In incomplementary partnership constellations, this might reflect an appreciation or insistence of the male-oriented female partner of genital involvement by the gender dysphoric partner. It appears that complementary partnership constellations are more often characterized by an avoidant approach of partner-related sexuality. Moreover, natal males in incomplementary partnerships mostly reported a more variable pleasure level of this behavior (42 %), while natal males in complementary constellations mostly found their genital sensations unpleasant (43 %).

References

1. American Psychiatric Association (2013) Diagnostic and statistical manual of mental disorders (Fifth edition, DSM-5). American Psychiatric Association, Washington, DC

2. World Professional Association for Transgender Health (2011) Standards of care for the health of transsexual, transgender and gender non-conforming people, 7th version. http://www.wpath.org
3. Cohen-Kettenis PT, Pfäfflin F (2010) The DSM diagnostic criteria for gender identity disorder in adolescents and adults. Arch Sex Behav 39:499–513
4. Socarides C (1969) The desire for sexual transformation: a psychiatric evaluation of transsexualism. Am J Psychiatry 125:1419–1425
5. Socarides C (1970) A psychoanalytic study of the desire for sexual transformation ('transsexualism'): the plaster-of-paris man. Int J Psychoanal 51: 341–349
6. Socarides C (1988) The preoedipal origin and psychoanalytic therapy of sexual perversions. International Universities Press, Madison
7. Volkan V, Greer W (1996) True transsexualism. In: Rosen I (ed) Sexual deviation, 3rd edn. Oxford University Press, Oxford, pp 158–173
8. World Health Organization (1975) ICD-9, international classification of diseases. World Health Organization, Geneva
9. American Psychiatric Association (1980) Diagnostic and statistical manual of mental disorders (Third edition, DSM-III). American Psychiatric Association, Washington, DC
10. American Psychiatric Association (1994) Diagnostic and statistical manual of mental disorders (Forth edition, DSM-IV). American Psychiatric Association, Washington, DC
11. Drescher J, Cohen-Kettenis P, Winter S (2012) Minding the body: situating gender diagnoses in the ICD-11. Int Rev Psychiatry 24:568–577
12. Stein DJ, Philips KA, Bolton D, Fulford KWM, Sadler JZ, Kendler KS (2010) What is a mental/psychiatric disorder? From DSM-IV to DSM-V. Psychol Med 40:1759–1765
13. Person E, Ovesey L (1974) The transsexual syndrome in males. Part I. Primary transsexualism. Am J Psychother 28:4–20
14. Person E, Ovesey L (1974) The transsexual syndrome in males. Part II. Secondary transsexualism. Am J Psychother 28:174–193
15. Pomeroy WB (1969) Transsexualism and sexuality: sexual behaviour of pre- and postoperative male transsexuals. In: Green R, Money J (eds) Transsexualism and sex reassignment. John Hopkins Press, Baltimore, pp 183–188
16. Cole C, O'Boyle M, Emory L, Meyer W (1997) Comorbidity of gender dysphoria and other major psychiatric diagnoses. Arch Sex Behav 26:13–26
17. à Campo J, Nijman H, Merckelback H, Evers C (2003) Psychiatric comorbidity of gender identity disorders: a survey among Dutch psychiatrists. Am J Psychiatry 160:1332–1336
18. Lawrence A, Zucker K (2012) Gender identity disorders. In: Hersen M, Beidel D (eds) Adult psychopathology and diagnosis, 6th edn. Wiley, London, pp 601–635
19. Heylens G, Elaut E, Kreukels BPC, Paap MSC, Cerwenka S, Richter-Appelt H, Cohen-Kettenis PT, Haraldsen I, De Cuypere G (2013) Psychiatric characteristics in transsexual individuals: multicentre study in four European Countries. Br J Psychiatry. doi:10.1192/bjp.bp.112.121954
20. Hoshiai M, Matsumoto Y, Sato T, Ohnishi M, Okabe N, Kishimoto Y, Terada S, Kuroda S (2010) Psychiatric comorbidity among patients with gender identity disorder. Psychiatry Clin Neurosci 64:514–519
21. Hepp U, Kraemer B, Schnyder U, Miller N, Delsignore A (2005) Psychiatric comorbidity in gender identity disorder. J Psychosom Res 58:259–261
22. Gómez-Gil E, Vidal-Hagemeijer A, Salamero M (2008) MMPI-2 characteristics of transsexuals requesting sex reassignment: comparison of patients in prehormonal and presurgical phases. J Pers Assess 90:368–374
23. Haraldsen I, Dahl A (2000) Symptom profiles of gender dysphoric patients of transsexual type compared to patients with personality disorder and healthy adults. Acta Psychiatr Scand 102:276–281
24. Miach PP, Berah EF, Butcher JN, Rouse S (2000) Utility of the MMPI-2 in assessing gender dysphoric patients. J Pers Assess 75:268–279
25. de Vries ALC, Kreukels BPC, Steensma TD, Doreleijers TAH, Cohen-Kettenis PT (2011) Comparing adult and adolescent transsexuals: an MMPI-2 and MMPI-A study. Psychiatry Res 186:414–418
26. Shiah I, Yang S, Shen L, Chang A, Gau Y, Chen Y, Chen C (2004) Psychopathology and dissociative experiences of male Taiwanese patients with gender identity disorder. J Med Sci 24:135–140
27. De Cuypere G, Jannes C, Rubens R (1995) Psychosocial functioning of transsexuals in Belgium. Acta Psychiatr Scand 91:180–184
28. Alonso J, Angermeyer MC, Bernert S, Bruffaerts R, Brugha TS, Bryson H et al (2004) Prevalence of mental disorders in Europe: results from the European Study of the Epidemiology of Mental Disorders (ESEMeD). Acta Psychiatr Scand Suppl 420:21–27
29. Murad M, Elamin M, Garcia M, Mullan R, Murad A, Erwin P et al (2010) Hormonal therapy and sex reassignment: a systematic review and meta-analysis of quality of life and psychosocial outcomes. Clin Endocrinol (Oxf) 72:214–231
30. Gallucci G, Hackerman F, Schmidt CW (2005) Gender identity disorder in an adult male with Asperger's syndrome. Sex Disabil 23:35–40
31. De Vries A, Noens I, Cohen-Kettenis P, van Berckelaer-Onnes I, Doreleijers T (2010) Autism spectrum disorders in gender dysphoric children and adolescents. J Autism Dev Disord 40:930–936
32. Pasterski V, Gilligan L, Curtis R (2014) Traits of autism spectrum disorders in adults with gender dysphoria. Arch Sex Behav. doi:10.1007/s10508-013-0154-5
33. Madeddu F, Prunas A, Hartmann D (2009) Prevalence of Axis II disorders in a sample of clients undertaking psychiatric evaluation for sex reassignment surgery. Psychiatr Q 80:261–267

34. Torgersen S (2012) Epidemiology. In: Widiger T (ed) The Oxford handbook of personality disorders. Oxford University Press, Oxford, pp 186–205
35. Smith Y, van Goozen S, Kuiper A, Cohen-Kettenis P (2005) Sex reassignment: outcomes and predictors of treatment for adolescent and adult transsexuals. Psychol Med 35:89–99
36. Smith Y, van Goozen S, Kuiper A, Cohen-Kettenis P (2005) Transsexual subtypes: clinical and theoretical significance. Psychiatry Res 137:151–160
37. Lawrence AA (2010) Sexual orientation versus age of onset as bases for typologies (subtypes) for gender identity disorder in adolescents and adults. Arch Sex Behav 39:514–545
38. Landén M, Walinder J, Hambert G, Lundstrom B (1998) Factors predictive of regret in sex reassignment. Acta Psychiatr Scand 97:284–289
39. Cohen-Kettenis PT, van Goozen SHM (1997) Sex reassignment of adolescent transsexuals: a follow-up study. J Am Acad Child Adolesc Psychiatry 36:263–271
40. Smith YLS, van Goozen SHM, Cohen-Kettenis PT (2001) Adolescents with gender identity disorder who were accepted or rejected for Sex reassignment surgery: a prospective follow-up study. J Am Acad Child Adolesc Psychiatry 40:472–481
41. Dhejne C, Lichtenstein P, Boman M, Johansson A, Langstrom N, Landen M (2011) Long-term follow-up of transsexual persons undergoing sex reassignment surgery: cohort study Sweden. PLoS One. doi:10.1371/journal.pone.0016885
42. Haas A, Eliason M, Mays V, Mathy R, Cochran S, D'Augelli A et al (2011) Suicide and suicide risk in lesbian, gay, bisexual, and transgender populations: review and recommendations. J Homosex 58:10–51
43. Terada S, Matsumoto Y, Sato T, Okabe N, Kishimoto Y, Uchitomi Y (2012) Suicidal ideation among patients with gender identity disorder. Psychiatry Res 200:469–474
44. Hirschfeld M (1991) Transvestites: the erotic drive to cross dress (trans: Lombardi-Nash MA). Prometheus Books, Buffalo (Original work published in 1910)
45. Lukianowicz N (1959) Survey of various aspects of transvestism in the light of our present knowledge. J Nerv Ment Dis 128:36–64
46. Randell JB (1959) Transvestism and transsexualism: a study of 50 cases. Br Med J 2:1448–1452
47. Benjamin H (1966) The transsexual phenomenon. Julian Press, New York
48. Bentler PM (1976) A typology of transsexualism: gender identity theory and data. Arch Sex Behav 5:567–584
49. Zucker KJ, Cohen-Kettenis PT, Drescher J, Meyer-Bahlburg HFL, Pfäfflin F, Womack WM (2013) Memo outlining evidence for change for gender identity disorder in the DSM-5. Arch Sex Behav 42:901–914
50. Blanchard R (1985) Typology of male-to-female transsexualism. Arch Sex Behav 14:247–261
51. Blanchard R (1988) Nonhomosexual gender dysphoria. J Sex Res 24:188–193
52. Blanchard R (1989) The classification and labeling of nonhomosexual gender dysphorias. Arch Sex Behav 18:315–334
53. Blanchard R (1994) A structural equation model for age at clinical presentation in nonhomosexual male gender dysphorics. Arch Sex Behav 23:311–320
54. Johansson A, Sundbom E, Höjerback T, Bodlund O (2009) A five-year follow-up study of Swedish adults with gender identity disorder. Arch Sex Behav 39:1429–1437
55. Nieder TO, Herff M, Cerwenka S, Preuss WF, Cohen-Kettenis PT, De Cuypere G, Haraldsen IRH, Richter-Appelt H (2011) Age of onset and sexual orientation in transsexual males and females. J Sex Med 8:783–791
56. Cerwenka S, Nieder TO, Briken P, Cohen-Kettenis PT, De Cuypere G, Haraldsen IRH, Kreukels BPC, Richter-Appelt H (2014) Intimate partnerships and sexual health in gender dysphoric individuals before the start of medical treatments. Int J Sex Health 26:52–65
57. Lawrence AA (2003) Factors associated with satisfaction or regret following male-to-female sex reassignment surgery. Arch Sex Behav 32:299–315
58. Money J, Gaskin RJ (1970–1971) Sex reassignment. Int J Psychiatry 9:249–269
59. Hastings DW (1974) Postsurgical adjustment of male transsexual patients. Clin Plast Surg 1:335–344
60. Lief HI, Hubschmann L (1993) Orgasm in the postoperative transsexual. Arch Sex Behav 22:145–155
61. Soli M, Brunocilla E, Bertacinni A, Palmieri F, Barbieri B, Martorana G (2008) Male to female gender reassignment: modified surgical technique for creating the neoclitoris and mons veneris. J Sex Med 5:2010–2216
62. Klein C, Gorzalka BB (2009) Sexual functioning in transsexuals following hormone therapy and genital surgery: a review (CMD). J Sex Med 6:2922–2939
63. Lawrence AA (2005) Sexuality before and after male-to-female sex reassignment surgery. Arch Sex Behav 35:147–166
64. Laumann EO, Gagnon JH, Michael RT, Michaels S (1994) The social organization of sexuality: sexual practices in the United States. University of Chicago Press, Chicago
65. Cerwenka S, Nieder TO, Cohen-Kettenis PT, De Cuypere G, Haraldsen IRH, Kreukels BPC, Richter-Appelt H (2013) Sexual behavior of gender dysphoric individuals before gender-confirming interventions: a European multi-center perspective. J Sex Marital Ther. doi:10.1080/0092623X.2013.772550

10 Endocrine Treatment of Transsexual Male-to-Female Persons

Alessandra Daphne Fisher and Mario Maggi

10.1 Background

In line with the emerging conceptualization of gender nonconformity [1] and the new view that proposes that passing for the opposite gender should not be assumed as the final goal for all non-conforming individuals [2, 3], hormonal treatment of gender dysphoric (GD) individuals should be individualized based on patient desires and outcomes [4]. In fact, therapy needs to be designed to address the specific needs of the patient who may not wish to live fully as an individual of the opposite gender [5]. Therefore, individuals with GD could benefit from flexibility in treatment, depending on their final goals with regard to aligning identity with body [5]. This is particularly the case when male-to-female (MtF) hormonal treatment is considered. In fact, different pharmaceutical options are available [4], and current guidelines [6] do not address the preferential order in which therapies should be chosen. In addition, it should be considered that follow-up data on the long-term side effects of cross-sex hormonal treatment (CHT) are still limited [7–10], and no randomized controlled trials are available. Therefore, ideal formulations and dosages of CHT are unknown to date. Current protocols for CHT are similar to those of hypogonadal individuals and aim at hormone values in the normal physiological range [6, 10]. Sustained supraphysiological levels of estrogen increase the risk for serious adverse reactions, such as thrombosis, whereas subphysiological levels may induce the effects known from hypogonadal states [10]. Moreover, patients' clinical characteristics and response should guide specialists in drugs and dose selection [4].

Endocrine treatment of gender dysphoric adults has two major goals: (1) to reduce the secondary sex characteristics of the natal sex and (2) to induce those of the desired gender [6] – as much as the client wishes [5].

In order to achieve these aims, it is needed to decrease endogenous hormone levels (androgens) and replace them with those of the reassigned sex [6]. Administration of estrogens alone will suppress gonadotropin secretion (and, consequently, androgen production). However, dual therapy, with both antiandrogens and estrogens drugs, is more effective to further reduce androgens and, consequently, to boost the feminizing effects of estrogens [4, 6].

10.2 Recommendations Before Starting Treatment

Before prescribing CHT, the treating endocrinologist needs to confirm that client fulfills diagnostic criteria for GD [11] and the eligibility and readiness criteria for hormonal transition (see Table 10.1) [1, 6].

A.D. Fisher, MD, PhD • M. Maggi, MD, PhD (✉)
Sexual Medicine and Andrology Unit, Department of Experimental, Clinical and Biomedical Sciences, University of Florence,
Viale Pieraccini 6, Florence 50139, Italy
e-mail: afisher@unifi.it; m.maggi@dfc.unifi.it

C. Trombetta et al. (eds.), *Management of Gender Dysphoria: A Multidisciplinary Approach*,
DOI 10.1007/978-88-470-5696-1_10, © Springer-Verlag Italia 2015

Table 10.1 Criteria for cross-sex hormone treatment as reported in Standards of Care of World Professional Association for Transgender Health 7th edition

1. Persistent, well-documented gender dysphoria
2. Capacity to make a fully informed decision and to consent for treatment
3. Age of majority in a given country
4. If significant medical or mental health concerns are present, they must be reasonably well controlled

Moreover, before starting treatment, it is recommended to evaluate and address conditions that can be exacerbated by this treatment, as thromboembolic diseases (*very high risk*), macroprolactinoma, severe liver dysfunction, breast cancer, coronary artery disease, cerebrovascular disease, and severe migraine headaches (*moderate to high risk*) [6]. Pretreatment schedule is reported in Table 10.2.

Cessation of tobacco use should be strongly recommended, in order to avoid an increased risk of cardiovascular complication and thromboembolism [6].

10.3 Cross-Sex Hormonal Regimens in MtF Individuals

10.3.1 Antiandrogens Treatment

Several agents are commercially available to inhibit androgen secretion or action. The most commonly used drug in Europe is cyproterone acetate (CPA, 50 mg once or twice daily, see also Table 10.3), a progestational agent with antiandrogenic properties [6, 12, 13]. Spironolactone (50–100 mg twice daily), a diuretic with antiandrogenic proprieties – mostly used in the United States (where CPA is not available) – has antiandrogenic effects by directly inhibiting testosterone secretion and androgen binding to the androgen receptor [14, 15].

GnRH agonists, injected monthly (3.75 mg) or every 3 months (11.25 mg), could be also considered a good alternative for their efficacy in reducing testosterone levels and their low risk of adverse effects [16]. However, they are extremely costly, and therefore their use is limited.

Table 10.2 Monitoring schedule for MtF GD individuals

Pretreatment
Physical examination: weight, blood pressure, waist, body mass index, hair distribution, balding pattern
Fasting lipid, renal and liver function, glucose, glycosylated hemoglobin, complete blood count, serum estradiol, testosterone, prolactin
For those taking spironolactone: electrolytes
If osteoporosis risk exists (previous fracture, family history, glucocorticoid use, prolonged hypogonadism), in older than 60 years: bone mineral density according to natal sex
During first year of treatment, every 3 months
Physical examination: weight, blood pressure, waist, body mass index, hair distribution, balding pattern, breast development
Fasting lipid and liver function, glucose, serum estradiol, testosterone, prolactin[a]
Electrolytes (for those taking spironolactone)
During second year of treatment, every 6 months
Physical examination: weight, blood pressure, waist, body mass index, hair distribution, balding pattern, breast development
Fasting lipid and liver function, glucose, glycosylated hemoglobin, complete blood count, hemoglobin, serum estradiol (ideal <200 pg/ml) and testosterone (ideal <55 ng/dl), prolactin[a]
Electrolytes (for those taking spironolactone)
PSA and digital rectal prostate exam (in older than 50 years)
After genital reassignment surgery (when requested), every 12 months
Physical examination: weight, blood pressure, waist, body mass index, hair distribution, balding pattern, breast development
Fasting lipid and liver function, glucose, glycosylated hemoglobin, complete blood count, hemoglobin, serum estradiol (ideal <200 pg/ml) and testosterone (ideal <55 ng/dl), prolactin[b]
Additional screening
Bone mineral density according to natal sex (if osteoporosis risk exists)
PSA, digital rectal prostate exam according to establish guidelines for biological sex
Mammogram/breast ultrasound according to establish guidelines for assigned sex

MtF male to female, *GD* gender dysphoria
[a]At least annually
[b]At least every 2 years

Nonsteroidal antiandrogen, such as flutamide (50–75 mg/day), which blocks binding of androgens to the androgens receptor, can be theoretically used; it induces gonadotropin secretion and, consequently, increases testosterone and estradiol

Table 10.3 Cross-sex hormone treatment protocols in MtF GD individuals

Antiandrogens regimens	
Cyproterone acetate	50–100 mg/d
Spironolactone	100–200 mg/d
GnRH analogs	3.75 mg sc/monthly or 11.25 mg sc/3 months
Estrogens regimens in MtF GD individuals	
Oral estradiol	2–6 mg/d
17-β estradiol patch	100–400 mcg/24 h (changing the patch as directed once or twice weekly)
17-β estradiol hemihydrate gel	2 mg twice daily
17-β estradiol gel	3–4.5 mg daily

levels (which can be desirable in this circumstance). However, for its liver toxicity and undemonstrated efficacy in GD population, its use is not recommended [6].

Finally, finasteride (5 mg daily) – which inhibits the conversion of testosterone to 5α-dihydrotestosterone – can be used as additional antiandrogen, particularly to slow male pattern balding.

10.3.2 Estrogens Treatment

A wide range of estrogenic compounds can be used (see also Table 10.3). Typical GD estrogen dosage needs to be two to three times as high as the recommended doses for hormone replacement therapy in postmenopausal women [14].

Oral or transdermal 17-beta-estradiol is the treatment of choice. As transdermal estradiol seems to have a lower thromboembolic risk, it should be particularly considered for individuals which are at highest risk for thromboembolic events (i.e., those older than 40 years, smokers, and/or with diabetes or liver disease) [6, 17, 18].

As oral ethinyl estradiol has been reported associated with a 20-fold increased risk of venous thrombosis – particularly in subjects over 40 years [19] – and with a threefold increase in cardiovascular mortality [9], it should be avoided. Moreover, the impossibility to monitor its blood levels represents an additional important and practical limitation for its use.

Many patients ask for injectable estrogens, but avoidance of intramuscular dosing is rationalized by the prolonged time to reach steady state and the potential for abuse of this formulation [14].

Moreover, often clients believe that progestins have a fundamental role for their feminization, particularly for breast development. However, they should have informed that progestagens' role is – in natal female – to prepare uterus for conception and breast for lactations. No evidences of additional feminization effects are available in transsexual populations [4, 7]. In addition, they have many side effects of which patients should be aware of, e.g., water retention and consequent elevation of blood pressure and weight gain, detrimental lipid changes, and depression [8]. Last but not least, breast cancer and cardiovascular diseases have been reported when used in postmenopausal women together with estrogens [20].

10.3.3 Approach in Specific Conditions

10.3.3.1 Partial Sex Reassignment

In clients wishing only partial sex reassignment, with only antiandrogens, it is fundamental to perform a careful medical supervision in order to mitigate the consequence of the induced hypogonadism, e.g., osteoporosis, obesity, loss of muscle mass and strength, cardiovascular risk, and depression.

10.3.3.2 After Genital Reassignment Surgery

On the other hand, if the patients choose to undergo genital reassignment surgery, estrogen treatment should be carried on, in order to avoid signs and symptoms correlated to hypogonadism and to avoid osteoporosis. Some subjects still complain for male typical sexual hair growth, and antiandrogens may remain effective, although their dose may be reduced compared to presurgery.

10.3.3.3 Prior and After an Elective Surgical Intervention

It is advisable to stop CHT 3–4 weeks prior to any elective surgical intervention, e.g., genital reassignment surgery. In fact, immobilization is a thrombogenic risk factor, and sex steroids may aggravate this risk. Once fully mobilized following the surgical procedure, the client may resume hormonal therapy [21].

10.3.3.4 Postmenopausal Age

Up to now, there is no consensus if CHT has to be stopped when client gets older, mirroring the postmenopausal milieu, and no data are available on this regard [7].

10.4 Adequacy Treatment Monitoring

According to the Endocrine Society guidelines [6], clinical and laboratory monitoring have to be performed every 3 months during the first year of CHT and then every 6–12 months, as reported in Table 10.2.

Routine cancer screening is recommended as in non-transsexuals individuals (breast, colon, prostate [6]).

Both estradiol and testosterone levels have to be monitored regularly in order to avoid supraphysiological levels and to minimize the risk of adverse effects [4].

Adequacy of estrogens levels could be monitored by measurement of serum estradiol levels when oral, transdermal, and intramuscular estradiol or its esters are used, but not with conjugated or synthetic estrogens. As daily stable levels are achieved after 1 week of therapy with transdermal or oral formulation, serum levels may be checked at any time during the treatment. When injectable formulations are used, serum levels have to be sampled in the middle between two injections [4]. Theoretically, serum estradiol should be maintained at the mean daily for premenopausal women (<200 pg/ml), and testosterone levels should be in the female range (<55 ng/dl) [6]. Treatment doses should be adjusted accordingly. Moreover, body feminization changes should be monitored in order to guide treatment [4].

10.5 Efficacy of CHT in MtF Individuals

10.5.1 Breast Formation

Increase in breast size usually begins within the first 3–6 months after initiation of CHT and achieves the maximum by 2 years of therapy [22]. It has been reported, from clinical experience, that only in one-third of patients it reaches cup B and that this is quantitatively satisfactory in 40–50 % of the subjects [23]. The remaining 50–60 % judge their breast formation as insufficient [23]. This may be also the consequence of the fact that the attained size could be disproportional to the male-typical chest and height of the subjects. Therefore, many clients ask for augmentation mammoplasty.

10.5.2 Skin

Often clients complain of dry skin and brittle nails, as a result of decreased sebaceous glands activity due to androgen deprivation [24].

10.5.3 Body Hair

CHT induces a reduction of sexual hair growth and hair shaft diameter. This decrease reaches a maximum after 4 months treatment with CHT, but then does not progress further [13]. Usually hair become thinner and less pigmented [24]. However, facial hairs are resilient to CHT particularly in Caucasian clients, and usually additional measures – electrolysis or laser treatment – to eliminate beard are almost always necessary. Electrolysis is effective but painful and potentially scarring. Laser is less uncomfortable but is most effective for people with dark hair.

Sexual hair on others parts of the body responds more satisfactorily, usually within 1–2 years of CHT, and, then, only waxing is required [24].

10.5.4 Body Composition

A decrease of lean body mass and an increase of subcutaneous fat deposits are observed [25]. It is therefore fundamental to encourage a healthy lifestyle.

10.5.5 Voice

CHT has no effects on voice on MtF individuals. Speech therapy can be considered an option to develop a voice within the frequency ranges for a biologic female [26]. Alternatively, laryngeal surgery may be considered in order to change the pitch of the voice, even it reduces its range.

10.5.6 Testes and Prostate

Testes and prostates become atrophy. Sometimes testis may cause discomfort as they enter in the inguinal canal.

10.5.7 Sexual Effects

Decrease of libido and spontaneous erections and male sexual dysfunction, often desired by patients, are usually observed within 1–3 months after starting CHT [6].

10.6 Adverse Effects of CHT

Serious adverse effects have been reported with long-term CHT.

10.6.1 Bone Health

Different studies have reported that estrogens are able to preserve adequately bone mineral density in MtF individuals [27, 28]. However, recently, some authors have observed a high prevalence of osteoporosis and osteopenia in their samples, which may be also related to an inadequate estrogenization of patients studied [9, 29].

An inverse relationship between serum luteinizing hormone levels and bone mineral density has been observed [7, 30]. Therefore, although based on limited evidence, a serum concentration of LH within the normal range may be a reliable marker of adequate dosing [7, 31].

10.6.2 Cardiovascular Health

In the general population, males have a higher cardiovascular risk when compared to females, and the risk in women increases only with cessation of estrogen production with menopause [23]. However, protective effects of exogenous estrogens have been refuted by the large randomized trials (Heart and Estrogen/Progestin Replacement Study (HERS) and the Women's Health Initiative) [32].

Data on cardiovascular effects of estrogens in MtF GD are still conflicting. A large morbidity and mortality study by van Kesteren et al. showed no increase in cardiovascular risk [17]. However, two more recent cohort studies reported an increase of mortality for cardiovascular diseases in MtF individuals [9, 33]. Interestingly, ethinyl estradiol use, as well as smoking habit and dyslipidemia were found in the Dutch study associated with cardiovascular events [9]. This result stresses the concept that transsexual individuals, under CHT, have to avoid ethinyl estradiol, as well as needs to be addressed to a healthy lifestyle.

Remarkably, in androgen-treated FtM subjects, no increased cardiovascular mortality was observed [9]. Therefore, CHT seems to have more deleterious effect on cardiovascular risk in MtF than in FtM subjects [10].

Regarding metabolic profile, it has been reported that estrogens induce in MtF clients favorable changes with increase of high-density lipoprotein cholesterol (HDL) and decrease of low-density lipoprotein cholesterol (LDL) [34]. However, the latter may be also associated with transition to smaller, denser, and more deleterious LDL (high in triglyceride content) [34]. In addition, CHT induces in MtF individuals an increase of weight, body mass index, total body, fat, blood pressure, triglycerides, and markers of insulin resistance [34–37]. Finally, oral therapy – but not the transdermal one – has been observed associated to an increase of inflammatory and hemostatic markers (such as interleukin-6, C-reactive protein, and factor IX) [38, 39].

10.6.3 Venous Thromboembolic Disease

An increased risk of venous thromboembolism (VTE) has been reported since 1989 in a large cohort of MtF transsexuals during CHT with ethinyl estradiol and CPA [18]. This result has been confirmed in some group later study, reporting a 20-fold increased VTE risk, even if a lower incidence was observed with transdermal estrogens [17]. Different studies have emphasized the more deleterious effect of ethinyl estradiol on VTE risk, probably linked to effects on activated protein C resistance and due to its molecular structure than first-pass liver effect [18]. It has also been reported that rates of thromboembolic events are higher in older than 40 years, similarly to figures seen in biological female treated with estrogens [18, 40, 41].

All these data taken together stress the point that the use of ethinyl estradiol has to be avoided, and transdermal preparations have to be preferred, particularly in those older than 40 years. In addition, according to the Endocrine Society Guidelines, thrombophilia screening in transsexual individuals starting CHT should be limited to those with a personal of family history of VTE [6, 42].

10.6.4 Hyperprolactinemia

Estrogens treatment can induce hyperplasia of pituitary lactotropic cells. Therefore, it should not surprise that prolactin increases to over 1,000 mU/l in up to 20 % of MtF persons during estrogen treatment, associated with enlargement of pituitary gland [17, 18]. Usually, levels of prolactin return to normal range after reducing or discontinuing estrogens. Despite several reports of prolactinomas in transsexuals persons are available [43–46], the overall risk of prolactinoma could be considered very low. Moreover, given the high frequency of occult prolactinoma formation and the apparent rarity of prolactinoma in genetic males during CHT, a direct link between exogenous estrogens and prolactinoma induction cannot be drawn [13].

However, it is suggested to check prolactin levels before starting CHT and then at least annually during the first year and, after, every 2 years (see also Table 10.2). If levels of prolactin are extremely high and increase despite stable or reduced levels of estrogens, a pituitary magnetic resonance imaging (MRI) has to be considered. In fact it should be taken into account that the majority of hyperprolactinemia symptoms (such as hypoactive sexual desire, sexual dysfunction, gynecomastia) are usually not apparent in MtF transsexual persons. Careful attention should be taken for those treated with psychotropic drugs, which can contribute to increase prolactin levels.

10.6.5 Cancer Risk

It is difficult to have a reliable figure of tumor prevalence in GD persons having received CHT for many years. Moreover, it is quite impossible to establish a potentially causal relationship because case–control analysis would be needed.

Breast cancer has been reported in relatively few cases of hormonally treated MtF transsexuals [47–51]. Therefore, the risk in MtF population seems to be quite low, even if a definite conclusion cannot be reached. As in biological women, routinely breast self-examination, as well as mammogram/breast ultrasounds, according to establish guidelines for assigned sex, should be suggested.

Despite what expected with the androgen deprivation therapy, prostate cancer has been observed in few MtF subjects receiving CHT treatment [52–55]. This happened specially – but not always – in those starting treatment after the age of 50 years, inducing some authors to doubt if the cancer was present before the initiation of CHT. Prostate-specific antigen (PSA) levels as well as digital rectal prostate exam should be checked according to establish guidelines for biological sex [6].

10.6.6 Reproductive Health

Regarding effect of CHT on male fertility, CHT leads to decreased spermatogenesis and eventually to azoospermia [56]. It has been reported that protracted exposure of the testes to estrogen is associated with testicular damage [57–59], and restoration of spermatogenesis after long-lasting treatment has not been studied [6].

Therefore, clients requesting hormonal reassignment need adequate information about options available to preserve (e.g., banking of spermatozoa) their fertility potential, before treatment takes place [6].

References

1. Coleman E, Bockting W, Botzer M, Cohen-Kettenis P, DeCuypere G, Feldman J, Fraser L, Green J, Knudson G, Meyer WJ, Monstrey S, Adler RK, Brown GR, Devor AH, Ehrbar R, Ettner R, Eyler E, Garofalo R, Karasic DH, Lev AI, Mayer G, Meyer-Bahlburg H, Hall BP, Pfäfflin F, Rachlin K, Robinson B, Schechter LS, Tangpricha V, van Trotsenburg M, Vitale A, Winter S, Whittle S, Wylie KR, Zucker K (2011) Standards of care for the health of transsexual, transgender, and gender-nonconforming people, version 7. Int J Transgenderism 13:165–232
2. Cohen-Kettenis PT, Pfafflin F (2010) The DSM diagnostic criteria for gender identity disorder in adolescents and adults. Arch Sex Behav 39:499–513
3. Bockting WO (2008) Psychotherapy and the real-life experience: from gender dichotomy to gender diversity. Sexologies 17:211–224
4. Knezevich EL, Viereck LK, Drincic A (2012) Medical management of adult transsexual persons. Pharmacotherapy 32:54–66
5. Fisher AD, Castellini G, Bandini E, Casale H, Fanni E, Benni L, Ferruccio N, Meriggiola MC, Manieri C, Gualerzi A, Jannini E, Oppo A, Ricca V, Maggi M, Rellini AH (2014) Cross-sex hormonal treatment and body uneasiness in individuals with gender dysphoria. J Sex Med 11(3):709–719. doi:10.1111/jsm.12413
6. Hembree WC, Cohen-Kettenis P, Delemarre-van de Waal HA, Gooren LJ, Meyer WJ 3rd, Spack NP, Tangpricha V, Montori V (2009) Endocrine treatment of transsexuals persons: an Endocrine Society clinical practice guideline. J Clin Endocrinol Metab 94:3132–3154
7. Gooren LJ, Giltay EJ, Bunck MC (2008) Long term treatment of transsexuals with cross-sex hormones: extensive personal experience. J Clin Endocrinol Metab 93:19–25
8. Gooren L (2011) Care of transsexual persons. N Engl J Med 364:1251–1257
9. Ascheman H, Giltay FJ, Megens J, de Ronde W, Trotsenburg MA (2011) A long term follow up study of mortality in transsexuals receiving treatment with cross-sex hormones. Eur J Endocrinol 164:635–642
10. Wierckx K, Mueller S, Weyers S, Van Canegem E, Roef G, Heylens G, T'Sjoen G (2012) Long term evaluation of cross-sex hormone treatment in transsexual persons. J Sex Med 9:2641–2651
11. American Psychiatric Association (2013) Diagnostic and statistical manual of mental disorders, Fifth Edition: DSM-5 tm. American Psychiatric Association, Washington, DC
12. Gooren L (2005) Hormone treatment of the adult transsexual patient. Horm Res 64:31–36
13. Levy A, Crown A, Reid R (2003) Endocrine intervention for transsexuals. Clin Endocrinol (Oxf) 59:409–418
14. Moore E, Wisniewski A, Dobs A (2003) Endocrine treatment of transsexuals people: a review of treatment regimen, outcomes, and adverse effects. J Clin Endocrinol Metab 88:3467–3473
15. Tangpricha V, Ducharme SH, Barber TW, Chiprkin SR (2003) Endocrinologic treatment of gender identity disorders. Endocr Pract 9:12–21
16. Dittrich R, Binder H, Cupisti S, Hoffmann I, Beckmann MW, Mueller A (2005) Endocrine treatment of male to female transsexuals using gonadrotropin-realinsing hormone agonist. Exp Clin Endocrinol Diabetes 113:586–592
17. van Kesteren PJM, Asscheman H, Megens JAJ, Gooren LJG (1997) Mortality and morbidity in transsexual subjects treated with cross-sex hormones. Clin Endocrinol (Oxf) 47:337–342
18. Asscheman H, Gooren L, Eklund P (1989) Mortality and morbidity in transsexual patients with cross-gender hormone treatment. Metabolism 38: 869–873
19. Toorians AW, Thomassen MC, Zweegman S, Magdeleyns EJ, Tans G, Gooren LJ et al (2003) Venous thrombosis and changes of hemostatic variables during cross-sex hormone treatment in transsexual people. J Clin Endocrinol Metab 88: 5723–5729
20. Chlebowski RT, Manson JE, Anderson GL, Cauley JA, Aragaki AK, Stefanick ML, Lane DS, Johnson KC, Wactawski-Wende J, Chen C, Qi L, Yasmeen S, Newcomb PA, Prentice RL (2013) Estrogen plus progestin and breast cancer incidence and mortality in the Women's Health Initiative Observational Study. J Natl Cancer Inst 105:526–535
21. Gooren LJ, Delemarre-van de Waal HA (2007) Hormone treatment of adult and juvenile transsexual patients. In: Ettner R, Monstrey S, Eyle E (eds) Principle of transgender medicine and surgery. The Haworth Press, Inc, New York
22. Meyer WJR, Webb A, Stuart CA, Finkelstein JW, Lawrence B, Walker PA (1986) Physical and hormonal evaluation of transsexual patients: a longitudinal study. Arch Sex Behav 15:121–138
23. Gooren L, Asscheman H (2013) Sex reassignment: endocrinological interventions in adults with gender dysphoria. In: Kreukels BPC, Steemsa T, De Vries A (eds) Gender dysphoria and disorders of sex development. Springer, New York/Heidelberg/Dordrecht/London, pp 27–297
24. Giltay EJ, Gooren LJ (2000) Effects of sex steroid deprivation/administration on hair growth and skin sebum production in transsexual males and females. J Clin Endocrinol Metab 85:2913

25. Elbers JM, Asscheman H, Seidell JC, Gooren LJ (1999) Effects of sex steroid hormones on regional fat depots as assessed by magnetic resonance imaging in transsexuals. Am J Physiol 276:E317–E325
26. de Bruin MD, Coert MJ, Greven AJ (2000) Speech therapy in the management of male to female transsexuals. Folia Phoniatr Logop 52:220
27. Mueller A, Dittrich R, Binder H, Kuehnel W, Maltaris T, Hoffmann I et al (2005) High dose estrogen treatment increases bone mineral density in male-to-female transsexuals receiving gonadotropin-releasing hormone agonist in the absence of testosterone. Eur J Endocrinol 153:107–113
28. Ruetsche AG, Kneubuehl R, Birkhaeuser MH, Lippuner K (2005) Cortical and trabecular bone mineral density in transsexuals after long-term cross-sex hormonal treatment: a cross sectional study. Osteoporos Int 16:791–798
29. Lapauw B, Taes Y, Simoens S, Van Caenegem E, Weyers S, Goemaere S, Toye K, Kaufman JM, T'Sjoen G (2008) Body composition, volumetric and areal bone parameters in male-to-female transsexual persons. Bone 43:1016–1021
30. van Kesteren P, Lips P, Gooren LJ (1998) Long-term follow-up of bone mineral density and bone metabolism in transsexuals treated with cross-sex hormones. Clin Endocrinol (Oxf) 48:347–354
31. Weyers S, Elaut E, De Sutter P, Gerris J, T'Sjoen G, Heylens G, De Cuypere G, Verstraelen H (2009) Long-term assessment of the physical, mental, and sexual health among transsexual women. J Sex Med 6:752–760
32. Grady D, Barrett-Connor E (2007) Postmenopausal hormone therapy. BMJ 334:860–868
33. Dhejne C, Lichtenstein P, Boman M, Johansson AL, Langstrom N, Landen M (2011) Long-term follow-up of transsexual persons undergoing sex reassignment surgery: cohort study in Sweden. PLoS One 6:e16885
34. Elbers JMH, Giltay EJ, Teerlink T (2003) Effects of sex steroids on components of the insulin resistance syndrome in transsexual subjects. Clin Endocrinol 58:562–571
35. Gooren LJ, Giltay EJ, Bunck MC (2004) Long-term treatment of transsexuals people. A review of treatment regimens, outcomes, and adverse effects. J Clin Endocrinol Metab 88:3467–3473
36. Elbers JM, Giltay EJ, Teerlink T, Scheffer PG, Asscheman H, Seidell JC, Gooren LJ (2003) Effects of sex steroids on components of the insulin resistance syndrome in transsexual subjects. Clin Endocrinol 58:562–571
37. Elamin MB, Garcia MZ, Murad MH, Erwin PJ, Montori VM (2010) Effect of sex steroid use on cardiovascular risk in transsexuals individuals: a systemic review and meta-analysis. Clin Endocrinol (Oxf) 72:1–10
38. Wilson R, Spiers A, Ewan J, Johnson P, Jenkins C, Carr S (2009) Effects of high dose oestrogen therapy on circulating inflammatory markers. Maturitas 62:281–286
39. Giltay E, Gooren L, Emeis J (2000) Oral ethinil estradiol, but not transdermal 17beta-estradiol, increases plasma C-reactive protein levels in man. Thromb Haemost 84:359–360
40. Scarabin P, Oger E, Plu-bureau G, on behalf of the Estrogen and Thromboembolism Risk (ESTHER) Study Group (2003) Differential association of oral and transdermal oestrogen replacement therapy with venous thromboembolism risk. Lancet 362: 428–432
41. Futterweit W (1998) Endocrine therapy of transsexualism and potential complications of long-term treatment. Arch Sex Behav 27–209:26
42. Otto J, Kaufmann U, Bentz E, Huber JC, Tempfer CB (2010) Incidence of thrombophilia and venous thrombosis in transsexuals under cross-sex hormone therapy. Fertil Steril 93:1267–1272
43. Gooren LJ, Assies J, Asscheman H, de Slegte R, van Kessel H (1998) Estrogen-induced prolactinoma in a man. J Clin Endocrinol Metab 66:444–446
44. Kovacs K, Stefaneanu L, Ezzat S, Smyth HS (1994) Prolactin-producing pituitary adenoma in a male-to-female transsexual patient with protracted estrogen administration. A morphologic study. Arch Pathol Lab Med 118:562–565
45. Serri O, Noiseux D, Robert F, Hardy J (1996) Lactotroph hyperplasia in an estrogen treated male-to-female transsexual patient. J Clin Endocrinol Metab 81:3177–3179
46. Garcia-Malpartida K, Martin-Gorgoko A, Rocha M, Gomez-Belaguer M, Hernandez-Mijares A (2010) Prolactinoma induced by estrogens and cyprogerone acetate in a male to female transsexual. Fertil Steril 94:1097.e13–1097.e15
47. Ganly I, Taylor EW (1995) Breast cancer in a transsexual man receiving hormone replacement therapy. Br J Surg 82:341
48. Pritchard TJ, Pankowsky DA, Crowe JP, Abdul-Karim FW (1988) Breast cancer in a male-to-female transsexual. A case report. JAMA 259:2278–2280
49. Symmers WS (1968) Carcinoma of breast in transsexual individuals after surgical and hormonal interference with the primary and secondary sex characteristics. Br Med J 2:83–85
50. Dhand A, Dhaliwal G (2010) Examining patient conceptions: a case of metastatic breast cancer in an African American male to female transgender patient. J Gen Intern Med 25:158–161
51. Grabellus F, Worm K, Willruth A, Schmitz KJ, Otterbach F, Baba HA et al (2005) ETV6-NTRK3 gene fusion in a secretory carcinoma of the breast of a male-to-female transsexual. Breast 14:71–74
52. Casella R, Bubendorf L, Schaefer DJ, Bachmann A, Gasser TC, Sulser T (2005) Does the prostate really need androgens to grow? Transurethral resection of the prostate in a male-to-female transsexual 25 years after sex-changing operation. Urol Int 75:288–290
53. Dorff TB, Shazer RL, Nepomuceno EM, Tucker SJ (2007) Successful treatment of metastatic androgen-

independent prostate carcinoma in a transsexual patient. Clin Genitourin Cancer 5(5):344–346
54. Thurston AV (1994) Carcinoma of the prostate in a transsexual. Br J Urol 73:217
55. van Haarst EP, Newling DW, Gooren LJ, Asscheman H, Prenger DM (1998) Metastatic prostatic carcinoma in a male-to-female transsexual. Br J Urol 81:776
56. Wierckx K, Stuyver I, Weyers S, Hamada A, Agarwal A, De Sutter P, T'Sjoen G (2012) Sperm freezing in transsexual women. Arch Sex Behav 41:1069
57. Lübbert H, Leo-Rossberg I, Hammerstein J (1992) Effects of ethinyl, estradiol on semen quality and various hormonal parameters in a eugonadal male. Fertil Steril 58:603–608
58. Schulze C (1988) Response of the human testis to long-term estrogen treatment: morphology of Sertoli cells, Leydig cells and spermatogonial stem cells. Cell Tissue Res 251:31–53
59. Thiagaraj D, Gunasegaram R, Loganath A, Peh KL, Kottegoda SR, Ratnam SS (1987) Histopathology of the testes from male transsexuals on oestrogen therapy. Ann Acad Med Singapore 16:347–348

11 My Personal Technique

Carlo Trombetta

11.1 Introduction

The challenging male-to-female sexual reassignment surgery requires good surgical technique and well-trained surgeons. My technique has been developed after 30 years of experience and after more than 400 patients treated. Herein are reported all preoperative, intraoperative and postoperative steps [1–5].

11.2 Preoperative Procedures

At the time of their first "surgical" visit, patients are prompted to get perineal laser hair removal to avoid hair growth inside the neovagina (Fig. 11.1) [6].

One month before surgery, patients must stop oestrogen therapy due to well-known potential cardiovascular risks, whereas the antiandrogenic therapy can be continued [7, 8].

If possible, patients undergo repeated self-bloodlettings for later personal use during surgery in case of excessive blood loss.

The day before the surgery, the patient starts antibiotic prophylaxis.

11.3 Position of the Surgeons

Since our initial experiences when we perform male-to-female surgery, we do so with two surgical teams who work in the same time and sometimes all together: two surgeons are placed on either side of the patient, and another two surgeons are positioned between the legs (Table 11.1; Fig. 11.2) [9, 10].

11.4 Markings

Before the beginning of the surgery, we start by marking on the pubic-umbilical line, which is done for correctly locating all the structures. Another drawing is done at the scrotal level, heart shaped with the apex pointing towards the anus, which represents the scrotal flap (Fig. 11.2). The correct distance between the anal verge and the apex of the "heart" is 1–2 cm. The length of the scrotal flap varies between 12 and 15 cm. It is crucial that when measuring the length of the scrotal flap, we take into consideration that there must not be tension at the apex of the skin flap after suturing. For the circumcision, another line is drawn in order to leave 1 cm of skin at the periglandular level.

The drawing is then continued for the length of the penis on the ventral side (Fig. 11.3).

11.5 Devices

The *sterile drop* that we put on the patient is provided with a hole to give the possibility of

C. Trombetta
Department of Urology, University of Trieste,
Cattinara Hospital, Trieste, Italy
e-mail: trombcar@units.it; trombcar@univ.trieste.it

C. Trombetta et al. (eds.), *Management of Gender Dysphoria: A Multidisciplinary Approach*,
DOI 10.1007/978-88-470-5696-1_11, © Springer-Verlag Italia 2015

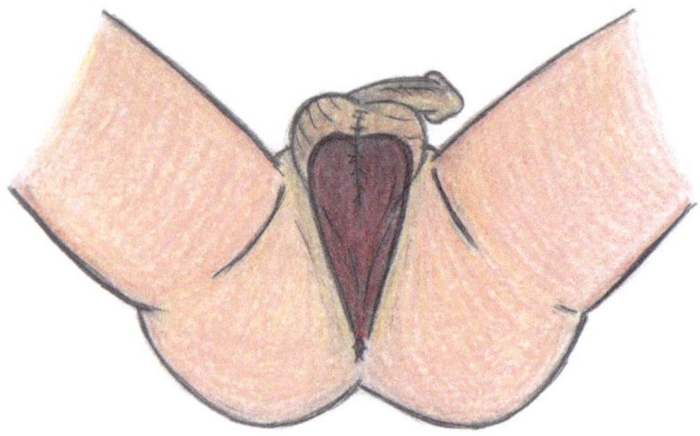

Fig. 11.1 The area shown in *red* corresponds to the scrotal and perineal skin that will definitely be shaved before surgery

Table 11.1 The steps of the preoperative procedure

Preoperative preparations
To stop oestrogen oral intake 1 month before surgery
Eventual autotransfusion
Laser perineal hair removal
Eventual antibiotic prophylaxis 1 day before surgery

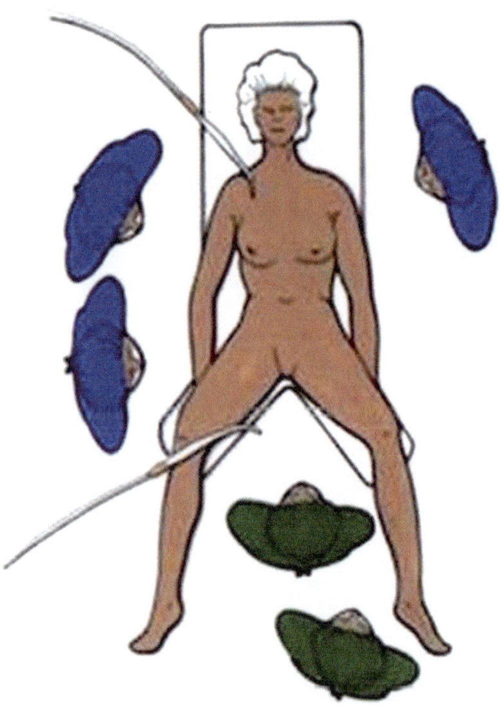

Fig. 11.2 Two surgeons are placed on either side of the patient, and another two surgeons are positioned between legs

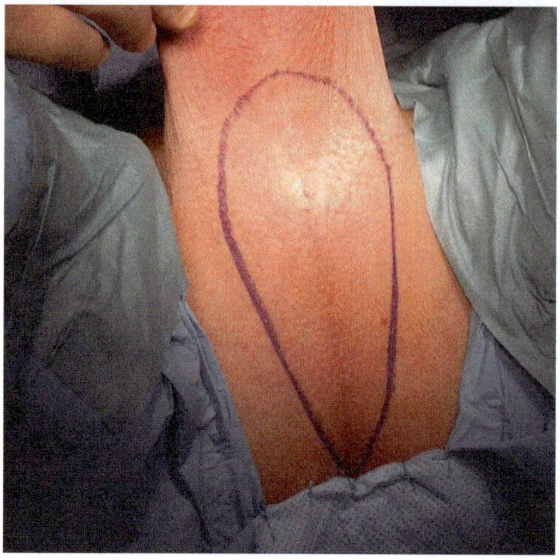

Fig. 11.3 Marking the scrotal, penile and perineal skin is an important step of this surgery for the construction of a symmetric neovagina and then to obtain a good aesthetic result

inserting a finger in the anus. This manoeuvre is determinant in avoiding rectal injuries during dissection. It consists of a water-repellent drape which can cover the legs and has also a fluid collection pouch.

Power star bipolar scissors (Johnson & Johnson Medical GmbH) are very useful especially to dissect the urethra.

The surgical illuminator provides cool, shadowless, deep cavity lighting. Flexible or malleable, it may be attached to most retractors or instruments, using two-side adhesives. Once attached to the instrument, its thin, low-profile takes minimal space.

When connected to an ACMI cable and standard, 300 Watt xenon light source, it lights the cavity as if a fluorescent light were switched on inside the patient. The LightMat® brings bright, cool light where it is needed – into the surgical cavity, improving visualisation, helping surgeons save time and avoid complications.

The V-Loc™ wound closure device (COVIDIEN) is a new technology that eliminates the need to tie knots, so you can close incisions up to 50 % faster without compromising strength and security. The V-Loc™ device offers secure, fast and effective incision closure for our patients: in particular, the absence of knots into the neovagina avoids painful dilatation manoeuvres in the postoperative period.

A medium (4×12 cm) or small (3×9.5 cm) *adjustable vaginal stent* (Porges) is important to maintain the neovaginal canal after our surgical procedures. It is a compression stylet for vaginal surgery, consisting of a sealed silicone shell filled with polyurethane foam, fully adjustable by inflation (Fig. 11.4; Table 11.2).

11.6 Perineal Surgery

The surgeon positioned between the legs incises the skin along the line drawned on the perineal area. The first step is the bilateral orchiectomy with dissection and suturing of both the spermatic cords at the level of the external inguinal rings. The peritesticular fat is preserved for later use as support for the labia majora. The dissection is extended through the subcutaneous tissue until reaching the corpus spongiosum, which is then isolated from the corpora cavernosa. The urethra is severed at the pubic simphysis, and the terminal portion is spatulated and longitudinally split on the ventral midline so as to obtain a Y-shape.

Only now do we insert the catheter (Fig. 11.5) [9].

The position of the neo-urethral meatus is ensured by applying a knot at the apex of the fork (Liguori's stitch). This becomes the reference point for positioning the neoclitoris, which will be surrounded by urethral mucosa. The urethral bulb is carefully removed in order to prevent its bulging during sexual arousal and pain during penetration. Running absorbable suture of the two margins of the urethra decreases the risk of postoperative bleedings.

Surgery continues with the removal of the corpora cavernosa's roots, facilitated by the placement of a traction point at the apex of the roots, paying attention to the vascular bundle. These manoeuvres allow the exposure of the perineal tendinous centre, which is then opened while monitoring the integrity of the rectal wall through the anal access provided by the sterile drop. At this point the surgeon creates in the

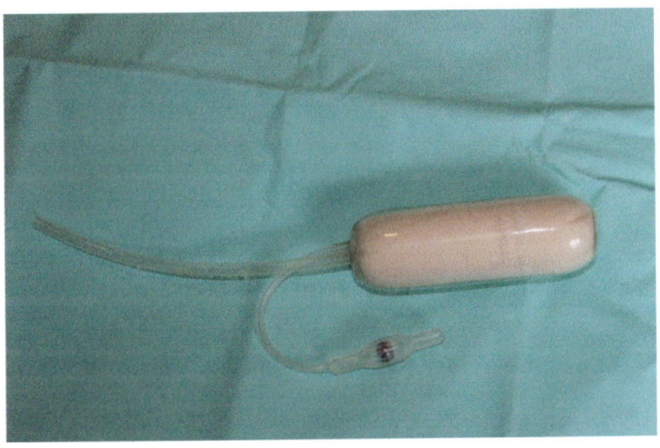

Fig. 11.4 Medium (4×12 cm) *adjustable vaginal stent* (Porges) is a compression stylet for vaginal surgery, consisting of a sealed silicone shell filled with polyurethane foam, fully adjustable by inflation. It is used to maintain the neovaginal canal after the surgery

Table 11.2 The steps to follow in the operating room

In operating room
Antiembolic stockings
Trendelenburg position
Skin disinfection
The sterile drop must allow the digital rectal exploration
Two surgical teams which operate simultaneously (two surgeons are placed on either side of the patient and another two surgeons are positioned between the legs)
To measure and to mark the scrotal skin for the packaging of the scrotal flap

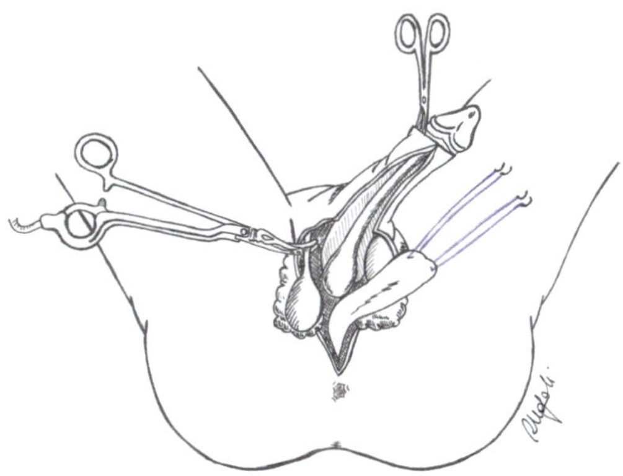

Fig. 11.5 During bilateral orchiectomy, the peritesticular fat must be preserved for later use as support for the labia majora

rectoprostatic space a neo-cavity which will accommodate the neovagina: we usually use a LigaSure device to sever the subcutaneous tissue, while sight is aided by an aspirator provided with a light source.

The knowledge of the rectoprostatic space has been acquired, thanks to a large number of pelvic postoperative MRIs administered in order to have a precise anatomical visualisation of all the structures involved in the surgery. These allow for measurements of inclination, length and distance of the neovagina and its neighbouring organs (Fig. 11.6) [11, 12].

When the catheter's balloon is palpated by the operator, it means that the neovagina is deep enough (Fig. 11.7). The fixation of the cul-de-sac in the rectoprostatic space is crucial to prevent the neovagina from prolapsing. Two Prolene double needle stitches are passed through the wall of the neo-cavity (anterior and posterior walls or the lateral walls), and both the ends of the sutures are passed through the penile-scrotal flap at the level of the cul-de-sac. In order to prevent prolapse, we also put another stitch through the scrotal flap and the subcutaneous tissue in proximity of the Denonvilliers' fascia incision (Table 11.3).

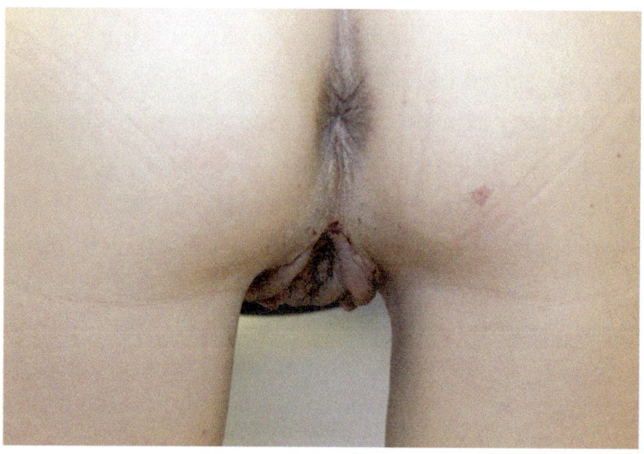

Fig. 11.6 The distance between the anus and the introitus of the neovagina must not exceed 3 cm

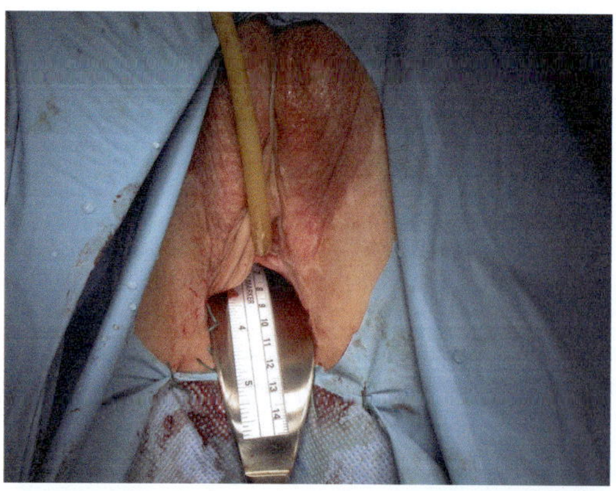

Fig. 11.7 Usually the depth of the neovagina is 13–15 cm

11.7 Penile Surgery

The two surgeons positioned on either side of the patient begin by performing incisions following the line previously drawn, and the penile flap is obtained by isolation from the corpora cavernosa, taking care to preserve vitality of the skin. By means of positioning a tourniquet around the corpora cavernosa and the urethra, it is possible to obtain a hydraulic erection using a butterfly needle and infusing saline solution into the corpora cavernosa. This is done to facilitate the blunt dissection of Buck's fascia from the tunica albuginea. Buck's fascia is identified and incised at paraurethral level to avoid damage of the dorsal nerves of the penis. This procedure is done in order to permit the creation of a sensitive neoclitoris.

These structures need to be manipulated with delicate instruments, such as anatomical

Table 11.3 The surgical steps of perineal surgery

Perineal surgery
Bilateral orchiectomy and careful sparing of the peritesticular fat
Isolation and section of the urethra at the level of the pubic simphysis
Y-section of the urethral stump
Urethral catheter insertion and Liguori's stitch placement
Isolation and amputation of the roots of the corpora cavernosa
Preparation of the perineal cavity
The neovagina must be deep enough to allow the palpation of the balloon urinary catheter
Prolene stitches are safely positioned at the level of the dome of the neovagina (to avoid any eventual postoperative prolapse)

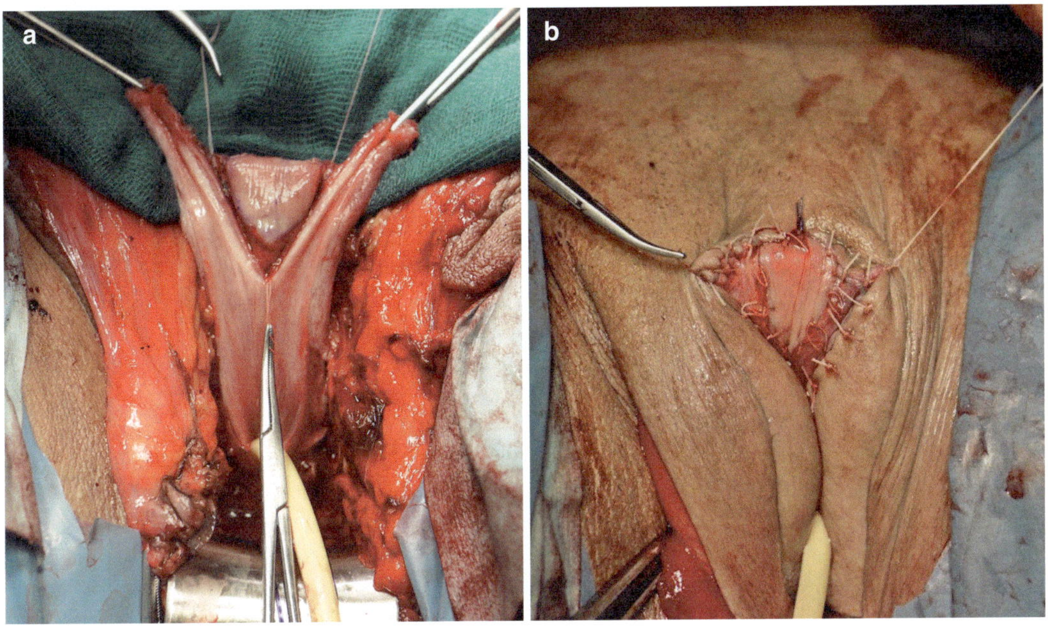

Fig. 11.8 (**a**, **b**) The creation of the urethra-clitoris complex gives to the neoclitoris a mucosal environment providing adequate lubrication; furthermore the two-layer suture permits a reciprocal vascular support, useful in case of urethral or clitoral ischemia

clamps, in order to reduce damage. For this same reason, bleeding is controlled with a bipolar coagulator.

After achieving the complete bilateral dissection of the neurovascular bundle we insert two open tourniquets up to favourite glandulectomy.

At the base of the penis, the dissection of the bundle is continued by positioning a Satinsky clamp at the level of the corpora cavernosa up to inhibit blood refilling so as to avoid wasting of blood.

Removal of all corpora cavernosa avoids an eventual residual erection that can cause dyspareunia.

The glans is reduced and remodelled preserving a good amount of spongiosum tissue to create a well-vascularised neoclitoris: the dimensions of the resulting button are greater than that of the female clitoris. This is done so as to oppose eventual excessive hypotrophy of the tissues.

The bundle is folded on itself and fixed with a stitch: in this way we create the mons pubis to better simulate the female form, and we also prevent the torsion of the flap avoiding neoclitoral ischemia.

Table 11.4 The steps of penile surgery

Penile surgery
Circumcision and degloving of the penis (taking care to preserve vitality of the skin)
Placement of a tourniquet around the base of the penis
Saline infusion into the corpora cavernosa up to obtain "hydraulic" erection
Longitudinal incision of Buck's fascia near the urethra
Blunt dissection of the penile bundle (bipolar coagulation!)
Remodelling of the glans
Complete removal of corpora cavernosa
The bundle is folded on itself (mons pubis)
Suture between the neoclitoris and urethral plate

The neoclitoris is now joined to the urethral plate at the forking previously created. The suture is done in two layers, at the level of spongiosum tissue and the other at the level of urethral mucosa and neoclitoris epithelium. It is interesting to underline that the two layers are both defined by the same histological characteristics (Fig. 11.8; Table 11.4) [13].

Creation of the urethra-clitoris complex is an innovative technique and presents two main advantages:

- It allows for the neoclitoris to be in a mucosal environment, providing adequate lubrication.
- The two-layer suture permits a reciprocal vascular support, useful in case of urethral or clitoral ischemia.

For a better comprehension please read the technical suggestions for better and lasting functional and aesthetic outcomes in creating the neoclitoris (Chap. 14).

11.8 Tubularisation of Penile-Scrotal Flap

At this point, the peritesticular fat is fixed at the perineal level.

Scrotal and penile skin is sutured, using Vicryl 3/0, only bilaterally leaving an opening at the apex.

We do this because no patient ever has enough skin to fully cover the entire length of the neocavity, and if we completely closed the neovaginal tube, there would be a possible loss of depth. Another option is to lengthen the penile-scrotal flap utilising redundant scrotal skin as a graft (Fig. 11.9) [14].

The two Prolene stitches we had put at prostatic and rectal level are now passed through the penile and scrotal flap.

A frank demarcation between the labia minora and labia majora is obtained by placing four stitches between the outside of the penile-scrotal

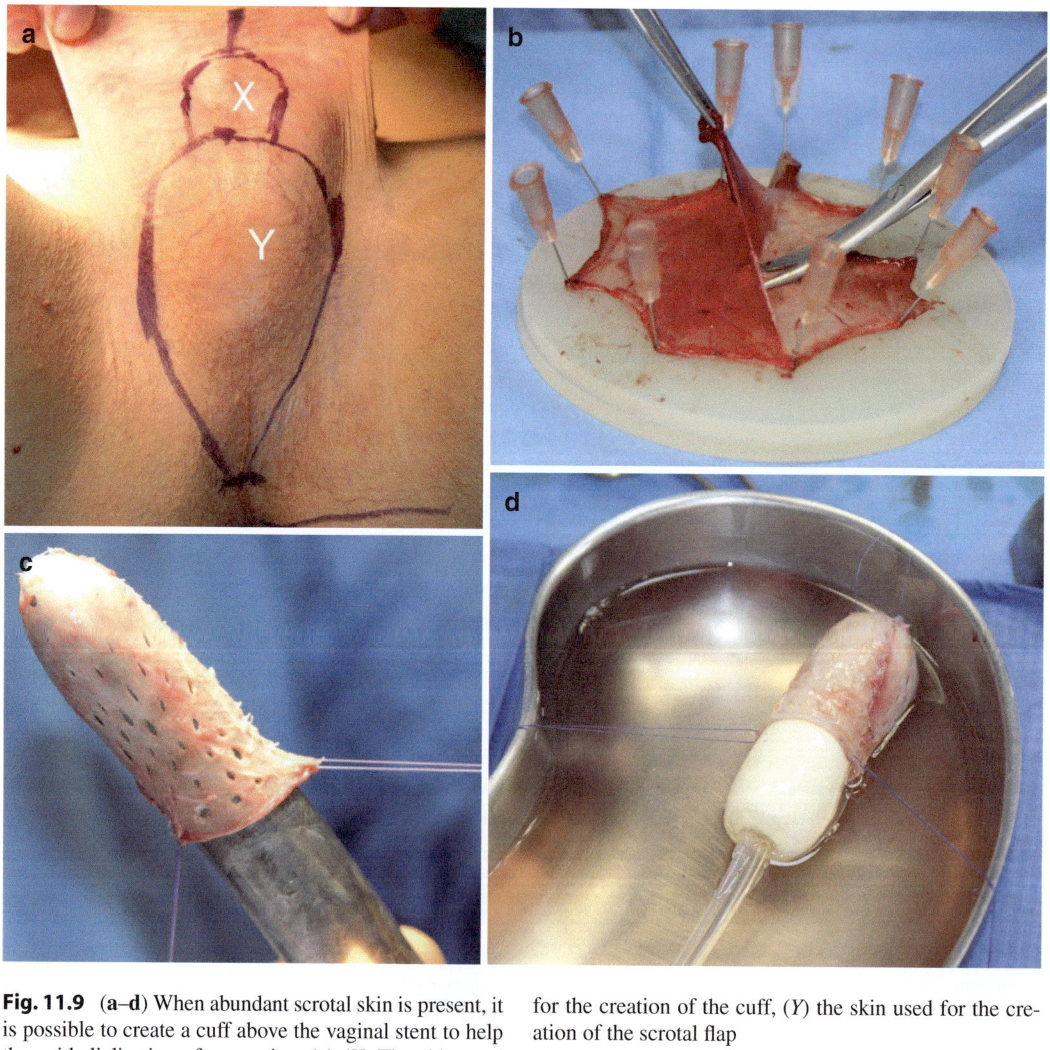

Fig. 11.9 (**a**–**d**) When abundant scrotal skin is present, it is possible to create a cuff above the vaginal stent to help the epithelialisation of neovagina. (**a**) (*X*) The skin used for the creation of the cuff, (*Y*) the skin used for the creation of the scrotal flap

cylinder and the crura. Eventual residual "dog ears" are excised.

A longitudinal midline incision on the penile flap is performed in order to allow the exteriorisation of the urethra-clitoris complex, catheter and Liguori's stitch.

In order to avoid hypersensitivity of the neoclitoris, a cap is created from the residual prepuce skin.

Now the penile-scrotal cylinder of skin is introduced into the neo-cavity, now forming the neovagina, and the two Prolene stitches are safely knotted to hold it in place and avoid any eventual prolapse (Fig. 11.10) [15]. We have to remember the presence of ureters when we pass the two stitches into the deep part of the neo-cavity [16].

The surgical incision at the end of the procedure appears as a wide "U" and is closed with a V-loc running suture (Table 11.5).

As the final step, a lubricated adjustable vaginal stent is inserted into the neovagina, making sure that it reaches the vault. The stent consists of a sealed silicone shell filled with polyurethane foam, fully adjustable by inflation. During insertion, the stent is deflated, only to be inflated once the position is satisfactory. After inflation, in order to avoid slipping due to the smooth surfaces of the stent, a cotton ball is always inserted in the vaginal meatus [17].

The usefulness of this vaginal stent is double: first it prevents the vaginal walls from collapsing, and second it is designed to permit the drainage of all secretions.

Table 11.5 The steps of the creation and the use of the penile-scrotal flap

The skin cylinder (penile-scrotal flap)
Fixation of peritesticular fat at perineal level
Suture between the penile and scrotal skin (Vicryl 3/0)
Placement of four stitches to better distinguish labia majora and labia minora
Longitudinal midline incision of the penile flap
Exteriorisation of the urethra-clitoris complex
Insertion of skin cylinder and closure of the two Prolene stitches
Eventual creation of a cutaneous cuff to place above the vaginal stent (when abundant scrotal skin is present)
Placement of the adjustable vaginal stent
V-lock running U-shaped suture of the external skin

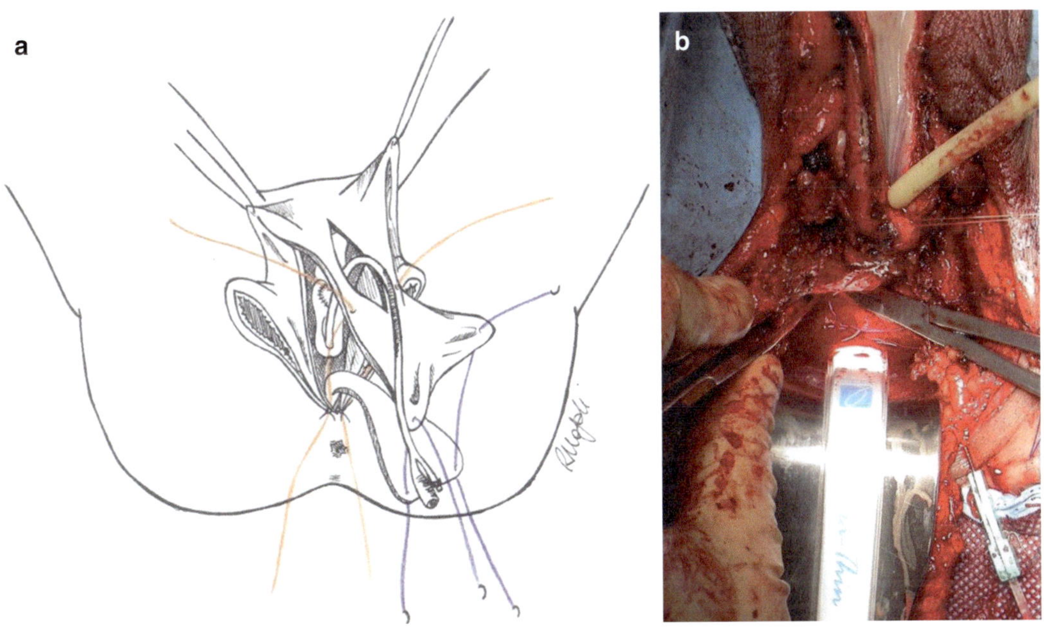

Fig. 11.10 (**a**) The longitudinal midline incision on the penile flap allows the exteriorisation of the urethra-clitoris complex and of the catheter. The stitches in orange and purple show how the penile flap is joined to the scrotal flap. (**b**) Two Prolene stitches knotted at prostatic and rectal level are passed through the penile and scrotal flap to hold it in place and avoid any eventual prolapse

A compressive packing is always done, in a criss-cross fashion, using a wide adhesive gauze. A good compression avoids postoperative bleeding and swelling and helps maintain the stent in place.

11.9 Postoperative Care

After surgery the patient must stay in a supine position, for the duration of 2 days. During this period of time, it is crucial to conduct thromboembolic prophylaxis (heparin, antiembolic stockings, mobilisation of the feet and legs).

The patient can begin eating again once bowels are open to gas: usually the *first* day she is restricted to a liquid diet, and during the second day she can begin a solid diet.

From the *second* day, washing of the neovagina is done by introducing a small amount of Betadine and/or saline solution into the stent.

On the *third* day, the stent is deflated and removed for the first time and disinfected with diluted Amuchina. Anti-swelling or heparin-based creams are applied on eventual haematomas.

After 4 days, the urethral catheter is removed, and the patient experiences urination as a woman for the first time.

Now dilatations with rigid vaginal stents begin, and the patient is taught the correct manoeuvres for insertion and care.

We usually adopt Amielle Comfort (Owen Mumford) vaginal dilators which have been designed for women experiencing vaginal discomfort and penetration problems from vaginismus, dyspareunia and gynaecological surgery.

The recommended position to insert into neovagina the lubricated dilators is to lie flat on back with the knees bent and legs slightly apart. Alternatively, the patient can stand with one leg raised on a chair.

Dilators can be washed in hot soapy water and dried thoroughly ensuring all traces of soap have been removed before their insertion into the neovagina.

Psychosexual therapists teach how [18]:

- To control breathing
- To relax the legs as much as possible
- To gently ease the lubricated dilator in an upward and backward direction as deeply as is comfortable
- To leave the dilator in position for up to 5 min

When a patient feels comfortable with using the smallest dilator, gradually move to the next size and so on (Fig. 11.11).

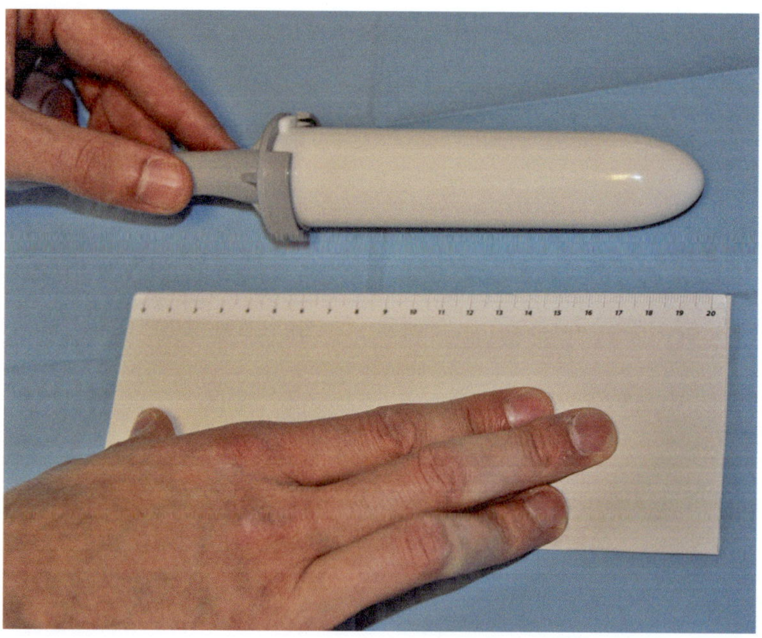

Fig. 11.11 Rigid vaginal stents are used for the periodic dilatations of the neovagina

Moreover during the first postoperative days, we suggest to use during the night the *adjustable vaginal stent* which allows a continuous dilatation of the neovagina during the night hours (Fig. 11.12).

In the first postoperative period, we suggest to repeat this procedure four to five times a day in a place that is comfortable and ensures her privacy.

When no complication occurs, the patient can be discharged 5–6 days after surgery.

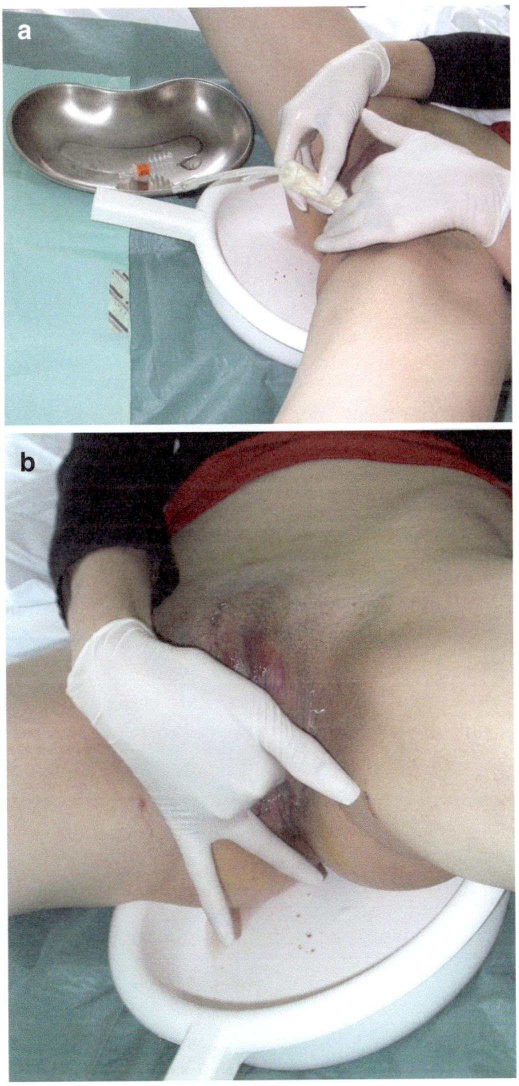

Fig. 11.12 (**a**, **b**) The patient learns to use the adjustable vaginal stent, which, during the first postoperative days, allows a continuous dilatation of the neovagina during the night hours

When patients feel comfortable with inserting the larger dilators, no secretion is evident and no pain is referred, they may be ready to attempt penetrative sexual intercourse.

Table 11.6 The postoperative steps

Postoperative timing
Supine position during the first night
Mobilisation of legs and feet asap
Restart nutrition once bowel movements have begun
Start washings through the stent with saline solution on second day p.o.
Patient can and should inspect herself with the use of a mirror
Removal of stent on the third day in order to wash it
Eventual application of heparin-based ointment on the skin
Removal of urethral catheter on the fourth day
On the fifth day, self-dilatation of the neovagina begins
Self-evaluation of the sensitivity of neoclitoris
Discharge on the seventh day after surgery
Follow-up visits after 1, 3 and 6 months

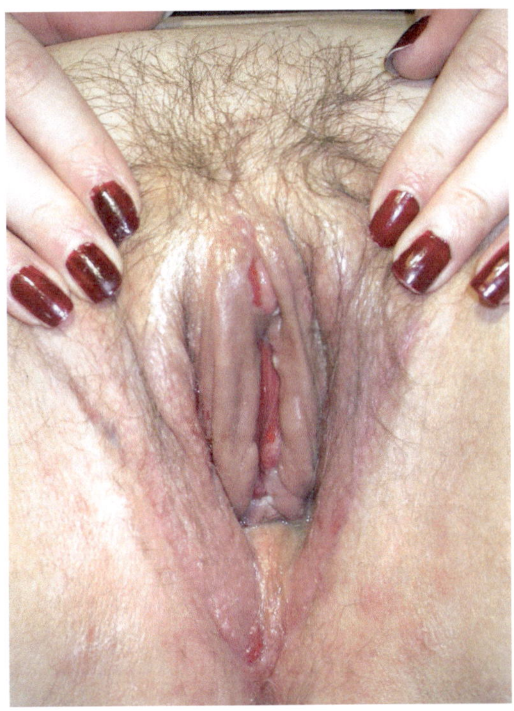

Fig. 11.13 After 3 months, the complete healing of surgical wounds is evident. Furthermore the clitoris appears pinkish and healthy

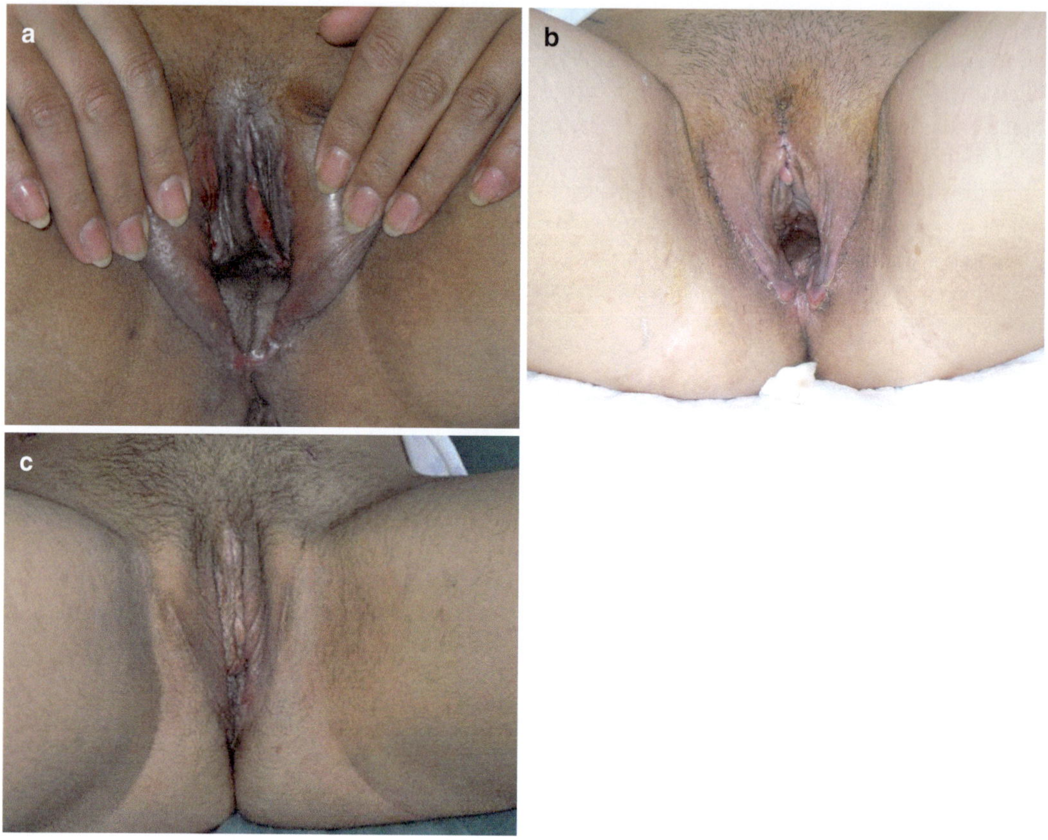

Fig. 11.14 (**a–c**) The goal of our surgery consists of creating a neovagina deep enough for intercourse and aesthetically acceptable

In our experience, the timing of the first intercourse is 45–60 days after surgery (Table 11.6; Figs. 11.13 and 11.14).

11.10 Possible Side Effects and Complications

A frequent side effect of this kind of procedure is the development of a haematoma of the labia of the neovagina which is more frequent in the presence of abundant skin and usually resolves spontaneously (Fig. 11.15).

If surgery lasts too much, BMI of the patient is too high, and patient's legs are not well positioned, a leg muscular contusion may develop due to the prolonged lithotomy position during operation: this rare event requires fasciotomy of the peronaeorum communis fascia to be performed as soon as possible (4–6 h after the first intervention) [19].

In our experience, an important critical step is the preparation of the neurovascular dorsal penile bundles. Injury to the arteries or nerves may result in an impaired blood supply or reduced sensation of the clitoris. Very rare is the eventuality of total necrosis of the neoclitoris.

Another possible complication is neo-meatal stricture or substenosis. In our opinion, it is extremely important to widely spatulate the urethra and to suture the neo-meatus with separate stitches.

Other possible major complications include the following:

- Partial necrosis of the penile or scrotal flap (Fig. 11.16)
- Bleeding from the urethra and the neoclitoris
- Shortening or substenosis of the neovagina

In case of partial or total prolapse of the neovagina, a second surgical treatment is necessary [20].

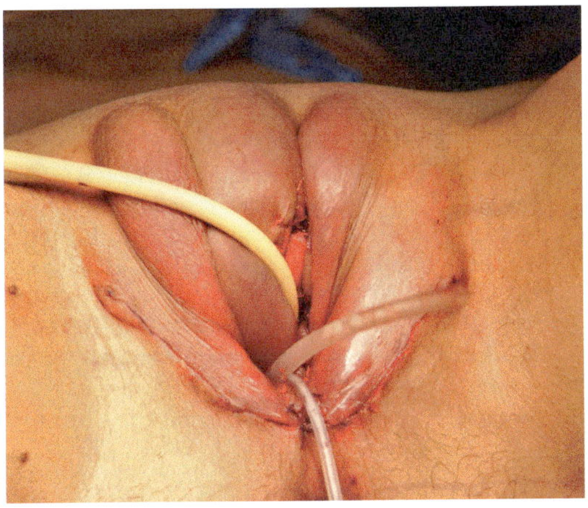

Fig. 11.15 Haematoma of the labia majora of the neovagina is a very frequent side effect especially in the presence of abundant scrotal skin. To avoid oedema, care must be taken to limit parenteral intraoperative intake of saline solution

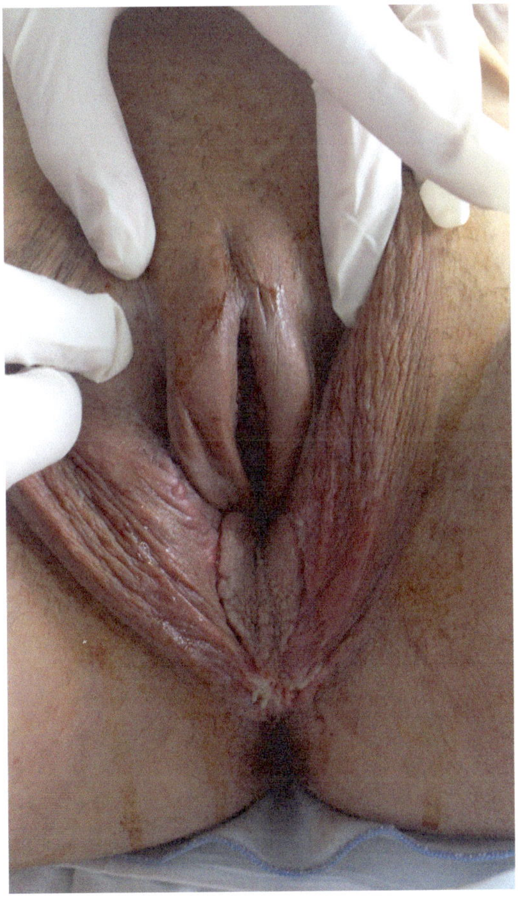

Fig. 11.16 Sometimes strong dilatations may create a little displacement of the stitches at 6 h

References

1. Belgrano E, Trombetta C, Repetto U, Pittaluga P, De Rose AF, Giuliani L (1986) Pseudoermafroditismo maschile con persistenza delle strutture mulleriane: descrizione di un caso. Atti 58° Congr. S.I.U.- Roma, 25–28 settembre 1985. Acta Urol Ital:429–433
2. Belgrano E, Repetto U, Trombetta C, Siracusano S, Bozzo W, Pittaluga P (1986) Persistenza delle strutture mulleriane: descrizione di un caso. Rassegna Ital Chir Pediatr XXVIII(2):120–123
3. Trombetta C, Siracusano S, Gabriele M, Belgrano E (1989) Hernia uteri inguinalis : un caso particolare di pseudoermafroditismo maschile. Atti 5° Corso Agg. Androl. di interesse chir.- Fiuggi Terme, 27–28 giugno 1988. Andrologia Chirurgica in Età Pediatrica. Acta Medica. 1989:77–82
4. Belgrano E, Trombetta C, Siracusano S, Desole S (1990) Creazione di neovagina in due casi di pseudoermafroditismo. Atti del 63° Congr. S.I.U. (Società Italiana di Urologia) – Ancona, 9–12 Settembre 1990
5. Trombetta C, Siracusano S, Desole S, Foddis G, Usai V, Belgrano E (1992) Creazione di una neovagina in caso di pseudoermafroditismo: presentazione di due soluzioni tecniche. Atti 40° Convegno S.U.I.C.M.I.- Alghero, 23–25 Maggio 1991. Acta Urol Ital (suppl. 5):231–234
6. Belgrano E, Fabris B, Trombetta C (1999) Il Transessualismo: identificazione di un percorso diagnostico e terapeutico. E. Kurtis, Milano, pp 1–374
7. Wierckx K, Elaut E, Declercq E, Heylens G, De Cuypere G, Taes Y, Kaufman JM, T'Sjoen G (2013) Prevalence of cardiovascular disease and cancer during cross-sex hormone therapy in a large cohort of trans persons: a case–control study. Eur J Endocrinol 169(4):471–478. doi:10.1530/EJE-13-0493
8. Van Kesteren PJ, Asscheman H, Megens JA, Gooren LJ (1997) Mortality and morbidity in transsexual subjects treated with cross-sex hormones. Clin Endocrinol (Oxf) 47:337–342
9. Trombetta C, Buttazzi L, Liguori G, Belgrano E (1998) Sex reassignment surgery: male-to-female transsexual operation. eUROtraining. International symposium on update on pelvic surgery. Genova, 5–7 Nov
10. Trombetta C, Liguori G, Buttazzi L, Belgrano E (1999) Surgical treatment of male-to-female transsexual patients: our experience. Urogynaecologia Int J 12(3):182–185
11. Trombetta C, Liguori G, Bucci S, Salamè L, Garaffa G, Cova M, Belgrano E (2004) Radiological evaluation of vaginal width and depth in male-to-female transsexuals by the use of magnetic resonance imaging. World J Urol 22(5):405–408
12. Trombetta C, Liguori G, Buttazzi L, Bucci S, Belgrano E (2000) Our technique for treatment of male-to-female transsexual patients. Br J Urol Int 86:202
13. Trombetta C, Liguori G, Benvenuto S, Petrovic M, Napoli R, Umari P, Rizzo M, Zordani A (2011) Neourethroclitoroplasty according to Petrovic. Urologia 78(4):267–273. doi:10.5301/RU.2011.8855

14. Trombetta C, Liguori G, Buttazzi L, Bucci S, Belgrano E (2002) Male-to-female sex reassignment surgery (SRS): urological technique. 100th AUA Orlando 25–30 Maggio 2002 – J. Urol. 167, 4 (suppl):149 (abstract no 597)
15. Stanojevic DS, Djordjevic ML, Milosevic A, Sansalone S, Slavkovic Z, Ducic S, Vujovic S, Perovic SV, Belgrade Gender Dysphoria Team (2007) Sacrospinous ligament fixation for neovaginal prolapse prevention in male-to-female surgery. Urology 70(4):767–771
16. Rezwan N, Basit AA, Andrews H (2014) Bilateral ureteric obstruction: an unusual complication of male to female gender reassignment surgery. BMJ Case Rep. doi:10.1136/bcr-2014-204894
17. Savoca G, Trombetta C, De Stefani S, Raber M, Siracusano S, Belgrano E (1995) Creazione di neovagina: presentazione di due soluzioni tecniche. Acts 9° Congress. S.I.A. – Ancona, 14–16 Sept "Andrologia 1995" Monduzzi Ed, pp 321–324
18. Trombetta C, Liguori G, Bucci S, Belgrano E (2003) Surgical therapy in transsexual patient: a multidisciplinary approach. 18° Congress of the European Association of Urology, Madrid, 12–15 March2003. Eur Urol 2(1):97
19. Raza A, Byrne D, Townell N (2004) Lower limb (well leg) compartment syndrome after urological pelvic surgery. J Urol 171:5–11
20. Selvaggi G, Bellringer J (2011) Gender reassignment surgery: an overview. Nat Rev Urol 8:274–282

12 Vaginoplasty in Male Transsexuals Using Penile Skin and Urethral Flap

Sava V. Perovic†

12.1 Introduction

Vaginoplasty presents the main problem in male-to-female surgery. There are many operative techniques [1–3] that can be used, but none is ideal. Therefore, continual challenge exists in search for new and better solutions. We have published our contribution to operative technique in male-to-female surgery [4]. Afterwards we continuously improved this technique, and now we present its latest variant.

12.2 Material and Methods

In the period from January 1994 to November 1999, 89 patients aged 18–56 years (mean 28 years) underwent vaginoplasty in male-to-female sex reassignment surgery. To create a new vagina, vascularized inverted penile skin and urethral flap were used in 85 patients. Nine of these had a disproportion between short inverted penile skin and a long vascularized urethral flap. Other four vaginas were created using a vascularized urethral flap and free penile skin grafts.

S.V. Perovic, MD
School of Medicine, University of Belgrade, Belgrade, Yugoslavia

12.2.1 Operative Technique

For the new vagina to be formed, the operative technique involves several procedures. After the usual bilateral orchidectomy, the penis is dissected into its anatomical entities: corpora cavernosa, the glans cap with the urethra and the neurovascular bundle and the vascularized penile skin. The corpora cavernosa are removed up to their attachments to the pubic bones. Remnants of the corpora cavernosa, i.e. erectile tissue, are destroyed in order to prevent their postoperative erection which can hinder sexual intercourse. The glans cap is divided into two parts: ventral and dorsal. Reduction of the dorsal part of the glans is performed by an excision of the central ventral tissue, leaving lateral sides of the glans intact. Lateral excisions on the glans are not recommended in order to avoid injury of the neurovascular bundle which enters into the glans cap lateroventrally. However, lateral sides are deepithelialized and sutured to obtain the conical shape of the neoclitoris. The ventral half of the glans, which remains attached to the urethra, is used to form the neocervix at the bottom of the new vagina. The urethra is spatulated, including the bulbous part, and used for creation of the mucosal part of the neovagina. The urethra of the female type is formed. The neoclitoris is fixed above the new urethral meatus. In reconstructing the new vagina, the skin of the penile

†deceased

C. Trombetta et al. (eds.), *Management of Gender Dysphoria: A Multidisciplinary Approach*,
DOI 10.1007/978-88-470-5696-1_12, © Springer-Verlag Italia 2015

body and prepuce (if present) are fashioned into a vascularized island tube flap. It is very important to obtain a very long vascularized pedicle of the tube. Therefore, the level of the incision is approximately 2 cm above the base of the mobilized penile skin. Only here, the existing loose subcutaneous tissue permits formation of a long vascularized pedicle. At the base of the pedicle, a hole is made for the transposition of the urethral flap. On the dorsal side of the skin tube flap, only the skin is incised, whereas the vascularized subcutaneous tissue remains intact. The urethral flap is embedded into the skin tube. The bottom of the tube is closed with the distal part of the urethra and the remaining ventral half of the glans cap after its inner side deepithelialization. The tube, consisting of skin and urethral flap, is inverted, thus forming the new vagina.

In cases of insufficient penile skin (a small and/or circumcised penis), there is a disproportion between the short skin tube and the long urethral flap. The vagina can then be formed in two ways. The proximal part at the bottom of the vagina is formed only from the urethral flap which initiates secondary epithelialization. If the length of the tube pedicle is insufficient for placing the tube into the perineal cavity, the new vagina is created using the vascularized urethral flap and free penile skin grafts. In this case, the vascularized urethral flap plays the key role in creating the new vagina. The new vagina is inserted into the previously prepared perineal cavity between the urethra, bladder and rectum. The neovagina is fixed to the sacrospinous ligament, usually to the right one. The sacrospinous ligament is palpated between the ischial spine and coccyx. After exposure of the ligament, long-handled Deschamps ligature carrier preloaded with 2-0 absorbable suture is used to pierce the ligament medially to the ischial spine. Care must be taken not to place the suture close to the ischial spine in order to prevent injury of the pudendal nerve and internal pudendal vessels.

Also, the suture must not be placed behind the ligament to prevent injury of the pudendal artery whose course is variable and may be found at any distance from the ischial spine. Both ends of the suture are brought out. One of them is passed through the skin part, while another one is passed

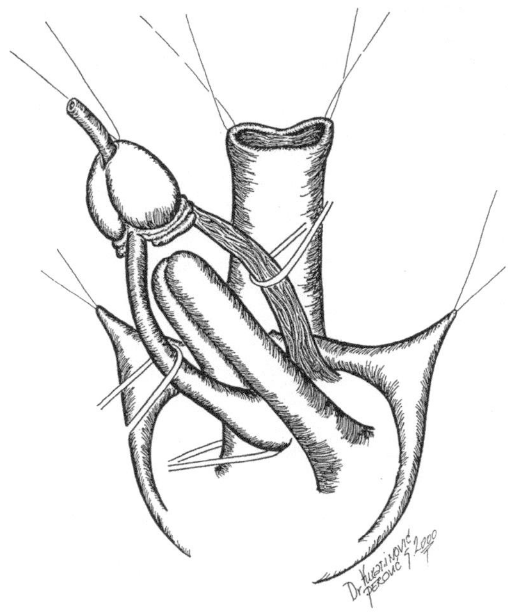

Fig. 12.1 The corpora cavernosa are completely dissected from the glans cap with the urethra and neurovascular bundle. Penile skin is completely mobilized in full thickness

through the urethral part of the neovagina and tied. This way, vaginopexy to the sacrospinous ligament is achieved and the neovagina is placed deeply in the perineal cavity.

Vulvoplasty involves creation of the labia minora and majora. The remaining part of the base of the penile skin is employed to form the labia minora, which are sutured to the deepithelialized area of the neoclitoris. This way the neoclitoris is hooded with the labia minora. The excessive scrotal skin is removed and the remaining part is used to form the labia majora.

Perivaginal Jackson-Pratt drain is left for 3 days. Urethral catheter and vaginal packing (condom filled with soft material) are removed on the 7th postoperative day. Vaginal stenting is dependent on the type of the new vagina. If the vagina is formed from sufficient penile skin, the vaginal stent is applied during the night for 6 weeks. If the vagina is formed from insufficient penile skin or from free penile skin flaps, the stent is applied continuously day and night for 3 months (Figs. 12.1, 12.2, 12.3, 12.4, 12.5, 12.6, 12.7, 12.8, 12.9, 12.10, 12.11, 12.12, 12.13, 12.14, 12.15, and 12.16).

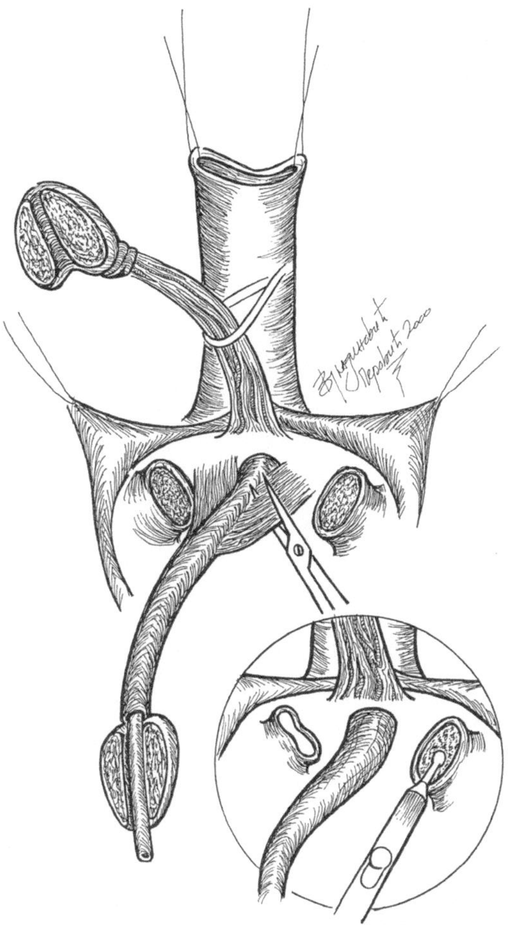

Fig. 12.2 The corpora cavernosa are removed up to their attachments to the pubic bones. Remnants of the corpora cavernosa, i.e. erectile tissue, are destroyed in order to prevent their postoperative erection (*inset*). The bulbospongiosus muscle is removed from the bulbous part of the urethra. The glans cap is divided into two parts: ventral with the urethra and dorsal with the neurovascular bundle

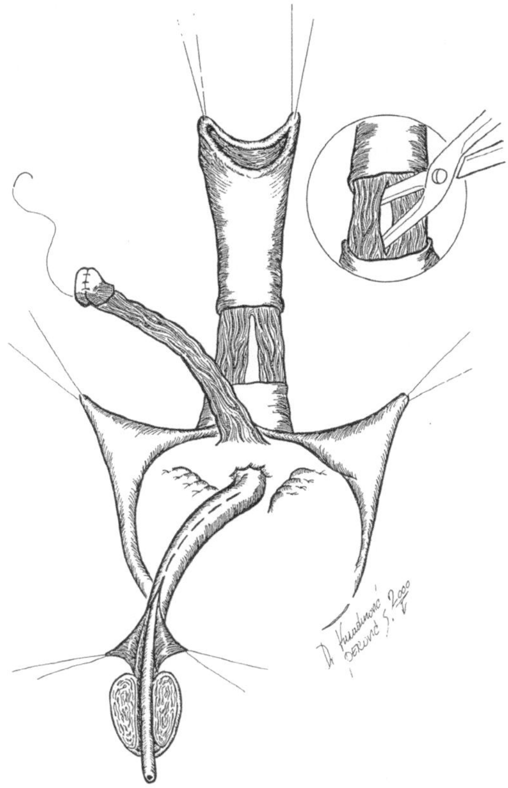

Fig. 12.3 Trimming of the glans to the size of a clitoris. Its lateral sides are deepithelialized. The urethra is spatulated dorsally including its bulbous part. Incision is made approximately 2 cm above the base of the mobilized penile skin. Loose subcutaneous tissue permits formation of a long vascularized pedicle. A hole is made on its base (*inset*)

12.3 Results

The follow-up ranged from 3 months to 6 years (mean 4.6 years). The most important features of the new vagina are depth and width. The depth ranges from 9 to 18 cm (mean 11.6 cm). Precise measuring of the vaginal width is difficult. In our patients it was estimated by the size of "Mentor" vaginal stent, according to which 8 vaginas were small, 67 were medium and 12 were large. Another important characteristic of the new vagina is moisture. It was satisfactory in 71 and unsatisfactory in 16 patients. By interviewing our patients we obtained data on sensitivity and orgasm. Sensitivity was good in 83, while 73 patients had orgasm. Aesthetically normal appearance of genitalia was achieved in 78 patients. In nine cases, additional aesthetic correction was necessary. Six months after surgery, 69 patients (79 %) had normal sexual intercourse. Despite having an adequate vagina, some patients abstained from intercourse (Figs. 12.17 and 12.18).

There was only one major complication, a rectovaginal fistula due to intraoperative injury to the rectum. Other postoperative complications were vaginal shrinking in two patients due to

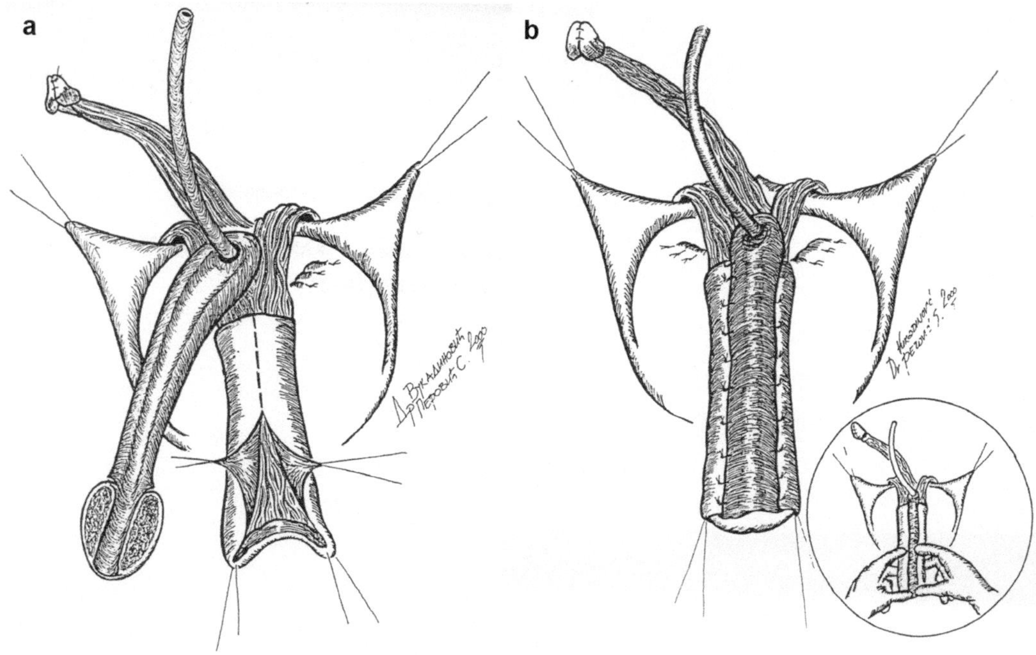

Fig. 12.4 (**a**) Transposition of the urethral flap dorsally through the hole on the base of the vascularized skin tube flap. On the dorsal side of the skin tube, only the skin is incised. Vascularized subcutaneous tissue remains intact. (**b**) The urethral flap is embedded at the place of the skin tube incision. Moisture and sensitivity of the new vagina are achieved by its mucous segment, the vascularized urethral flap. The bottom of the tube is closed using the ventral part of the glans cap. Epithelial surface of the glans remains outside. The skin tube with urethral flap is invaginated (*inset*)

insufficient length of the vaginal pedicle (vaginopexy under high tension), which were resolved with rectosigmoid vaginoplasty. Stenosis of the vaginal introitus was in six patients, late stenosis of the urethral meatus in one patient due to injury during sexual intercourse, urethral prolapse in two patients which was easily resolved by simple excision and posterior vaginal wall rupture during intercourse in one patient but without injury to the rectum.

12.4 Comment

Surgery of male transsexuals still presents a major challenge of the new vagina. Thus we have improved our operative technique previously published by having introduced several refinements [5]. The crucial point of our technique is introducing the complete penile disassembly which ideally enables the usage of all penile entities except the corpora cavernosa in the construction of the new vulva, clitoris and vagina. By this principle, the penis is completely disassembled into its anatomical parts: the corpora cavernosa and glans cap with the urethra and neurovascular bundle. This way, the corpora cavernosa are ideally exposed for their removal at the level of their attachment to the pubic rami. Remnants of the corpora cavernosa, i.e. erectile tissue, are additionally destroyed in order to prevent their postoperative erection which can hinder sexual intercourse. Lifting of the glans with neurovascular bundle, dorsally, and urethra, ventrally, from the tips of the corpora cavernosa is made together with Buck's fascia. In this way, these penile entities are completely preserved. Since the glans cap is divided into two parts, dorsal one is used for creation of

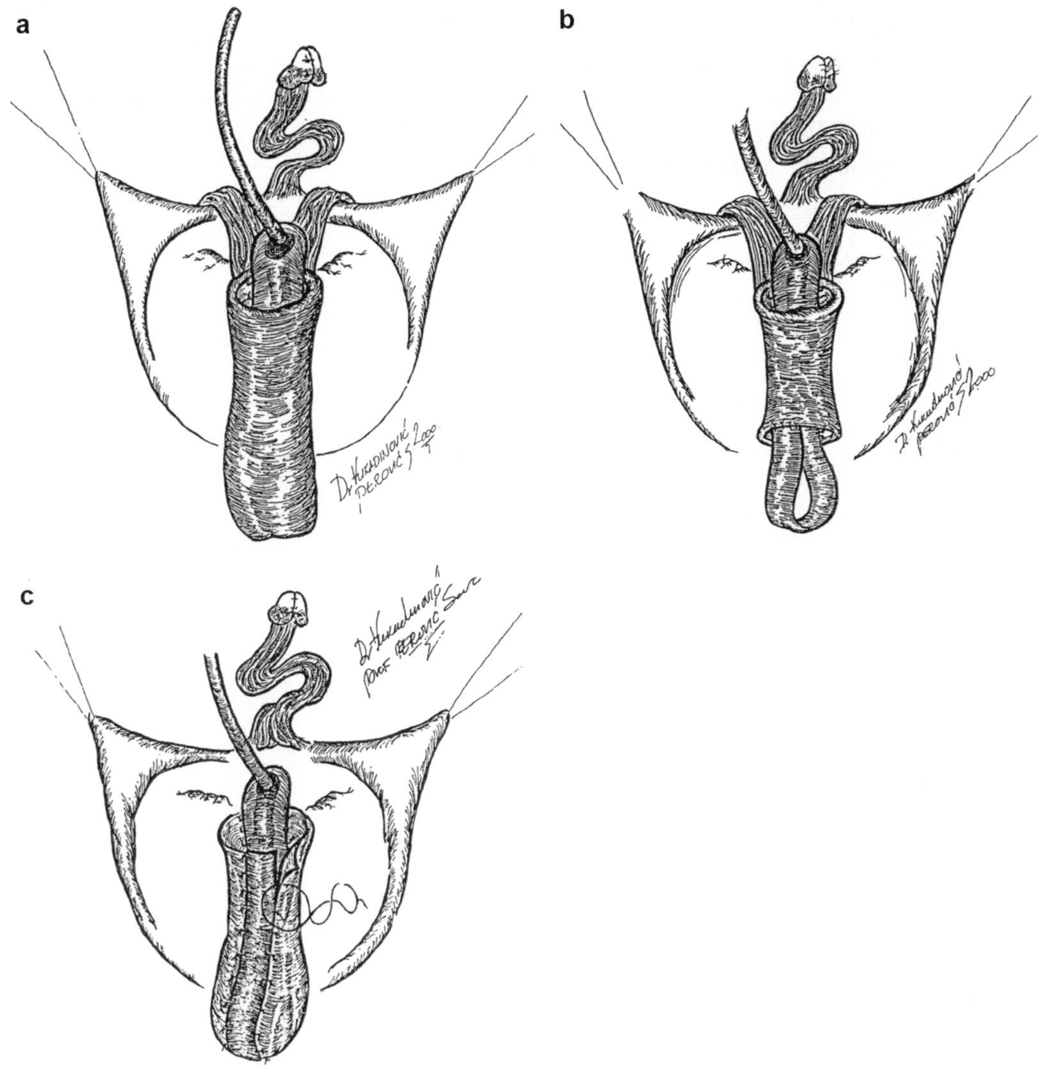

Fig. 12.5 (**a**) A neovagina is created. The new urethral meatus of female type is in continuity with the urethral flap. The new vagina is composed from the vascularized penile skin and vascularized urethral flap. (**b**) When there is insufficient penile skin, the proximal part and bottom of the new vagina are formed only with vascularized urethral flap. (**c**) When the skin tube pedicle is of sufficient length, the new vagina is made from the vascularized urethral flap and free penile skin flaps

the neoclitoris. Care must be taken to perform reduction of the dorsal part of the glans which is made by excision of its central ventral tissue, leaving lateral sides of the glans intact. Lateral excisions on the glans are not recommended in order to avoid injury of the neurovascular bundle which enters into the glans cap lateroventrally. Finally, the newly formed clitoris has small dimension and excellent vascularization and sensitivity.

In our technique, the new vagina is composed of an inverted pedicled island penile skin and vascularized urethral flap. Success in vaginoplasty depends on the available amount of skin. The essential part in the usage of penile skin is to

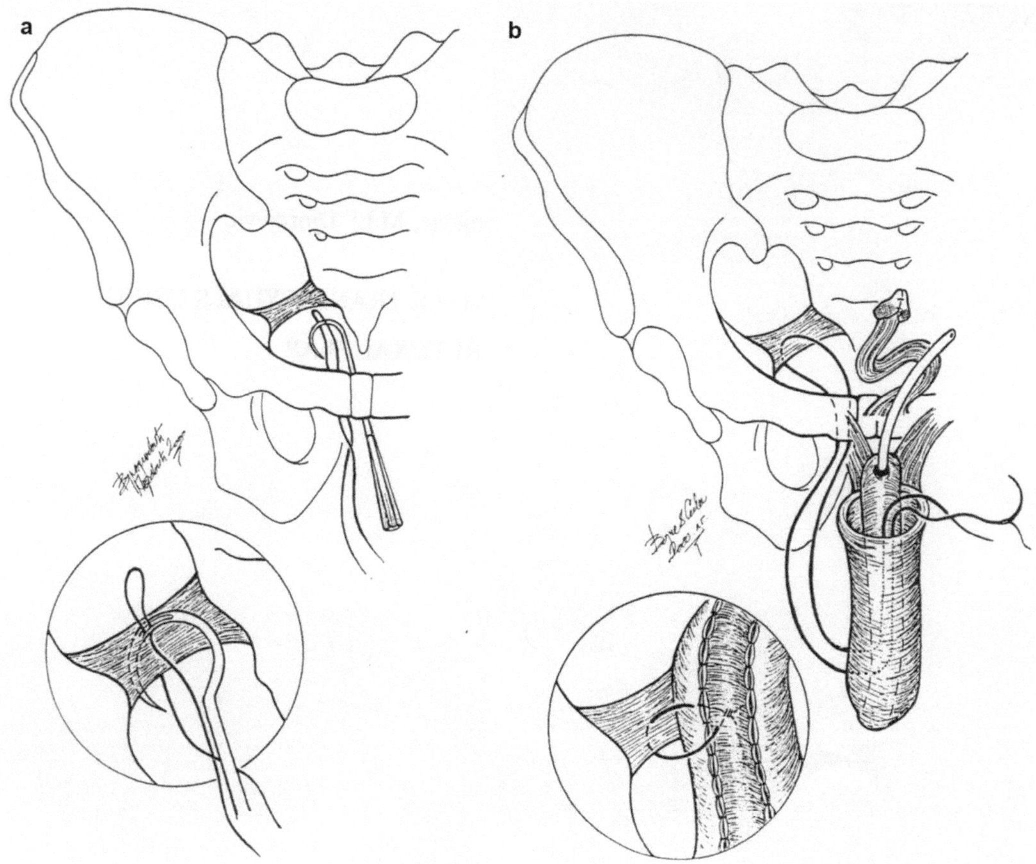

Fig. 12.6 (**a**) The neovagina is fixed to the sacrospinous ligament, usually to the right one. Deschamps ligature carrier preloaded with 2-0 absorbable suture is used to pierce the ligament medially to the ischial spine. Both ends of the suture are brought out. (**b**) One of them is passed through the skin part, while another one is passed through the urethral part of the neovagina and tied. The new vagina is usually fixed in its distal third in order to provide good placement and to avoid its prolapse

obtain a long pedicle, allowing the penile skin flap to be brought into the new vaginal space without tension. If there is insufficient skin, the question is what to do? There are two possibilities. One is to use the penile skin in order to create only the distal part of the vagina, avoiding tension. In this case, the proximal part and the bottom of the vagina are formed from the urethral flap and secondary epithelialization. If the length of the tube pedicle is insufficient for placing the tube into the perineal cavity, the new vagina is created using the vascularized urethral flap and free penile skin flaps. Thus, the technique may also be used in patients with a small and/or circumcised penis.

In our vaginoplasty, the vascularized urethral flap plays the essential role. It is always of adequate length and never presents the limiting factor in vaginoplasty. By penile disassembly technique, the corpus spongiosum is completely preserved and ensures excellent blood supply. Also, the urethral flap makes the new vagina wider, especially the introitus. If penile skin is insufficient, the creation of the vagina completely

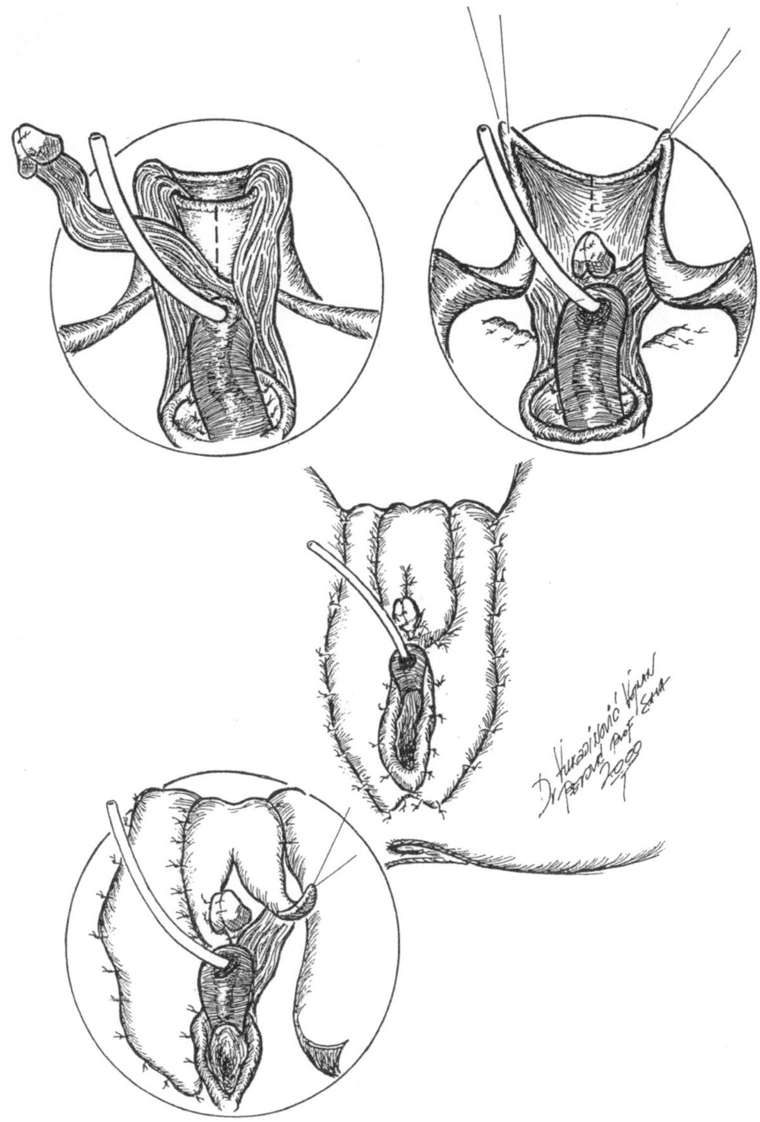

Fig. 12.7 Vulvoplasty. The remaining penile skin is split ventrally and incised partially on the dorsal side forming two sliding penile skin flaps for the creation of the labia minora. The labia minora are sutured to the deepithelialized area of the neoclitoris

depends on the urethral flap. Additionally, it gives moisture and sensitivity to the new vagina. Data obtained by interviewing showed that orgasm mainly depends on the urethral flap. Pseudocervix, made from the ventral part of divided glans cap, contributes to the sensitivity of the neovaginal bottom. Prolapse of the urethral part of the vagina, which we observed with Stamey fixation procedure, is completely solved with vaginal fixation to the sacrospinous ligament. This prolapse and exaggerated posterior vaginal fourchette are avoided. Contrary to the transvaginal sacrospinous ligament fixation for the treatment of vaginal prolapse in females [6], there are significant difficulties to perform this procedure in male transsexuals. Good exposure

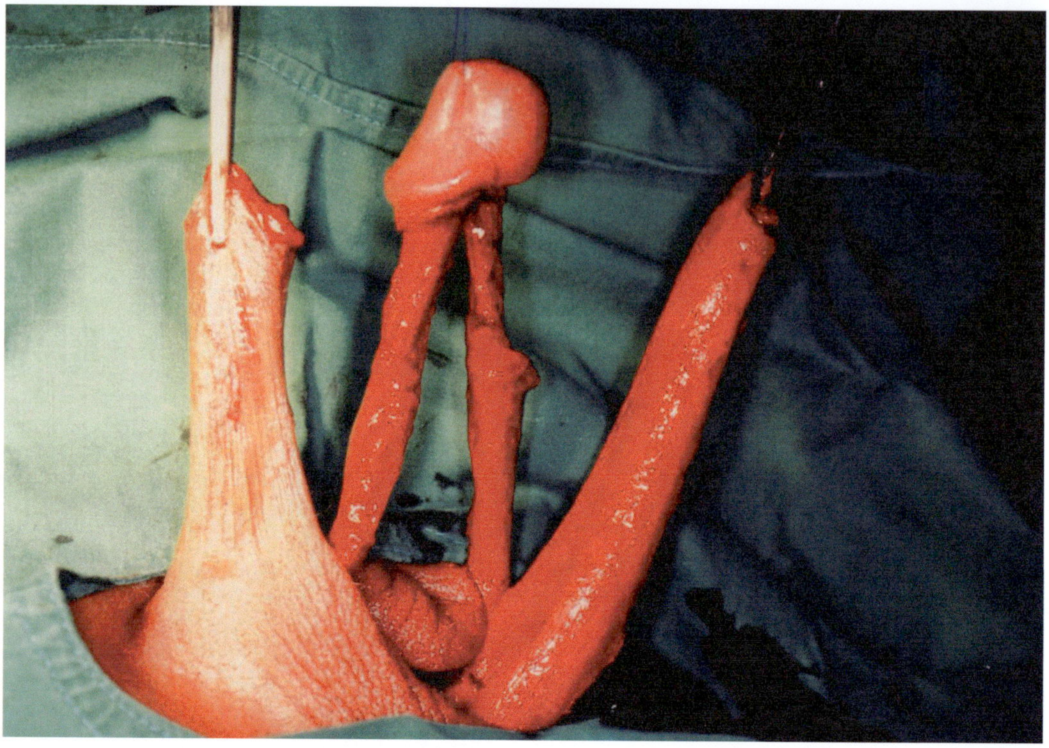

Fig. 12.8 The penis is completely disassembled into its anatomical parts: penile skin, corpora cavernosa and glans with the urethra and neurovascular bundle. All penile entities, except the corpora cavernosa, are used for vaginoplasty

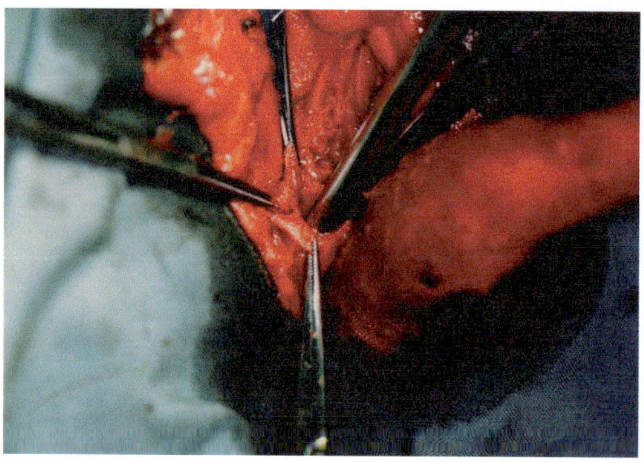

Fig. 12.9 Remnants of the corpora cavernosa, i.e. erectile tissue, are destroyed

and direct visualization of the sacrospinous ligament are crucial in order to prevent injury of the rectum, pudendal nerve and internal pudendal artery and vein. For this, great experience on male pelvic surgery is required. Shifting of the vagina to the fixed side does not have any clinical consequences in male transsexuals since the distance between the two sacrospinous ligaments is shorter than in females.

Vulvoplasty involves creation of the labia minora and majora. The labia minora, formed from remaining part of the base of the penile skin, are sutured to the deepithelialized area

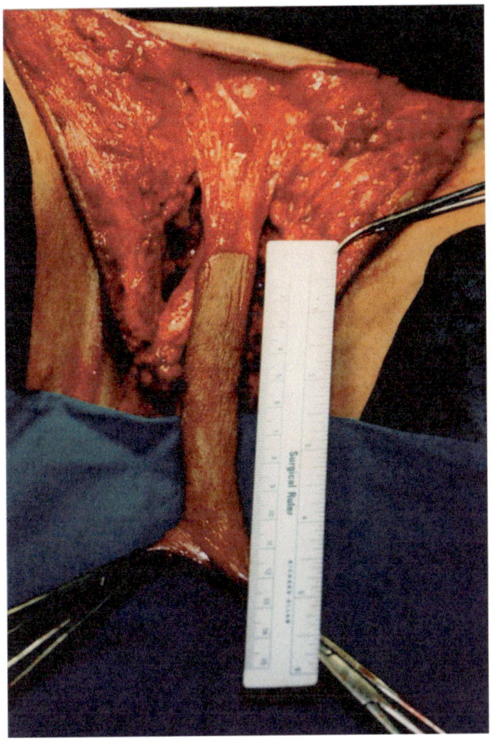

Fig. 12.10 A vascularized island penile skin flap is created on a very long vascularized pedicle

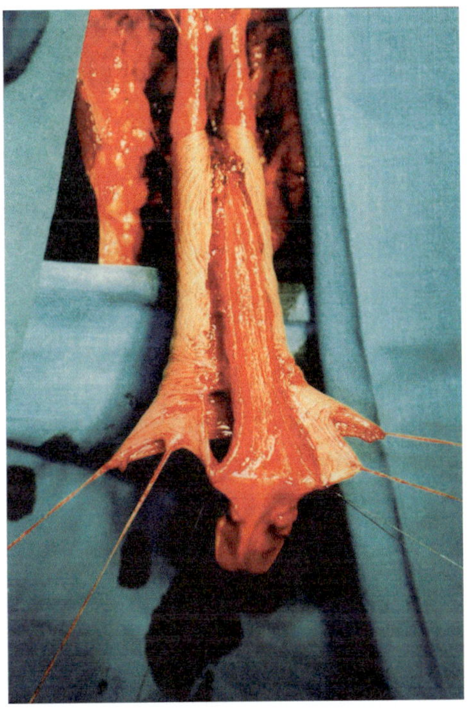

Fig. 12.11 Urethral flap is inserted into the island skin tube flap. The ventral half of the glans will be used to form a pseudocervix at the base of the new vagina

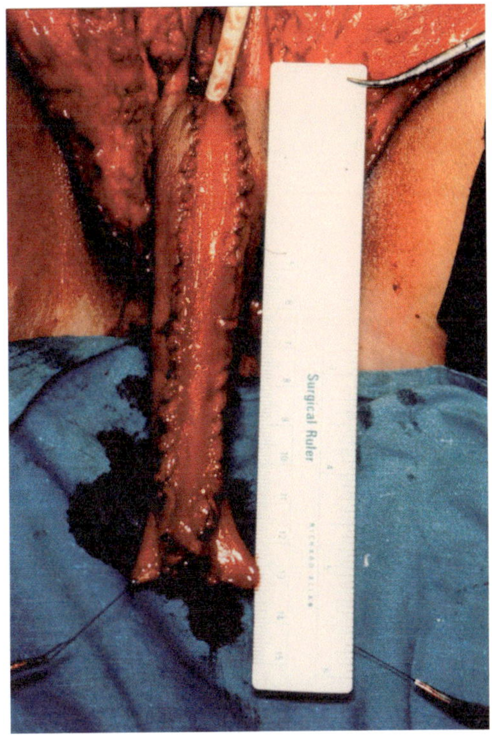

Fig. 12.12 A 12-cm-long tube is created. It consists of the vascularized penile skin and vascularized urethral flap

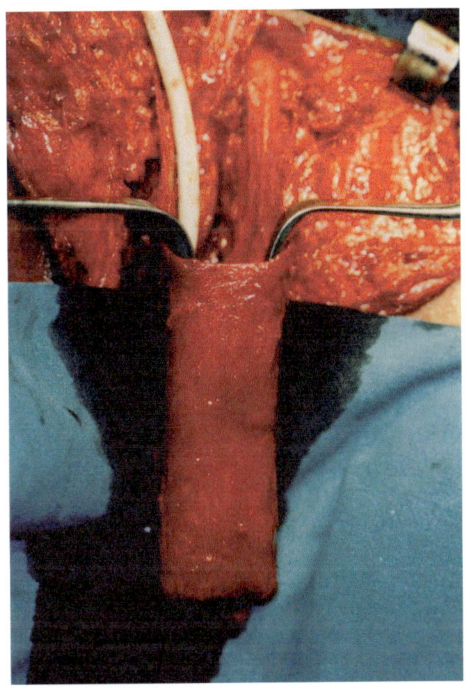

Fig. 12.13 The new vagina is formed after invagination of the tube. Wounded surfaces are outside

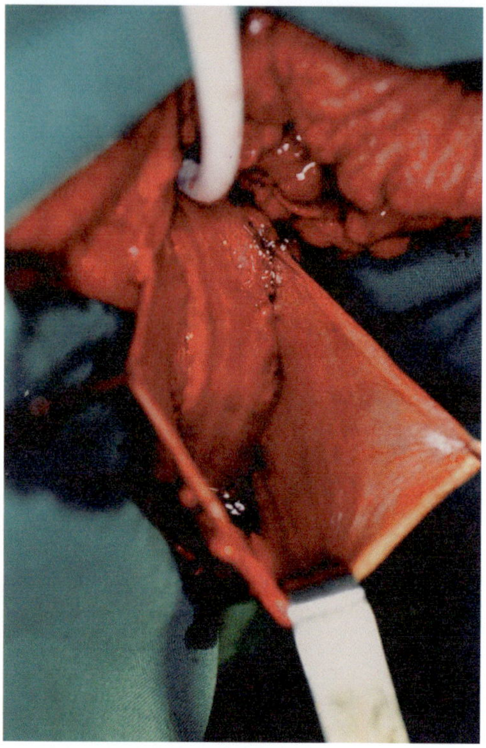

Fig. 12.14 Creation of the new vagina using the vascularized urethral flap and free penile skin grafts

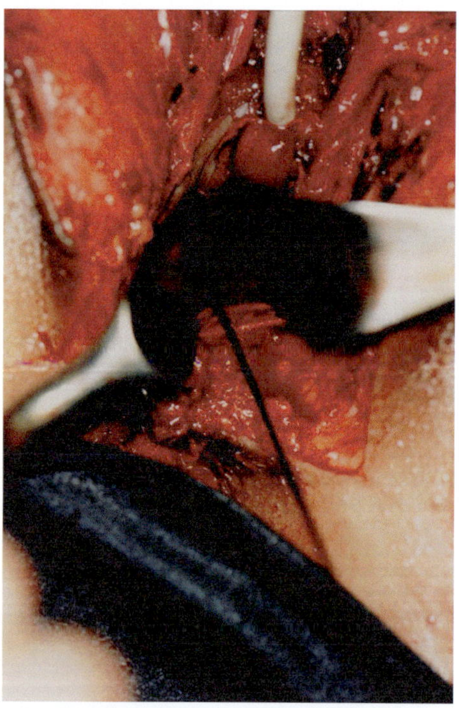

Fig. 12.15 The new vagina is deeply placed into the perineal cavity and fixed to the sacrospinous ligament. The urethra of the female type is visible

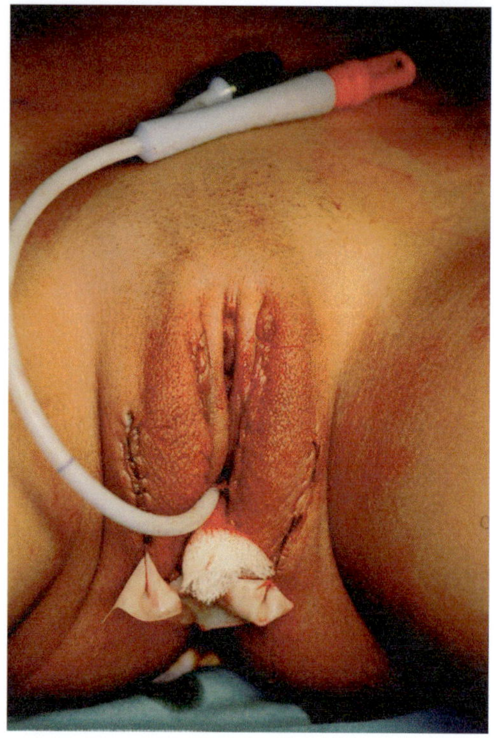

Fig. 12.16 Aspect at the end of the surgery. The labia minora cover the neoclitoris (hooded clitoris)

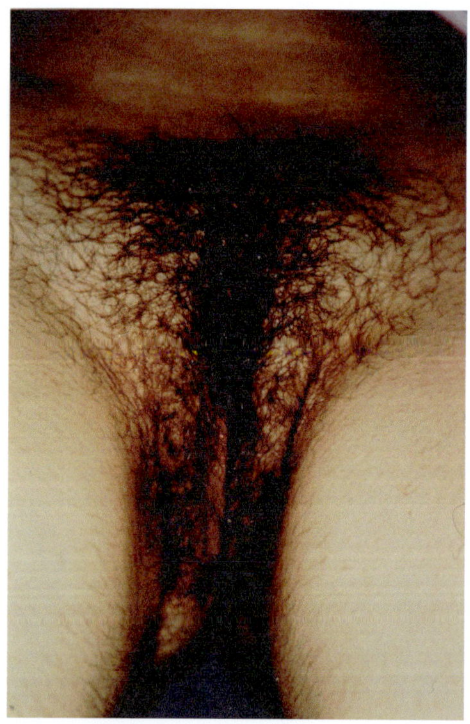

Fig. 12.17 Appearance of the vulva 1 year after surgery

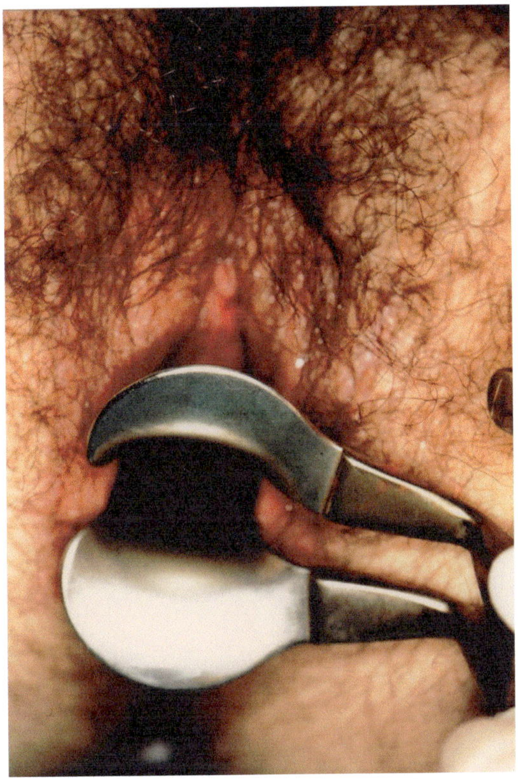

Fig. 12.18 A speculum inserted into the new vagina shows adequate depth and width

of the neoclitoris and covered it creating a hooded clitoris. Also, sensitivity of the labia minora and neoclitoris enables better-quality intercourse.

The question regarding the vaginal stent is raised. We recommend usage of the vaginal stent in all cases, to enable the patient to have intercourse as soon as possible. Duration of its application depends on the type of vaginoplasty. If the new vagina is fashioned from sufficient penile skin, the vaginal stent should be applied only during the night, while in other cases it should be continuously applied day and night until sexual intercourse is regularly practised. Sexual intercourse should be started as soon as possible, even though bleeding may occur from the mucosal part of the new vagina. This is transitory and patients should continue their sexual activity

Conclusions

The technique provides results that have the most of normal anatomical and physiological characteristics, in comparison to other methods, since all penile entities, except the corpora cavernosa, are used to form almost normal external female genitalia. It presents an advance in male-to-female surgery, but it cannot be regarded as a final solution. Only through continuous improvement of old solutions should we be in quest of new and better ones.

References

1. Meyer R, Kesselring UK (1980) One-stage reconstruction of the vagina with penile skin as an island flap in male transsexuals. Plast Reconstr Surg 66:401–406
2. Belgrano E, Lissiani A (1999) La femminilizzazione dei genitali esterni e la creazione della neovagina. In: Belgrano E, Fabris B, Trombetta C (eds) Il Transessualismo. Editrice Kurtis, Milano, pp 87–97
3. Hage J (1999) Vaginoplasty in male to female transsexuals by inversion of penile and scrotal skin. In: Ehrlich RM, Alter GJ (eds) Reconstructive and plastic surgery of the external genitalia. W.B. Saunders Company, Philadelphia, pp 294–300
4. Perovic S (1993) Male to female surgery. A new contribution to operative technique. Plast Reconstr Surg 91:703–712
5. Perovic SV (1998) Vaginoplasty in male transsexuals using penile skin and the urethral flap. J Urol 159(suppl 5):314
6. Sauer HA, Klutke CG (1995) Transvaginal sacrospinous ligament fixation for treatment of vaginal prolapse. J Urol 154:1008–1012

13 Surgical Therapy: Construction of the Neovagina Using the Pelvic Peritoneum

Alenka Fetih, Andreja Štolfa Gruntar, and Miloš Petrović

The creation of a neovagina is usually necessary in cases of vaginal agenesia, i.e. Mayer-Rokitansky-Kuster-Hauser syndrome, and in some forms of male pseudohermaphroditism such as androgen insensitivity syndrome. The described technique using pelvic peritoneum can also be applied in cases of transsexualism.

The first technique learned and used by the author was vaginal reconstruction with the sigmoid colon, which had been used in our hospital since 1955. The principal advantages with the utilisation of the colon are that after operation there are very few patients with introital stenosis, there is no need for vaginal dilation since the vaginal cavity is the sigmoid lumen itself, and the length of the neovagina is always over 10 cm and remains constant. The main disadvantages though are the following: a complex surgical intervention, involving resection of the intestine in otherwise healthy women; mucoid secretions, which can cause great discomfort to the patients; vaginal prolapse; and adenocarcinoma of the neovagina. The utilisation of bowel vaginoplasty is not suitable for patients with a short sigmoid colon, chronic inflammatory bowel disease, and renal ptosis.

Because of so many disadvantages, sigmoid colon vaginoplasty was stopped to be performed for vaginal reconstruction and the technique using pelvic peritoneal transposition has been started since 1983. It has many advantages in comparison to other vaginoplasty techniques [1–5]:

1. Compared to skin graft vaginoplasty, which is extensively used, with the use of pelvic peritoneum, there are no scars on the body from graft harvesting and there is no postoperative vaginal shrinking and/or stenosis of the newly constructed vagina.
2. The dilations and application of the mould needed to stabilise the diameter and depth of the neovagina are only temporary, since the vaginal cavity is after a certain period of time covered with normal vaginal epithelium.
3. Mostly only the perineal/vaginal approach is sufficient and there is no visible postoperative scar. There is only very rarely a need for additional abdominopelvic surgery.
4. With no bowel surgery there are no bowel-related complications. Only very rarely it happens that the rectum is opened during the formation of the vaginal cavity and is sutured as any other bowel injury.

A. Fetih, MS (✉) • A. Štolfa Gruntar, MD
Department of Obstetrics and Gynecology, University Medical Centre Ljubljana, Slajmerjeva 3, 1000 Ljubljana, Slovenia

M. Petrović, MD
General Hospital Izola, Polje 40, 6310 Izola, Slovenia

C. Trombetta et al. (eds.), *Management of Gender Dysphoria: A Multidisciplinary Approach*, DOI 10.1007/978-88-470-5696-1_13, © Springer-Verlag Italia 2015

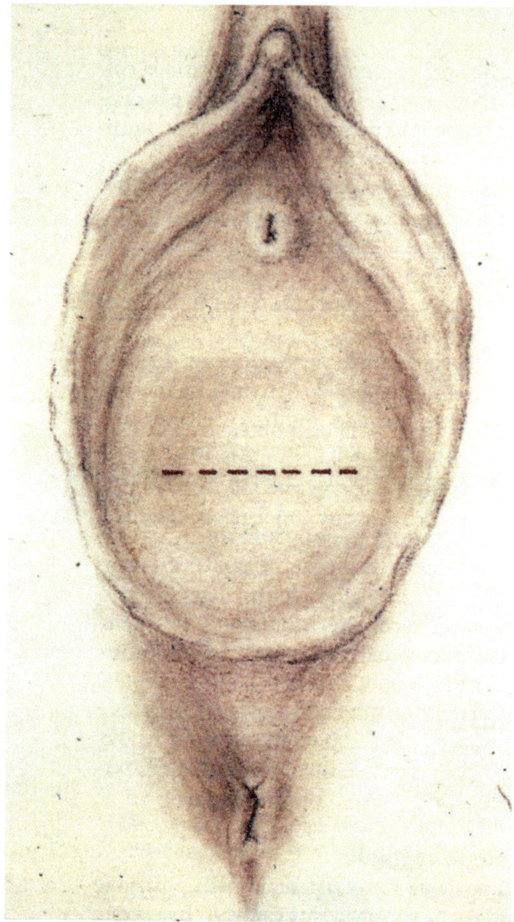

Fig. 13.1 Transverse incision line of the vaginal introitus

13.1 Preoperative Laparoscopy

It is advisable to perform an exploratory laparoscopy before peritoneal vaginoplasty. This way the surgeon is able to identify any intraperitoneal abnormality and it enables him to evaluate the depth of the pouch of Douglas. The infusion of 200 ml of sterile saline solution into the pouch of Douglas is very useful. It helps us identify the peritoneal reflection when operating perineally.

13.2 Perineal Surgery

The patient is positioned as usually when performing vaginal surgery in a dorsal lithotomy position with widened lower extremities. A Foley catheter is inserted into the bladder and filled with methylene blue. A transverse incision is made at the site of the future neovaginal introitus in the vestibular part of the vagina (Fig. 13.1), between the two little dots, that mark the exit of the Mullerian ducts. The dissection of the vaginal opening/cavity is performed mainly bluntly with small and then larger instruments and fingers in the plane between the bladder and urethra ventrally and the rectum dorsally. This step is usually performed without difficulty, but it must be kept in mind that the direction is between the bladder and the rectum. Dissection by scissors is then utilised to advance the cavity cranially until the peritoneal reflection is met. It is important to widen the diameter of the newly formed cavity between the bladder and rectum to accommodate the neovagina, which is usually done with extension laterally to avoid damage of the near structures: the bladder, urethra, ureters, and rectum; this is why great care is necessary

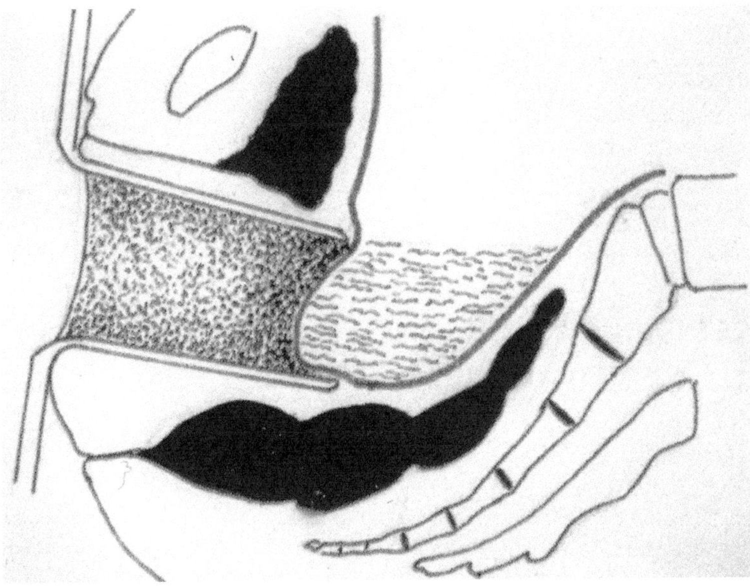

Fig. 13.2 Identification of fluttering of the peritoneum

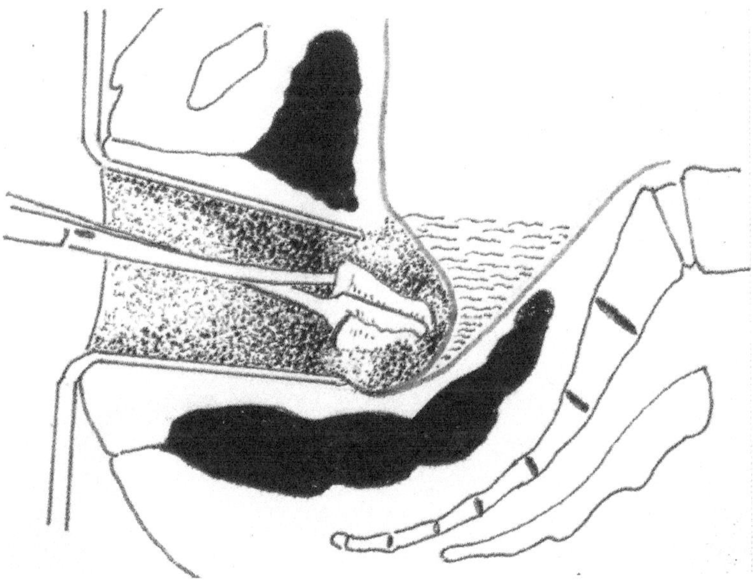

Fig. 13.3 Blunt preparation with a hard tampon of a large peritoneum field

when performing the dissection. Meticulous haemostasis is utilised at every step to control bleeding, which usually poses no problem.

The pouch of Douglas is identified with typical fluttering of the peritoneum that can be appreciated with the use of sterile saline which is infused in the peritoneal cavity laparoscopically (Fig. 13.2). The prepared field of peritoneum between the bladder and rectum should be as large as possible. Blunt preparation with a hard tampon seems to be the most efficient (Fig. 13.3).

A long aspiration needle is then introduced at the site of fluctuation into the peritoneal cavity. Aspiration of fluid confirms that the peritoneal

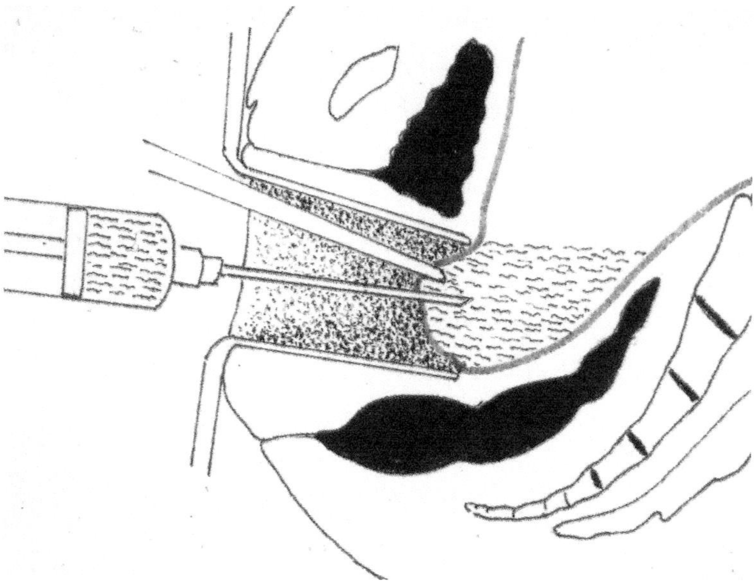

Fig. 13.4 Aspiration of the saline fluid from the pouch of Douglas

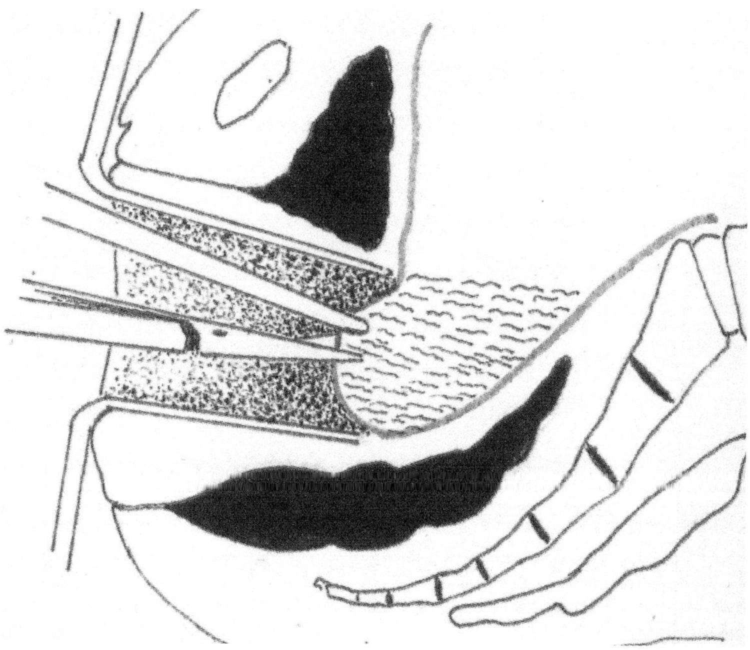

Fig. 13.5 Incision of the peritoneum at the point of fluid aspiration

reflection reached is the pouch of Douglas, because the saline infused accumulates at the lowest point of the peritoneal cavity (Fig. 13.4). The peritoneum is grabbed with two pincers, and an incision is performed in between and the peritoneum opened allowing the fluid evacuation down the preformed perineal cavity (Fig. 13.5). The incision is enlarged and with the aid of

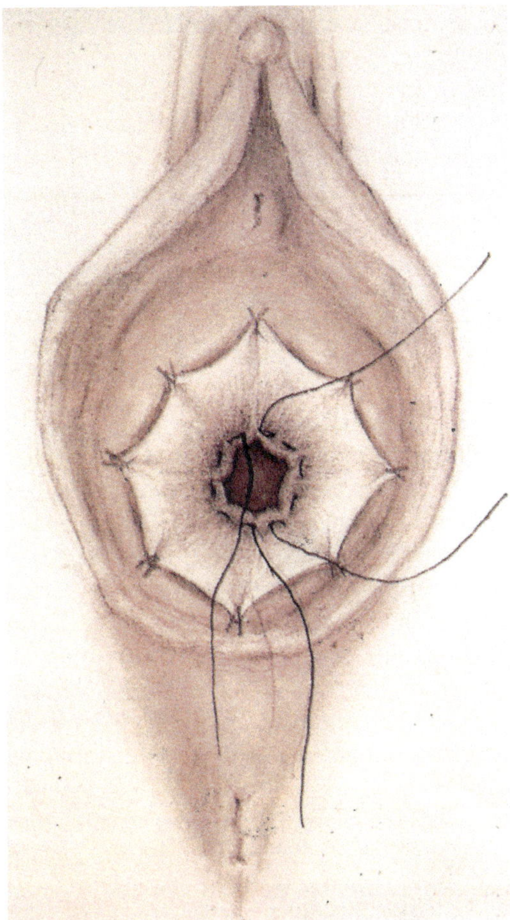

Fig. 13.6 The two semicircular continuous sutures closing the top of the neovaginal cavity

traction the incised peritoneum is then transposed and brought down the preformed perineal cavity and finally sutured to the introitus of the neovagina with 4–6 sutures that are placed on the margins of the incised peritoneum. Cranially the peritoneal lining of the neovagina is closed at the level of appropriate depth, which is usually around 10–12 cm deep. Two semicircular continuous sutures of absorbable material 2-0 are used for closure as shown (Fig. 13.6), and making these sutures is the most difficult step in the operative procedure because of the depth of the workplace.

At the end of the operation, a self-made vaginal mould is inserted into the neovagina that fits in the vaginal cavity but is placed above the pelvic floor structures. It is fixed with some stitches to the skin of the vulva. Foley catheter remains in place.

13.3 Abdominal Surgery

When performing peritoneal vaginoplasty for vaginal aplasia, i.e. Mayer-Rokitansky-Kuster-Hauser syndrome, abdominal surgery is usually avoided. Although some particular cases do need abdominal surgical approach, i.e. difficulty in dissection and small size of the space between the bladder and rectum and gonadectomy in cases of androgen insensitivity syndrome, a laparoscopic approach can be used (if difficult, Pfannenstiel incision or median laparotomy can be used). The preformed vaginal cavity is packed with a sterile gauze. When the pouch of Douglas is identified, the caudal part of the peritoneum is incised over the gauze previously packed in the neovaginal cavity. Stay sutures are placed on the borders of the incision which are then pulled down through the perineal opening; the procedure goes on exactly the same way as previously described with fixation of the peritoneum to the neovaginal introitus. The fundus of the neovagina is finally closed transabdominally in a similar manner (like from the perineum) and a vaginal mould inserted.

13.4 Intraoperative Complications

During the procedure of forming the vaginal cavity, the integrity of the rectum and bladder has to be preserved. This is why the bladder is filled with methylene blue before starting the intervention. This enables the surgeon to notice if the bladder is injured during the procedure. The Foley catheter and balloon also serve as guides during dissection. With a gloved finger put into the rectum, it is possible to displace the rectum dorsally and protect it from injury. Even if the bladder or rectum is opened during the procedure, the opening is closed with a double-layered suture. In our hospital there had never been complications associated with fistula formation after the damage was immediately recognised and fixed. The percentage of intraoperative lesions is small: less than 3 % for bowel and bladder injury together.

13.5 Postoperative Period

The Foley catheter and vaginal mould are removed on the fifth to seventh postoperative day. The neovagina is then washed with sterile saline solution, and a new vaginal mould is inserted. Anaesthesia is not necessary though the procedure – removing stitches – can be painful. Afterwards the vaginal mould has to be removed, and the procedure repeated daily, twice during the first month and after that once a day. It is advisable to clean the neovagina with antiseptic solution. The vaginal tutor has to be washed by tap water every time before it is reinserted into the neovagina. Estrogenic ointment can also be applied on the tutor. The patient is taught by the nurses to perform this procedure by herself in just a few days. It is important that the patient is mature enough and that she is in a relationship and wanting to start with sexual intercourses. If not, the compliance is not good enough and it may affect the success of the operation.

After the patient is discharged from the department, she is instructed to wear the vaginal mould in place all day long, except when the cleaning of the neovagina and mould have to be done. The patient is followed up monthly until epithelialisation of the neovagina is completed. It is advisable to start with sexual intercourses after 2 months.

If after some time the patient has no regular sexual intercourses, she is advised to wear the vaginal mould during night for some period. She is also instructed to perform vaginal dilations daily. This way the vaginal width and depth can be preserved, otherwise neovaginal shortening can occur. After the neovagina is fully epithelialised, manual dilations and vaginal moulds are not necessary anymore.

The neovagina becomes epithelialised and covered with pluristratified non-keratinised epithelium over a period of 2–12 months. It is not known why there is such a difference in epithelialisation time among patients (the factors affecting growth rapidity of vaginal epithelium is not known).

13.6 Vaginal Moulds

After the operation is finished, a self-made vaginal mould is used, which is made of sponge. It is measured and fashioned according to vaginal width and depth obtained for the actual patient. Usually it measures 10–12 cm in length and 3.5–4 cm in width. Before it is inserted into the neovagina, it is covered with a preservative (condom) and lubricated.

On the fifth to seventh postoperative day, the sponge mould is removed and substituted with a custom-made silicone vaginal tutor. It is pear shaped and the size is measured according to neovaginal size. The usual size is 6–7 cm in length and 3–3.5 cm in width. When properly inserted it is situated superior to the perineal musculature. This way it does not produce any discomfort to the patient, not even in sports or other activities, similarly as the menstrual tampon (Figs. 13.7 and 13.8).

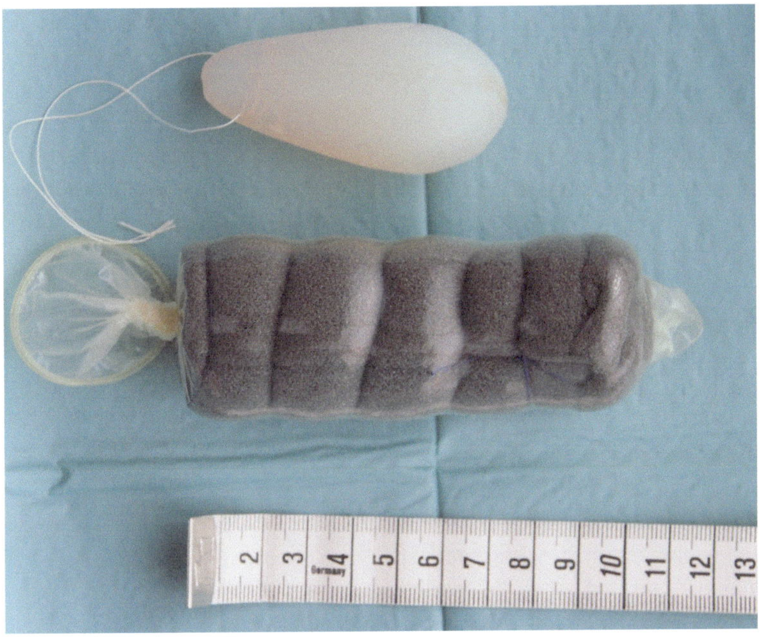

Fig. 13.7 Photograph of a permanent silicone mould used by patients till the vagina is epithelialised and a sponge mould covered with condom put into the neovagina immediately after the operation

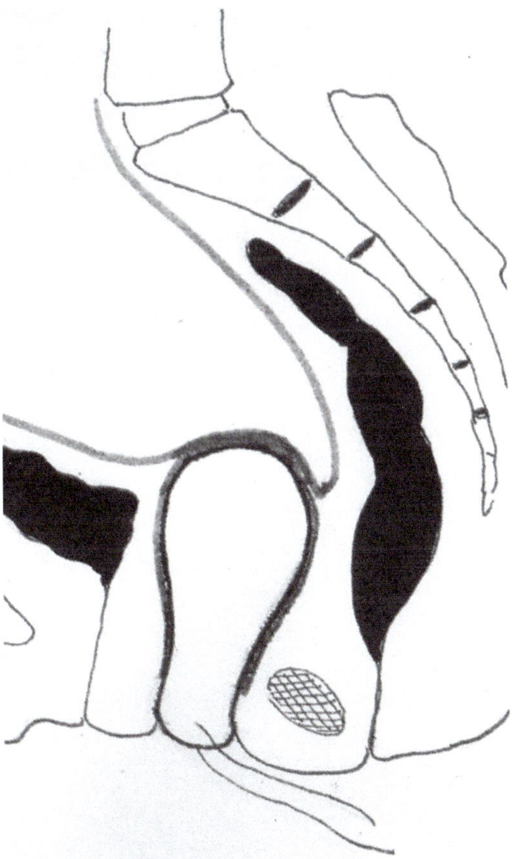

Fig. 13.8 After being fully epithelialised, the neovagina is covered with normal stratified squamous epithelium

13.7 Other Techniques

In the patients that have at least some centimetres of vaginal cavity, it is possible to perform Frank's dilation. Frank described the method in 1938 and it is used worldwide with modifications. Sometimes even the patients themselves not knowing about their condition have successful sexual life and with regular vaginal intercourses prolong the vaginal cavity till it is sufficiently long. In the era of easier surgical interventions, we sometimes forget the method and recruit a patient, in whom the Frank's method would be successful, to surgery. Nevertheless the vaginal dilation and prolongation method should be offered as the first-line treatment to chosen patients, and surgical treatment becomes a choice only when long-term dilation is refused or fails and the surgical technique is fully explained to the patient.

There are numerous surgical techniques described, each of them with its advantages and disadvantages, and the best method is not determined yet, because the case series are usually too small. With no standardised indications and treatment results (regarding also the satisfaction of patients with the different technique outcomes), it is not possible to compare different techniques.

In the review article published in 2013, it is stated that a patient with vaginal aplasia does not get the best treatment for herself but is treated with the technique used in the hospital to which she is referred [6].

In the past one of the most widely used techniques was vaginoplasty with the sigmoid colon, which was abandoned for its disadvantages in most of the centres, but with a minimally invasive laparoscopic approach, it continues to be performed in others [7].

Vaginoplasty using vulvoperineal flaps is a technique that leaves too many scars, and the skin grafts pose a lot of problems after – the length and width of the vagina diminish with time – so continuous dilation is needed when the patient has no sexual intercourses [8].

Many different techniques used in creating a neovagina have been introduced and used till now: Abbe-McIndoe's modification of split thickness graft, Williams vaginoplasty (and Creatsas' modification), the Vecchietti operation with postoperative daily dilation till successful result is achieved, and then techniques using amnion, buccal mucosa graft [9], or skin graft. There are numerous other modifications of already known techniques with little case series [10, 11]. As many surgeons are more capable of laparoscopic than vaginal approach, laparoscopy has become an excellent help for presenting the right route during the creation of neovaginal cavity and thus preventing intraoperative complications and shortening the intervention time.

With modified Davydov's technique, very good results are obtained so it is the first choice in our hospital.

Conclusion

Peritoneal vaginoplasty is a relatively safe procedure for the patient. The complication rates are low. The outcome is satisfactory since the size of the neovagina tends to remain constant. Even when shortening or loss of width occurs, the neovagina and introitus can be dilated to sufficient size so as to permit the patient to have intercourse. After being fully epithelialised, the neovagina is covered with normal stratified squamous epithelium, which provides natural lubrication to the neovagina and is hormonally responsive.

References

1. Fetih A (1999) Creazione di vagina artificiale dal peritoneo pelvico. Il transessualismo, Editrice Kurtis, Milano: 107–112
2. Davydov SN (1980) 12 Jahre Erfahrung mit Kolpopoesis unter Verwendung von Peritoneum. Gynakologe 13:120–121
3. Fetih A (1990) Plastika neovagine s transpozicijo pelveoperitoneja. Diplomska naloga za akademsko specializacijo, Ljubljana: Medicinska fakulteta (Surgical therapy of congenital vaginal aplasia with pelveo-peritoneum transpositional methods. Master of Science Thesis, Medical Faculty, Ljubljana, 1990)
4. Radzuweit H (1990) Das phallusphantom – ein uberflussige Relikt bei der Korektur der Vaginal aplasie. Zbl Gyn 102:519–526
5. Willemsen WNP (1982) Neovagina-plastiek met peritoneum transpositie. Krips repro meppel, Nyjmegen
6. McQuillan SK, Grover RS (2014) Dilation and surgical management in vaginal agenesis: a systematic review. Int Urogynecol J 25(3):299–311. doi:10.1007/s00192-013-2221-9. Epub 2013 Oct 10
7. Zhong CX, Wu JX, Liang JX et al (2012) Laparoscopic and gasless laparoscopic sigmoid colon vaginoplasty in women with vaginal agenesis. Chin Med J (Engl) 125:203–208
8. Lanza H, Balestrelli J, Pastoni D et al (2013) Vaginoplasty technique using vulvoperineal flaps. Aesthetic Plast Surg. doi:10.1007/s00266-013-0220-3
9. Lin WC, Chang CYY, Shen YY et al (2003) Use of autologous buccal mucosa for vaginoplasty: a study of eight cases. Hum Reprod 18:604–607
10. Miyahara Y, Yoshida S, Shirakawa T et al (2012) Less invasive new vaginoplasty using laparoscopy, atelocollagen sponge, and hand-made mould. Kobe J Med Sci 58:E138–E144
11. Sang WK, Dong YK, Deuk YO et al (2013) Use of a silicone gel sheet vaginal mould in McIndoe vaginoplasty. Arch Plast Surg 40:652–655

14 Technical Suggestions for Better and Lasting Functional and Aesthetic Outcomes in Creating the Neoclitoris

Carlo Trombetta, Fulvio Colombo, Paolo Umari, Giovanni Liguori, Michele Rizzo, Miloš Petrović, and Giorgio Gentile

14.1 Introduction

Sex reassignment surgery (SRS) is a very complex field of reconstructive surgery. Among many reconstructive solutions already described, urethral and clitoral reconstruction remains one of the most challenging fields. This is a very difficult and demanding step of the intervention, often followed by complications that have a grave impact on long-term results, quality of life and general patient satisfaction.

The expectations of individuals undergoing male-to-female SRS are often very high, especially as regards cosmetics and functionality. To reach these expectations and make the patient satisfied, a great knowledge of reconstructive surgery techniques and aesthetic refinements is required.

Since then many experts, as Rubin, Pandya, Malloy, Perovic, Eldh and so on, are trying to construct a genitalia resembling that of the female with the aim of forming a functioning neovagina that enables patients to have sexual intercourses, a patent and stenosis-free urethral neomeatus and a sensitive neoclitoris [1–5].

The standard procedure for neoclitoral reconstruction in male-to-female sex reassignment surgery is generally considered as the use of the dorsal portion of the glans penis with a pedicled island neurovascular flap. This flap was initially described by Hinderer for intersex anomalies and later by Brown specifically for neoclitoroplasty in transsexuals. The neoclitoris is usually exposed through a small cutaneous incision at the midline of the posteriorly advanced penopubic area, the latter being the pedicle of the skin flap [6, 7].

Hage et al. described a new technique applying Eicher's method using a free glandular graft and a shortening of the neurovascular bundle. The neoclitoris is created using a free graft of the tip of the glans incorporating the urethral orifice [8].

Giraldo et al. proposed a modification of clitoroplasty based on the possibility of elevating a bifid coronal flap from the glans penis for configuration of the neoclitoris. The authors called this method the "corona glans clitoroplasty" to differentiate it from the well-known "dorsal glans clitoroplasty" [9].

Some authors evaluated the sexual function results in patients after 3 months from surgery. Selvaggi et al. measured neoclitoral orgasmic sensitivity 4 years after male-to-female sex reassignment surgery demonstrating that sexual

C. Trombetta (✉) • P. Umari • G. Liguori • M. Rizzo
Department of Urology, Cattinara Hospital,
Strada di Fiume 447, Trieste 34100, Italy
e-mail: trombcar@units.it; paoloumari@alice.it; mik.rizzo@gmail.com

F. Colombo • G. Gentile
Department of Urology, Policlinico S. Orsola Malpighi, Via Albertoni 15, Bologna 40138, Italy
e-mail: dr.giorgio.gentile@gmail.com

M. Petrović
Department of Urology, General Hospital of Izola, Via Polje 40, Izola 6310, Slovenia
e-mail: 5rovic.milos@gmail.com

C. Trombetta et al. (eds.), *Management of Gender Dysphoria: A Multidisciplinary Approach*,
DOI 10.1007/978-88-470-5696-1_14, © Springer-Verlag Italia 2015

arousal is not present in all patients. The authors suggest that keeping the pedicled, reshaped and replaced glans for creation of the clitoris is fundamental for preservation of sensitivity. They also supposed that pain during sexual intercourse (due to unlubricated neovagina) could cover sexual sensation coming from the stimulation of the neoclitoris [10].

In this chapter, we minutely describe two different techniques that permit to construct a functional and aesthetically pleasing neoclitoral complex emphasising the most important and critical steps.

The two techniques have been applied in Italy in a great series of patients by two different surgical equipment in Trieste and Bologna.

Both techniques entail the use of a small part of the dorsal aspect of the glans penis, with preservation of the dorsal neurovascular bundle (DNVB). The main features that distinguish these two techniques are the modality of the DNVB dissection (with or without the preservation of the underlying tunica albuginea) and the utilisation of the urethral tissue.

The first technique is *the neourethroclitoroplasty with microsurgical dissection of the DNVB*; the urethral flaps are used in continuity with the previously spatulated urethral plate in order to surround the neoclitoris and construct a neourethroclitoris covered by the urethral neoprepuce. On the contrary, in the second technique, *the dorsal part of the tunica albuginea is preserved*, acting as a framework for the attached DNVB. The neoclitoris is configured maintaining the inner foreskin mucosa attached to the glans and the remaining subglandular urethral part is used for the creation of the epithelial lining between the neoclitoris and the urethral neomeatus.

14.2 Surgical Technique

14.2.1 Neourethroclitoroplasty with Microsurgical Dissection of the DNVB: "Trieste Technique"

This technique can be clearly explained in three main steps: the dissection of the neurovascular bundle, the preparation of the urethra and the urethral plate formation; the construction of the neomeatus; and the assembly of the neoclitoral hood.

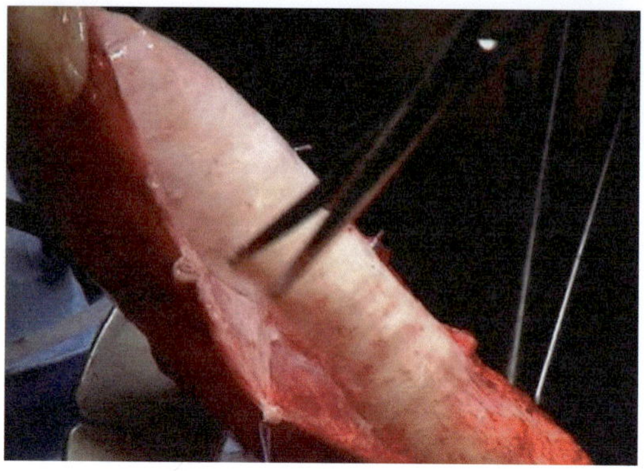

Fig. 14.1 DNVB dissection from the underlying tunica albuginea is performed starting from the sides of the urethra bilaterally

14.2.1.1 Neurovascular Bundle Dissection and Neoclitoris Formation

The neoclitoris is created from the dorsal part of the glans penis. A glans island should be carefully isolated preserving the neurovascular bundle that contains nerves and blood vessels.

A tourniquet is placed at the base of the degloved penile shaft and hydraulic erection is established. The DNVB dissection from the underlying tunica albuginea is performed starting from the sides of the urethra bilaterally (Fig. 14.1). The use of microsurgical loupes may help the surgeon during this manoeuvre. The neurovascular bundle is meticulously dissected within Buck's fascia along the entire penile shaft. It sometimes happens that the DNVB appears particularly hypotrophic and thin due to prolonged hormonal therapy. At this point, the risk of injury is high, so it is preferred to perform a partial microsurgical dissection of the DNVB. The glans penis is entirely dissected from the corpora cavernosa of the penis maintaining continuity with the DNVB (Fig. 14.2). At this point, the neoclitoris' shape is outlined and dissected from the dorsal part of the glans penis along the previously marked lines. The amount of spongiosal tissue may be greater than a real female clitoris, thus avoiding postoperative loss of sensitivity. The urethral tissue should be removed from the neoclitoris flap ventrally.

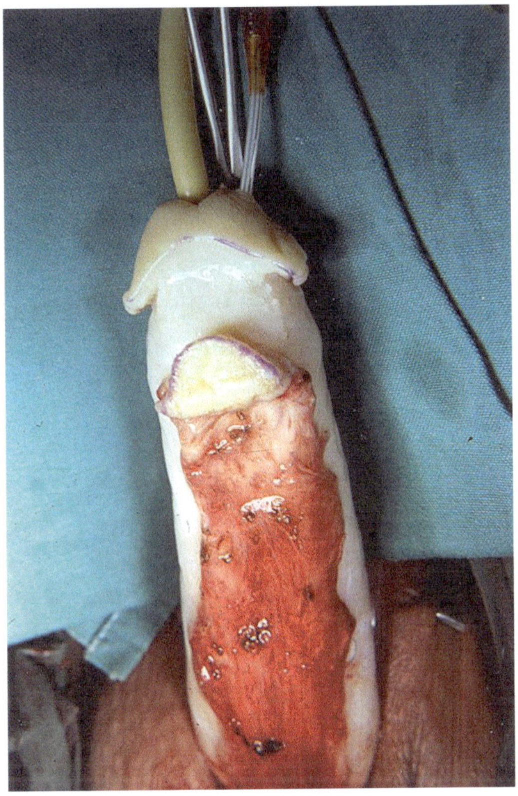

Fig. 14.2 The glans penis is entirely dissected from the corpora cavernosa of the penis maintaining continuity with the DNVB

14.2.1.2 Urethral Dissection and Spatulation of the Urethral Plate with Removal of the Bulbs

The urethra is carefully dissected from the corpora cavernosa within Buck's fascia and shortened approximately 7 cm distally from the bulbous urethra. It is then spatulated ventrally all down to the bulb where the neourethral meatus will be formed (Fig. 14.3a, b). The spongiosal tissue of the bulbous urethra is carefully removed, in order to prevent bulking sensation during sexual arousal and consequently difficult and painful penetration [11]. For this step the utilisation of Ligasure or a similar surgical instrument is a good solution since profuse bleeding can be difficult to control. The urethral plate is further incised dorsally on the distal end following the median line to form a forking (Fig. 14.4a, b). It is very important to avoid damage of the urethral circulation which runs laterally on both sides of the urethral plate.

14.2.1.3 Urethral Neomeatus Construction and Neourethroclitoral Complex with Neoclitoral Hood Assembly

The neoclitoris is unified with the urethral plate at the level of the bifurcation, between both urethral flaps. The neoclitoris is joined with urethral flaps in two layers: spongiosum tissue of the urethral flap is sutured with the spongiosal tissue of the neoclitoris and the urethral mucosa is sutured with the neoclitoris epithelium (Fig. 14.5a, b). Urethral flaps are fixed around the neoclitoris (Fig. 14.6a, b). At this point the newly created neourethroclitoris complex is transposed ventrally through the incision in the penile skin flap, which runs above it. The urethral plate with the urethra-clitoris complex is joined and sutured to the surrounding penile skin flap.

14.2.2 Neoclitoroplasty with the Preservation of the Tunica Albuginea: "Bologna Technique"

Here, the two longitudinal incisions are made directly onto the tunica albuginea, without the need of isolation of the DNVB. The albuginea is incised longitudinally parallel to the urethra, care being taken to reduce the width of its terminal by 2 cm. By this way, a strip of albuginea is prepared, running from the glans to the common portion of the corpora cavernosa, carrying the neurovascular bundle on it (Fig. 14.7). This surgical step is completed by the resection of the residual cavernous tissue from the ventral aspect of the albugineal strip.

The neurovascular bundle and the underlying albuginea is bended on itself and fixed in the suprapubic area in order to create the mons veneris. According to the technique proposed by Perovic, the neoclitoris is configured/built maintaining the inner foreskin (mucosal) attached to the glans [12]. The urethra is divided 4–5 cm proximally from the meatus and the glans is opened ventrally. Glans reduction is done medially, leaving its sides intact, in order to preserve the vascular support of both the neoclitoris and the foreskin that will become the neolabia minora.

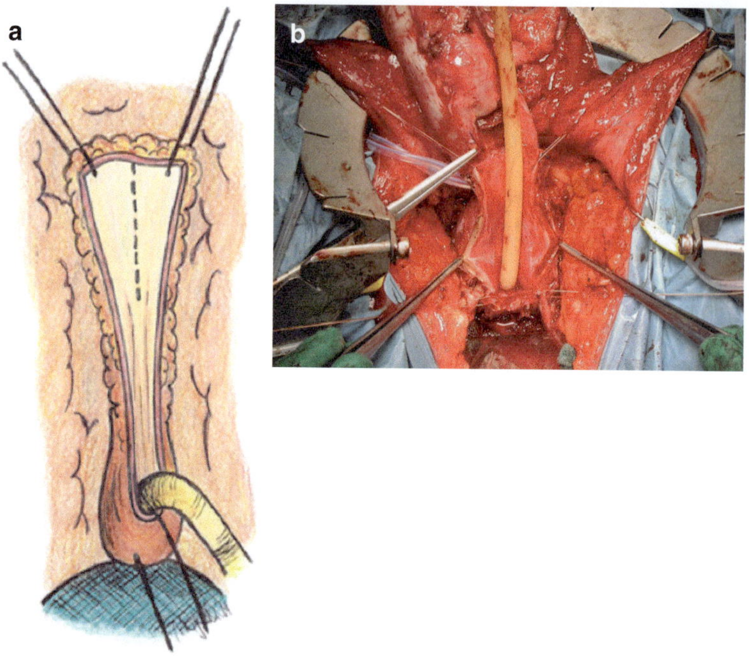

Fig. 14.3 (**a**, **b**) The urethra is shortened approximately 7 cm distally from the bulbous urethral and it is spatulated ventrally

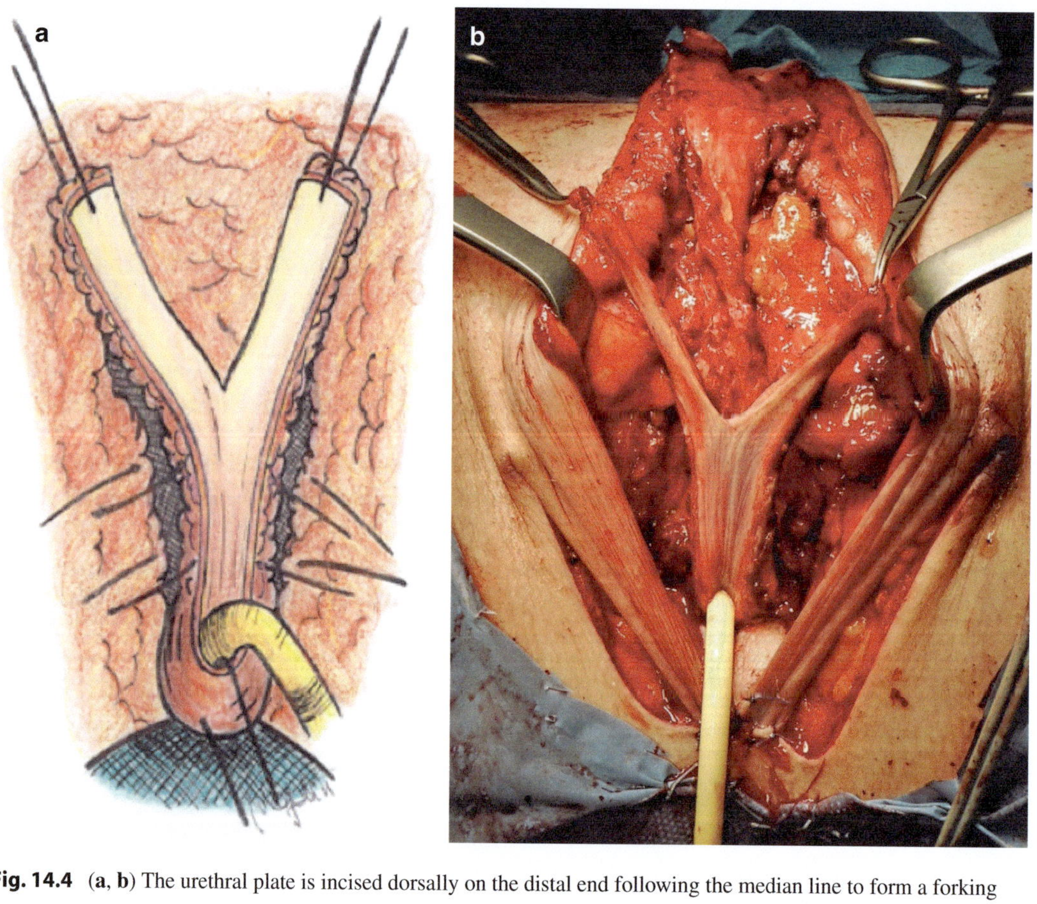

Fig. 14.4 (**a**, **b**) The urethral plate is incised dorsally on the distal end following the median line to form a forking

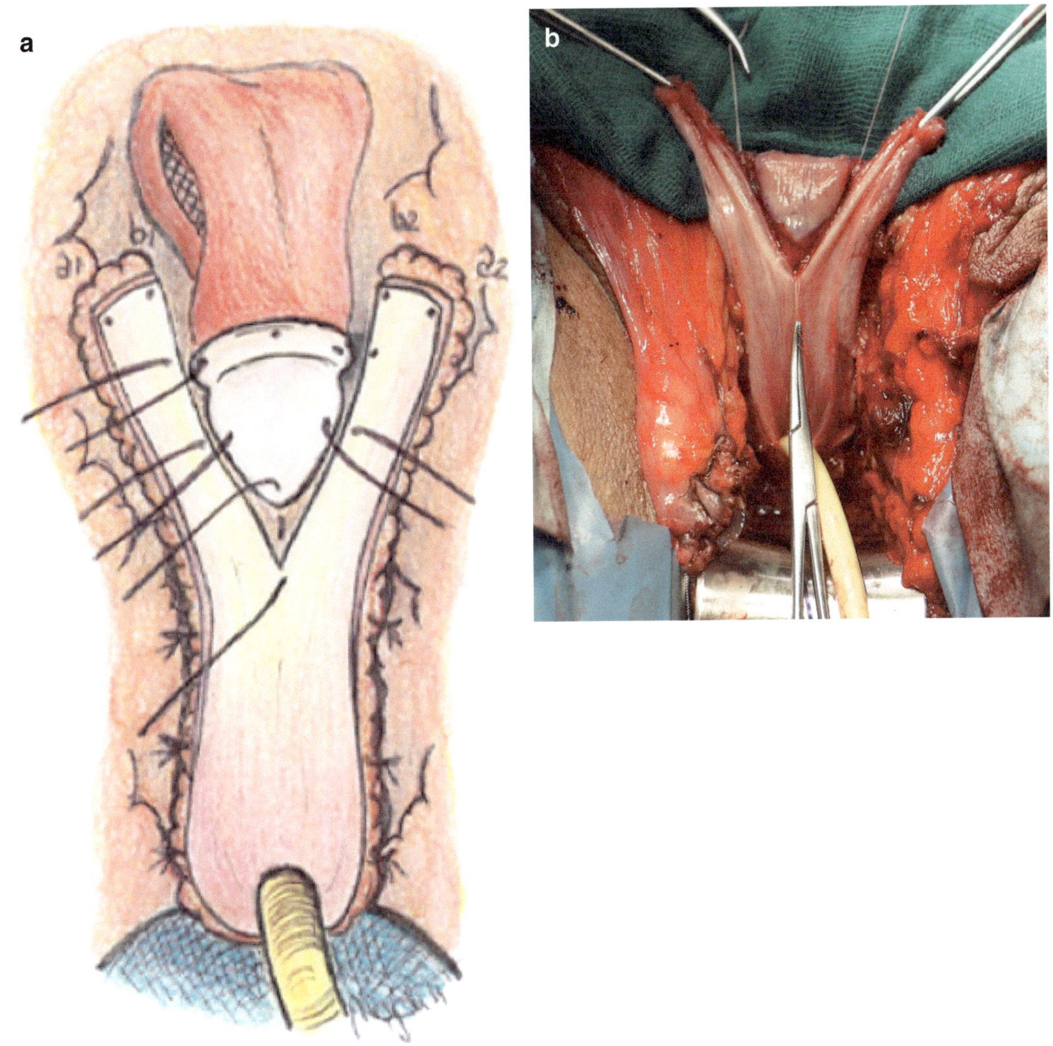

Fig. 14.5 (**a**, **b**) The neoclitoris is unified with the urethral plate at the level of the bifurcation and sutured in two layers

The neoclitoris and its preputial hood are then positioned and fixed in a proper distance from the new urethral meatus. The remaining subglandular urethral part is used for the creation of the epithelial lining between the neoclitoris and the urethral meatus (Fig. 14.2).

14.3 Postoperative Care

In the immediate postoperative period, intensive monitoring of the neourethroclitoris complex is of essential importance. In the absence of major bleeding, the dressing is removed and changed 48 h after surgery. After that the neourethra and neoclitoris area should be adequately medicated at least once a day to maintain adequate hygiene and avoid infections. It is recommended to use antiseptic dressing. The application of antibiotic ointments is not indicated routinely. Prompt discovery of necrotic or infected areas should be followed by surgical therapy with debridement and dressing.

The catheter should be frequently mobilised to avoid formation of decubitus ulcer on the neomeatus and neoclitoris. It should be left in place until the wound edges looked properly closed in order to avoid contact with urine that slows the healing process. Usually the catheter is left in place approximately until the 5th postoperative day.

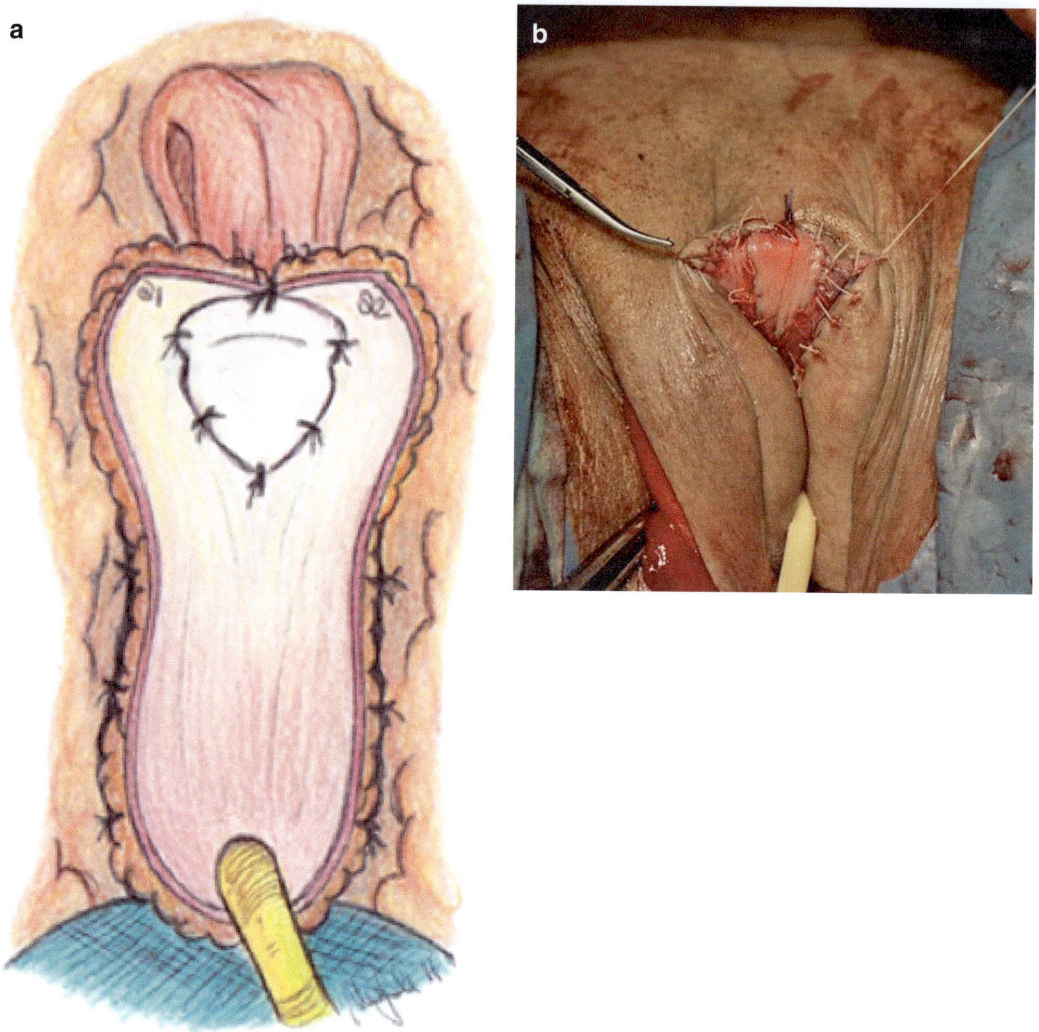

Fig. 14.6 (**a**, **b**) Urethral flaps are fixed around the neoclitoris

Some patients may experience pain due to hypersensitivity of the neoclitoris. In that case, lidocaine ointments can be useful.

A psychosexological support is essential since the first postoperative day to start learning about new anatomy, function and appearance of the genitalia. In the past a group of patients have been evaluated by means of preoperative and postoperative biothesiometry [13].

14.4 Complications

Complications can be divided into intraoperative (lesion of the neuromuscular bundle, lesion of the urethra, haemorrhage), early postoperative (partial or total neoclitoris, urethral plate and skin flap necrosis) and late postoperative (urethral stenosis, neoclitoral atrophy, hyposensitivity or insensitivity).

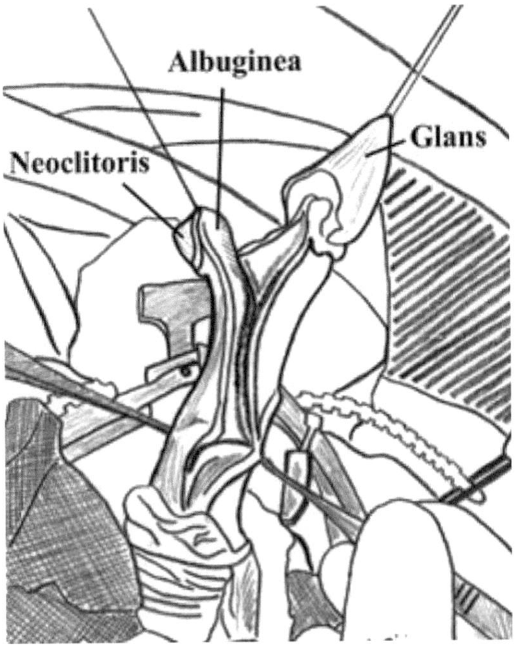

Fig. 14.7 Neoclitoroplasty with the preservation of the tunica albuginea; a strip of albuginea carrying the neurovascular bundle is prepared

14.4.1 Intraoperative Complications

Neoclitoris ischaemia is possible but avoidable with meticulous technique of dissection and in selected cases with partial microsurgical dissection of the DNVB. When ischaemia occurs, it is usually recognised early intraoperatively. A clitoris that becomes pale during the isolation of the neurovascular bundle or during the fixation means that probably there is an ischaemia. The most common sites of neurovascular bundle injuries are the site of insertion into the glans, the origin at the level of ligamentum suspensorium and between the crura of the corpora cavernosa. It is extremely important to maintain as much as possible the blood supply of the urethra while making the dissection between the urethra, bladder and rectum and also during the detachment of corpora cavernosa. At the same time, an accurate haemostasis of the potential sources of significant bleeding is mandatory. The surgeon may decide to put a soft drainage if considered necessary.

14.4.2 Early Postoperative Complications

Early postoperative complications associated with bleeding and necrosis of the urethral flaps surrounding the neoclitoris are rare. Necrotised tissue should be removed and appropriate dressing applied. Complications associated with wound or urinary tract infections are more common and are often successfully treated with appropriate antibiotic therapy. Rarely there is a prolonged bleeding from the operative site (neourethra, neovagina), and occasionally blood transfusion is needed.

14.4.3 Late Postoperative Complications

Neoclitoris atrophy and loss of sensation are serious but fortunately rare complications. It can be avoided with a good surgical technique and preservation of a neoclitoris of adequate size.

Stenosis of the urethral neomeatus is also rare because of the large spatulation of the urethra.

14.5 Discussion

The configuration of a neoclitoris with good aesthetic and functional results is mandatory to achieve complete postoperative satisfaction in transgender patients. Unfortunately a surgical technique that enables to construct a neoclitoris and neovulva that are indistinguishable from female's does not exist until now. A long learning curve and a high dexterity of the surgeon positively influence the outcome of the intervention.

Since the first surgical procedures of male-to-female SRS, many surgeons have used the glans penis to create a neoclitoris. Edgerton et al. and Marten Perolino et al. suggested preserving all the glans penis and the neurovascular bundle with the overlying penis cutis placed at the bottom of the neovagina [14, 15]. Some authors prefer to leave the glans penis intact, with excision of the urethral tissue ventrally. The risk of postoperative atrophy and loss of sensation is lower, but the size of the neoclitoris is aesthetically unacceptable

[1]. A solution to avoid this problem is a wide disepithelisation of the glans penis, with exclusion of the neoclitoris area. In this way, the skin can be sutured around the neoclitoris area previously disepithelisated, hiding the remaining part of the glans penis underneath [16]. The glans pedicled flap is accepted to be the most important key point in maintaining erogenous sensations and its use becomes the standard procedure for clitoroplasty in male-to-female SRS [17, 18].

The techniques for clitoral reconstruction in transsexuals with glans reduction we've described above are relatively widely used and safe [19, 20]. Postoperative complications as neoclitoral atrophy and loss of sensation are not frequent but can occur. We described two modalities of DNVB dissection that can be chosen considering the habits and the preferences of the surgeon. DNVB dissection preserving the tunica albuginea may offer some advantages in certain cases: it is time saving, in fact the reduction in operating time is about 30 min and a further reduction to about 45 min can be obtained if the albuginea is cut without isolating the Buck fascia, it is safer because there are less possibilities to damage the DNVB and it offers a satisfactory appearance of the pubic area that mimics a natural mons veneris. The microsurgical dissection of the DNVB is a more time-consuming procedure, but in our experience it does not significantly change the overall time of the intervention if it is performed by two surgical teams simultaneously, one operating on the penis and one on the perineum. The use of loupes may reduce the risk of DNVB injury and increase the dissection accuracy. In cases of hypotrophic DNVB due to prolonged hormonal therapy, the surgeon should take into consideration the partial microsurgical dissection.

The urethral tissue can be utilised in different ways. It can be used to increase the diameter of the neovagina and provide more moisture, as proposed by Passerini in paediatric intersex surgery [21]. The same principle was then applied to male-to-female reassignment surgery described by Perovic [12]. Pain sensation during sexual intercourse is often referred by patient who underwent this kind of surgery.

In most "standard" SRS techniques, a wide portion of the penile urethra is removed. The urethral neomeatus is then performed simply by suturing the urethral stump to a preformed hole in the penile skin flap. This is a relatively simple approach but is usually associated with postoperative meatal stenosis, urinary dysfunction and unnatural appearance. The creation of the urethral meatus combined with a wide spatulation of the urethra, like we've described above (neourethroclitoroplasty with microsurgical dissection of the DNVB), decreases the risk of postoperative meatal stenosis. In this way the newly created urethral meatus is anatomically correctly positioned and aesthetically acceptable.

With neourethroclitoroplasty the urethral flaps surrounding the neoclitoris form a prepuce that covers the neoclitoris. The urethral flaps around the clitoris provide some moisture, and there is no hair growth around the clitoris.

The urethral flaps can be sometimes damaged during urethral plate incision and suturing. The midline incision has to be done very carefully and precisely in order to preserve as much as possible the urethral vascularisation that runs laterally. During suturing, as less as possible tissue should be damaged with tension-free sutures. It is also very important to preserve the vascularisation of the urethral plate during the removal of the spongiosal tissue. A complete removal avoids difficult and painful penetration during sexual intercourses [11].

While sectioning the centrum tendineum and advancing the dissection between the rectum and urethra and also while removing the corpora cavernosa from their attachments, care should be taken not to injure the urethral arteries that run laterally at the base of the bulbar part of the urethra.

References

1. Rubin SO (1993) Sex-reassignment surgery male-to-female. Review, own results and report of a new technique using the glans penis as a pseudoclitoris. Scand J Urol Nephrol Suppl 154:1–28
2. Pandya NJ, Stuteville OH (1973) A one-stage technique for constructing female external genitalia in male transsexuals. Br J Plast Surg 26(3):277–282

3. Malloy TR, Noone RB, Morgan AJ (1976) Experience with the 1-stage surgical approach for constructing female genitalia in male transsexuals. J Urol 116(3): 335–337
4. Perovic SV, Stanojevic DS, Djordjevic ML (2000) Vaginoplasty in male transsexuals using penile skin and a urethral flap. BJU Int 86:843–850
5. Eldh J (1993) Construction of a neovagina with preservation of the glans penis as a clitoris in male transsexuals. Plast Reconstr Surg 91(5):895–900; discussion 901–3
6. Hinderer UT (1989) Reconstruction of the external genitalia in the adrenogenital syndrome by means of a personal one-stage procedure. Plast Reconstr Surg 84:325
7. Brown J (1976) Creation of a functional clitoris and aesthetically pleasing introitus in sex conversion. In: Marchac D, Hueston JT (eds) Transactions of the sixth international congress of plastic and reconstructive surgery. Masson, Paris, pp. 654–655
8. Hage JJ, Karim RB, Bloem JJ, Suliman HM, van Alphen M (1994) Sculpturing the neoclitoris in vaginoplasty for male-to-female transsexuals. Plast Reconstr Surg 93(2):358–364
9. Giraldo F, Esteva I, Bergero T, Cano G, González C, Salinas P, Rivada E, Lara JS, Soriguer F, Andalusia Gender Team (2004) Corona glans clitoroplasty and urethropreputial vestibuloplasty in male-to-female transsexuals: the vulval aesthetic refinement by the Andalusia Gender Team. Plast Reconstr Surg 114:1543–1550
10. Selvaggi G, Monstrey S, Ceulemans P et al (2007) Genital sensitivity after sex reassignment surgery in transsexual patients. Ann Plast Surg 58:427–433
11. Karim RB (1991) The importance of near total resection of the corpus spongiosum and total resection of the corpora cavernosa in the surgery of male to female transsexuals. Ann Plast Surg 26(6):554–556
12. Perovic S (1993) Male to female surgery: a new contribution to operative technique. Plast Reconstr Surg 91:703–711
13. Buttazzi L, Trombetta C, Liguori G, Bucci S, Belgrano E (2001) Valutazione della sensibilità del neoclitoride in seguito ad intervento di conversione androginoide. Atti del 74° Congresso della Società Italiana di Urologia (S.I.U.), Cagliari, 9–12 maggio 2001, pp 40–41, abstract book
14. Edgerton MT, Knorr NJ, Callison JR (1970) The surgical treatment of transsexual patients: limitations and indications. Plast Reconstr Surg 45:38–46
15. Marten-Perolino R, Cocimano V, Marino G (1990) Male-female transsexualization with glandular preservation. Arch Ital Urol Nefrol Androl 62(1):101–105
16. Spehr C (2007) Male-to-female sex reassignment surgery in transsexuals. Int J Transgenderism 10(1):25–37
17. Fang RH, Chen CF, Ma S (1992) A new method for clitoroplasty in male-to-female sex reassignment surgery. Plast Reconstr Surg 89(4):679–682
18. Rubin SO (1980) A method of preserving the glans penis as a clitoris in sex conversion operations in male transsexuals. Scand J Urol Nephrol 14(3):215–217
19. Trombetta C, Liguori G, Benvenuto S, Petrovic M, Napoli R, Umari P, Rizzo M, Zordani A (2011) Neo-urethroclitoroplasty according to Petrovic. Urologia 78(4):267–273
20. Soli M, Brunocilla E, Bertaccini A, Palmieri F, Barbieri B, Martorana G (2008) Male to female gender reassignment: modified surgical technique for creating the neoclitoris and mons veneris. J Sex Med 5(1):210–216
21. Passerini-Glazel G (1989) A new procedure for clitorovaginoplasty in severely masculinized female pseudohermaphrodites. J Urol 142:565–568, 572

15 Feminization Laryngoplasty: Surgical Therapy

Andrea Luigi Cavalot and Diego Cossu

15.1 Phoniatric Evaluation

People looking for an alleged gender identity disorder (GID) must begin a complex path.

The fundamental purpose of the standards of care is to articulate the consensus among different organized professionals to management regarding psychological, medical, and surgical treatment of GID. These standards provide guidance for professional practice, providing the minimum requirements for the treatment procedure. An accurate diagnosis (*diagnostic criteria for GID according to DSM-IV TR, 2000*) is structured in:

- A real life experience, preferably along with psychotherapy
- Hormonal therapy
- Surgical therapy (especially sex reassignment surgery and others including voice modification)

The female speech is very different from the male speech. Markers of female speech are [1] as follows:

- Higher fundamental frequency than in male.
- Intonation range and pitch variability are higher in female.
- Females tend to have more vocal expression, variety of pitch, and emphasis than males.
- Females tend to have rising intonation after sentences containing statements suggesting uncertainty.
- Females tend to have an overall breathy voice quality and some degree of dysphonia can be considered as attractive.
- The use of feminine modalities of phrasing.
- Nonverbal visual markers including maintaining eye contact, use of more hand/arm and upper body gestures, sitting closer, and occasionally touching the listener.

Because of differences in laryngeal size and mass, average fundamental frequency (f0) for females is higher (220 Hz) than for males (110 Hz). The perceived pitch of the laryngeal fundamental has long been accepted as an acoustic cue to speaker's sex. Thus, for male-to-female transsexuals, in order to be perceived as female voice, fundamental frequency must change.

An f0 of 165 Hz represents the borderline frequency above which a voice is perceived as female [2]. In case of androgynoid conversion (MtF), the use of female hormones can determine a smoother, thinner, and glabrous skin; it can cause moderate mammary gland hypertrophy, and overall it can offer a more feminine look.

A.L. Cavalot (✉) • D. Cossu (✉)
Department of ENT and Phoniatric, Santa Croce Hospital, Moncalieri, Tourin, Italy
e-mail: info@cavalot.it; diegocossu61@gmail.com

C. Trombetta et al. (eds.), *Management of Gender Dysphoria: A Multidisciplinary Approach*,
DOI 10.1007/978-88-470-5696-1_15, © Springer-Verlag Italia 2015

Intake of female hormones has *mild effects* on the vocal cords, larynx, and laryngeal skeleton *but has no effect on the vocal tract in general* [3].

So, with the intake of hormonal therapy, the f0 does not undergo a significant increase.

Consequently, these patients maintain a male voice type.

To increase the value of f0 before the MtF conversion, speech therapists pay attention to the following:

- Emphasize the pronunciation of consonants.
- Use a tone more gentle and subdued, even falsetto.
- Reduce the rounding of the mouth opening, contracting the length of the vocal tract by raising the tongue and the larynx.

This reduces the volume of the vocal tract amplifying the higher frequencies of the voice.

15.1.1 Methods to Change the Voice: FtM

The therapy is more simple when we transform a voice from female to male gender: testosterone administration produces an increase in the volume of the vocal cords and a consequent lowering of the voice, which normally follows a speech therapy rehabilitation.

In particular, an alternative method is represented by the injection of silicone or hydroxyapatite microgranules or autologous fat into the vocal cord to obtain the same effect (increase of the vibrating mass).

15.1.2 Methods to Change the Voice: MtF

The therapy is more complex in case of change from man to woman: as already mentioned, the hormones do not modify the laryngeal structure; surgery is needed in order to modify the structural aspects of the vocal cords, *tension, mass, and length*, and consequently the f0.

The fundamental frequency (f0) is a specific characteristic of each person, and it varies with age and gender. f0 at birth is the same in male and female. This value changes dramatically during puberty up to the values that allow to perceive a voice as female or male. The limit of perceptual discrimination between male and female voice is 165 Hz.

The f0 (fundamental frequency) is expressed by the following formula:

$$f0 = (1/2L)\sqrt{T/P}$$

where:

- *L* is the length of the vocal cord.
- *T* is the medium longitudinal tension.
- *P* is the density of tissue.

Then the three variables are as follows:

- Length
- Mass
- Tension

So, the f0 depends on the variation of these three parameters. The pitch (and specifically the f0) is directly proportional to the tension and inversely proportional to vocal cord length and mass.

It means that it is possible to elevate the fundamental frequency of glottal vibration (f0) by increasing the tension and/or reducing the mass and/or the length of vocal cords. It can be achieved by three different surgical procedures:

1. Mass reduction of the vocal folds
2. Tension increase of the vocal folds
3. Shortening the length of the vibrating portion of the vocal folds

15.1.3 Surgical Techniques to Increase the f0

15.1.3.1 Injection into the Vocal Muscle of Triamcinolone Acetate Depot

The procedure consists in the injection with triamcinolone into the vocal muscle, which can be performed under local anesthesia in fiberendoscopy or in direct microlaryngoscopy.

Triamcinolone is a long-lasting corticosteroid which has a side effect of the atrophy of soft tissues at the point of intramuscular injection. This side effect is used to reduce the mass of the vocal folds. This technique produces a temporary muscle hypotrophy and the f0 raising of approximately 25–40 Hz. It is an easy technique to perform but with conflicting and sometimes unpredictable results.

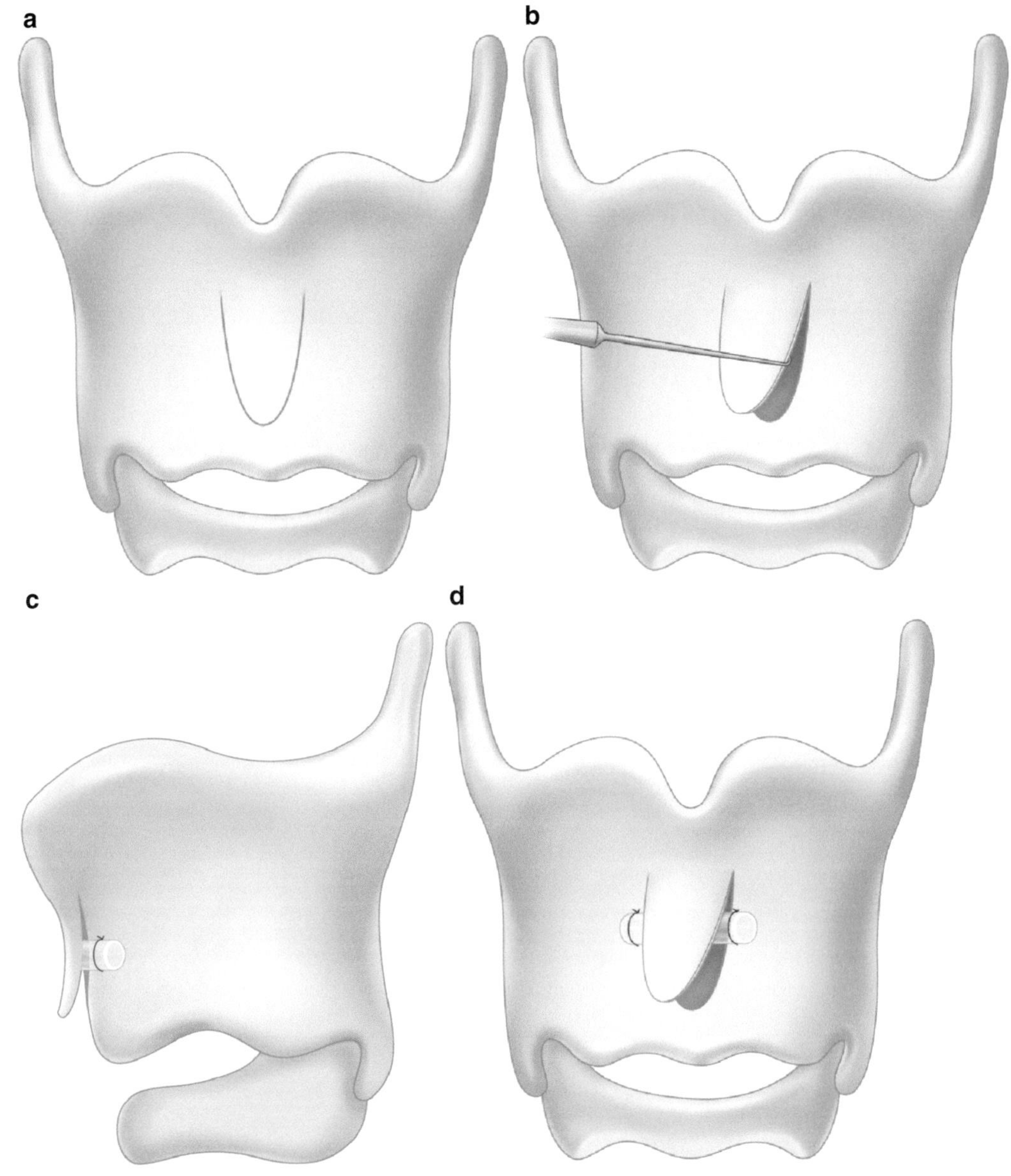

Fig. 15.1

15.1.3.2 Advancement of the Anterior Glottic Commissure

This surgery, proposed by Tucker in 1985, is difficult to achieve.

It requires the incision in the thyroid cartilage at the level of the anterior glottic commissure and the insertion of a silicone thickness to keep it advanced. In these cases, So the vocal cords, as well as increase their tension, become longer and thinner and the tension increases. It produces an action on the vocal cord length.

Despite the good results on the speech signal, this surgical technique is not acceptable to the patient because it creates a second Adam's apple and is not aesthetically acceptable (Fig. 15.1a–d).

15.1.3.3 Endoscopic Anterior Commissure Backward

This procedure, proposed by Wendler, is performed in direct microlaryngoscopy under general anesthesia, and it involves the laser decortication of the anterior third (or often the front half) of the vocal cords.

The purpose of this intervention is to reduce the length of the vibrating portion of the vocal cord and to simulate the dimension of a female glottis. This action creates an anterior synechia, peeling the anterior third of the vocal cords with the laser and then approaching them with a surgical suture; the synechia is also closed using biological glue to avoid any opening. Sometimes, especially if the surgery is not properly performed, synechia can be opened with the use and give a bad voice (Fig. 15.2a–c).

This is the procedure that can lead to the best results in f0 elevation, but it is also the one that is associated with the greatest surgical and postsurgical complications.

15.1.3.4 Cricothyroid Approximation or Thyroplasty Type IV

The procedure is based on an external laryngoplasty with cricothyroid approximation (laryngoplasty type IV). This procedure, proposed by Isshiki in 1980, is the most widespread approach, and it is associated, in most cases, with a surgical remodeling of the Adam's apple.

This is the surgical technique used by the authors and described in the Sect. 15.2.

It consists in lengthening of the vocal cords (action on the length) performed by attaching the cricoid cartilage to the thyroid cartilage through non-resorbable sutures, simulating a continued spasm of the cricothyroid muscle with a consequent increase of the tension and of the length of the vocal folds (Fig. 15.3a, b).

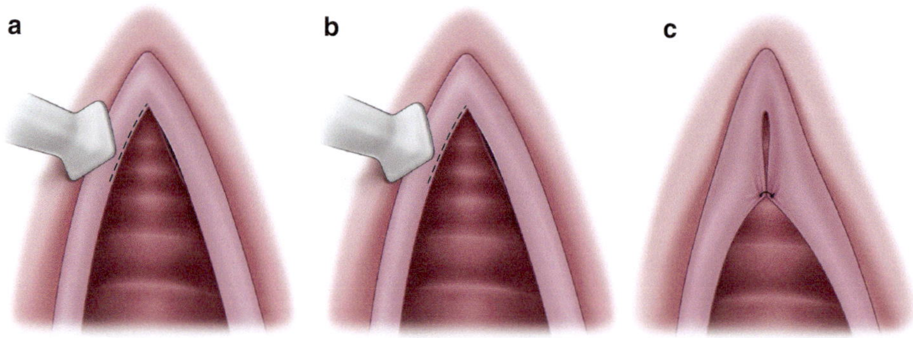

Fig. 15.2

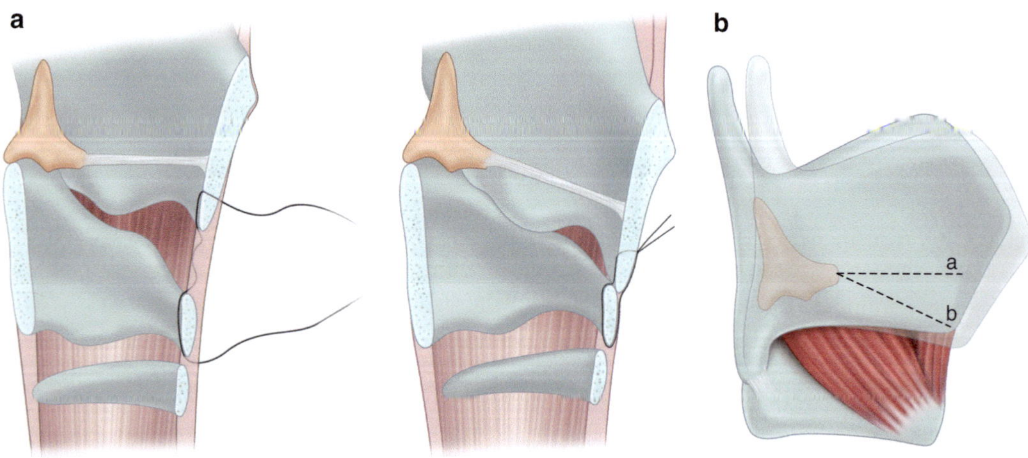

Fig. 15.3

Radiologic studies confirm that by reducing the distance between the thyroid and cricoid cartilage, the pitch increases (about 18 Hz for each mm of approaching).

15.1.4 The Preoperative Phoniatric Evaluation

- Counseling
- Laryngostroboscopy
- Functional examination
- Acoustic spectrum of the speech
- Manual approximation test

15.1.4.1 Counseling

Counseling in the MtF patient candidate for thyroplasty type IV is the most important and delicate moment in phoniatric presurgical evaluation.

In addition to assessing the substantial appearance of the female candidate (somatic and vocal), the phoniatrician has to objectively assess the quality and the manner of speech (through the use of instruments such as GIRBAS and CAPE-V).

The phoniatrician should inform the patient about the surgical approach, should illustrate where the incision will be made, and should inform about the various steps of surgery and postsurgical phases, including the treatment of the postsurgical scar.

The phoniatrician invites later the candidate to explain the reasons that have led him to the surgical choice, their doubts, and their expectations about the surgery, trying to establish a constructive and honest relationship with the patient.

So he should remind the patient that surgery can only act on one of the voice-generating factors, the vocal cords, and remember that the ventilatory function and the cavity of resonance will remain unchanged (i.e., male). After surgery, patients will have to readjust all their body-voice patterns to find the best coupling between vibrator and resonator, also through a modification of Psub.

And this is why speech therapist is essential before and after surgery. It is very important during counseling to suggest the use of speech therapy to the transgender patient.

The aims of speech therapy are as follows:

- Removal of mostly incorrect spontaneous forms of compensation
- Maintenance of postsurgical results.
- Modification of the acoustic parameters of the spoken voice:
  Fundamental frequency (f0)
  First and second formant (F1, F2)
- Modification of suprasegmental features of speech:
  Pitch (prosodic contour), intonation, and duration
- Pragmatic skills and communicative behavior

In addition, speech therapy, by changing the attitude of the supraglottic structures and tongue, helps to elevate f2. This increase is as important as the elevation of the f0 because vocal tract resonance characteristics may be the second most important acoustic cue to speaker identification.

Later modified test TSEQ of Davies et al. [4] (Italian version to 14 items by the writer) and the VHI-10 are administered.

The use of both these tests is due to the fact that the VHI has been shown to be a valid tool used to assess psychosocial handicap of voice disorders representing the breadth of pathology seen in most clinical settings and a moderately strong relationship was found between the patient's self-perceived severity and VHI scores.

Individuals seeking vocal feminization may or may not have vocal pathology and often have concerns not addressed on the VHI (e.g., my laughing, coughing, and sneezing sound like a man). The Transgender Self-Evaluation Questionnaire (TSEQ) is a subjective measure of voice handicap tailored to the transgender population.

Hancock et al. [5] demonstrated a significant relationship ($r=0.89$) between VHI and TSEQ scores when administered to male-to-female transgender individuals presenting as females 100 % of the time, indicating criterion validity of the TSEQ.

Additionally, a strong correlation ($r=0.97$) indicated test-retest reliability of the TSEQ. Although the VHI and TSEQ may be correlated, they are not identical; therefore, using a measure with greater content validity will provide the clinician with a richer picture of the client's feelings and may be helpful in directing treatment.

Already in the 1950s, Peterson and Barney [6] and Ladefoged and Broadbent [7] found that females have higher average vowel formant frequencies than males.

The importance of vocal tract resonances as a cue to speaker sex identification was shown by Coleman [8].

He reported that listeners correctly identified speaker's sex in 88 % when listening to the sound produced by an artificial laryngeal source with a fundamental of 85 Hz of both sexes. In 1976, Coleman further investigated the importance of vocal tract resonance and fundamental frequency related to gender identification.

In one experiment, male and female speakers produced speech samples using normal voice, and in another they used an artificial larynx.

When speakers used normal voice, vocal tract resonance and fundamental frequency were both important to male vs. female identification.

When they used artificial voice and when vocal tract resonance characteristics of one sex were combined with f0 characteristics of the opposite sex, listeners generally identified the speaker as male. This was true both when a male f0 was combined with female vocal tract resonance and when a female f0 was combined with male vocal tract resonance.

These cumulative findings lead to the hypotheses that in MtF transsexuals, raising the f0 alone will likely result in perception of male voice and simultaneously raising the f0 and the vocal tract resonance will likely result in the perception of female voice. So, we use a speech therapy focused on changing both the laryngeal tone and its resonance.

During the speech therapy, the patient's natural abilities were used to produce voluntarily a higher laryngeal f0 and to enhance it by forward carriage of the tongue, thereby raising f2 vowel frequency.

So, key elements of success are as follows:

- Adjustment of vocal parameters (f0, f1, f2)
- Use of correct verbal communicative signals (linguistic code)
- Use of correct nonverbal communicative signals (tone, duration, intensity, pitch)
- Use of correct nonlinguistic communicative signals (facial expressions, gestures)

15.1.4.2 Laryngostroboscopy

We use this technique to investigate the following:

- General morphology
- Pathological findings (cysts, nodules, polyps, tumors, inflammation, edema)
- Involuntary muscle activity (fasciculations, myoclonus, tremor)
- Vocal cord motility
- Glottic closure
- Attitude of the supraglottic structures

15.1.4.3 Acoustic Spectrum of the Speech (Yang)

We use this technique to evaluate the following:

- f0 of vowel /a/ sustained for at least 4 s (CSL 4500)
- f0 on a standardized test of reading (VRP)
- Vocal range in semitones (VRP)
- Evaluation of voice signal
- Perturbation indexes (jitter-shimmer)

15.1.4.4 Manual Approximation Test

During phonation, the cricoid and the thyroid cartilages are manually approached: the right index finger lifts the bottom edge of the cricoid while the left index finger pushes down the thyroid cartilage (Fig. 15.4). In this way, we can check the approximation length between the cricoid and thyroid cartilages and simultaneously listen to a "preview" of the postoperative voice result. A modest result is usually due to excessive mass.

A low pitch (due to vocal cord hypertrophy) is not significantly raised with cricothyroid approximation only.

In this case, after the surgical approximation, one or more injections of triamcinolone inside the vocal muscle can be performed, in order to decrease its mass.

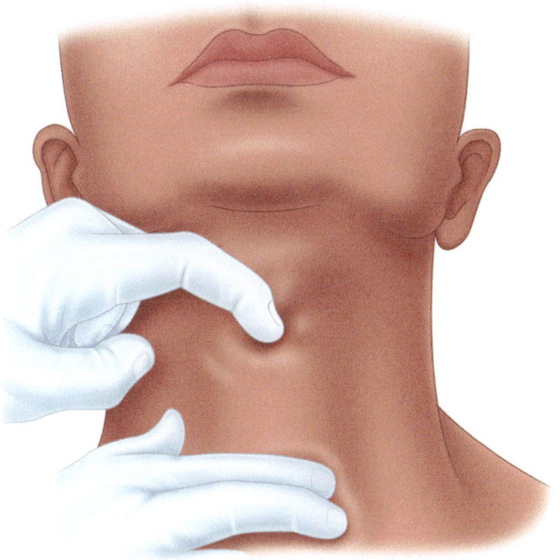

Fig. 15.4

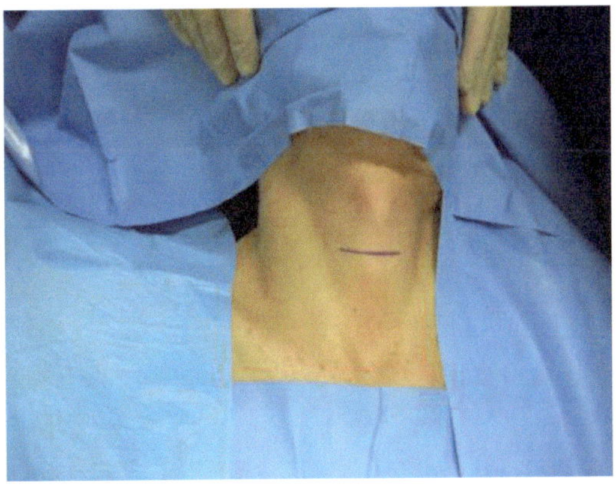

Fig. 15.5

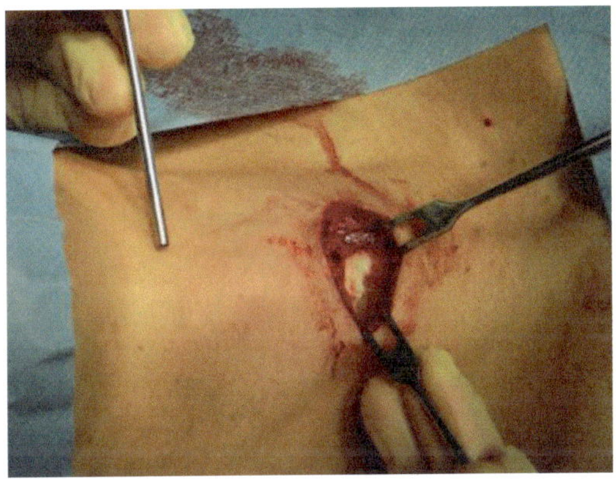

Fig. 15.6

15.2 Surgical Procedure

15.2.1 Thyroplasty Type IV: Surgical Technique

The surgery begins with a careful choice of the surgical incision site, trying to match the surgical wound with a preexisting skinfold.

For this purpose, the neck is mobilized with extension and flexion to identify the most suitable fold, possibly coinciding with the cricothyroid membrane.

A dermographic pencil is used to mark the incising line. Later a subcutaneous infiltration is done with 10 cc of Carbocaine 2 % with epinephrine (Fig. 15.5).

The incision of the skin and subcutaneous tissue is done, removing the excess fat until reaching the level of the prelaryngeal muscles.

Here you can see large-caliber venous vessels, consisting of the anterior jugular and its collateral branches.

If the caliber is greater than 3 mm, they must be tied and cut.

The cervical "linea alba" is identified, and the muscles are lateralized, carefully avoiding to dissect them, to identify the membrane between the cricoid and thyroid, to the upper edge of the cricoid cartilage and the lower edge of the thyroid (Fig. 15.6).

In this phase, after careful hemostasis, we must carefully avoid to cut the membrane between the cricoid and thyroid, avoiding even its damage, which would expose the patient to bleeding and subcutaneous emphysema.

Later we proceed carefully to subperiosteal dissection of the internal side of the lower edge of the thyroid cartilage and the upper one of the cricoid cartilage by the use of a surgical instrument used in septoplasty.

This allows the sliding of the cricothyroid membrane that is folded into the internal side, favoring a good healing (Fig. 15.7).

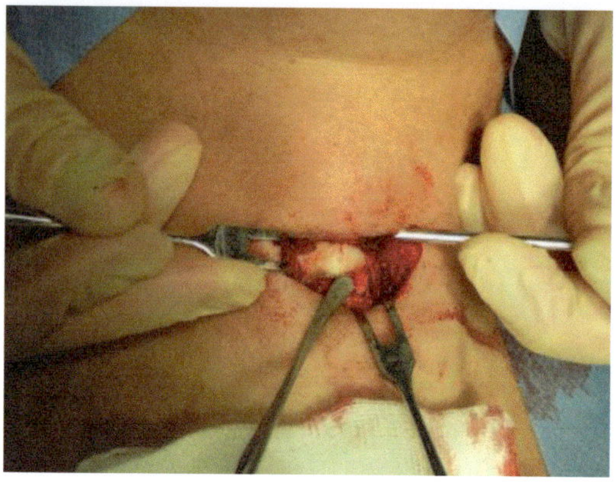

Fig. 15.7

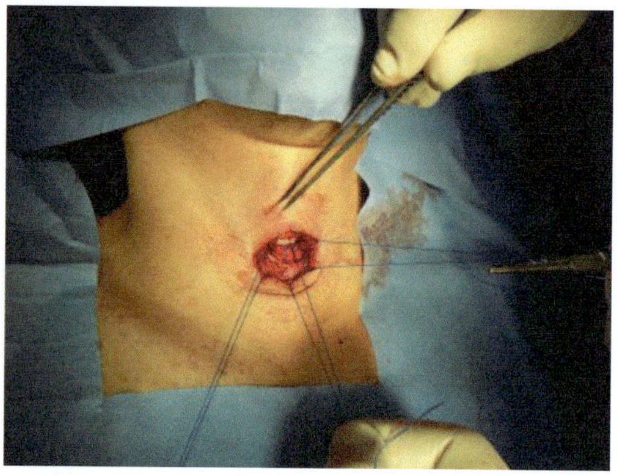

Fig. 15.8

After checking again the correct hemostasis and after measuring the space between the two cartilaginous edges to have a prediction on frequency increase, we proceed to surgical fastening between the two cartilages.

We usually use three large-size (0/1) Prolene wire and we suture starting from the central point (Fig. 15.8).

The lower suture does not pass through the cricoid cartilage to prevent its rupture, but below it. Regarding the thyroid cartilage, the needle must enter 4–5 mm from the bottom edge. When the cartilage is not yet ossified, as occurs in young patients, drilling is quite easy. When this is not possible due to cartilage ossification is necessary to prepare three holes by using the drill. Once the Prolene wires are positioned, these are tightened starting from the central wire (Fig. 15.9).

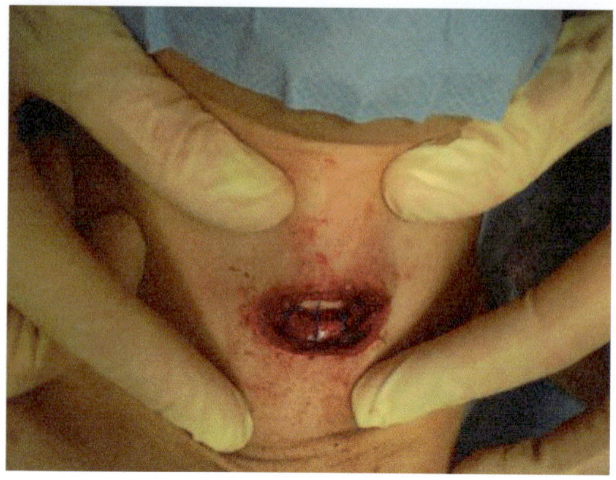

Fig. 15.9

It may happen that, due to the hormonal action, cartilages become particularly fragile. In this case, the risk to tear the cartilage at time of traction of the sutures is very high.

In this case, it may be helpful to use wires with little "wings" on the side (e.g., Quill). In this way, there is no need to tie knots.

In this case, the "hoist" effect is used. Of course, we will have to increase the number of steps with respect to sutures with Prolene.

After, the muscles are joined in the midline, and subcutaneous and intradermal suture is executed.

No drains are placed, and the wound is treated with a flat plaster.

The reduction of the Adam's apple, if requested, will be made only after finishing the thyroplasty.

This is particularly important because the approximation between the cartilages tilts down and forwards the front angle of the thyroid cartilage which is precisely the Adam's apple.

We must therefore remove the perichondrium to expose the cartilage.

At this point, the anterior dihedral angle can be modeled initially with an aggressive bur and further with a diamond bur.

The goal is to modify the anterior angle, from an acute angle to an angle as close as a straight angle, taking great care not to penetrate the larynx and to avoid damaging the anterior tendon (Broyles tendon).

The aesthetic result is usually very satisfactory (Fig. 15.10a, b).

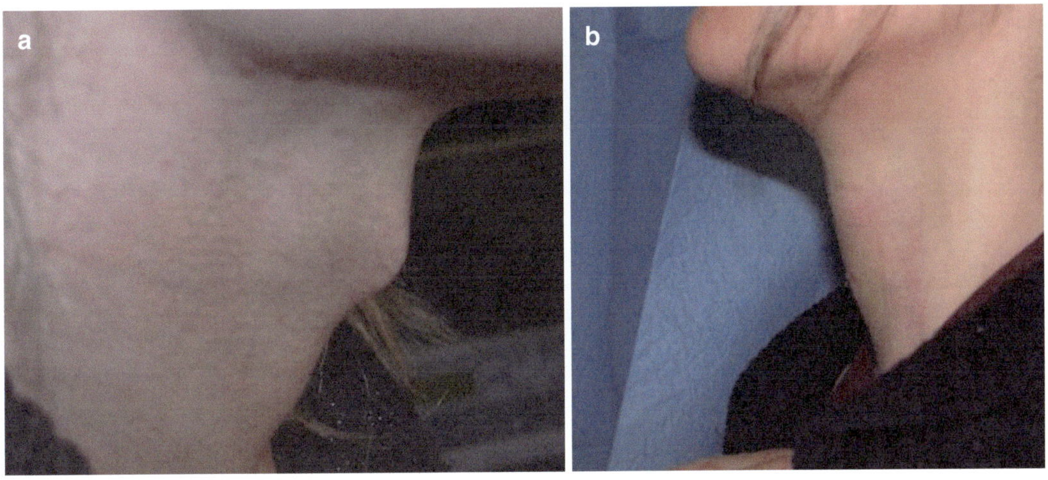

Fig. 15.10

15.3 The Postoperative Phoniatric Evaluation

15.3.1 Postsurgical Process

It is not necessary to place a drain; a bandage which is a little bit compressive, maintained for 24 h, is sufficient to prevent a hematoma.

The patient must be maintained with the head slightly bent forward and is recommended absolute vocal rest for a week.

No complications were reported when the patient maintained absolute silence for a week. Note that in the first week of postsurgery, the patient is almost voiceless and should not strive to speak (use of alternative communication: SMS, e-mail, block notes, etc.).

15.3.2 Postsurgical Evaluations

15.3.2.1 Laryngostroboscopy

Evaluation of the vocal fold anatomy and in particular paying special attention to potential blood spills and the integrity of the anterior commissure and free edge, especially after an Adam's apple reduction.

Analysis of the vocal cord motility for a physiological reduction of breathing space.

Following careful monitoring of the recovery and quality of mucosal wave.

15.3.2.2 Acoustic Spectrum of the Speech

f0 of vowel /a/ sustained for at least 4 s (CSL 4500).
f0 evaluated on a standardized reading test (VRP).
Vocal range in semitones (VRP).
Evaluation of indexes of voice signal perturbation (jitter%).
Voice analysis detects a substantial elevation of the pitch of sustained speech (fundamental frequency) and of reading, immediately after surgery and 6–8 months later.

Finally, are the results stable?

Generally yes. For a stable result some operator binds the cricoid and thyroid cartilage with the classical three stitches and, in addition, peels the perichondrium of the upper border of the cricoid and the lower one of the thyroid to facilitate, through contact, the process of neochondrogenesis and fusion of the two cartilage surfaces.

However, this process is practically not used because *it is not reversible.*

The instability of the result due to loosening or breakage of sutures isn't acceptable.

There is a physiological adaptation of the vocal cord to the new state of tension, with a slight decrease of f0. This value will stabilize over time and always be above the threshold of perception for the female voice.

Although a rehabilitation (speech therapy) it's always preferred after phonosurgery, the results, even without proper rehabilitation (often patients don't come back to controls!) appeared good, capable of raising a significant and lasting pitch.

References

1. Davies S, Goldberg JM (2006) Clinical aspects of transgender speech feminilization and masculinization. Int J Transgenderism 9(3–4):167–196
2. Spencer LE (1988) Speech characteristics of male-to-female transsexuals a perceptual and acoustic study. Folia Phoniatr (Basel) 40:31–42
3. Wolfe VI, Ratusnik DL, Northrop G (1980) Vocal characteristics of male transsexuals on a masculinity-femininity dimension. In: The proceedings of the Congress of the International Association of Logopedics and Phoniatrics, vol 1. pp 469–474
4. Dacakis G, Davies S, Oates JM, Douglas JM, Johnston JR (2013) Transsexual voice questionnaire (male-to-female). J Voice 27(3):312–320
5. Hancock A, Owen K, Siegfriedt L, Brundage S (2009) Reliability and validity of the transgender self-evaluation questionnaire. Paper presented at: Voice Foundation's Annual Symposium, Philadelphia
6. Peterson GE, Barney HL (1952) Control methods used in a study of the vowels. J Acoust Soc Am 24:175–184
7. Ladefoged P, Broadbent D (1957) Information conveyed by vowels. J Acoust Soc Am 29:98–104
8. Coleman RO (1971) Male and female voice quality and its relationships to vowel formant frequencies. J Speech Hear Res 14:565–577

Surgical Therapy: Mastoplasty 16

Giovanni Papa, Vittorio Ramella, and Michele Pascone

Chest wall contouring is material in male to female (MtF) transsexual treatment since the patient's social rehabilitation goes through the acceptance of body image; thus, breast is the main external indicator of gender. After a period of hormonal therapy (at least 12 months [1, 2]), during which the patient has to live in her new sex identity, she will be candidable for sex reassignment surgery (SRS). The hormonal therapy induces mammogenesis [3] and the breast appears like a puberal female breast, but a complete development is rarely reached [4]. Maximum volume growth is usually obtained after 18–24 months and is permanent. General side effects are gaining weight, galactorrhea, decreased red cell mass, lower libido, and infertility [5]. Some patients achieve a good mammary size (cup B), but not all of them are satisfied with this volume [6]. In those cases it is necessary to perform breast augmentation mammoplasty, selecting the appropriate technique among those described for genetic female patient [1] based on patient's anatomical condition. In breast reshaping, the surgeon has to take into account the differences between male and female anatomy. The female figure is generally characterized by rounded shapes and flowing contours, with a more represented fat component above the muscle edges [7]. The female chest is shorter with a conical shape, and the breast prominence extends from the II or III rib to the VI or VII. The nipple is usually located at the level of the most projected portion, at the midpoint of the humerus length. According to Ramselaar [8], the cross-sectional shape of the female breast can be represented ideally by a cone with a spherical surface. The sagittal shape is that of a drop with a concavity in the upper level up to the areola and a convexity that runs from below the areola until the inframammary fold. An axillary tail extends backward along the outer margin of the pectoralis muscle. The entire shape of the breast is also very dependent on age, volume of the breast, attachment to the parenchymal-muscle interface, and mobility of the gland [9]. The male breast consists predominantly of fat and supporting tissue with very little glandular tissue; the nipple areola complex (NAC) is in the same position of the female breast [4] if it is not ptotic; and it is qualitatively identical [10] and differs only in size [11]. Before changing the breast shape from male to female phenotype, it is very important to be able to produce high-quality aesthetical and functional results [12]. This is the only way to reduce risks for the patient and costs of treatment [10].

G. Papa, MD, PhD (✉) • V. Ramella
Department Plastic and Reconstructive Surgery, Cattinara Hospital,
Strada di Fiume 447, Trieste 34100, Italy
e-mail: giovanni.papa@aots.sanita.fvg.it; vittorio.ramella@aots.sanita.fvg.it

M. Pascone
Department of Plastic and Reconstructive Surgery, Policlinico, piazza G. Cesare 11, Bari 70100, Italy
e-mail: michele.pascone@uniba.it

C. Trombetta et al. (eds.), *Management of Gender Dysphoria: A Multidisciplinary Approach*, DOI 10.1007/978-88-470-5696-1_16, © Springer-Verlag Italia 2015

16.1 Surgical Issues

Timing of augmentation mammoplasty in the history of this kind of surgery has often been arbitrary and depending on the different theories of various authors. It could be performed either concurrently with genital surgery or in a precedent or subsequent procedure [7]. In our gender team guidelines, the procedure of gender reassignment begins, after the disorder identity gender diagnosis confirmation, with penovaginal surgery that is usually performed before the mammoplasty augmentation because it is covered by the National Health Insurance. In order to perform breast augmentation, the plastic surgeon can implement several techniques. Many types of injectable substances have been used in the past with adverse effects and complications, and in the literature there are not long-term evidence-based medicine studies about permanent fillers. Lipofilling technique can be used in cases of moderate volume augmentation, but several surgical operations are required. Moreover, the effects and the presence of stem cells in the injected centrifuged adipose tissue are still debated. More significant augmentation with fewer surgical procedures can be obtained combining lipofilling with the Brava system.

Nowadays the gold standard technique in MtF mammoplasty is implant breast augmentation.

Generally speaking, surgical planning deals with skin incision, implant selection, and positioning for breast augmentation.

16.2 Skin Incision

The emiperiareolar incision is one of the approaches in breast augmentation. Despite its popularity, it is not recommended as the incision of the gland increases the risk of infection, and pocket dissection and implant positioning are challenging due to the small dimension of the male NAC.

Furthermore, also the axillary incision is not a valuable option. The strong muscle and the conformation of the inferior pole of the male breast cause a difficult submuscular dissection and risk of implant displacement. With a little incision and an endoscopical approach, it is not possible to detach the gland from the muscular plane. In addition, the little scar, the vertical or the s shaped even more, is visible when raising the hands and also wearing any kind of bra.

The access route preferably selected for the insertion of the prosthesis is at the level of the inframammary fold as it allows good visibility, easy dissection of all pocket location (subglandular, submuscular, and combination of both), and placement of all kinds of implant, silicon texturized as well.

The scar normally is linear and is hidden in the inframammary fold, and it is not visible wearing the bra, even with arms laying down.

In any case, scar becomes much more visible if pathological scarring occurs.

16.3 Implant Selection

With reference to prosthesis selection, saline ones are not frequently used, as they do not give a natural feeling like gel-filled implants. Their insertion is easier because the saline solution is inflated in a second time, but the implants become more rigid and the risk of loss of volume of the implant and skin wrinkling is higher.

Nowadays, smooth implants are not a good choice as well because their surface does not integrate to the surrounding tissue.

For all of these reasons, silicone gel-filled implants with textured surface are the most frequently used. Moreover, gel cohesivity prevents gel leakage in case of implant rupture.

The main complaint of MtF patients after surgery is an insufficient breast volume, as their aim is to achieve a clearly feminine appearance.

For this reason, where possible, consider a prosthesis that is slightly bigger than the one chosen by the patient preoperatively (usually by 250 cc) [3].

The male chest is usually larger than the female's, so this often involves obtaining an aesthetic result which is not satisfactory with the prosthesis sizes commonly used in female patients. The transsexual patients often require more extensive prostheses to reach a higher-level filling medially, but however this may result in symmastia and other complications.

Because of male chest conformation and lateral position of the NAC, it is often difficult to fill the wide cleavage between the two breasts and this point has to be stressed with the patient.

It is also important to pay attention to the positioning of the NAC that must be placed centrally above the prosthesis to avoid the divergence of the nipples. This is the reason why prosthesis selection is very important. The implant size has to be related to the nipple-inframammary fold distance in order not to risk scar malpositioning or shape alteration of the breast.

The distance between the inframammary fold and the lower edge of the areola increases after surgery. This effect seems to be related to skin tightening and the recruitment of skin from the abdominal region and inframammary fold. Therefore, it is preferable to make the incision for the insertion of the prosthesis 7 cm below the lower edge of the areola. Immediately after the surgery, the scar can be positioned lower relative to the fold and could appear too low, but after a few months, the scar goes back toward the inframammary fold.

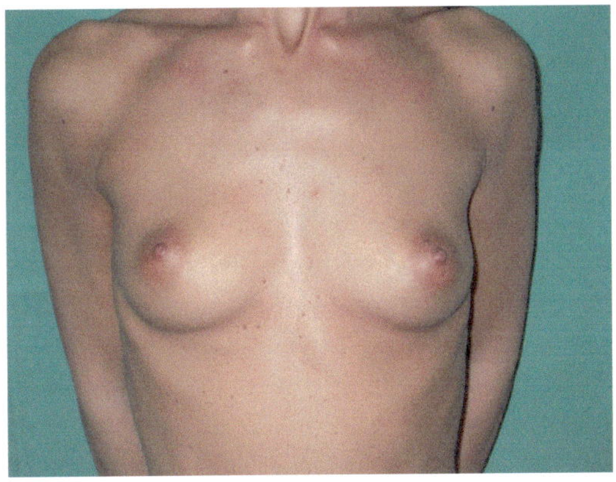

Fig. 16.1 Preoperative view

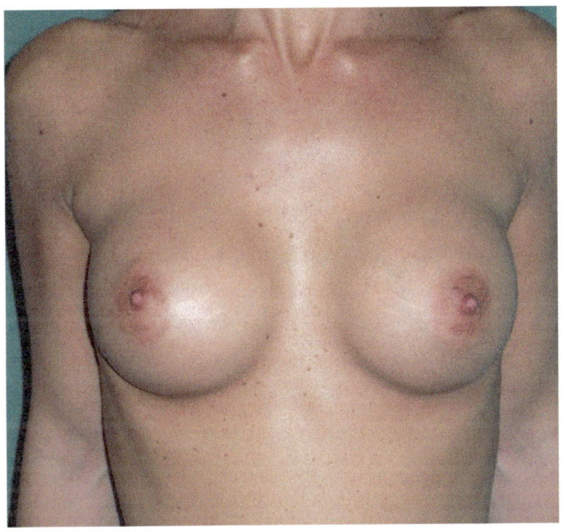

Fig. 16.2 Postoperative view

16.4 Implant Position

Surgical technique and pocket selection have to be planned also in light of the glandular amount. A subglandular pocket can be harvested if there is enough glandular tissue in order to provide a complete coverage of the implant.

If doable, this is the best technique as it increases the control of breast shape and inframammary fold position and postoperative recovery is more rapid.

The implants placed in subglandular position can give problems often related to the lack of glandular tissue and fat. In fact, these being underrepresented give limited protection and poor coverage of the prosthesis, with greater risk of visibility and palpability and a more evident capsular contracture (Figs. 16.1 and 16.2).

The pinch test in the upper pole of the breast can also give additional information in choosing between subglandular or submuscular pocket. If the pinched tissue of upper pole is less than 2 cm, a submuscular dissection should be performed. In MtF patients, total and partial submuscular pocket is not indicated. The stiffness and the strength of the pectoralis muscle due to its development under the influence of testosterone can cause implant displacement in a lateral position or upward when inferior pectoralis origins across the inframammary fold are not divided, even if the risk of capsular contracture is lower than in the case of subglandular pocket. With partial retropectoral (only pectoralis major) or total submuscular (pectoralis major and serratus) location, there is also more postoperative tenderness and a more prolonged recovery.

In order to ensure that greater force does not push the prosthesis below and parenchymal attachment does not give shape distortion like "double-bubble" deformity, it is necessary to detached the lower portion of the pectoralis from the chest wall combined with a subglandular dissection, as described in dual-plane technique [13].

Dual-plane breast augmentation usually allows greater coverage in a wide range of breast in women and gives better cosmetic result in terms of volume and projection. The possibility of the implant going downward is preserved too.

In male patients it is more difficult to identify the muscular plane and prepare the pocket, because the planes are less defined. Bleeding can be a problem. It is also important to fix the space between the two breasts to extend the subglandular pocket more medially toward the sternum.

In our clinical experience, when the gland is firm and more conspicuous, dual-plane type I is more indicated; if it is mobile on the muscular surface (rarely in male), we should choose a type II.

The difference between these two techniques is that in type I, the surgeon creates the pocket only dissecting the muscle at the inframammary fold while in type II, also the glandular tissue is mobilized to the NAC.

In MtF patients, the gland, even if adequately represented, is usually firm on the muscle; this is the reason why dual-plane II is rarely performed.

In MtF the lower pole is often not well represented so the suggested technique is dual-plane type III, in which the mammary gland is elevated from the pectoralis major muscle more cranially. This allows a better downward mobilization of the gland ensuring an adequate coverage of the lower pole of the implant (Figs. 16.3, 16.4, 16.5, and 16.6)

To redistribute the parenchyma and widen the base of this kind of breast, radial or concentric parenchymal scoring is often required. To put pressure on the scored parenchyma and to expand the lower pole, more projecting anatomical implants have to be used.

In those cases of dual-plane type III where the inferior pole of the prosthesis has an insufficient coverage, the use of acellular dermal matrix should be considered. This matrix is sutured in its upper part to the inferior border of the muscle and in its inferior part to the chest wall at the inframammary fold. This technique provides

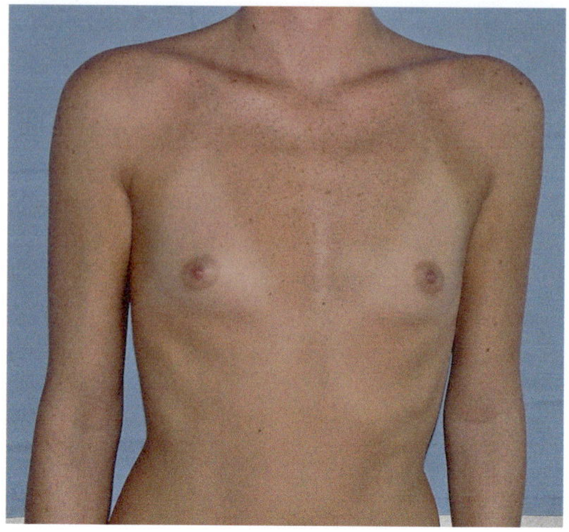

Fig. 16.3 Preoperative view

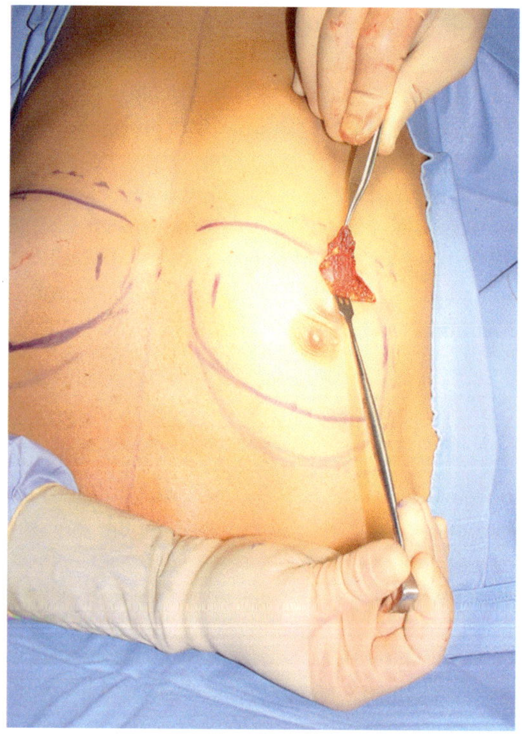

Fig. 16.4 Intraoperative detail: type III dual plane

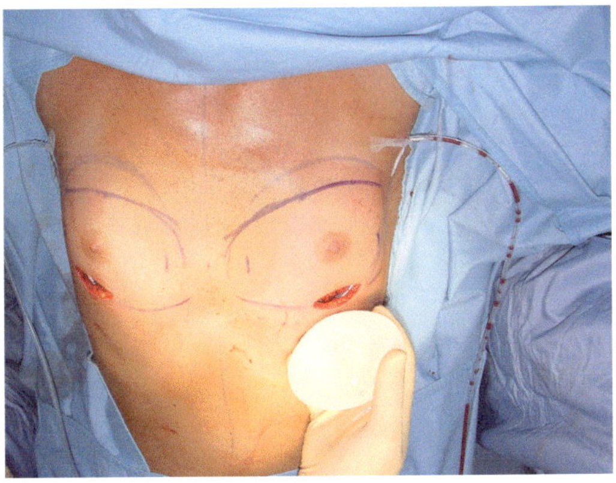

Fig. 16.5 Intraoperative detail: before prosthesis implantation

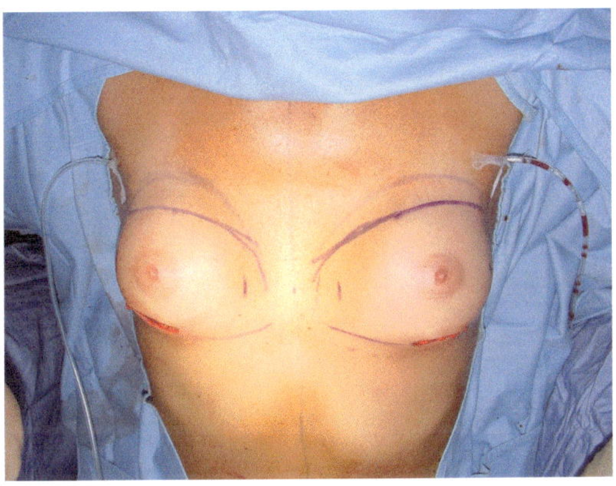

Fig. 16.6 Intraoperative detail: after prosthesis implantation

good coverage and protection of the prosthesis and a better cosmetic outcome as the skin flaps become thicker, preventing skin wrinkling.

16.5 Surgical Approach

In subglandular technique, pocket plane is created through a dissection on top of the pectoralis major beyond the gland.

In subpectoral technique, the dissection is below the pectoralis major but above the pectoralis minor and does not disrupt the inferior attachments of the pectoralis if total subpectoral dissection is performed.

In dual plane, pectoralis is released along the inframammary fold in addition to subpectoral dissection; three types of dual-plane technique can be used; the difference is represented by the grade of pectoralis separation from the parenchyma (no separation in type I, to the level of inferior NAC in II, and to the level of superior NAC in type III). Subpectoral coverage of upper pole, less implant displacement at rest and during pectoralis contraction, increases implant-parenchymal interface, which expands the lower pole and prevents double-bubble deformity.

In all of these cases, after pocket dissection, the surgeon performs careful hemostasis and inserts a suction drain in the pocket. A sizer is used before definitive implant positioning in order to see the definitive result in a laying but also in a standing position (the patient is secured to the operating table adequately to be put in a sitting position during surgery). After that, subcutaneous and cutaneous tissues are sutured and a compressive medication is applied.

In light of all these considerations, our team developed an algorithm for the planning of augmentation mammoplasty in MtF patients (Fig. 16.7).

Particular techniques have been described for the treatment of MtF affected by Poland's syndrome or tuberous breast [14, 15].

16.6 Results and Complications

The literature does not provide for specific results of breast augmentation in MtF patients.

Patients who undergo this kind of surgery must be properly informed about the risks and complications related to the procedure.

The most frequent complications are capsular contracture, implant rupture (that in 90 % of cases is intracapsular), hematoma, seroma, infection, implant exposure, chronic pain, skin flaps, and NAC necrosis and wound dehiscence.

The risk of developing breast cancer due to long-term hormonal therapy is unclear, even if many studies confirm that this risk in biological women and MtF patients is the same. In light of these considerations, transsexual women should undergo regular screening examination by mammography and ultrasounds [6].

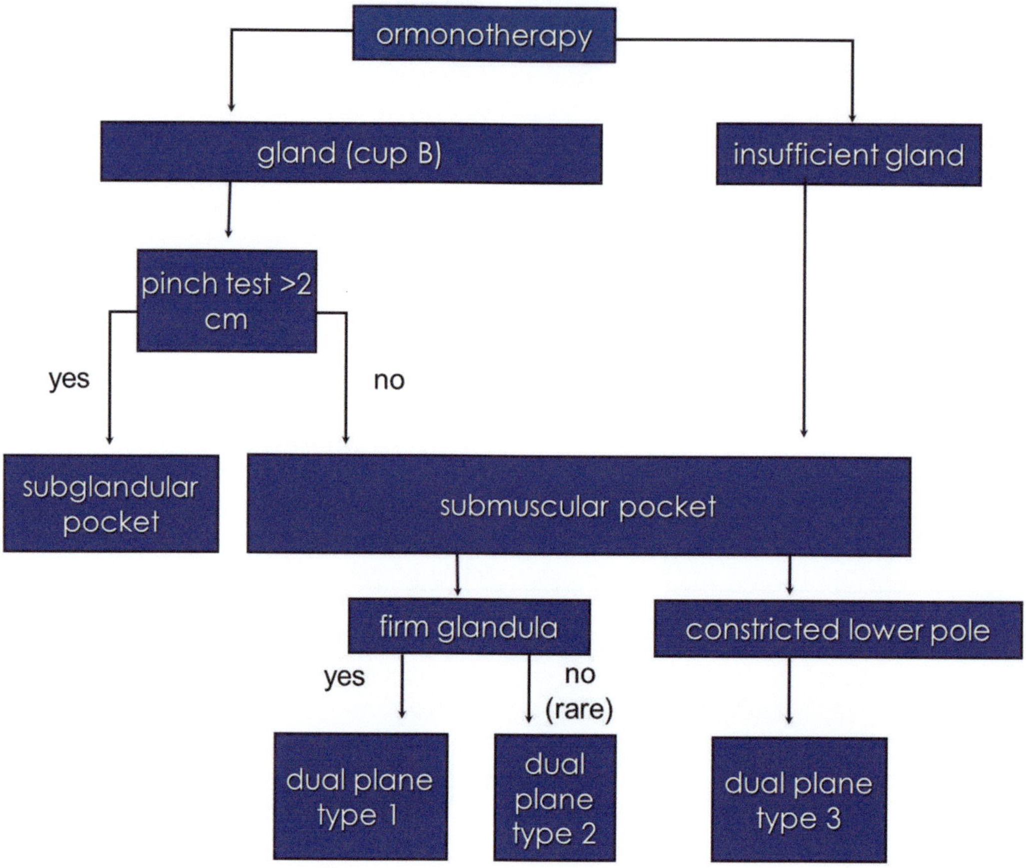

Fig. 16.7 Flow chart of the algorithm for the surgical approach

References

1. Coleman E, Bockting W, Botzer M, Cohen-Kettenis P, DeCuypere G, Feldman J, Fraser L, Green J, Knudson G, Meyer WJ, Monstrey S, Adler RK, Brown GR, Devor AH, Ehrbar R, Ettner R, Eyler E, Garofalo R, Karasic DH, Lev AI, Mayer G, Meyer-Bahlburg H, Hall BP, Pfaefflin F, Rachlin K, Robinson B, Schechter LS, Tangpricha V, van Trotsenburg M, Vitale A, Winter S, Whittle S, Wylie KR, Zucker K (2011) Standards of care for the health of transsexual, transgender, and gender-non-conforming people, version 7. Int J Transgenderism 13:165–232
2. Orentreich N, Durr NP (1974) Mammogenesis in transsexuals. J Invest Dermatol 63(1):142–146
3. Seal LJ, Franklin S, Richards C, Shishkareva A, Sinclaire C, Barrett J (2012) Predictive markers for mammoplasty and a comparison of side effect profiles in transwomen taking various hormonal regimens. J Clin Endocrinol Metab 97(12):4422–4428. doi:10.1210/jc.2012-2030
4. Dahl M, Feldman JL, Goldberg JM, Afshin J (2006) Physical aspects of transgender endocrine therapy. Int J Transgenderism 9:111–134
5. Lawrence AA (2007) Transgender health concerns. In: Meyer IH, North Ridge ME (eds) The health of sexual minorities: public health perspectives on lesbian, gay, bisexual and transgender population. Springer, New York, pp 437–555
6. Weyers S, Villeirs G, Vanherreweghe E, Verstraelen H, Monstrey S, Van den Broecke R, Gerris J (2010) Mammography and breast sonography in transsexual women. Eur J Radiol 74(3):508–513. doi:10.1016/j.ejrad.2009.03.018
7. Montagna W, Macpherson EE (1974) Some neglected aspects of the anatomy of human breasts. J Invest Dermatol 63(1):10–16
8. Ramselaar JM (1988) Precision in breast reduction. Plast Reconstr Surg 82(4):631–643
9. Edgerton MT (1974) The surgical treatment of male transsexuals. Clin Plast Surg 1(2):285–323
10. Kuiper B, Cohen-Kettenis P (1988) Sex reassignment surgery: a study of 141 Dutch transsexuals. Arch Sex Behav 17(5):439–457

11. Kanhai RC, Hage JJ, Mulder JW (2000) Long-term outcome of augmentation mammaplasty in male-to-female transsexuals: a questionnaire survey of 107 patients. Br J Plast Surg 53(3):209–211
12. Kanhai RC, Hage JJ, Karim RB (2001) Augmentation mammaplasty in male-to-female trans-sexuals: facts and figures from Amsterdam. Scand J Plast Reconstr Surg Hand Surg 35(2):203–206
13. Tebbetts JB (2001) Dual plane breast augmentation: optimizing implant-soft-tissue relationships in a wide range of breast types. Plast Reconstr Surg 107(5):1255–1272
14. Majdak-Paredes EJ, Shafighi M, Fatah F (2009) Unilateral hypoplastic breast in a male-to-female transsexual with Poland syndrome after gender reassignment–reconstructive considerations. J Plast Reconstr Aesthet Surg 62(3):398–401. doi:10.1016/j.bjps.2008.01.017
15. Argenta LC, VanderKolk C, Friedman RJ, Marks M (1985) Refinements in reconstruction of congenital breast deformities. Plast Reconstr Surg 76(1):73–78

Complications of MTF Vaginoplasty

17

Allison S. Glass and Marci L. Bowers

17.1 Complications of Male-to-Female Sex Reassignment Surgery

Many transgendered individuals desire surgical procedures as a component of their individual gender transition. Such surgical procedures are generically described as sexual reassignment surgery (SRS). More recently, with respect to genital surgical procedures in male-to-female (MTF) transsexuals, such procedures are also described as "gender/genital reassignment surgery" (GRS) or "gender affirming surgery." Vaginoplasty, also referred to as neocolporrhaphy (Latin for creation of new vagina), is nearly synonymous with SRS in MTF individuals.

The specifics of the surgical technique utilized for SRS/GRS vary widely across the globe but have evolved dramatically since the "world's first sex change" was performed on Einar Wegener (later named Lili Elbe) in 1931 Berlin. For Ms. Elbe, who ultimately died as a result of complications attributed to the operation, her surgical sex change was the culmination of more than two decades of research and interest in transsexualism [1] in pre-WWII Germany. In fact, the term transsexual was first coined by Magnus Hirschfeld, a gay sexologist, whose transsexual laboratory was among the first casualties following Adolf Hitler's ascent to power in 1933 [1]. Unvanquished, the transgender movement smoldered. Newer surgical techniques eventually followed and gradually showed improvements in cosmetic and functional outcomes. Complications have also reduced precipitously.

Although uncommon, complications of SRS/GRS/vaginoplasty still occur. This chapter will discuss categories of complications that can occur with contemporary vaginoplasty techniques with an emphasis on recognition, strategies of prevention, and treatment. Complications specific to colovaginoplasty will not be considered in this discussion.

The role of primary care providers (PCP) in the management of postoperative complications of SRS/GRS cannot be overemphasized. Although the number of qualified surgeons is growing worldwide, most surgical care is offered regionally in large metropolitan areas. Patient preference for certain surgeons, variance and inconsistency among surgical techniques, and differing eligibility criteria in national health plans and among insurers mean that most patients

A.S. Glass, MD
Department of Urology,
University of California-Davis, 2315 Stockton Blvd,
Sacramento, CA 95817, USA
e-mail: Allison.s.glass@gmail.com

M.L. Bowers, MD (✉)
Department of Gynecology and Obstetrics,
Mills-Peninsula Hospital,
1501 Trousdale Drive, Burlingame,
CA 94010, USA
e-mail: Marcibdoc@man.com

C. Trombetta et al. (eds.), *Management of Gender Dysphoria: A Multidisciplinary Approach*,
DOI 10.1007/978-88-470-5696-1_17, © Springer-Verlag Italia 2015

travel great distances to access surgical care. Fortunately, with current approaches, the incidence of complications is increasingly rare and relatively minor. This current model of care delivery consequently shifts the postoperative care burden to PCPs.

17.1.1 Acute Postsurgical Complications

Acute postsurgical complications include those inherent to any major surgical procedure such as blood loss, wound-related complications (infection or hematoma), and thromboembolic events (e.g., venous thrombosis or pulmonary embolism). Complications unique to this advanced procedure may include tissue necrosis (e.g., flap, urethral, or neoclitoral), neovaginal graft expulsion, or urinary complications such as stricture, fistula, or misdirected stream. Surprisingly, urinary incontinence is not commonly reported following MTF reassignment due to surgical activity confined distally to the internal urinary sphincter. Finally, and most significantly, there is also intraoperative risk of entry into viscus structures such as the bladder, urethra, or rectum.

17.1.2 Late Postsurgical Complications

Most complications related to GRS occur outside of the acute postsurgical period and include sensory loss, problems related to tissue healing (e.g., granulation or scar tissue), pelvic or genital pain, scarring, vaginal stenosis or stricture, vaginal prolapse, or development of fistula (Fig. 17.1). Fistulous complications in particular can be devastating as they can require multiple surgical interventions and result in a compromised or potentially nonfunctional neovagina. Recognition of each complication and strategies for prevention and solution become critical for both the surgeon and primary care provider. Poor cosmetic outcomes as well as many functional complications can be corrected at a second surgery or "labiaplasty." The timing and exposure required for labiaplasty likewise allow correction of issues with pain or urologic problems.

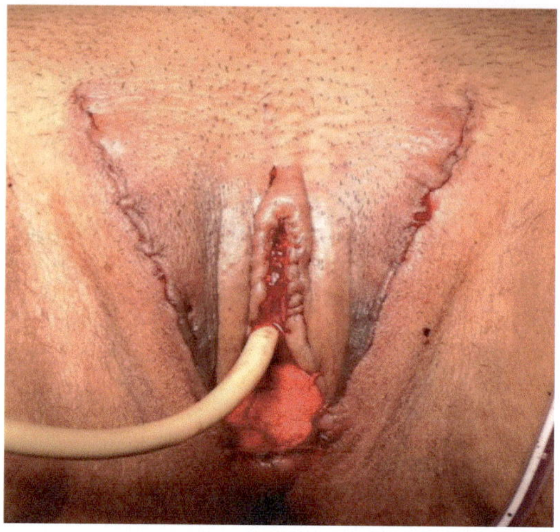

Fig. 17.1 Immediate, uncomplicated post-op MTF vaginoplasty appearance. Foley, vaginal packing, and JP drain (on right) visible

17.1.3 Blood Loss

Average blood loss for male-to-female SRS is minimal. However, pelvic blood flow is impressive and blood loss can quickly exceed 600 cc even among experienced surgeons. Risk of hemorrhage increases with BMI >30, in younger patient age, and in patients who experience tumescence (erection) at the time of surgery. Less blood loss is seen in older patients, in those with prior orchiectomy, and in patients with medical problems that compromise microvascular blood flow (e.g., diabetes and hypertension) [2]. A 2012 German study involving 332 patients who underwent single-stage vaginoplasty reported an average of 150 mL blood loss with very low need for blood transfusion (2 %) [3]. For most surgeons, modest blood loss normally does not result in transfusion. The author's experience was that transfusion was necessary in just 7 of 1,135 (0.6 %) GRS procedures (Bowers ML, 2014, MTF vaginoplasty blood loss, unpublished data). Surgeons typically no longer have blood on site, favoring a type and screen as opposed to type and cross. Threshold criteria for blood transfusion have also changed and become increasingly selective. In general, a hematocrit of greater than 22 % (hemoglobin 7.0 g/dL) immediately postoperatively, in the absence of symptoms and significant cardiac risk factors, is well tolerated by patients and does not require transfusion.

17.1.4 Surgical Site Infection (SSI)

Infection of tissue, whether grafted, a flap, or adjacent to the surgical site, is unusual but may arise because of compromised blood supply and tissue stretching. One study reported a 5 % rate of SSI (superficial abscesses, largely labial) that was successfully managed with incision and drainage and cephalosporin-based antibiotics [3]. A Detroit center reported on 43 patients who underwent genital reconstructive operations between years 1984 and 2008 and found a 21 % rate of SSI in those who underwent male-to-female GRS. Importantly, SSIs were independently associated with increased frequency of total operative procedures [4]. Other authors have suggested that development of SSI, particularly severe infection, contributed to complications such as loss of vaginal depth or stricture requiring additional surgical revision [3]. In general, the incidence of SSI is lower with increased surgeon experience and reduced operative time [5].

17.1.5 Tissue Necrosis

The etiology of this complication relates to devascularization of tissues secondary to ligation of arterial supply, compression of arterial structures, or poor host blood supply. Medical history (presence or absence of comorbidity) and nutritional status can also play a significant role in determining outcome and successful healing. Diabetes, while not a contraindication to GRS per se, is associated with greater risk for tissue necrosis. Selective debridement of tissues, wet-to-dry dressings, and "a tincture of time" are the best allies in treatment of these issues. Reopening of a portion of the incision and drainage is indicated for abscess but is rarely necessary. Pelvic and perineal circulation tends to be excellent and resilient, allowing many of these losses to ultimately resolve with such conservative management.

17.1.6 Clitoral Necrosis

*Necrosis of the neoclitoris*is, fortunately, is uncommon. Most surgeons report an incidence of 1–3 % [3, 6–9], but rates as high as 10 % were noted in one review series [10]. Even in these cases, the outlook remains reasonably positive, as most patients can achieve orgasm with or without clitoral sensation. The best evidence for this comes from earlier techniques for GRS (Drs. Biber and Schrang) where clitoral preservation using homologous tissues was not done. In those procedures, amputation of the dorsal nerves and arteries at the crus meant that postoperative sensation arising from the neoclitoris was not possible. Despite a lack of sensory innervation from the dorsal nerves, cavernosa, and glans, most of these patients – via innervations from residual spongiosum tissue, retained in these surgeons' patients as the neoclitoris – were able to orgasm. When clitoral necrosis does occur, the necrosis is most often partial with neovascularization and some residual sensation possible. Finally, for the rare patient whose clitoris loses both blood supply and innervation, the other areas retaining erectile or erogenous sensation (spongiosum, G-spot, prostate, etc.) can provide enough stimuli to allow orgasm. If patients remain anorgasmic after 1 year, topical testosterone cream (1 % compounded) can be helpful.

Labial necrosis is uncommon, with *wound dehiscence* being a more frequently reported problem [3]. Dehiscence is generally focal and localized and, in such cases, is best managed with local wound care and healing by secondary intention. Cosmetic complaints or scarring can be addressed at subsequent labiaplasty. Labiaplasty is normally not offered until at least 3 months following primary GRS to permit optimal healing and restoration of blood flow in flaps. For surgeons who perform a so-called two-stage procedure, this secondary cosmetic procedure is routine. In patients who have undergone vaginoplasty in a single stage, labiaplasty and/or scar revision could be offered as an additional surgical procedure but is rarely necessary due to the remarkable healing capacity of this area of the body.

17.1.7 Venous Thromboembolism (VTE)

Major surgery predisposes patients to a risk of *deep venous thrombosis or pulmonary embolism.* The pathophysiology relates to acute inflammatory reaction caused by tissue trauma, activation of clotting cascade, and venous slowing or stasis created by prolonged immobility [10]. Risk is further compounded by certain comorbidities such as age, obesity, tobacco smoking, malignancy, and certain medications. While long-term use of cross-gender hormones appears to be safe [11–13], these patients, theoretically, may be at greater risk of VTE due to use of exogenous hormones during the perioperative period. Rare reports of nonfatal VTE associated with GRS are found in the literature [14].

To reduce the risk of thromboembolic complications, most clinicians have advocated discontinuation of exogenous hormones several weeks prior to plastic surgery procedures [12, 15]. In fact, half of British plastic surgeons who responded to a survey advocated discontinuation of hormone replacement therapy prior to surgery, with most recommending a hormone-free interval of 5–6 weeks prior to reassignment [13]. Although a dose-related risk assessment of HRT does not exist, these recommendations have been accepted as fact, although route of administration and type of hormone rather than presence or absence of HRT may be more important in terms of risk assessment for VTE. Transdermal application of estrogens appears to hold a lower risk for VTE than oral administration [16]. Additionally, ethinyl estradiol is known to increase VTE risk by 20-fold in MTF transsexuals on cross-sex HRT and is no longer recommended [11, 13]. Recent data suggests that *reduction* of estrogens prior to surgery, rather than outright discontinuation, may improve perioperative feelings of well-being without increasing the risk of VTE. Accordingly, not all surgeons who perform GRS consistently recommend discontinuation of exogenous hormones prior to surgery [17]. Early postoperative mobilization, sequential compression devices, and prophylactic anticoagulant therapy may be sufficient prophylaxis for the majority of low-risk clientele.

17.1.8 Hollow Viscus Injury

Inadvertent entry into the bowel, bladder, or urethra is an inherent risk of MTF vaginoplasty. Although rare and not disastrous in experienced hands, these complications need immediate recognition and repair if major fistulous sequelae are to be avoided. A fistula represents the gravest of potential complications and can occur even with expert repair. A mechanical bowel prep with or without antibiotic is recommended preoperatively by most surgeons when embarking upon perineal dissection to create the neovaginal cavity. The key anatomic landmark followed is the central tendon of the perineum immediately beneath the urethra, a route similarly taken in perineal prostatectomies. Urologic structures are normally well protected with the use of a handheld retractor (Ferreira Breast Retractor 95 × 25 mm, smooth end with fiber-optic light) held squarely in the midline. For rectal protection, aside from assiduously following the central tendon, keeping a portion of it posterior to the dissection field, surgeons variably use other methods. This can include the use of a Lowsley retractor placed transurethrally to retract the urologic structures anteriorly to allow the rectum to drop as dissection advances cephalad. Others employ an assistant's finger or dilator in the rectum, retracting posteriorly in addition to the anterior retraction. This allows the surgeon an additional palpable posterior backstop as dissection proceeds. Thermal injury is a potential problem but does not appear to be a significant factor in viscous injury [18]. Some have also advocated blunt dissection as opposed to sharp or cautery dissection, although this surgical philosophy remains debatable. Fistula rates after viscous injury are rarely reported but should not occur if a tension-free repair of the viscous injury has been performed [19].

17.1.9 Rectovaginal Fistula

Rectovaginal fistula presents with passage of stool or rectum through the neovagina.

Presentation later than 6 weeks post-op is unusual, although reports of late RV fistula in patients with inflammatory bowel disease have been reported. Aside from RV fistula arising de novo secondary to inflammatory bowel disease, the etiology of most other RV fistulas is likely surgical. Dilator related injuries causing RV fistula have been reported. Cautery injuries do not appear to be causative. Most injuries occur within 3 cm of the vaginal introitus, although a higher injury is possible. Diagnosis is best confirmed by Gastrografin enema. Referral to a colorectal surgeon is indicated for repair.

17.1.10 Hematoma

Hematoma is often recognized as labial asymmetry or as a firm, often fluctuant swelling beneath the neolabia majora. Postoperative induration is normally present but can easily be confused with hematoma. Ultrasound can be extremely helpful in clarifying the nature of the swelling and in estimating size. A hematoma of less than 4 cm is best managed conservatively with time and pressure. For larger hematomas, needle aspiration can result in significant reduction in size. Reopening the incision and evacuation of the hematoma can also be helpful and will relieve symptoms quickly. The reopening incision can be quite small if expressed, packed, and allowed to drain (Table 17.1).

17.1.11 Granulation Tissue

Granulation tissue results from tissue nonunion or dehiscence. It appears late in healing as bright-red, fleshy tissue that is tender and bleeds easily. It can originate along either incision, beneath the clitoral hood, or vaginally. For persistent complaints of bleeding beyond the usual recovery period (6–12 weeks), assume there is treatable granulation tissue. Granulation tissue can be managed by application of silver nitrate, although this may require several applications and multiple visits. Best practice is to simply excise the tissue at its base and treat residual bleeding with silver nitrate.

17.1.12 Urologic Complications

Urologic complications are uncommon and can be as simple as an adhesion band deviating the urinary stream. Other urologic complications are surprisingly rare. *Urethral stenosis* is particularly rare with modern approaches to vaginoplasty which splays open the posterior length of urethral spongiosum to line the inner labia. This technique not only lines the labia with mucosal, non-hair-bearing tissue but also makes urinary stricture theoretically impossible. "Fishmouthing" the neourethra can also allay the possibility of stenosis (Figs. 17.2 and 17.3). *Urinary incontinence* is not associated with

Table 17.1 Sources of postoperative vulvar swelling in MTF vaginoplasty

Induration	Hematoma	Seroma	Abscess
Neolabial swelling unilateral or bilateral	Neolabial swelling unilateral or bilateral	Neolabial swelling, tends to be unilateral	Neolabial swelling, almost always unilateral
Weeks to months in duration	Weeks to months in duration	Weeks to months in duration	Weeks to months in duration
Non-tender	Moderately tender	Non-tender unless large	Extremely tender
	Variable size to 20 cm or more	Variable size corresponding to preexistent hematoma	Usually small 2–5 cm
Self-limiting	Can evolve to abscess or seroma if undrained		
Drainage unlikely	Spontaneous dark bloody drainage possible	Spontaneous clear amber fluid drainage possible	Spontaneous purulent drainage possible
Expectant management and/or pressure	Aspiration or incision and drainage or time and pressure for 5 cm or less	Aspiration or incision and drainage	Incision and drainage, packing and antibiotics, +/− culture

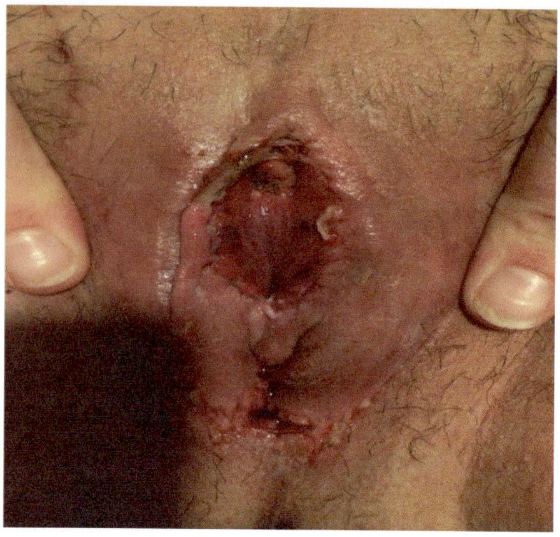

Fig. 17.2 Neoclitoris with superficial necrosis, bilateral labial necrosis, and slight posterior incisional dehiscence. Patient recovered without debridement or additional intervention

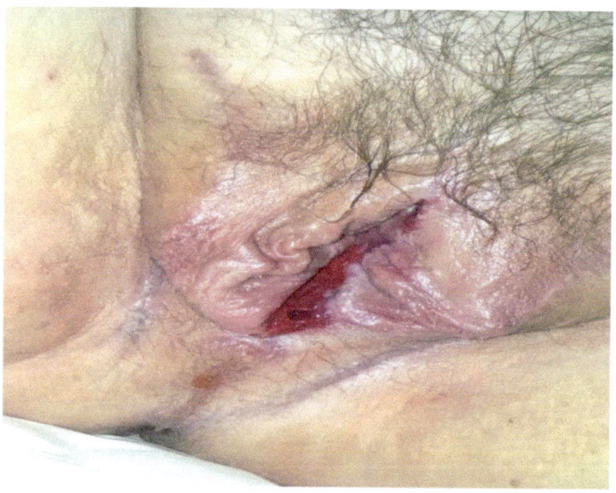

Fig. 17.3 Large area of labial granulation easily excised with scissors. Bleeding treated with silver nitrate. A smaller area located near the vaginal apex was also identified in this patient and treated

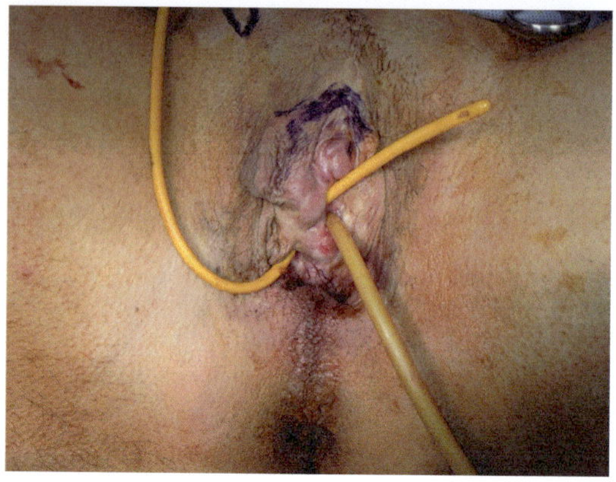

Fig. 17.4 Multiple urethrocutaneous fistulae, the largest of which is identified here at the time of consultation in preparation for corrective surgery

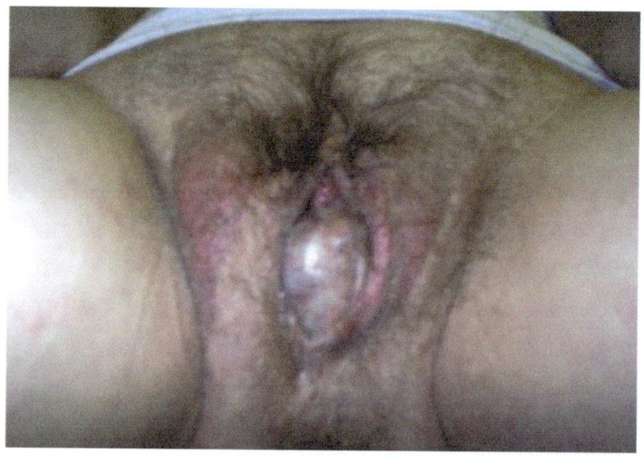

Fig. 17.5 Large residual spongiosum preventing dilation. Corrected at surgical resection

neocolporrhaphy due to limitations of the dissection field which do not extend above the internal urethral sphincter.

17.1.13 Vaginal Stenosis

Vaginal stenosis or lack of depth can be attributed to one of several technical problems: (a) surgical omission, (b) failure to dilate, or (c) infection, dehiscence, or pain which prevents a patient from suitably maintaining a satisfactory dilation regimen. In most cases, dilation is always recommended in order to maintain depth and diameter following vaginoplasty. When this is omitted, particularly during the first year following GRS/SRS, the body tends to narrow the caliber of the vaginal introitus with fibrosis and scarring (Figs. 17.4 and 17.5). Treatment options include: (a) reengaging the patient in the dilating process, (b) releasing scar tissue that has narrowed the introitus, (c) surgically reopening the area along the original lining scar along the original dissection plane and repacking the vagina, then resumption of dilation, or (d) vaginal deepening with a relining of some or all of the neovagina. Estrogen cream can be a helpful addition to this process.

17.1.14 Psychological Regret

Although not a complication of SRS per se, *regret or remorse* following genital surgery is frequently thrown up as a precautionary red flag by practitioners and outsiders who are not familiar with the technique or outcome results. Regret is exceedingly uncommon among patients who have undergone MTF vaginoplasty, perhaps less than for any surgery available in any specialty [6]. This fact alone, despite risks and variable outcomes, supports the long-standing, deeply held convictions that most trans persons hold when contemplating irreversible genital surgery. Current and evolving "standards of care" requiring psychological assessment and a period of time living in the role of the intended gender also contribute to a low, but not zero, likelihood of dissatisfaction with operative results.

In summary, vaginoplasty for MTF transsexuals is a relatively safe procedure with important but relatively rare complications. Most *major* complications present in the immediate postoperative period. Current trends of remote surgical care and recovery over weeks and months mean that the majority of postsurgical care will continue to fall to primary care providers to recognize and treat or refer. With more education of surgeons and increasing standardization of operative techniques, outcomes should continue to improve (Fig. 17.6).

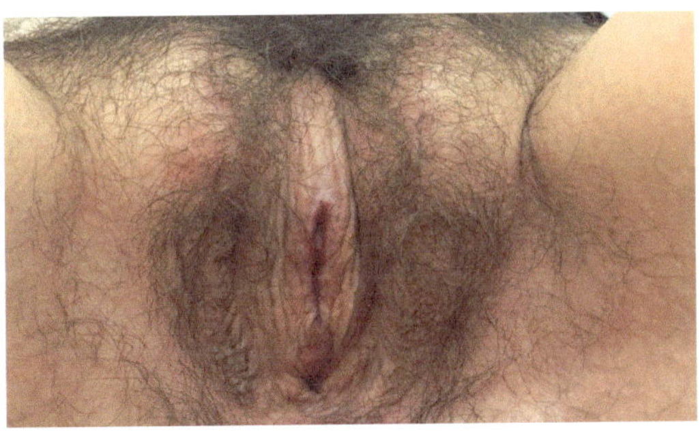

Fig. 17.6 MTF single-stage vaginoplasty, 4 months post-op uncomplicated. Note clitoris, labia major, and labia minor

References

1. Meyerowitz J (2004) How sex changed: a history of transsexuality in the United States. First Harvard University Press, Cambridge. ISBN: 9780674013797
2. Jaap AJ, Shore AC, Tooke JE (1994) The influence of hypertension on microvascular blood flow and resistance to flow in the skin of patients with non-insulin-dependent diabetes. Diabet Med 11(9):883–887
3. Rossi Neto R, Hintz F, Krege S, Rubben H, Vom Dorp F (2012) Gender reassignment surgery–a 13 year review of surgical outcomes. Int Braz J Urol 38:97–107
4. Zhao JJ, Marchaim D, Palla MB, Bogan CW, Hayakawa K, Tansek R, Moshos J, Muthusamy A, Kotra H, Lephart PR, Wilson AN, Kaye KS (2013) Surgical site infections in genital reconstruction surgery for gender reassignment, Detroit: 1984–2008. Surg Infect (Larchmt). doi:10.1089/sur.2012.225
5. Uckay I, Harbarth S, Peter R, Lew D, Hoffmeyer P, Pittet D (2010) Preventing surgical site infections. Expert Rev Anti Infect Ther 8(6):657–6701
6. Lawrence AA (2006) Patient-reported complications and functional outcomes of male-to-female sex reassignment surgery. Arch Sex Behav 35:717–727. doi:10.1007/s10508-006-9104-9
7. Eldh J (1993) Construction of a neovagina with preservation of the glans penis as a clitoris in male transsexuals. Plast Reconstr Surg 91:895–900; discussion 901–893
8. Rehman J, Melman A (1999) Formation of neoclitoris from glans penis by reduction glansplasty with preservation of neurovascular bundle in male-to-female gender surgery: functional and cosmetic outcome. J Urol 161:200–206
9. Krege S, Bex A, Lummen G, Rubben H (2001) Male-to-female transsexualism: a technique, results and long-term follow-up in 66 patients. BJU Int 88:396–402
10. Baranyi A, Piber D, Rothenhausler HB (2009) Male-to-female transsexualism. Sex reassignment surgery from a biopsychosocial perspective. Wien Med Wochenschr 159:548–557. doi:10.1007/s10354-009-0693-5
11. Desciak MC, Martin DE (2011) Perioperative pulmonary embolism: diagnosis and anesthetic management. J Clin Anesth 23:153–165. doi:10.1016/j.jclinane.2010.06.011
12. Shiffman MA (2003) Estrogen and thromboembolic disorders: should patients stop hormones prior to cosmetic surgery? J Womens Health (Larchmt) 12:853–855; discussion 855. doi:10.1089/154099903770948078
13. Toorians AW, Thamassen MC, Zweegman S, Magdelyns EJ, Tans G, Gooren LJ, Rosing J (2003) Venous thrombosis and changes of hemostatic variables during cross-sex hormone treatment in

transsexual people. J Clin Endocrinol Metab 88:5723–5729. doi:10.1210/jc.2003-030520
14. Asscheman H, Giltay EJ, Megens JA, de Ronde WP, van Trotsenburg MA, Gooren LJ (2011) A long-term follow-up study of mortality in transsexuals receiving treatment with cross-sex hormones. Eur J Endocrinol 164:635–642. doi:10.1530/EJE-10-1038
15. Asscheman H, Gooren LJ, Eklund PL (1989) Mortality and morbidity in transsexual patients with cross-gender hormone treatment. Metabolism 38:869–873
16. Laliberte F, Dea K, Duh MS, Kahler KH, Rolli M, Lefebvre P (2011) Does the route of administration for estrogen hormone therapy impact the risk of venous thromboembolism? Estradiol transdermal system versus oral estrogen-only therapy. Menopause 18:1052–1059. doi:10.1097/gme.b013e3182175e5c
17. Johnson RL, Hemington-Gorse SJ, Dhital SK (2008) Do cosmetic surgeons consider estrogen-containing drugs to be of significant risk in the development of thromboembolism? Aesthetic Plast Surg 32:743–747. doi:10.1007/s00266-008-9156-4
18. Wu M-P, Ou CS, Chen SL, Yen EY, Rowbotham R (2000) Complications and recommended practices for electrocautery in laparoscopies. Am J Surg 179: 67–73
19. Levine JH, Longo WE, Pruitt C, Mazuski JE, Shapiro MJ, Durham RM (1996) Management of selected rectal injuries by primary repair. Am J Surg 172(5):575–578; discussion 578–579

18 Surgery in Complications: Colon Vaginoplasty

Paolo Verze, Davide Arcaniolo, Marco Franco, Roberto La Rocca, and Vincenzo Mirone

An intestinal transplant for vaginoplasty in a non-transsexual patient was reported for the first time in 1892 by Sneguireff using the rectum 40 and in 1904 by Baldwin using the ileum 41. The first application of the technique in a transsexual patient was described only in 1974 by Markland and Hastings that performed a one-stage vaginoplasty with the use of both cecum and sigmoid transplants 42. The advantages of using a rectosigmoid transplant are its length and texture and appearance similar to a natural vagina 48, 49. In addition, it is the only method that provides a vaginal lining with natural lubrication 43, 48.

Although this technique could be used to create a neovagina in naïve transsexual patients, many authors agree that it is the best choice for transsexual patients who have previously undergone penectomy and orchidectomy and that it is also the best technique for patients with an unfavorable previous vaginoplasty.

In fact, in about 10–20% of patients who underwent sex reassignment surgery with penoscrotal flap or penile skin inversion, the one-stage operation fails, usually because of inadequate perineal dissection or flap necrosis or infection, leading to loss of vaginal depth and introital stenosis. In these cases, a corrective operation is then indicated. Although further skin grafting procedures may be considered, they are often subject to the same factors as the initial procedure. To remedy such complications, the technique of vaginal bowel reconstruction evolved [1–4].

18.1 Surgical Technique

The development of this technique was possible as the sigmoid mesocolon has a long and easily mobilized mesentery that allows the selected tract to reach the perineum in a satisfactory way. The sigmoid segment is isolated by division of the sigmoid mesocolon so that the most distal long sigmoid branch of the inferior mesenteric artery is preserved to function as the main segmental blood supplier. The more proximal branches are divided. The blood supply then, depending on the primary arterial arcade, runs on the mesenteric side of the bowel. The sigmoid is reverted so the previous proximal end can be brought down for the perineal-cutaneous anastomosis. In this way, considerable length can be achieved without generating unnecessary tension in the mesenteric blood supply, thus reducing chances of ischemic necrosis.

The surgical procedure should be preferably performed under both general anesthesia and epidural analgesia. The epidural catheter is left in

P. Verze • D. Arcaniolo (✉) • M. Franco
R. La Rocca • V. Mirone
Department of Urology, University of Naples _ Federico II, Via S.Pansini 5, Naples 80131, Italy
e-mail: pverze@gmail.com; davide.arcaniolo@gmail.com; marcofranco87@gmail.com; robertolarocca87@gmail.com; mirone@unina.it

C. Trombetta et al. (eds.), *Management of Gender Dysphoria: A Multidisciplinary Approach*, DOI 10.1007/978-88-470-5696-1_18, © Springer-Verlag Italia 2015

place for a better postoperative analgesia. The preoperative preparation included full mechanical preparation of the colon and prophylactic administration of heparin. The patient is placed in an extended lithotomy position with the buttocks slightly elevated. The lithotomy position guarantees a wide access to the perineum, with excellent intra-abdominal exposure.

Through a Pfannenstiel incision (semicircular, slightly above the mons pubis – Fig. 18.1), the descending colon is mobilized down to, and including, the sigmoid colon. Then, a sigmoid segment was isolated with its vascular pedicle (Figs. 18.2 and 18.3). It is of paramount importance that before choosing the definitive sigmoid colon segment, surgeons should assess the length of the sigmoid and its mesentery in order to determine whether it can reach the perineum. Usually, a tension-free rectosigmoid vagina can be made up if the lowest point of the sigmoid can be pulled down to reach easily the pubic symphysis. The length of the isolated rectosigmoid segment should range from 8 to 12 cm, to avoid excessive postoperative mucus production. Rectosigmoid is harvested with its blood supply originating from sigmoidal arteries and/or superior hemorrhoidal vessels. Preferably, it should be divided distally first in order to check its mobility and determine the correct site for its proximal division. The proximal end of the isolated segment was closed in two layers using absorbable sutures. Bowel continuity was restored with a hand-sewn single-layer anastomosis with 3-0 silk sutures. The mesenteric defect is closed with the neovagina and its mesentery at the left side of the field (Figs. 18.4 and 18.5). Afterwards, an H-shaped incision is performed in the perineum, and a blunt dissection is performed between the urethra and rectum to create a space for the allocation of the neovaginal colon conduit. In salvage intervention for female transsexuals, scarred and nonfunctional vagina is completely excised to provide adequate space to position the sigmoid loop.

Then isolated sigmoid is brought down to the perineal canal without tension to create a tension-free coloperineal anastomosis. In order to prevent

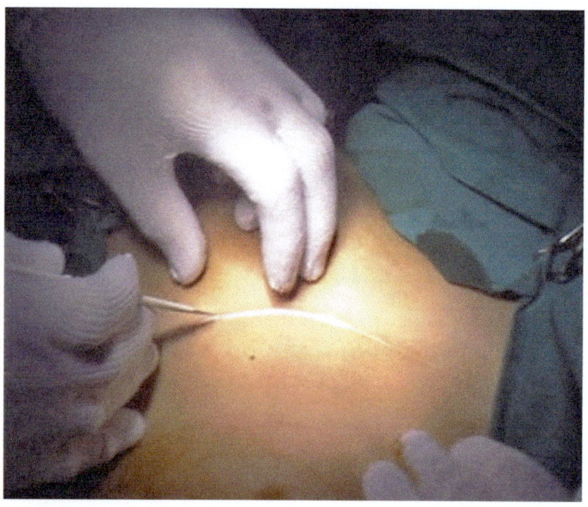

Fig. 18.1 Abdominal incision

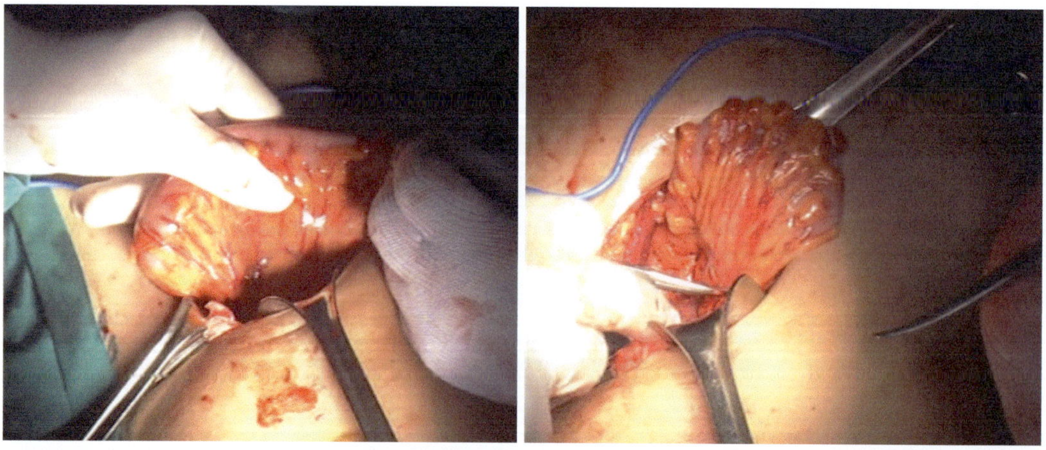

Figs. 18.2 and 18.3 Isolation of the sigmoid segment

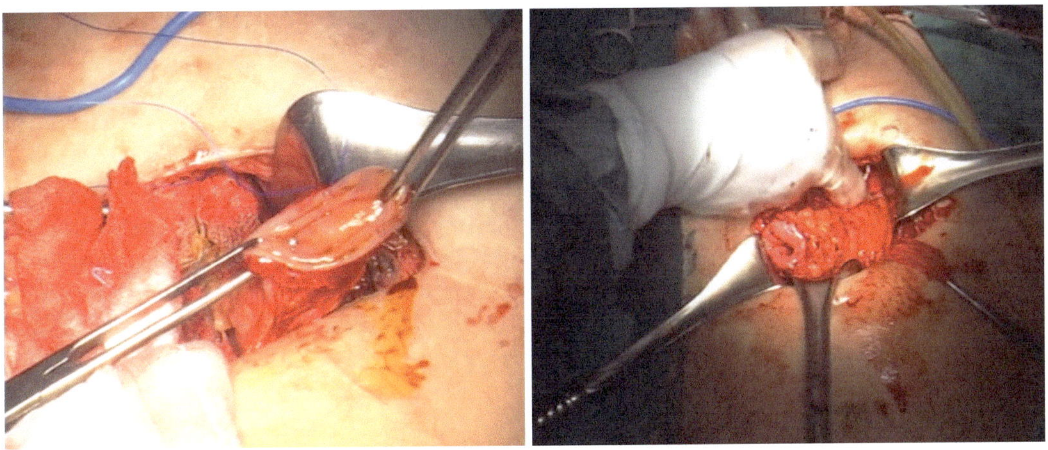

Figs. 18.4 and 18.5 Creation of neovagina

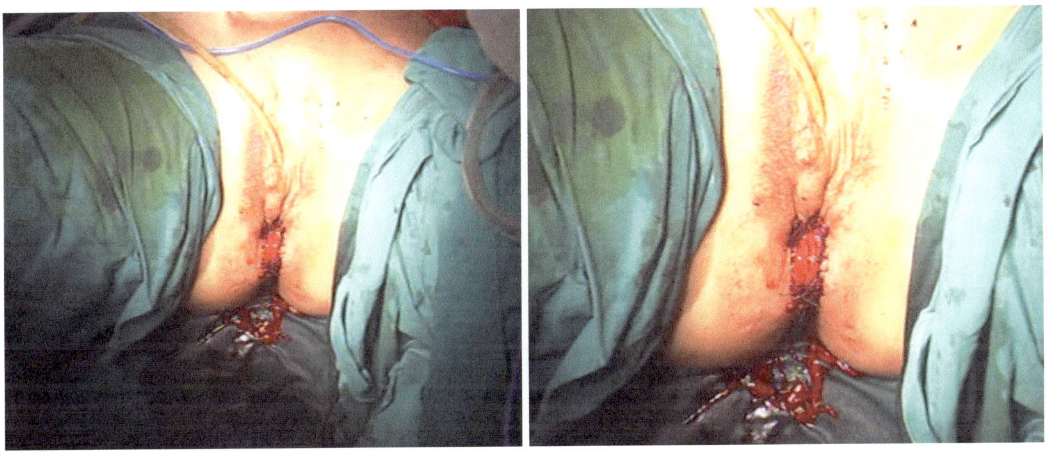

Figs. 18.6 and 18.7 Final result

purse-string scarring, introital or perineal skin flaps are formed and approximated to the sigmoid vagina. In order to avoid prolapse, some authors perform a "U"-shaped incision posterior to the urethra and complete it with two lateral vascularized introital flaps. Vascularized flaps are completely mobilized to push the neo-introital opening as high as possible to prevent mucosal prolapse and to yield better aesthetic results with the anastomosis deeply hidden. Some other surgeons prefer to fix the proximal end of the neovagina to the sacral promontory.

Then the neovagina was packed with a compressive dressing for about 7 days, and a Foley catheter is placed and removed 4–5 days after surgery, in order to facilitate the fixation of the rectosigmoid graft to the surrounding tissues. Patients are instructed on how to perform self-dilation of the neovaginal introitus and irrigation of the neovagina for mucus removal, daily for 8 weeks and weekly thereafter.

The final result is showed in Figs. 18.6 and 18.7 [2–9].

The maintenance of hormonal therapy after surgery allows to aid the feminine aspect of external genitalia (hair and fat distribution) rectosigmoidal vaginoplasty.

As described more successfully for ileal vaginoplasty, some authors present the possibility of a combined laparoscopic and perineal approach for rectosigmoidal vaginoplasty. A three-port transperitoneal approach is used for the complete vaginal isolation and mobilization, for rectosigmoid segment isolation, and for vaginal anastomosis [10–11].

Furthermore, Kim et al. presented a case of a robot-assisted sigmoid vaginoplasty in a woman with vaginal agenesia. To date, this operation has never been performed for transsexual surgery [12].

18.2 Complications

The advantages of rectosigmoid vaginoplasty are summarized in Table 18.1. Although the neovaginal length is usually regarded as an advantage, it can also lead to stasis and dehydration of mucus in the deepest portion of the vagina. Further disadvantages of this technique are the need for additional abdominal surgery and occasional disappointing long-term results. Furthermore, the colonic mucosa is more vulnerable and thus more accessible to sexually transmitted diseases including human immunodeficiency virus infection.

Peri- and postoperative complications usually occur only in a small proportion of patients (incidence lower than 10 %). The most frequent complications are excessive mucosal discharge and malodor. Diversion colitis (inflammation that occurs in the bypassed colonic tissue related to diversion of the fecal stream), ulcerative colitis, peritonitis, intestinal obstruction, junctional neuroma, adenocarcinoma, introital stenosis, mucocele, and constipation have been reported to occur more rarely but are deserving of more attention by the clinicians.

Usually, patients who had partners are able to have sexual intercourse starting 6 months after surgery, and only a small percentage of patients (<5 %) used lubricants or dilators before intercourse for more than a year postoperatively. During intercourse, a high amount of M-to-F transsexual patients experienced orgasm [13–14].

Table 18.1 Advantages of sigmoid neovagina

1. Rare contraction of the reconstructed vagina
2. Vaginal width and depth maintained without long-term vaginal stent
3. Spontaneous mucus production facilitating sexual intercourse
4. Avoidance of the malodor frequently accompanying skin graft
5. Texture and appearance similar to that of the natural vagina
6. Suitable as a rescue intervention after neovagina stenosis or necrosis

References

1. Sneguireff WF (1904) Zwei Falle von Restitutio Vaginiae per Transplantationen. Ani Recti Zentralbl Gynakol 28:772
2. Baldwin JF (1904) The formation of an artificial vagina by intestinal transplantation. Ann Surg 40:398–403
3. Markland C, Hastings D (1974) Vaginal reconstruction using cecal and sigmoid bowel segments in transsexual patients. J Urol 111:217
4. Vecchietti G (1965) Neovagina nella syndrome di Rokitansky-Kuster-Hauser. Annu Ostet Gunecol 11:131–147
5. Creatsas G, Deligeoroglou E, Makrakis E, Kontoravdis A, Papadimitriou L (2001) Creation of a neovagina following Williams vaginoplasty and the Creatsas modification in 111 patients with Mayer-Rokitansky-Kuster-Hauser syndrome. Fertil Steril 76:1036–1040
6. Davies MC, Creighton SM, Woodhouse CR (2005) The pitfalls of vaginal reconstruction. BJU Int 95:1293–1298
7. Jarolím L, Sedý J, Schmidt M, Nanka O, Foltán R, Kawaciuk I (2009) Gender reassignment surgery in male-to-female transsexualism: a retrospective 3-month follow-up study with anatomical remarks. J Sex Med 6:1635–1644
8. Hensle TW, Reiley EA (1998) Vaginal replacement in children and young adults. J Urol 159:1035–1038
9. Djordjevic ML, Stanojevic DS, Bizic MR (2011) Rectosigmoid vaginoplasty: clinical experience and outcomes in 86 cases. J Sex Med 8(12):3487–3494
10. Liguori G, Trombetta C, Bucci S, Salamè L, Bortul M, Siracusano S, Belgrano E (2005) Laparoscopic mobilization of neovagina to assist secondary ileal vaginoplasty in male-to-female transsexuals. Urology 66(2):293–298
11. Wedler V, Meuli-Simmen C, Guggenheim M, Schneller-Gustafsson M, Künzi W (2004) Laparoscopic technique for secondary vaginoplasty in male to female transsexuals using a modified

vascularized pedicled sigmoid. Gynecol Obstet Invest 57(4):181–185
12. Kim C, Campbell B, Ferrer F (2008) Robotic sigmoid vaginoplasty: a novel technique. Urology 72(4): 847–849
13. Kapoor R, Sharma DK, Singh KJ, Suri A, Singh P, Chaudhary H, Dubey D, Mandhani A (2006) Sigmoid vaginoplasty: long-term results. Urology 67(6): 1212–1215
14. Kwun Kim S, Hoon Park J, Cheol Lee K, Min Park J, Tae Kim J, Chan Kim M (2003) Long-term results in patients after rectosigmoid vaginoplasty. Plast Reconstr Surg 112(1):143–151

19 Surgery in Complications: Ileal Vaginoplasty

Giovanni Liguori, Carlo Trombetta, Bernardino De Concilio, Gaetano Chiapparone, Michele Rizzo, and Emanuele Belgrano

19.1 Introduction

As concluded by Karim [1] in 1996, "the surgical aim of *genital reassignment* in MF-TS is to create a perineogenital complex as feminine in appearance and function as possible. The perineogenital area should be free of poorly healed areas, scars, and neuromas. The neovagina should ideally be lined with moist, elastic, and hairless epithelium. Its depth should be at least 10 cm and its diameter should be 30 mm."

Today, the penile-scrotal skin flap technique is considered the technique of choice for vaginoplasty in MTF transsexualism [2].

Unfortunately, secondary corrections are often needed (up to 30 % of cases) to improve the function in case of stenosis when patients are not compliant with dilation or simply following a shrinkage of the skin lining the vagina which often causes a reduction in the caliber and the length of the vagina with associated undesirable symptoms [3].

The surgical management of *neovaginal stenosis* in a transsexual patient is a complex problem and constitutes a significant technical challenge. As a matter of fact, although urologic treatment of the male transsexual is becoming more common, few follow-up studies have been reported and a standardized follow-up is particularly difficult in this group because of the anatomical differences and large range of surgical approaches. Moreover, international reports have generally lacked consistent published information about the surgical management of postoperative neovaginal stenosis in transsexual patients.

G. Liguori, MD, PhD (✉) • C. Trombetta
B. De Concilio • G. Chiapparone • M. Rizzo • E. Belgrano
Department of Urology, University of Trieste,
Strada di Fiume 447, Trieste 34144, Italy
e-mail: Gioliguori33@gmail.com;
trombcar@univ.trieste.it;
bernardinodeconcilio@hotmail.com;
g.chiapparrone@gmail.com; mik.rizzo@gmail.com;
emanuelebelgrano@gmail.com

19.2 Conservative Management

The key to success in the management of vaginal strictures is the punctual diagnosis. It is imperative to identify strictures early in the disease process. Preventative procedures against vaginal stenosis development constitute conservative management. The approach is similar in all patients and is based on the underlying condition causing the development of stricture. The mainstay in conservative treatment is the use of *rigid dilators* for treatment as well as prevention. As a matter of fact, the habitual use of vaginal dilators has been suggested by many authors in order to prevent vaginal stenosis [4, 5].

19.3 Surgical Management

Successful sexual intercourse should be the primary end point when choosing the method for savage vaginoplasty. As a matter of fact, an ideal

C. Trombetta et al. (eds.), *Management of Gender Dysphoria: A Multidisciplinary Approach*,
DOI 10.1007/978-88-470-5696-1_19, © Springer-Verlag Italia 2015

method for vaginal replacement should provide a cosmetically acceptable, low-maintenance vaginal substitute with minimal morbidity and excellent long-term function.

When conservative treatment yields insufficient results, a secondary *vaginoplasty* using intestinal segments is the first-choice treatment for vaginal reconstruction [6].

Achieving a satisfactory result is influenced by many factors, including the underlying condition and previous pelvic surgery, as well as the surgeon's skills and technique elected. Moreover, the increasing recognition of the efficacy of vaginal dilation [7] means that those patients needing secondary vaginoplasty are usually complex patients with previous failed surgical intervention and in whom dilator treatment is not possible [8].

However, a standardized treatment does not yet exist [9], and many techniques have been described for vaginal reconstruction. Other surgical options have included skin transplants [10–12] and myocutaneous transplants [13] or epithelialization from the outer skin layer (the Vecchietti method) [14].

In our opinion, the *split-thickness skin graft* is indicated only in cases of small reconstructions of the distal vaginal tract because it requires lubrication, prolonged vaginal dilations, or sexual intercourses to maintain patency. Moreover, contracture, shortening, bleedings, and dyspareunia are frequent [15].

19.3.1 Bowel Vaginoplasty

Where a primary vaginoplasty, combining inversion of the penile and scrotal skin flaps, yields unsatisfactory functional results, a secondary vaginoplasty using the pedicled intestinal segments represents an elegant means to achieve a functional improvement.

The use of bowel has been revisited in the last few decades because of concerns about complications associated with grafting and flap techniques: today the majority of surgeons favor a technique using a pediculated isolated sigmoid colon segment [9, 12]. The advantages of intestinal transplant methods include adequate vaginal length, natural lubrication, early coitus, and a lack of shrinkage [16].

In 1904, Baldwin [17] first described a vaginoplasty performed with an isolated *ileum loop* and suggested a possible use of the sigmoid colon for the same purposes. Wallace, in 1911, referred the first sigmoid colon vaginoplasty.

The sigmoid colon has been popular because of its proximity and its easily mobilized vascular pedicle [18]. On the other hand, the ileum is technically the least demanding of the conduits to create, and it has become the segment of choice over colon in conduit diversion in urological practice [19].

19.3.2 Ileal Vaginoplasty

19.3.2.1 Preoperative Evaluation

The preoperative evaluation included detailed counseling, physical examination, full hormone profile, magnetic resonance imaging, and detailed explanation with possible risks of the planned procedures to the patients.

19.3.2.2 Preoperative Preparation

Preoperative preparation included full mechanical preparation of the colon and prophylactic administration of heparin and perioperative antibiotics. Under general anesthesia, the patient is positioned in supine lithotomy position in order to achieve a good intra-abdominal exposure as well as wide access to the perineum and introitus.

19.3.2.3 Technique of Ileal Vaginoplasty

The patient is positioned for surgery in supine lithotomic position in order to achieve a good intra-abdominal exposure as well as wide access to the perineum and introitus. A simultaneous abdominal perineal approach is used. Through a midline or Pfannenstiel approach, after inspection of the abdomen and pelvis, the pouch of Douglas is accessed.

19.3.2.4 Perineal Phase

Different kinds of perineal incision shapes are used depending on the case: H-shaped incision in the perineum posterior to the urethra, transverse incision in the vaginal groove between the urethra and the posterior commissure, or circular incisions are viable options.

Then dissection of the neovaginal cavity is performed, and the perineo-abdominal tunnel is created by blunt finger dissection. A tunnel with two or three finger width is developed until the peritoneum is reached.

19.3.2.5 Abdominal Phase

A *Hegar* sound is inserted in the distal vaginal segment, and the peritoneal reflection is opened while pushing the sound as a marker. The vaginal vault is then isolated completely. This step of the operation is generally very difficult after previous surgery because scars and fibrosis obliterate the natural tissue planes. Using this method, with blunt dissection, a surgical plane was developed between the urethra and rectum. Careful attention must be paid to prevent damage to the surface of the rectum and urethra. It is important to create a space large enough for the bowel segment to fit easily and enable mobilization of the vaginal vault to allow a capacious, well-vascularized, and tension-free anastomosis.

19.3.2.6 External Configuration of the Neovagina

The ileum is extracted, and an ileal loop of 15–20 cm that more easily reaches the pelvis is chosen, at about 20 cm from the ileocecal valve. Vascularization of the loop is preserved using the standard transillumination technique.

The advantages of the distal ileum is its intrapelvic location: for this reason, it can be transposed to the pelvic floor without causing tension on the blood vessels that supply the region and without jeopardizing tissue survival. Furthermore, equilibrium between liquid resorption and mucus secretion in the distal ileum provides optimal lubrication of the neovagina.

Although transplantation of straight ileal segments is a possible option, this technique is limited by the inadequate lumen size. In order to overcome this drawback and increase the lumen size, vaginoplasty is usually performed with ileum segments grafted with different folding techniques. The segment of the ileum, once isolated, can be opened along its anti-mesenteric border (Fig. 19.1) and reconfigured into a "U" shape (Fig. 19.2a, b) or "J" shape and tubularized to create the vagina (Fig. 19.3). This is commonly performed over a 20-F Hegar dilator to approximate an adequate caliber. The pouch is then opened in the fold to form the vaginal introitus. Care is taken to create a *tension-free anastomosis* that is recessed at the introitus.

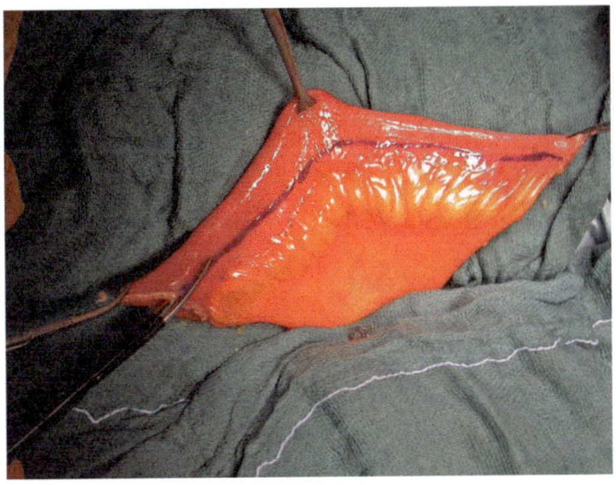

Fig. 19.1 The segment of the ileum, once isolated, is opened along its anti-mesenteric border

Another surgical option is the application of the *Monti* principle to ileal vaginoplasty: the isolated segment is detubularized and transversally retubularized in order to configure the roof of the neovagina. The proximal end of the conduit is closed with two layers of absorbable suture material (Fig. 19.4).

The ileal segment is then brought to the perineum with as little tension as possible in order to allow a tension-free anastomosis. Ileocutaneous anastomoses with interrupted absorbable sutures (Monocryl 3-0) are finally performed through the perineal approach.

An inflatable silicon vaginal tutor is introduced in the vaginal cavity and is maintained all day long for 7 days. The catheter is removed after 5 days.

19.3.2.7 Postoperative Management

It is important to avoid washing the neovagina with substances that can damage or irritate the ileum: utilization of sterile saline solution is recommended in the first postoperative month. After

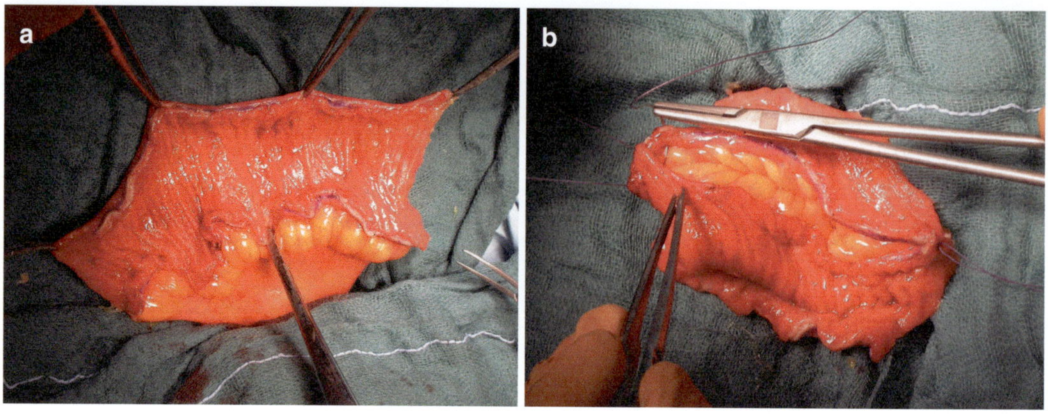

Fig. 19.2 (**a**) The intestinal segment is folded and reconfigured into a "U" shape and (**b**) anastomosed with the anti-mesenteric sides toward each other

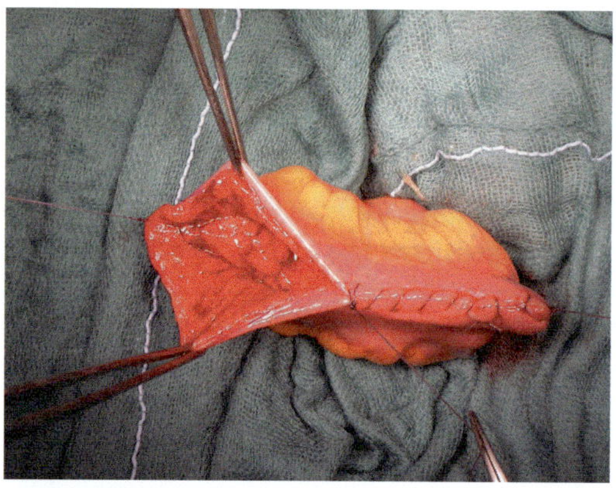

Fig. 19.3 The neovagina is constructed from an ileal U-pouch anastomosed to the vaginal stump

removal of the inflatable silicon vaginal tutor, patients are instructed to insert a lubrified dilator in the neovagina to prevent stenosis of the introitus and in order to achieve a correct modeling of the cavity. In our opinion, prolonged stenting of the neovagina is mandatory when neovagina creation is performed after failure of a previous surgical method.

19.4 Discussion

Many techniques have been described for secondary vaginal reconstruction [9], but disadvantages are in all of them. The nonoperative techniques for vaginal dilation rely on repeated pressure against the vaginal dimple to create the vagina [20]. Results of this technique have not been universally satisfactory [21]: this procedure has the disadvantages of requiring long-term dilations, which may be not well accepted by all patients. *Vecchietti* developed a laparotomic surgical variant which has been widely used for many years [14]. It consists of implantation of a device designed to increase the depth of the vaginal cupola. The technique does not require vesicorectal dissection and has a good success rate. However, a daily application of a vaginal probe is required for a long time, and the resulting depth of the neovagina is limited. A laparoscopic modification of this technique has been done successfully but still requires the use of dilators [22].

The most popular technique for vaginal replacement has been the split-thickness free graft or *McIndoe* procedure. Advantages of the technique are the ease of surgery, but it requires continuous and frequent home dilation and the wearing of a vaginal stent during the night. In addition, there is a high rate of incidence of inadequate vaginal length, vaginal stenosis, and dyspareunia [10].

Several series now have shown the utilities of intestinal vaginoplasty for reconstruction [23, 24]. Reconstruction with bowel can be done at any age, and the risk of flap necrosis or lack of graft take is minimal. Moreover, the reconstructed vagina has a natural axis for sexual intercourse. Other advantages of using bowel segments

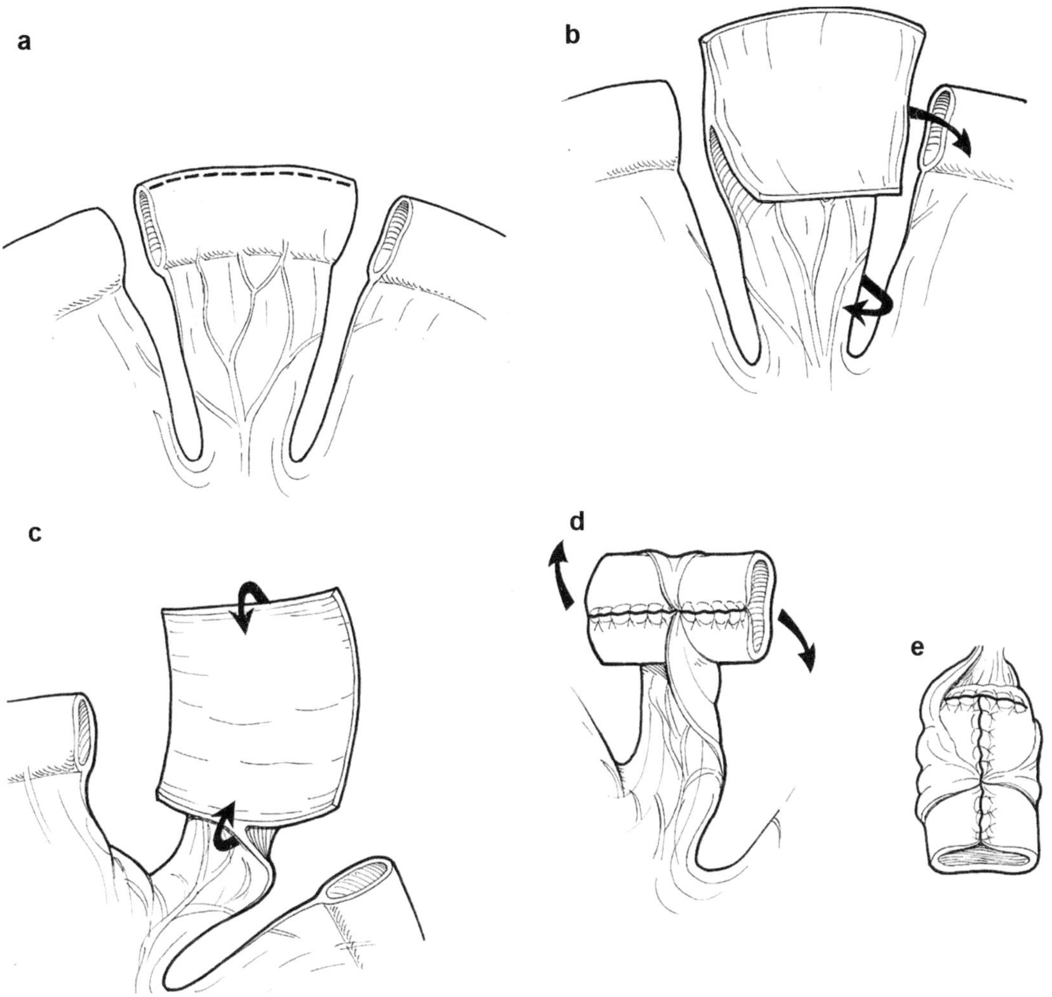

Fig. 19.4 Detubularization-and-retubularization technique. (**a**) A 12-cm ileal segment is isolated, (**b**) detubularized through longitudinal incision halfway on the anterior side. (**c**) The flap is then rotated and (**d**) transversally retubularized with total running suture. (**e**) The vault of the neovagina is then configured and prepared for the anastomosis with the perineum or the distal

include the limited need for dilations in the postoperative period, the relatively stronger resistance of the mucosa to trauma, and the ability of the intestinal mucus to act as lubrifier.

In the last years, many authors have reported their successful experience in the use of the sigmoid colon for vaginal replacement in children and adults [12, 23]. The sigmoid colon has been popular because of its proximity and its easily mobilized vascular pedicle [8]. Use of the ileum and cecum has been described too, but reports are more rare [25]. As a matter of fact, when ileum is used, its smaller diameter and its mesentery's origin make construction more challenging, and extra care must be taken to ensure the distal segment will reach the perineum tension free [18].

Formation of an ileo-neovagina by longitudinal *detubularization* and transverse retubularization has many advantages: small intestinal segments are necessary; the mesentery remains in the central portion of the tube leaving the two branches free; in this manner the conduit is highly mobile, with the opportunity to reach the perineum and provide a tension-free anastomosis: as a matter of fact, the ileum has a low vascular loops and short mesenterium; standard ileal vaginoplasty requires isolation of long segments (20–30 cm at least) to reach the perineum safely, without tension. Furthermore, the diameter of the conduit can be selected according to individual needs and allows sufficient drainage of mucus; the tube is cylindrical, regular, and of an adjustable length so as to achieve a correct modeling of the cavity [26].

Moreover, dehiscence, necrosis, and late complications such as stenosis and perforation of the tube have not been reported so far in the Monti channel [27].

Alternatively, a 12- to 15-cm segment of the ileum, once isolated, can be opened along its anti-mesenteric border, reconfigured into a "U" shape, and tabularized to create the vagina. This is commonly performed over a 20-F Hegar dilator to approximate an adequate caliber. Care is taken to create a *tension-free anastomosis* that is recessed at the introitus, similar to sigmoid repair [18].

More recently, a J-pouch of the distal ileum was constructed pedicled on the ileocolic artery and accompanying nervous plexus, transferred into the lower pelvis, and sutured to the vaginal stump. One-year follow-up showed a highly satisfied, sexually active patient, with adequate vaginal size, optimal lubrication, and no molesting fecal odor [28].

As far as we are concerned, there are several reasons to prefer the ileum instead of sigmoid colon for vaginal reconstruction. First of all, the ileum is technically the least demanding of the conduits to create, and this is why it has become the segment of choice in conduit diversion in urological practice [29]. Secondly, the ileum has a lower mucus production as compared to the large bowel, and last but not least, the urologist has a general familiarity with the small bowel used for reconstructive surgery. In a recent review on intestinal vaginoplasty, Bouman analyzed surgical procedures performed by gynecologists, urologists, and plastic surgeons. Although no rationale was provided for choosing either the ileum or sigmoid as the graft donor site, he observed that ileal graft was mostly used by urologists, perhaps because of their experience with the use of ileal grafts in bladder reconstruction. Gynecologists and plastic surgeons tended to use sigmoid grafts [25].

Furthermore, the ileal segment has the advantages of satisfactory neovaginal function similar to a normal vagina with self-lubrication, which decreases the incidence of dyspareunia; less secondary deformity in the perineum [30]; and a natural axis for sexual intercourse [31].

Moreover, there are several potential chronic complications of the use of sigmoid segments that must be underlined. Sigmoid segment isolation may induce diversion colitis: this pathology may be more common than suspected and may take as long as 7 years to develop [32–34]. The mucous discharge commonly seen after colon vaginoplasty is possibly secondary to asymptomatic diversion colitis in most patients.

We have described a case in which mucus production within the neovaginal continued and the introital stenosis led to stasis of the mucus, which ultimately perforated the neovagina and caused acute peritonitis [35].

Moreover, patients may develop gastrointestinal disease such as ulcerative colitis or hereditary polyposis [36]. Primary adenocarcinoma in sigmoid neovagina has been reported too [37, 38].

In accordance with Syed et al. [34], in patients who need an *enterovaginoplasty*, the use of small bowel should be assessed as an alternative to the sigmoid colon. If the colon is used, the risk of diversion colitis should be explained and long-term surveillance should be recommended because of the theoretical increased risk of malignant change.

Today, the use of bowel segments for vaginoplasty is becoming more frequent, as in some centers (e.g., Free University, Amsterdam), younger patients are being treated with hormonal treatment, which is arresting the puberty; consequently, less amount of penile skin is available for lining the neovagina and bowel vaginoplasty is primarily indicated [39].

For best results, in our opinion, prolonged stenting of *the neovagina* is mandatory when vaginoplasty is performed after failure of a previous gender surgery: in these patients, an inflatable silicon vaginal tutor is introduced in the vaginal cavity and is maintained all day long for

7 days in order to achieve a correct modeling of the cavity, and then the patients are encouraged to perform dilation of the vagina using a rigid stent 15 min every day over a 1-month period or until they became sexually active. Functional results were also encouraging: all patients are sexually active after neovagina repair and are happy with their sexual functioning. Moreover, there is an evident difficulty in the objective evaluation of patients' satisfaction after SRS: as a matter of fact, transsexual patients are a completely different group of patients in which validated questionnaire is not available.

References

1. Karim RB, Hage JJ, Cuesta MA (1996) Rectosigmoid neocolpopoiesis for male-to-female transsexuals: Amsterdam experience. Ann Plast Surg 36(4): 388–391
2. Selvaggi G, Ceulemnas P, De Cuypere G (2005) Gender identity disorder: general overview and surgical treatment for vaginoplasty in male-to-female transsexuals. Plast Reconstr Surg 116:135e–145e
3. Nowier A, Esmat M, Hamza RT (2012) Surgical and functional outcomes of sigmoid vaginoplasty among patients with variants of disorders of sex development. Int Braz J Urol 38(3):380–386
4. Decruze SB, Guthrie D, Magnani R (1999) Prevention of vaginal stenosis in patients following vaginal brachytherapy. Clin Oncol (R Coll Radiol) 11:46–48
5. Robinson JW, Faris PD, Scott CB (1999) Psychoeducational group increases vaginal dilation for younger women and reduces sexual fears for women of all ages with gynecological carcimona treated with radiotherapy. Int J Radiat Oncol Biol Phys 44:497–506
6. Selvaggi G, Bellringer J (2011) Gender reassignment surgery: an overview. Nat Rev Urol 8(5):274–282
7. Laufer MR (2002) Congenital absence of the vagina: in search of the perfect solution. When, and by what technique, should a vagina be created? Curr Opin Obstet Gynecol 14:441–444
8. Davies MC, Creighton SM, Woodhouse CRJ (2005) The pitfalls of vaginal construction. BJU Int 95:1293–1298
9. Hensle TW, Chang DT (1999) Vaginal reconstruction. Urol Clin North Am 26:39–47
10. Adamson CD, Naik BJ, Lynch DJ (2004) The vacuum expandable condom mold: a simple vaginal stent for McIndoe style vaginoplasty. Plast Reconstr Surg 113:664–666
11. McIndoe A (1950) Treatment of congenital absence and obliterative conditions of vagina. Br J Plast Surg 2:254–267
12. Parsons JK, Gearhart SL, Gearhart JP (2002) Vaginal reconstruction utilizing sigmoid colon: complications and long-term results. J Pediatr Surg 37:629–633
13. McCraw JB, Massey FM, Shanklin KD (1976) Vaginal reconstruction with gracilis myocutaneous flaps. Plast Reconstr Surg 58:176–183
14. Vecchietti G (1980) Neovagina in Rokitansky-Küster-Hauser syndrome. Gynakologe 13:112–115
15. Lima M, Ruggeri G, Randi B, Dòmini M, Gargano T, La Pergola E, Gregori G (2010) Vaginal replacement in the pediatric age group: a 34-year experience of intestinal vaginoplasty in children and young girls. J Pediatr Surg 45(10):2087–2091
16. Luis-Sylvestre C, Haddad B, Paniel BJ (1997) Creation of a sigmoid neovagina: technique and results in 16 cases. Eur J Obstet Gynecol Reprod Biol 75:225–229
17. Baldwin JF (1904) The formation of an artificial vagina by intestinal transplantation. Ann Surg 40:398
18. O'Connor JL, DeMarco RT, Pope JC IV, Adams MC, Brock JW III (2004) Bowel vaginoplasty in children: a retrospective review. J Pediatr Surg 39(8):1205–1208
19. Madersbacher S, Schmidt J, Eberle JM, Thoeny HC, Burkhard F, Hochreiter W, Studer UE (2003) Long-term outcome of ileal conduit diversion. J Urol 169(3):985–990
20. Frank RT (1938) The formation of an artificial vagina without operation. Am J Obstet Gynecol 35:1053–1055
21. Rock JA, Reeves LA, Retto H, Baramki TA, Zacur HA, Jones HW Jr (1983) Success following vaginal creation for Mullerian agenesis. Fertil Steril 39(6):809–813
22. Fedele L, Bianchi S, Zanconato G, Raffalli R (2000) Laparoscopic creation of a neovagina in patients with Rokytansky syndrome: analysis of 52 cases. Fertil Steril 74:384–389
23. Rajimwale A, Furness PD III, Brant WO, Koyle MA (2004) Vaginal construction using sigmoid colon in children and young adults. BJU Int 94(1):115–119
24. DeMarco RT, Pope JC IV, Adams MC, Brock JW III (2003) The use of bowel in vaginal reconstruction. Curr Urol Rep 4(6):409–411
25. Bouman MB, van Zeijl MC, Buncamper ME, Meijerink WJ, van Bodegraven AA, Mullender MG (2014) Intestinal vaginoplasty revisited: a review of surgical techniques, complications, and sexual function. J Sex Med 11(7):1835–1847
26. Trombetta C, Liguori G, Siracusano S, Bortul M, Belgrano E (2005) Transverse retubularized ileal vaginoplasty: a new application of the Monti principle–preliminary report. Eur Urol 48(6):1018–1023
27. Monti PR, de Carvalho JR, Arap S (2000) The Monti procedure: applications and complications. Urology 55(5):616–621
28. Schneider W, Nguyen-Thanh P, Dralle H, Mirastschijski U (2009) Ileal J-pouch vaginoplasty: reconstruction of a physiologic vagina with an ileal J-pouch. Am J Obstet Gynecol 200(6):694.e1–4

29. Farnham SB, Cookson MS (2004) Surgical complications of urinary diversion. World J Urol 22(3):157–167
30. Zhao YZ, Jiang DZ, Jiang H, Qiu M, Lin ZH, Zhu XH (2006) Laparoscopic small intestinal flap colpopoiesis. Chin J Plast Surg 22:339–342
31. Ismail IS, Cutner AS, Creighton SM (2006) Laparoscopic vaginoplasty: alternative techniques in vaginal reconstruction. BJOG 113:340–343
32. Toolenaar TA, Freunt I, Huikeshoven FJ, Drogendijk AC, Jeekel H (1993) The occurrence of diversion colitis in patients with a sigmoid neovagina. Hum Pathol 24:846–849
33. Abbasakoor F, Mahon C, Boulos PB (2004) Diversion colitis in sigmoid neovagina. Colorectal Dis 6(4):290–291
34. Syed HA, Malone PS, Hitchcock RJ (2001) Diversion colitis in children with colovaginoplasty. BJU Int 87(9):857–860
35. Liguori G, Trombetta C, Buttazzi L, Belgrano E (2001) Acute peritonitis due to introital stenosis and perforation of a bowel neovagina in a transsexual. Obstet Gynecol 97:828–829
36. Malka D, Anquetil C, Ruszniewski P (2000) Ulcerative colitis in a sigmoid neovagina. N Engl J Med 343(5):369
37. Hiroi H, Yasugi T, Matsumoto K, Fujii T, Watanabe T, Yoshikawa H (2001) Mucinous adenocarcinoma arising in a neovagina using the sigmoid colon thirty years after operation: a case report. J Surg Oncol 77(1):61–64
38. Ursic-Vrscaj M, Lindtner J, Lamovec J, Novak J (1994) Adenocarcinoma in a sigmoid neovagina 22 years after Wertheim-Meigs operation. Eur J Gynaecol Oncol 15(1):24–28
39. Wroblewski P, Gustafsson J, Selvaggi G (2013) Sex reassignment surgery for transsexuals. Curr Opin Endocrinol Diabetes Obes 20(6):570–574

20 Surgery Complications: Management of Neovaginal Prolapse

Stefano Bucci, Giorgio Mazzon, Giovanni Liguori, Nicola Pavan, and Carlo Trombetta

The goal of male-to-female sex reassignment surgery (SRS) is to create a perineogenital complex as feminine in appearance and function as possible and free of poorly healed areas, scars, and neuromas. The neovagina should ideally be lined with moist elastic and hairless epithelium. Its depth should be at least 10 cm and its diameter should be 30 mm [1].

During the past decades, several techniques has been proposed but no operative standards of care are available in this surgical field, as suggested by Sutcliffe et al. in a systematic review [2].

These procedures expose patients to several possible early and late complications leading to loss of aesthetic and functional satisfaction.

In particular, partial or total neovaginal prolapse, after sexual reassignment surgery in male-to-female transsexuals, is a distressing complication for both the patient and surgeon, leading to poor aesthetic and functional outcomes, and sometimes difficult to correct. The frequency of this complication is difficult to ascertain, and literature reports single cases (since the anatomic circumstances preceding the operation and the postoperative course are often not known) (Figs. 20.1 and 20.2).

Several authors have reported their casuistics after SRS, but all of them involved a low number of patients, though the real incidence of neovaginal prolapse is not well known.

Perovic SV et al. in 89 consecutive transsexual M to F patients using penile skin and urethral flap had no reported cases of neovaginal prolapse [3].

Moreover, Krege S et al. reported two cases in 66 patients who had undergone male-to-female SRS by penoscrotal flap vaginoplasty. However, the authors did not specify if prolapse were partial or total [4].

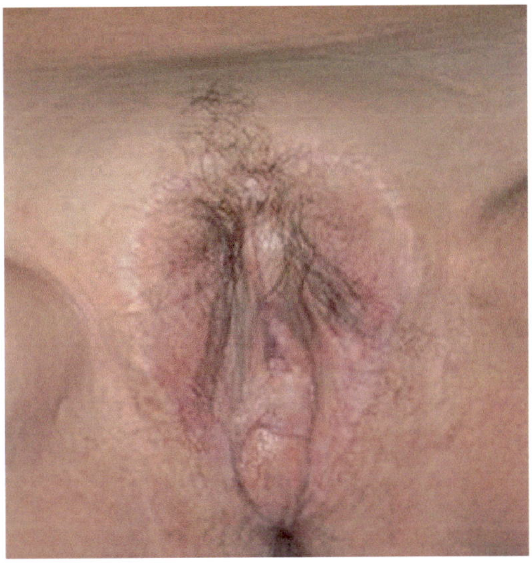

Fig. 20.1 Partial neovaginal prolapse. In this picture, the prolapse of the posterior vault is evident

S. Bucci • G. Mazzon, MD, FEBU (✉) • G. Liguori
N. Pavan • C. Trombetta
Department of Urology, Ospedale di Cattinara, University of Trieste, Strada di Fiume 447, Trieste 34100, Italy
e-mail: urostef@yahoo.it; giorgio_mazzon@libero.it; gioliguori@libero.it; nicpavan@gmail.com; trombcar@units.it

C. Trombetta et al. (eds.), *Management of Gender Dysphoria: A Multidisciplinary Approach*, DOI 10.1007/978-88-470-5696-1_20, © Springer-Verlag Italia 2015

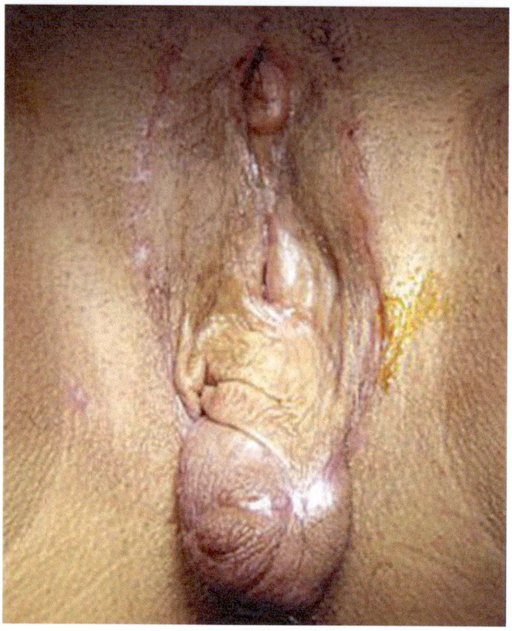

Fig. 20.2 Total neovaginal prolapse

Finally, Djordjevic et al. [5] reported a series of 86 consecutive rectosigmoid vaginoplasties; in their experience seven cases (8.1 %) of partial vaginal prolapse had been observed. However, this series comprise transsexual patients as well as females affected by vaginal agenesia or who had undergone vaginectomy for genital trauma. All vaginal prolapse were repaired by minor surgery.

We herein report the incidence in our experience of total and partial neovaginal prolapse, how we prevent it, and what's the optimal way to correct it.

We have retrospectively analyzed the prevalence of partial and total neovaginal prolapse after androgynoid sexual reassignment surgery between December 1994 and January 2012 in our institute, performed using a single surgical equipment. Our procedure includes bilateral orchiectomy, removal of corpora cavernosa, creation of the urethrostomy, neovaginoplasty, creation of neoclitoris with preservation of neurovascular bundles, and neovulvoplasty. Since the end of 2010, we had adopted an original technique, which consists of creating a neoclitoris embedded in the urethral mucosa using a urethral flap [6]. In the refinement the urethra is carefully dissected from the corpora cavernosa within Buck's fascia and shortened approximately 7 cm distally from the bulbs. It is then spatulated on its ventral side all down to the bulbs where a neomeatus is then created at the level of the female-type urethra. Urethral bulbs are removed carefully and entirely, because their remnants may cause painful penetration and bulky sensations during erection [4]. At this point, the urethral plate is further incised on the distal end following the median line to form a bifurcation, which surrounds the neoclitoris.

To create the neovagina, a penile and scrotal skin inversion technique has been adopted. We prefer to not close the apex of the neovaginal cylinder; in this way, the penile and scrotal skin covers spontaneously the cavity where the cylinder is located, ensuring a deeper neovagina.

During the years, two different techniques were adopted with the aim of fixing the neovaginal cylinders:

In the first, two absorbable stitches (Vicryl 3-0, which requires 35 days to be absorbed) are positioned at the top of the penoscrotal cylinder with the aim of fixing it to the prerectal fascia (old technique) (Fig. 20.3). In the second technique, we decided to fix the neovagina using four sutures: two absorbable stitches were fixed from the top of the penoscrotal cylinder to the Denonvilliers fascia and the other two from the midpart of the scrotal flap (which will constitute the posterior neovaginal wall) to the prerectal fascia (new technique) (Fig. 20.4).

When the suture is passed through the Denonvilliers fascia, we often decide to incorporate in the suture even some prostatic tissue or seminal vesicles, with the aim of strengthening the suture.

At the end of procedure, an inflatable silicon vaginal tutor is introduced in the neovaginal cavity and maintained for 3 days and during nighttime for 3 months. This guarantees that the penoscrotal flap well adheres to the cavity, facilitating recovery. Four days after the procedure, patients have been educated by a specialized nurse to self-dilate the neovagina with progressive larger dilators. Neovaginal self-dilatation is a fundamental step for a good long-term

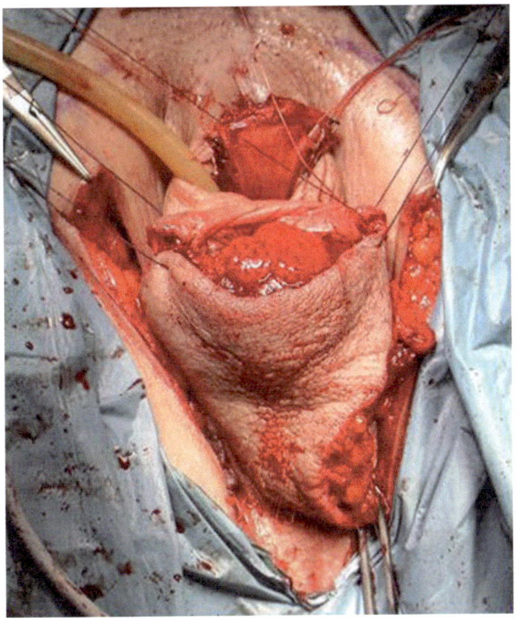

Fig. 20.3 Penile and scrotal skin flaps are sutured to each other forming a skin tube, two absorbable stitches are fixed from the top of the penoscrotal cylinder to the Denonvilliers fascia and the cylinder is inverted

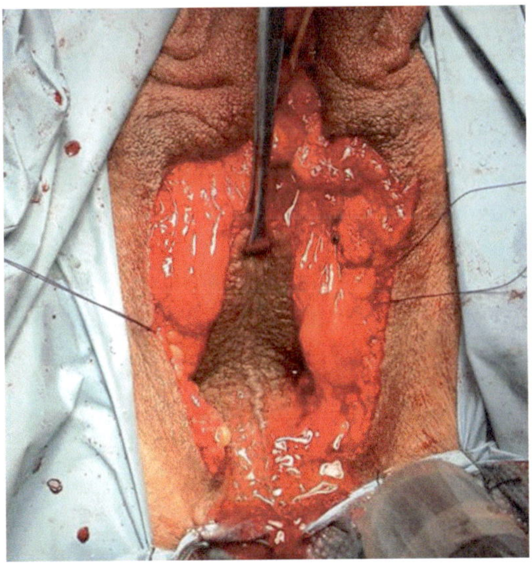

Fig. 20.4 Two additional stitches are fixed from the mid-part of the cylinder to the prerectal fascia. In our opinion, this fixation reduces the risk of prolapse of the posterior vault

result – first, a deep neovagina and second, prevention of vaginal prolapse. Patients must well learn how to perform it without straightening the penoscrotal flap.

After surgery, patients had been evaluated 6 and 12 months after the procedure.

We included in our casuistic 282 consecutive male transsexuals who had undergone to male-to-female SRS.

Sixty-five (23.04 %) of 282 were treated with our old technique and the remaining 217 (76.96) with the new technique.

Furthermore, since we had started sexual reassignment procedure, inverted penile skin vaginoplasty was used for the first nine patients, while in the remaining cases penile and scrotal skin inversion technique was adopted.

In the old technique casuistic, on 65 patients, 8 patients presented a neovaginal prolapse (12.30 %). One case (1.53 %) of total prolapse and seven cases (10.76 %) of partial prolapse had been observed, while in the next 217 patients treated with the new technique, only nine cases of partial prolapse were observed (4.14 %) and no cases of total prolapse. Considering partial prolapse, ten occurred in the posterior vault and six in the lateral vault. All prolapse occurred within 6 months after the procedure. Results are shown in Table 20.1; differences between two groups were statistically significant.

In our casuistic, only one patient has developed a total neovaginal prolapse. In this case, the old technique was used.

Different methods for suspension of the neovagina have been described:

Stanojevic et al. proposed sacrospinous ligament fixation of neovaginal to prevent prolapse. The authors haven't referred prolapse after 62 consecutive patients treated with this technique [7]. We prefer to not use this procedure because it requires consideration of the anatomic relationship to pudendal vessels and nerve, sciatic nerve, ureter, and rectum.

Table 20.1 Incidence of partial and total neovaginal prolapse in our casuistic. A lower incidence in the new technique group was observed

	Old technique	New technique	
Patients	65 (23.04 %)	217 (76.96 %)	P
No prolapse	57	208	0.026
Prolapse	8 (12.30 %)	9 (4.14 %)	0.031
Partial	7 (10.76 %)	9 (4.14 %)	0.019
Total	1 (1.53 %)	0 (0 %)	0.025

Other authors propose nonsuture fixation of neovagina with pliable lubricated [8] intravaginal packing that is left in place for 5 days postoperatively.

In our technique, prolapse of the neovaginal vault is exceptionally rare since using four stitches: two to suture the vault under the prostate and two over the rectum in the lateral part of the neocavity.

We believe that fixing the apex of penoscrotal flap with Denonvilliers fascia avoids the risk of total prolapse, while suturing the midpart of cylinder considerably reduces the risk of partial prolapse.

Sacropexy with synthetic mesh should be the most valid approach to neovaginal prolapse as the correct neovaginal axis is restored and neovaginal function is preserved. This technique guarantees an adequate neovaginal depth and an excellent physical result. The risk of detachment of stitches from the neovaginal wall, the main cause of suspension failure, is also reduced, not only because of the large vagina mesh contact area but also the nontraction suspension. This is possible because the length of the mesh is regulated by the distance between the neovagina and sacral promontory.

Long-term outcomes of prolapse treatment in transsexual patients are not available in literature. A review of literature including 40 studies which provide an update of surgical management of pelvic organ prolapse in women was published in 2011 [9]. The first dilemma is clarifying what's the best surgical choice for prolapse treatment. The authors compared the outcomes of abdominal sacropexy versus those of vaginal sacrospinous colpopexy. Abdominal sacral colpopexy was better than vaginal sacrospinous colpopexy with a lower rate of recurrent vault prolapse (RR 0.23, 95 % CI 0.07–0.77) [10, 11], even if it is associated with a longer operating time and more expensive.

A second question is if colpopexy must be performed with absorbable or nonabsorbable graft. One trial compared abdominal sacral colpopexy using either absorbable cadaveric fascia lata graft (Tutoplast) or nonabsorbable monofilament polypropylene mesh (Trelex). In either group there were no recurrences of vaginal prolapse, but the objective failure rate for recurrence at any other vaginal site was significantly worse (32 % in the fascial graft group versus 9 % in the mesh group) [12].

In our knowledge, in transsexual patients only single cases are reported, and transvaginal sacrospinous colpopexy or abdominal colposacropexy has been reported to restore the neovagina, with good functional results [13, 14]. In all of these cases, an open approach was used.

The same intervention has been already described laparoscopically. This procedure was reported for the first time in 2006 [15] with the aim of restoring the neovagina without compromising its function.

The optimal choice for treating partial prolapse is not clear, but probably even in these cases colposacropexy is the best choice. In 6 of 17 patients affected by partial prolapse, we decided to reposition the two sutures in the midpart of the cylinders but the risk of recurrence was very high; in fact four of them referred a partial prolapse again. In these cases, no other surgical procedures had been performed.

In our casuistic we had a case of total neovaginal prolapse; in this case we decided to correct it with an open colposacropexy considering that she had a history of surgery for acute local peritonitis 7 years before.

We believe that a crucial role in prolapse prevention is performed by patients. In order to avoid stenosis and prolapse of the neovagina, it is very important to use the vaginal tutor regularly after the intervention.

In fact, they must be adequately informed about the management of their neovagina after the surgical procedure. Daily dilatations are mandatory to maintain depth and avoid stenosis, as well as the use of abundant lubrication with the aim of reducing friction during dilatations and intercourses which in our opinion may cause detachment of the skin cylinder and prolapse onset.

In our experience, a more proximal position of the sutures to fix the penoscrotal apex with Denonvilliers fascia guarantees a lower risk of prolapse. In particular, total neovaginal prolapse has been no more observed and partial prolapse has a lower incidence.

Positioning 4 suture stitches is a short procedure and guarantees excellent functional outcome.

Moreover, we believe that the postoperative management, in particular the use of a vaginal dilator for self-dilatation and adequate lubrication, is mandatory as well as timing and compliance of the patients in order to achieve a good aesthetic and functional result.

References

1. Karim RB, Hage JJ, Mulder JW (1996) Neovaginoplasty in male transsexuals: review of surgical techniques and recommendations regarding eligibility. Ann Plast Surg 37(6):669–675
2. Sutcliffe PA et al (2009) Evaluation of surgical procedures for sex reassignment: a systematic review. J Plast Reconstr Aesthet Surg 62(3):294–306; discussion 306–308
3. Perovic SV, Stanojevic DS, Djordjevic ML (2000) Vaginoplasty in male transsexuals using penile skin and a urethral flap. BJU Int 86(7):843–850
4. Krege S et al (2001) Male-to-female transsexualism: a technique, results and long-term follow-up in 66 patients. BJU Int 88(4):396–402
5. Djordjevic ML, Stanojevic DS, Bizic MR (2011) Rectosigmoid vaginoplasty: clinical experience and outcomes in 86 cases. J Sex Med 8(12):3487–3494
6. Trombetta C et al (2011) Neo-urethroclitoroplasty according to Petrovic. Urologia 78(4):267–273
7. Stanojevic DS et al (2007) Sacrospinous ligament fixation for neovaginal prolapse prevention in male-to-female surgery. Urology 70(4):767–771
8. Karim RB et al (1995) Refinements of pre-, intra-, and postoperative care to prevent complications of vaginoplasty in male transsexuals. Ann Plast Surg 35(3):279–284
9. Maher CM et al (2011) Surgical management of pelvic organ prolapse in women: the updated summary version Cochrane review. Int Urogynecol J 22(11): 1445–1457
10. Benson JT, Lucente V, McClellan E (1996) Vaginal versus abdominal reconstructive surgery for the treatment of pelvic support defects: a prospective randomized study with long-term outcome evaluation. Am J Obstet Gynecol 175(6):1418–1421; discussion 1421–1422
11. Maher CF et al (2004) Abdominal sacral colpopexy or vaginal sacrospinous colpopexy for vaginal vault prolapse: a prospective randomized study. Am J Obstet Gynecol 190(1):20–26
12. Culligan PJ et al (2005) A randomized controlled trial comparing fascia lata and synthetic mesh for sacral colpopexy. Obstet Gynecol 106(1):29–37
13. Loverro G et al (2002) Repair of vaginal prolapse following penoscrotal flap vaginoplasty in a male-to-female transsexual. Gynecol Obstet Invest 53(4): 234–236
14. Frederick RW, Leach GE (2004) Abdominal sacral colpopexy for repair of neovaginal prolapse in male-to-female transsexuals. Urology 64(3): 580–581
15. Condous G, Jones R, Lam AM (2006) Male-to-female transsexualism: laparoscopic pelvic floor repair of prolapsed neovagina. Aust N Z J Obstet Gynaecol 46(3):254–256

21 Evaluation of Lower Urinary Tract Function After Surgery

Salvatore Siracusano, Stefano Ciciliato, Francesco Visalli, and Laura Toffoli

21.1 Introduction

It is well known that sex reassignment surgery is considered to be the gold standard in the treatment of gender dysphoria [1]. In this context, the surgical approach of male-to-female transsexuals (MTF) is the resection of the penis shaft and the removal of the testes allowing the use of the penile and scrotum skin to create a neovagina while the urethra is shortened and the prostate stays in situ. Therefore, from a functional point of view, this surgical technique, not involving the sphincter complex in its proximal and distal component, should not lead to problems concerning urinary continence, while conversely, a reduction of the total length of the urethra should lead to a reduction of the resistance to urine flow with a consequent decrease in the total time needed to empty the bladder.

In this chapter, therefore, we cannot avoid dealing with some aspects about the pathophysiology of continence that will allow us to make a reasoned assessment of the useful path leading to the identification of a possible diagnostic algorithm in these patients. In this context, we will also discuss the evidence provided by literature in this respect and the opportunity of identifying new diagnostic pathways.

S. Siracusano (✉) • S. Ciciliato • F. Visalli
L. Toffoli
Department of Urology, Cattinara Hospital, Trieste University, Via Strada di Fiume 447, Trieste 34100, Italy
e-mail: siracus@units.it; stefanociciliato@gmail.com; Visa83@virgilio.it; lauratoffoli1@yahoo.it

21.2 Aspects of the Pathophysiology of Continence and Micturition

The discussion of these aspects is somewhat difficult because the patients undergoing a MTF surgical approach possess the neuroanatomical characteristics of a male subject in which the urethra is shortened with an obvious modification of urethral resistance while the native anatomic sphincter area remains unchanged.

In this way, in order to assess the continence parameters in these subjects, we considered that it is essential to start from the assumptions that characterize continence in the normal male.

Normally, continence in male is guaranteed by the integrity of the proximal urethral sphincter (PUS) and by the integrity of the distal urethral sphincter (DUS) (Fig. 21.1). The PUS extends from the bladder neck up to the verumontanum with innervation from the sympathetic nervous system through the fibers of the pelvic nerve. The external sphincter contributes to the mechanism of continence due to the integration between the smooth and striated muscle fibers which are in turn closely related to the striated muscles of the pelvic floor muscles (rectourethral muscle and puboprostatic ligaments). The external sphincter contributes to the mechanism of continence

C. Trombetta et al. (eds.), *Management of Gender Dysphoria: A Multidisciplinary Approach*, DOI 10.1007/978-88-470-5696-1_21, © Springer-Verlag Italia 2015

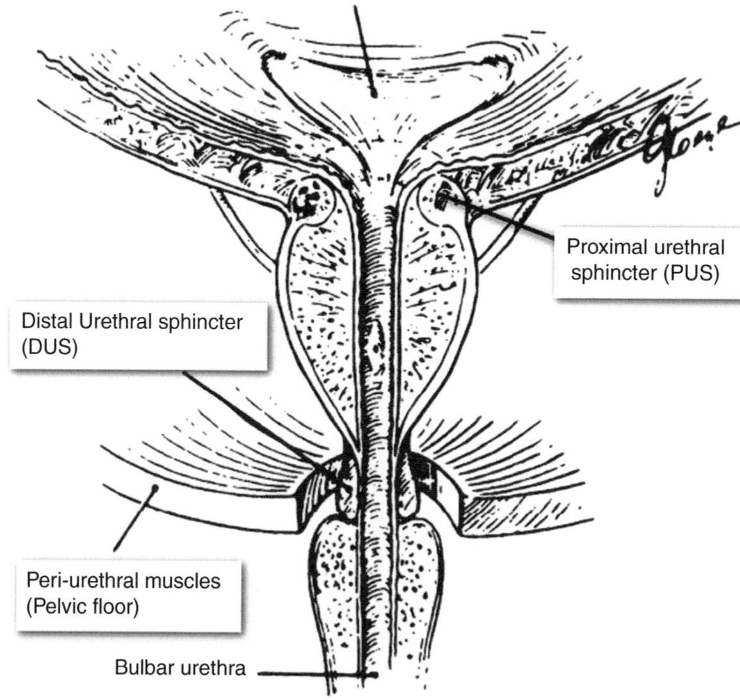

Fig. 21.1 Male urethral sphincter complex. PUS extends from the bladder neck through the prostatic urethra above the verumontanum. DUS extends from the prostatic urethra below the verumontanum through the membranous urethra surrounded by the periurethral skeletal muscle (pelvic floor)

thanks to the integration between the smooth and striated muscle fibers which are in turn closely related to the striated muscles of the pelvic floor muscles.

The innervation of the DUS runs along the walls of the urethra in posterolateral fashion and has both a sympathetic and a somatic component. In patients undergoing MTF surgical approach, the DUS should not suffer any alteration, and in any case even if there was a lesion of the latter continence should be kept intact for the persistence of integrity of PUS, since male continence can be maintained even with the integrity of a single sphincter (PUS or DUS).

In this context the filling phase of the bladder should in any case be preserved even if it is believed by some that the prolonged administration of estrogen may lead to a reduction of the protective effect on the escape of urine during the increase of abdominal pressure due to a reduction of the functional length of the urethra. Of particular interest, however, is the relief of the urgency and urge incontinence in some cases. Surely, the obstructive component could be responsible for this symptomatology even if some assume that the creation of the neovagina can determine a variation of the anatomical position of the bladder with the consequent appearance of detrusor overactivity [2]. With regard to the emptying phase, it appears obvious that the shortening of the urethra is relative to the component under the sphincteric area and it is identifiable with the urethra fixed which contributes passively to empty the bladder. In any case, however, the patient changes its condition of bladder emptying both for the assumption of a no longer standing but sitting body position and finally because the reduction of urethral resistance requires a reduction of the detrusor contractility and of mechanical energy required to ensure the complete emptying of the bladder.

21.3 Diagnostic Aspects and Evidence from the Literature

The evaluation of LUT after MTF surgical approach is closely connected with the PHASES of the bladder that are specifically represented by stress urinary incontinence (SUI) or the urge/urge incontinence (UI) in the first case and the series of symptoms that normally characterize the condition of cervico-urethral obstruction in the second case.

As regards the SUI or urgency associated or not with IU, the data in the literature are very scarce especially with reference to a limited number of patients. In particular, the King's Health Questionnaire showed that hyperactive bladder was the main problem in SUI [3] although both not interfering with QoL. In this study, Kuhn et al. [4] described that 12/18 (66 %) of patients are affected by overactive bladder, 6/18 (33 %) by SUI, and finally 6/18 (33 %) by symptoms compatible with bladder outlet obstruction (BOO).

Both Kuhn and Hoebeke in this context, however, report the presence of these symptoms solely on the basis of the evaluation of the questionnaires utilized and not on the basis of instrumental analysis except for uroflowmetry that may be specific for the assessment of the symptoms of the emptying phase.

It is therefore clear that the proposal for a diagnostic algorithm could be useful to try to assess MTF patients suffering from disorders of the filling and voiding phases in a more analytical way. In particular, we propose the following recommendations following at least 6 months after surgery:

HISTORY OF INCONTINENCE

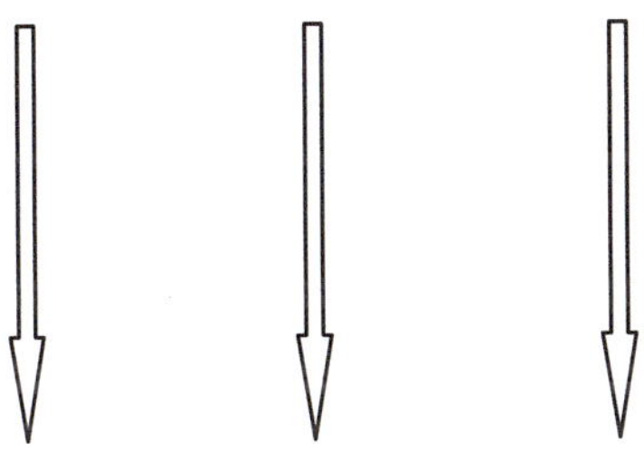

SUI

MIXED INCONTINENCE

URGENCY/URGE INCONTINENCE

- Urinary symptoms assessment by King's Health Questionnaire
- Urinalysis (if positive for infection, treat and reassess)
- Pelvic and perineal examination (evaluation of possible vaginal descensus and TROPHISN of the neovagina)
- Cough test
- Assessment of pelvic floor muscle strength
- Assessment of post-void residual urine

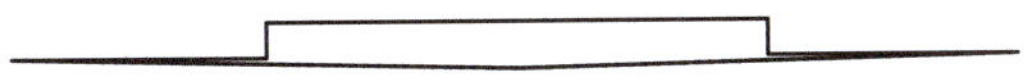

DIAGNOSIS OF SUI

DIAGNOSIS OF MIXED INCONTINENCE

DIAGNOSIS OF OAB WITH OR WITHOUT INCONTINENCE

HISTORY OF BLADDER OUTLET OBSTRUCTION

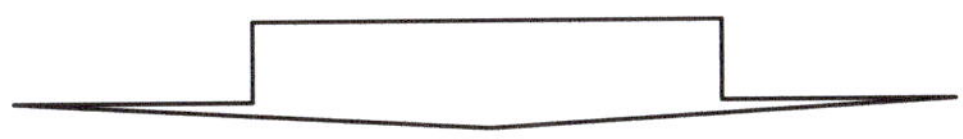

- Urinary symptoms assessment by King's Health Questionnaire
- Urinalysis (if positive for infection, treat and reassess)
- Pelvic and perineal examination (evaluation of possible vaginal descensus and TROPHISN of the neovagina)
- Assessment of pelvic floor muscle strength
- Assessment of post-void residual urine (if positive uroflow and cystoscopy)

21.4 Future Directions

The evaluation of the LUT function after surgery in MTF patients is still undefined. In particular, an in-depth study of the changes that surgery induces in these patients during bladder filling and emptying phases is absolutely necessary, as to date there is no evidence of clinical judgment. In this respect, the design of a uroflow nomogram would be helpful as well as PET and fMRI evaluations of the new bladder function control in the brain.

References

1. Laub DR, Fisk N (1974) A rehabilitation program for the gender dysphoria syndrome by surgical sex change. Plast Reconstr Surg 53:388–403
2. Hampel C (1997) Definition of overactive bladder and epidemiology of urinary incontinence. Urology 50(Suppl 6A):4–14
3. Hoebeke P, Selvaggi G, Ceulemans P et al (2005) Impact of sex reassignment surgery on lower urinary tract function. Eur Urol 47:398–402
4. Kuhn A, Hiltebrand R, Birkhäuser M (2007) Do transsexuals have micturition disorders? Eur J Obstet Gynecol Reprod Biol 131:226–230

22 Follow-Up of Patients After Male-to-Female (Mtf) Sex Reassignment Surgery (SRS)

Girolamo Morelli, Giorgio Pomara, Cinzia Traversi, Domenico Canale, and Filippo Turri

Following surgery and legalization of the gender reassignment, long-term physical, sexual, hormonal, and psychological follow-up is necessary to establish and maintain the success of the procedure. Since persistent regret after sex reassignment surgery must be considered, along with suicide, as the worst conceivable outcome of SRS [1], it is crucial to know the opinion of patients when evaluating the cosmetic and functional results of the surgery [2].

It is difficult to define a standard level of care for these patients since the evidence of published studies is of very low quality due to the following shortcomings: (1) the nature of the procedure itself prevents double-blind randomized controlled studies of the result; (2) transsexualism is rare and many of the follow-ups described in literature present small numbers of patients; (3) high dropout rates due to relocation of the patients or decline in participation; and (4) often limited follow-up periods [1].

G. Morelli (✉) • G. Pomara • C. Traversi
Urologia 2, Azienda Ospedaliero-Universitaria, Pisa, Italy
e-mail: girolamomorelli@gmail.com

D. Canale
Clinica Endocrinologica, Università di Pisa, Pisa, Italy

F. Turri
Clinica Urologica, Università di Pisa, Pisa, Italy

With scarcely any doubt, the following areas must be addressed when evaluating the results of SRS:

1. Surgical outcomes
2. Quality of life
3. Sexual outcomes
4. Micturition outcomes
5. Global health
6. Mental health

22.1 Surgical Outcomes [2]

Short-term postoperative complications:

- Rectal lesion during creation of the neovaginal canal: 1.5 %
- Bleeding from the urethral stump in the first 48 h postoperatively requiring secondary suturing: 4.5 %
- Temporary urinary retention: 5.2 %
- Healing of the suture between the perineum and the posterior aspect of the vaginal introitus by secondary intention: 5.2 %

At our institution, in order to prevent some of these complications, we have developed a hydrodissection technique of the prostato-rectal space.

Hydrodissection was first adopted by radiation oncologists in order to develop a plane

C. Trombetta et al. (eds.), *Management of Gender Dysphoria: A Multidisciplinary Approach*, DOI 10.1007/978-88-470-5696-1_22, © Springer-Verlag Italia 2015

in between the prostate and rectum where a hydrogel aimed at protecting the rectum from high-dose prostate EBRT is injected [3].

To the best of our knowledge, we have been the first to adopt this procedure in SRS as a preoperative step after general anesthesia induction.

Under TRUS guidance with a linear probe, through a perineal puncture, a 14G needle is advanced till the prostate apex, injecting 5–10 ml of saline as it proceeds. Once the needle has reached the prostate apex, more saline is injected, in order to develop a safe space through which the needle is further advanced till the mid-gland. At this point 50–70 ml of saline is injected, and a wide dissection plane is created.

This is extremely helpful given the small size of the MtF patients' prostates due to androgen deprivation and the consensual difficulties encountered in tissue dissection.

In our experience, we have noticed a great decrease in operative time, reduction of bleeding, and less incidence of rectal injury: the 10–15 min needed for this procedure is therefore widely regained during the following dissection step of the operation.

Long-term postoperative complications:

- Vaginal stenosis
- Scarce urethral spatulation, leading to unsatisfactory aesthetic outcomes and/or stenosis of the urethral neo-meatus
- Urethral fistulae following urethral perforation
- Hair in the neovagina
- Neovaginal prolapse
- Unsatisfactory cosmetic appearance (e.g., edema and/or asymmetry of the labia majora)

22.2 Satisfaction After SRS and Quality of Life

There is growing consensus that subjective criteria may provide a more meaningful basis for evaluating sex reassignment surgery than the use of so-called objective criteria such as employment, choice of "appropriate" sexual partners, or anatomic aspects assessed by the medical professionals [4]. The following areas should therefore be addressed: social life, partnerships, sexual relationships, and family relationships, always comparing them to the preoperative setting. De Cuypere et al., on a long-term follow-up of 55 patients (32 MtF, 23 FtM), found how transsexual person's expectations were met on the physical, emotional, and social level and less on the sexual level, with satisfaction rates of 81.5, 99.4, 90.7, and 66.7 %, respectively [5].

The most employed tools used to assess these aspects are:

- VAS (visual analogue scale): a validated tool to assess health and satisfaction, with 0 as the greatest dissatisfaction and 10 as the greatest possible satisfaction.
- King's health questionnaire: a validated tool to assess quality of life, widely adopted in incontinence care. It specifically addresses the following domains: general health perception, incontinence impact, role limitations, physical limitations, social limitations, personal relationships, emotions, sleep/energy, and severity measures with scores between 0 and 5 and 1 and 5, respectively, and a change of at least 5 points is considered significant.

At our institution, we employ a brief questionnaire, here presented, addressing the main areas of patient satisfaction and eventually the presence of regret and dissatisfaction.

Patient data

Name:

Last name:

Age:

Date of SRS:

Mastoplasty:

Hormonal therapy:

Post-operative complications (if any) and/or ulterior surgical procedures:

Global satisfaction

1) How would you rate yourglobal satisfaction?

   0______________________10

2) How would you rate your satisfaction about your body aesthetic aspect?

   0______________________10

3) How would you rate your satisfaction about genitals' aesthetic aspect?

   0______________________10

Sexual function

1) Vaginal sensitivity, both deep and superficial
2) Clitoral sensitivity
3) Pain at intercourse (or any form of penetration)
4) Pain at clitoral stimulation
5) Level of vaginal lubrication
6) Ability to reach orgasm, both with intercourse and/or masturbation
7) Aesthetic aspet of the vulva
8) Aesthetic aspect of pubic hair

Urinary function

1) Have you experienced any form of urinary leakage in your daily activities? If so, has it the characteristics of a stress (associated with physical activity) or an urge (impellent need to urinate without being able to reach the toilet in time) incontinence?
2) Have you experienced any loss of urine during sexual activity?
3) Have you uncontrolled urinary leakage during defecation?
4) Have you ever experienced incomplete bladder emptying?
5) Do you need to strain to urinate?
6) Have you ever experienced irritative urinary symptoms?
7) Have you ever done urinalysis and/or urine culture? If so, which were the results?

Regret may be defined as follows [6]: (a) definite regret (patient openly regrets SRS and has applied for retransformation to original sex), (b) some regret (indirectly expressed regret and signs of ambivalence about SRS), and (c) no regret. Dissatisfaction and regret have been reported to be associated with the following factors: age over 30 at first request of surgery, personality disorders, personal and social instability, secondary transsexualism, heterosexual sexual orientation, poor surgical results, and poor support from the family [7]. The self-perception the patient has of her body after the surgery needs to be as close as possible to that of a true female. That is why it is often necessary to consider aesthetic surgical procedures, both for the genital area and the body figure, following SRS, to reach this goal. Poor results of SRS that remind the patient and partner of the patient's transsexual background are an important risk factor for regret [1]. It is therefore of milestone importance to adequately counsel and follow the patient both in the preoperative and postoperative setting, being able to identify and modify the abovementioned factors as soon as they are noticed.

22.3 Sexual Outcomes

What the patients expect from SRS is that the surgery be performed with such skills that the sensitivity of his/her genitals would be preserved and the results would be true to nature both in appearance and function. The evaluation of patients' sexual function after SRS is therefore of great importance to fully define success of the operation. In a Brazilian cohort of 19 patients (18 MtF, 1 FtM), sexual satisfaction was considered improved by 83.3 % of the patients, while it was rated poor or very poor by 11.2 % [7]. A Swedish population-based controlled study over 30 years [1] on 324 patients (191 MtF and 133 FtM) found a 60 % satisfaction rate and a 22 % dissatisfaction rate. In order to grade sexual satisfaction, one should address the following: overall sexual satisfaction after SRS, frequency of sex after SRS, pleasure with the neovagina, frequency and degree of pleasure with anal sex, and frequency and degree of pleasure with masturbation [5, 7]. It is interesting to note how the majority of patients report a more intense, smoother, and longer orgasm and two thirds of them report secretion of fluid in the neovagina [5].

In this setting, an aspect that needs to be stressed out is that of vaginal dilatation. Postoperatively a soft vaginal tutor is left continuously in place for 15 days, thereafter only at night until it comes out spontaneously. When this happens, it means that the neovagina is wide enough to stop using it. At this point the patient is encouraged to use, three times a day (morning, midday, evening), rigid tutors with gradual increase in diameter and length. This maneuver is essential, at least twice a day, to ensure neovaginal depth and elasticity. It is obvious how these maneuvers need to be performed with the aid of lubricating and moisturizing creams. A possible complication of rigid vaginal tutors is urethral neo-meatus stenosis. We have observed this circumstance in one patient, and it was successfully managed with progressive urethral dilatations.

At our institution, we push the patients to engage in sexual activity as soon as the neovaginal conditions allow safe intercourse, and we evaluate this area with the same questionnaire presented above plus a thorough gynecological examination.

22.4 Micturition Outcomes

SRS carries a high risk of micturition problems. Next to the change of urethral length, becoming it shorter, there is also a change in voiding habits, like voiding while seating. About 32 % of the patients undergoing MtF surgery reported changes in voiding, with 19.3 % of them affirming it was better, 12.9 % it was worse, and 67.8 % neither worse nor better [7]. The problems reported are incontinence, hesitancy, spraying, decreased or diverted stream, post-voiding dribbling, and UTIs. The most frequently presented changes are, however, incontinence (19.3–33 %) and UTIs (32 %) [8, 9].

As for incontinence, appearing as stress incontinence, urge incontinence, or mixed incontinence, various hypotheses have been proposed to justify it. First of all, we need to consider that the sphincter complex, the pelvic muscles, and the pudendal nerves are in the dissected area, so some of the stress incontinence might be due to surgical trauma. Another concurrent cause might be the reduction in prostate size. Obstruction, i.e. due to urethral scarring, as well as nerves damage, could also explain the increased incidence of overactive bladder (OAB) and urge incontinence in this population. Another proposed cause is the presence of a neovagina behind the bladder, thus altering its normal anatomic position and filling [8, 9].

Infections are another important issue, most of them being observed in the immediate postoperative period. The more plausible explanation is the shortening of urethra leading to an easier penetration of pathogens, especially after intercourse [8, 9].

Uroflowmetries have been done, showing a not statistically significant reduction in the mean Qmax (18 ml/s), without significant post-voidal residue in any of the patients [8, 9].

Interestingly, it is important to note how for the majority of the patients changes in micturition, including incontinence, which is by far the worst problem, were not considered as a problem, with only 11 % of them being unhappy or socially disturbed, and no correlation was noted between visual analogue scale and micturition symptoms given by the King's health questionnaire [8, 9]. Despite these comforting data, we need not to forget to give appropriate information about these possible consequences before SRS.

In order to establish how SRS affects overall bladder functioning, besides using the same questionnaire reported above, we have recently started to study MtF patients with urodynamic assessment both before and after the surgery.

From a clinical point of view, these are the main observations we did on our patients:

- No modification in defecation.
- No dysuria nor difficulties during micturition; the majority of patients reported a spraying urinary stream.
- No stress nor urge incontinence.
- Mild to low irritative bladder symptoms in the immediate postoperative days.

We have performed urodynamic evaluation before and after SRS on six patients. What we have noticed so far, with regard to the different part of the functional studies performed, is:

- Uroflowmetry: similar traces with no significant difference in maximum and average flows
- Cystomanometry: no signs of overactive bladder nor modifications in bladder compliance and capacity
- Urethral pressure profile: no significant alterations in urethral closure pressure, with reduced height and length of prostatic plateau

What we can infer from the previous results is:

- Androgen blockage preoperatively, causing prostate shrinkage, results in a reduced "prostate effect" during voiding with regard to the urethral pressure profile.
- The urinary stream modifications (i.e., spraying), caused by new relationships of the external urethral meatus with the neo-vulva, or even its own morphology (i.e., neo-labia majora) does not alter significantly the uroflowmetry trace.
- The reported increased frequency of micturition in the first postoperative days does not alter significantly cystomanometric traces.

22.5 Global Health

In order to prevent loss of secondary characteristics of the reassigned sex, transsexual subjects need to continue hormone therapy lifelong, thus leading to potential complications. There is still no worldwide consensus regarding which is the best treatment regimen.

In the protocol for diagnosis and treatment of gender dysphoria established by Tuscany region, a strict follow-up is expected. This follow-up starts in the immediate postoperative setting and requires the presence of psychological support at anesthesia awakening. From a strict medical point of view, besides routine perioperative care, patients restart hormonal therapy at discharge. Since orchiectomy was performed, MtF patients do not need androgen blockage therapy anymore. Estrogen replacement therapy is usually the same given preoperatively. We have always preferred transdermal preparations given their ability to avoid hepatic first-pass effect. It is also preferable to use "pure" estradiol since it allows an easier monitoring of its circulating levels. Monitoring for thromboembolic clinical and biochemical manifestations is required and performed with serial evaluation of coagulation parameters. Other parameters to monitor are bone status with bone mineral densitometry, hepatic function, and lipid profile. At our institution we usually perform these examinations 1 month after discharge and then once every 6 months.

No matter the hormonal treatment scheme and the doses used, the patients become indeed at risk for the following conditions:

A. Cardiovascular diseases: hypertension, hyperlipidemia, and atherosclerosis are well-known consequences of estrogen-substitutive therapy in postmenopausal women. In a recent extensive meta-analysis by M.B. Elamin [10] on the published literature evaluating main cardiovascular outcomes (myocardial infarction, stroke, VTE, and death) in transsexuals undergoing hormonal treatment, no definitive conclusions could be drawn. This is mainly due to low-quality evidence, downgraded due to methodological limitations of included studies, imprecision, and heterogeneity, suggesting that cross-sex hormone therapies increase serum tryglycerides in MtF and FtM and have a trivial effect on HDL-cholesterol and systolic blood pressure in FtM, with sparse and inconclusive data about patient important outcomes.
B. Osteoporosis: 2–6 % of MtF transsexuals are diagnosed with low bone mass. Compared to healthy males in the same age range, transsexuals are to be considered in a state of prolonged androgen deficiency, a well-known risk factor for decreased bone mass [11] .
C. Thrombophilia and venous thromboembolism (VTE): there is a 6–8 % risk of VTE in MtF transsexuals using ethinyl estradiol [12]. We know from oral contraception in women about this risk. It is well accepted that in the general female population a screening strategy for thrombophilia is not cost-effective [12]; a recent study showed how, also in the transsexual population, general screening is not recommended and should be restricted to individuals with a personal or family history of VTE.
D. Emotional lability and depression: it is a common observation, especially in premenopausal women, how hormonal status modifications correlate with dysphoria disorders.
E. Liver malfunctioning [13].
F. Hypothyroidism [5].
G. Hyperprolactinemia: estrogens act as potent stimulants of the synthesis and liberation of prolactin from the lactotroph cells, given their antidopaminergic and lactotroph cell proliferation-stimulating actions; they are therefore capable of producing hyperprolactinemia, lactotroph hyperplasia, and, eventually, prolactinoma [13]. Periodic blood samples are therefore necessary to monitor prolactinemia and detect as early as possible this condition.
H. Hormon-related tumors: patients who have undergone SRS remain at risk of some male-related conditions, such as BPH or prostate cancer, because the prostate is left intact during the procedure [2]. It is true that androgen-suppression therapy should drastically reduce these possibilities, but we need to keep that in mind as our patients will be aging with their prostate in situ, considering a thorough urological evaluation as needed. One thing needs to be stressed: if prostate cancer arises, it is, by definition, a castrate-resistant disease, the patient being already castrated [13].

   Another condition we need not to forget is the risk of breast cancer favored by estrogen-circulating levels [13].
I. Minor adverse effects: weight gain, migraine, asthenia, irritability, vertiginous disorders, and edemas [13].

Talking about global health, we also need to remember that some of these patients, considering their sexual background and habits, are at risk for HIV and hepatitis B and C and need therefore to be screened for these infections.

22.6 Mental Health

One of the most extensive works in this sense is that published by Dhejne et al., who evaluated 324 patients (191 MtF and 133 FtM) in a long-term population-based controlled study over a 30-year period (1973–2003) in Sweden [1]. They investigated: mortality (all-cause mortality, death by definite/uncertain suicide, death by cardiovascular disease, death by tumor), psychiatric morbidity (any psychiatric disorder (excluding gender identity disorders), alcohol/drug misuse and dependence, definite/uncertain suicide attempt), and accidents and crime (any criminal violence, any violent offense). This study found substantially higher rates of overall mortality, death from cardiovascular disease and suicide, suicide attempts, and psychiatric hospitalizations in sex-reassigned transsexual individuals compared to a healthy control population. No differences were noted with regard to crime. This highlights that postsurgical transsexuals are a risk group that needs long-term psychiatric and somatic follow-up. Even though surgery and hormonal therapy alleviate gender dysphoria, it is apparently not sufficient to remedy the high rates of morbidity and mortality found among transsexual persons, thus demanding an improved long-term care.

References

1. Dhejne C, Lichtenstein P, Boman M et al (2011) Long-term follow-up of transsexual persons undergoing sex reassignment surgery: cohort study in Sweden. PLoS One 6(2):e16885
2. Jarolim L, Sedy J, Schmidt M et al (2009) Gender reassignment surgery in male-to-female transsexualism: a retrospective 3-months follow-up study with anatomical remarks. J Sex Med 6(6): 1635–1644
3. Susil RC, McNutt TR, DeWeese TL et al (2010) Effects of prostate-rectum separation on rectal dose from external beam radiotherapy. Int J Radiat Oncol Biol Phys 76(4):1251–1258
4. Kuhn A, Bodmer C, Stadlmayr W et al (2009) Quality of life 15 years after sex reassignment surgery for transsexualism. Fertil Steril 92(5):1685–1689
5. De Cuypere G, T'Sjoen G, Beerten R et al (2005) Sexual and physical health after sex reassignment surgery. Arch Sex Behav 34(6):679–690
6. Olsson SE, Moller A (2006) Regret after sex reassignment surgery in a male-to-female transsexual: a long-term follow-up. Arch Sex Behav 35(4): 501–506
7. Lobato MI, Koff WJ, Manenti C et al (2006) Follow-up of sex reassignment surgery in transsexuals: a Brazilian cohort. Arch Sex Behav 35(6):711–715
8. Hoebeke P, Selvaggi G, Ceulemans P et al (2005) Impact of sex reassignment surgery on lower urinary tract function. Eur Urol 47(3):398–402
9. Kuhn A, Hiltebrand R, Birkhäuser M (2007) Do transsexuals have micturition disorders? Eur J Obstet Gynecol Reprod Biol 131(2):226–230
10. Elamin MB, Garcia MZ, Murad MH et al (2010) Effect of sex steroid use on cardiovascular risk in transsexual individuals: a systematic review and meta-analyses. Clin Endocrinol (Oxf) 72(1):1–10
11. T'Sjoen G, Weyers S, Taes Y et al (2009) Prevalence of low bone mass in relation to estrogen treatment and body composition in male-to-female transsexual persons. J Clin Densitom 12(3):306–313
12. Ott J, Kaufmann U, Bentz EK et al (2010) Incidence of thrombophilia and venous thrombosis in transsexuals under cross-sex hormone therapy. Fertil Steril 93(4):1267–1272
13. García-Malpartida K, Martín-Gorgojo A, Rocha M et al (2010) Prolactinoma induced by estrogen and cyproterone acetate in a male-to-female transsexual. Fertil Steril 94(3):1097.e13–5

23 Quality of Life After Sexual Reassignment Surgery

Luigi Rolle, Carlo Ceruti, Massimiliano Timpano, Marco Falcone, and Bruno Frea

23.1 Introduction

Quality of life (QoL) is a multidisciplinary and transversal topic that includes a variety of aspects related to medical, social, political, and economic sciences. It is a broad concept that concerns the well-being of a person or a community, comprehending physical and mental health, occupational satisfaction, social integration and economic welfare.

Sex reassignment surgery (SRS) in patients with gender dysphoria affects not only physical modifications in the aesthetics and function of the genitalia, but also allows many changes in lifestyle and sexual behaviour and, last but not least, allows a complete transition to another social, familiar and sexual role. Therefore, taking into account QoL means treating not only the surgical issues, but also the psychological and social aspects. Many factors can be considered to be determinants of QoL after SRS. We can distinguish between physical/biological factors, directly depending on the surgical procedure and its functional outcomes, and social/relational factors.

L. Rolle • C. Ceruti (✉) • M. Timpano
M. Falcone • B. Frea
Clinica Urologica, Università di Torino – Citta della Salute e della Scienza, C.so Bramante, Turin 10126, Italy
e-mail: luigi.rolle@unito.it; Carlo.ceruti@unito.it; Massimiliano.timpano@gmail.com; marcofalcone1986@gmail.com; bruno.frea@unito.it

23.1.1 Physical Determinants of Quality of Life

The first factor influencing QoL is satisfaction with the outcomes of treatment, which is intended to be a meeting of expectations. Objective results have no absolute value, but have to be considered in relation to the patient's expectations, and it is important to consider not only the results of the surgical procedure, but also the effects of hormonal treatment, which is the main factor influencing the general aspect of the subject [7, 14, 17]. Therefore, before surgery it is mandatory for the whole inter-disciplinary medical team to give the patient exhaustive and clear information about results that are reasonably achievable from both an aesthetic and a functional point of view.

In the immediate postoperative period QoL mainly depends on the presence of complications and aesthetic imperfections; even if severe complications are quite rare, many subjects present with mild imperfections that require minor interventions, in a few cases repeated, performed on an outpatient basis. In some cases, other surgical procedures, in both the genital and extragenital areas, are scheduled ab initio after SRS. All these procedures, despite their minimal invasiveness, can increase the "medicalisation" of the subject and delay the resumption of a normal and satisfying life.

SRS procedures have a major component of reconstructive surgery. As after other reconstructive procedures, SRS requires care and maintenance in the postoperative period, but also

C. Trombetta et al. (eds.), *Management of Gender Dysphoria: A Multidisciplinary Approach*,
DOI 10.1007/978-88-470-5696-1_23, © Springer-Verlag Italia 2015

in the long term, that in some cases can be negatively perceived by the subject, thus affecting QoL. In the long term, the acquisition of good genital function, allowing intercourse to the satisfaction of the subject and their partner, is the major determinant of QoL among factors related to the biological outcomes of surgery.

23.1.2 Social and Relational Determinants of Quality of Life

Among the determinants of quality of life after SRS, a key role is played by social and labour integration. The level of integration depends mainly on the subjective disposition of the patient, but also undoubtedly on society. Still, nowadays, despite there being less prejudice in most countries, full integration and total acceptance by society do not occur in all cases. In subjects with more pronounced social rejection marginalisation, loss of self-esteem and depression can occur and, in some extreme situations, cases of suicide have been reported. Equally important is the construction of a stable sexual relationship or family nucleus.

The acquisition of genital and body appearance consistent with the psychological sex is not always an adequate condition to establish a stable relationship (heterosexual or homosexual based on the sexual orientation of the subject). The physical changes of the genitalia provided by SRS can induce psychological reactions in the subject or in the partner that in some cases can lead to the termination of a relationship already present before surgery or make it difficult to start a new relationship. These situations, described in the literature, are mostly transient and tend to normalise, but they can have a negative impact on quality of life.

In general, we can say that complete immersion in the new gender role, good social and labour integration and a satisfactory sexual life are essential determinants of overall self-satisfaction with the new body image and thus of a high quality of life. Normally, good identification of the new phenotype that is completely appropriate to the psychological sex requires a good psychological balance and the completion of a structured course in tandem with specific multidisciplinary experience in the field. The dissertation on the determinants of quality of life, especially biological determinants, needs a separate approach for male to female and female to male transsexuals.

23.2 Quality of Life After Male to Female Sexual Reassignment Surgery

23.2.1 Physical Determinants of Quality of Life After Male to Female SRS

Sex reassignment surgery in male to female (MtoF) transsexuals is extremely important for people who undergo it, and also for the expectations and satisfaction they have with regard to surgical intervention [45]. The transsexual patient, during his path toward intervention, creates in his imagination a “virtual vagina”, a sort of “how I wish it were”, that is often far from the reality of what can reasonably be achieved; generally, she refers to the surgeon before surgery an idea and a desire for perfection in the symmetry of the anatomy, an obsession regarding the depth of the neovagina and the need to have sensitivity so as to experience orgasm that can also clash with reality. Therefore, it is crucial to carry out a preoperative interview with these people in order to clarify the possibilities and limitations of genital reconstructive surgery in order to formulate some credible expectations. In the chapters below are discussed the aspects that should be pointed out during preoperative interview, with a particular regard to the real possibilities of surgery, to prevent those misunderstandings that are often at the basis of postoperative unsatisfaction and poor quality of Life.

23.2.2 The Aesthetic Appearance of the Neovulva

From an anatomical point of view, the vulva of female 46, XX is characteristically pear-shaped and begins with a raised area, called the mound of Venus, in the upper part of the pubic symphysis and it extends downwards along the ischio-pubic branches, ending about 1 cm from the anus. The mound of Venus, formed by a thick pad of skin and adipose tissue, continues downward with two skin folds that are generally equal and symmetrical, called the labia majora. The mound of Venus and the labia majora have a well-developed covering of hair. Below, there are two other skin folds, equal but not always symmetrical, that are free of follicles, thinner than labia majora, and called the labia minora; these converge and are joined at the top by a small tubercle formation representing the female erectile organs, known as the clitoris. After sexual development, the labia minora can be contained by the labia majora, but more frequently they protrude. This anatomical premise of the female anatomy emphasises that in principle, surgery aims to satisfy all the morphological aspects of a "true" vulva, making the mound of Venus using the dorsal part of the tunica albuginea of the penis, the labia majora using scrotal skin, the labia minora using the foreskin and a portion of the glans, and the neoclitoris, reconfiguring the glans, whose vascularisation and innervation (the dorsal neurovascular bundle) are preserved to ensure that sensitivity is maintained [16, 18]. However, it is not always so simple to reconstitute the perfect anatomy, there may be limits for anatomical reasons. For example, in people who are overweight or even obese, the mound is not so prominent; in the presence of a small amount of scrotal skin or underweight people, the labia may be poorly represented. It is very important to talk about the hair distribution of the vulva. Often, MtoF transsexuals use permanent hair removal to prevent growth of hair in the neovagina. It is important to emphasise pre-operatively that hair removal should affect only the penile and scrotal areas, obviously avoiding the pubic area, as the regrowth of hair there helps to hide any scars that are created [35].

23.2.3 Maintaining a Sensitive Neo-clitoris

An important goal of surgical intervention is to make a neoclitoris with sensitivity. The neoclitoris can be reconfigured from the glans, which is disassembled from the tip of the corpora cavernosa of the penis, taking care to save its vascular supply and nerve connections, which run in the dorsal penile neurovascular bundle. This specification, namely the extreme respect of the neurovascular bundle, is mandatory in order to ensure and maintain the sensitivity of the neoclitoris [36, 39]. It is important to point out to people who are undergoing surgery that the neoclitoris may be subject to change in size during the first few months postoperatively; this is to prevent them from requiring to a reduction of a neoclitoris that is considered hypertrophied too soon. It is sometimes possible that the surgical trauma leads to the formation of small, but very hard eschars of neoclitoris. Patients are often scared by this temporary outcome, and this may lead to an anxious status with worsening of QoL if the surgical team has not informed the patient that it is generally a partial necrosis of the mucosa of the neoclitoris (as can happen to the glans after plaque surgery with a prosthetic penis implant for induratio penis plastica [IPP] in men) that resolve spontaneously within a few weeks. Both the patient and the surgical team have to keep calm and avoid any therapeutically aggressive behaviours.

23.2.4 Micturiction in Sitting Position

A typical aspect that differentiates a man from a woman is the possibility of voiding in standing position. It is important for the QoL of MtoF patients to be able to achieve micturition in a sitting position; from a surgical point of view this goal can be achieved by placing the urethral neomeatus in the orthotopic position. Most of the penile urethra is sacrificed, but a portion of about 4 cm in length is spared, spatulated and fixed to the pelvic floor so as to contribute to the effect of the mucous neovulva and to prevent the stenosis of the urethral neomeatus, which constitutes one of the most frequent complications of this surgery. A forwarded neomeatus can cause a horizontal stream and lead to considerable discomfort postoperatively.

23.2.5 Capacity of the Neovagina

One of the major concerns of MtoF transsexuals is having the deepest vagina possible. A psychosocial consideration: the obsession with size is a typically male concern. Perhaps, this is a “genetic” reminder that remains in genetically XY neo-women? That said, there are anatomical and anthropometric limits that affect the neovaginal depth. The neovagina is obtained by opening a hole in the prostato rectal space, after cutting the central tendon of the perineum, and then developing a plane to the front of the rectum that stops at the peritoneal reflection, above the prostate and seminal vesicles. This part of the surgery, often very challenging owing to tissue adhesions and the small size of the prostate because of oestrogen administration and androgen-suppressive therapy is not the only conditioning element: in fact, the cavity created needs to be covered with penoscrotal skin. Thus, when we are facing penoscrotal hypoplasia, with a scarce amount of usable skin, there is a risk of obtaining a cutaneous channel shorter than surgical dissection would allow; this defect can be overcome by creating a skin graft, recovering scrotal skin not used to make up labia majora. The final outcome of the intervention is important for adequate neovaginal depth to ensure satisfactory intercourse, but not all; in fact, there are some aspects of peri- and postoperative management of the neovagina by the neowomen that are critical to the long-term maintenance of surgical results. At the end of the intervention, a cylindrical silicone expander is positioned in the neovaginal cavity, to drain any secretions through a central channel, but especially to maintain the skin lining of the neovaginal wall and contribute to haemostasis [38]. This expander is kept in place for the first 5 postoperative days and is then removed. At this point, it is crucial that the person becomes autonomous in the management and placement of the expander, as for the first month after surgery the subject has to keep it in place during the night and occasionally, but regularly, during the day. Then, the patients has to carry out self-dilation twice a day with four cylinders of plastic material, that are rigid, increasing in calibre and length, with a generally flat tip, so as to add tension to even the most distal part of the neovagina.

The “maintenance” of the neovagina is an important task given to the patient, and this can be perceived as a limitation of the QoL in the first few weeks after surgery, but the patient should learn that her neovagina requires continuous care that has to be seen as a sort of personal hygiene protocol rather than as a long medicalisation period.

23.2.6 Complications and Imperfections

For many aspects related to QoL, SRS is the main goal for those who have undergone it. On the other hand, it is also a starting point, as the new condition can be a source of small or large problems to avoid with appropriate behaviours, to retouch or to repair. In fact, in a variable but still considerable percentage of cases (58 % in our series), the intervention of conversion is not unique and definitive, but is followed by other procedures that are more or less complex, performed for a wide range of imperfections, and the more frequent of them are listed below.

Asymmetry of the labia majora: this is the most evident problem for neowomen, although it is not very frequent. Before any retouching, which can be performed in a one-day surgery setting, at least 6 months must have passed since SRS, so that tissues and scars are suitably stabilised.

Hypertrophy of the neoclitoris: sometimes, the neoclitoris is too large and too protruding from the floor of the labia minora. In this condition, the continuous tactile stimulation due to the contact with underwear can be annoying. Therefore, a small revision needs to be carried out under local anaesthesia to reduce its size or to provide further cover with the creation of a so-called clitoral hood.

Stenosis of the urethral neomeatus: this is the most frequent functional complication. A technical device that we have adopted and which permitted a significant reduction in its incidence was a large urethral spatulation (which is used as a plate of the vulvar neovestibulus), associated with the fixation of the free half of the neomeatus to the skin with everting sutures. Any use of small urethral dilators postoperatively allows this risk to be minimised. If it is necessary to correct a stenosis, meatoplasty with a vertical incision at 6 o’clock complete with everting sutures to the skin provides a perfect resolution.

Micturition complications: it may happen infrequently that the urethral neomeatus is too high or too far forwards, so that it affects the urinary stream in a horizontal direction. The practical consequences are obvious. The retraction of the urethral neomeatus is a simple and rapid procedure that is performed with a vertical incision of the further neomeatus and spatulation of the urethra down to the orthotopic position. Stress incontinence due to sphincteric lesions is extremely rare.

Introital stenosis: the stenosis of neovaginal introitus is a bad functional complication that does not allow patients to have satisfactory coital sexual activity. It is mostly due to a lack of compliance with the neovaginal expansion programme, which is not performed with the right frequency or for the period of time required daily; sometimes, they can be the result of hypertrophic scar healing, which affects the appearance of retracting keloids. The management of this complication is essentially surgical, sectioning the scar tissue and retracting the introitus (usually, two lateral incisions are sufficient); sometimes the correcting procedure requires the interposition of autologous tissue (skin in an island flap) or heterologous grafts (small intestine porcine sobmucosa) to provide a better enlargement of the introitus. Essential to keep the introitus open during the healing process is the use of a vaginal expander for approximately 5 days postoperative before returning to the regular expansion programme.

Stenosis of the neovagina: this represents the most feared complication for both the surgeon and transsexual people. For this reason, it is absolutely imperative before surgery to emphasise the importance of postoperative dilatation, which represents, in fact, the only way of preventing this dramatic complication, provided that the intervention has given adequate depth. In our series, this complication is present in 3 of the patients on whom we operated, which had not complied with the requirements given to them on vaginal dilatation. Over the last few years, growing experience has been taken up by several centres on the use of MRI to diagnose, objectivate and evaluate the severity of neovaginal stenosis [4, 8, 38]. The importance of the recommendations on the expansion can be better understood in the light of what needs to be done to repair the stenosis; a new vaginoplasty means undergoing a major operation via a combined vaginal–abdominal pathway, to reconfigure the vaginal canal with an ileal loop or colon.

23.2.7 Postoperative Rehabilitation and Sexual Activity

The ability to have satisfactory sexual intercourses is definitely one of the major factors conditioning the QoL. To achieve this goal, the proper management of the neovagina in the peri- and postoperative period is essential, and the surgeon must be very clear and incisive in making the neowoman understood in the need to be regular and consistent with the expansions that are performed even every day for the first few months after surgery. These expansions can be replaced by sexual activity: approval at the start of sexual activity is generally given 2 months after surgery. From this point of view, in our series, regular sexual activity is reported by 52 % of our transsexuals; more than half of these have reported reaching orgasm.

We have recently reported that MtoF transsexuals, who underwent SRS as well as genital surgical feminisation, tend to assume female cerebral features. In our opinion this study underlines the beneficial effects of SRS to the patients, who react to the genital surgery conversion with a cerebral femininisation. These two effects tend to solve the typical conflict of this disorder: the discrepancy between cerebral and physical features leading to an effective improvement of their QoL [33].

23.2.8 Social and Relational Determinants of Quality of Life After Male to Female SRS

23.2.8.1 Social and Labour Integration After SRS

Gender dysphoria patients may encounter many social and relational problems in their lives; these problems do not necessarily disappear after SRS. The most difficult obstacle to overcome, from the beginning of the Real Life Test, is the social re-integration of transsexual patients. During this phase, in fact, the individual must adapt his life, social and professional aspects, according to the definitive transitional genre. The ambiguity that characterises these patients, their physical appearance and the way they relate to the world around them induce reactions of unease, discrimination and exclusion in society. In fact, in the general population a need to protect the status quo and the psychological and social balance is often present, that can support discriminatory attitudes towards those who disturb the norm. Discrimination and exclusion influence the overall QoL of transsexual patients and specifically all areas of everyday life, such as work, study, relational life and housing research. From a social point of view, data from the available literature argue that SRS gives rise to a significant general improvement in the QoL of transsexual patients compared with their condition before surgery (approximately 70–90 % of patients are socially satisfied) [29, 32]. After SRS, data also show a marked improvement in self-destructive and antisocial behaviours frequently found in patients who have not undergone surgery [32]. However, comparing the patient's QoL after SRS with that of the general population, it is evident that the QoL of the former is still lower [10, 25, 29]. In particular, from the available literature data it is evident how MtoF patients have a more difficult and troubled process of socio-professional reintegration. These obstacles in part derive from a difficulty in establishing interpersonal relationships and perhaps from a minor ability to adapt themselves to the society; these difficulties are compounded by the fact that these people often feel singled out and observed for their outward appearance [29]. In the field of labour integration, discrimination and social rejection towards transsexuals (sometimes due to feelings of fear) often interfere with the objective evaluation of their real abilities and skills, shifting more attention to their "different" condition. This can make it difficult to search for employment, leading to non-assumption/unemployment phenomena, and for those who do have a job, to mobbing, unequal treatment through to dismissal. The available literature data are conflicting regarding the effects of SRS on the scope of employment. Some studies support the notion that after surgery there is no significant improvement in the employment situation and consequently with job satisfaction. Others, however, reported an improvement (30–60 % of cases), in terms of patient satisfaction, with regard to this area [22, 29, 32]. In some series, up to 90 % of patients in stable employment reported that they have not been the victim of any prejudice, but, on the contrary, they have been understood and supported by colleagues both before and after surgery [22]. On the other hand, there are published data that represent more difficulties integrating into the workplace: up to 20 % of patients reported that they were forced to change jobs because of personal embarrassment from colleagues or because of discrimination and isolation phenomena. These dynamics seem to be more frequent among MtoF patients [32].

23.2.8.2 Sexual Relationships After SRS

Among the determinants of the social QoL, an important position is occupied by the possibility of achieving a satisfying sexual life and a stable relationship. Many authors reported that most MtoF patients are able to resume an active sexual life after surgical intervention [26]. Moreover, they report having a partner more frequently. However, data strongly differ in the different series reported in the scientific literature. The percentage of patients who report having experienced sexual intercourse with at least one partner after surgery varies from 54 % [24] to 73 % [31] to 90 % [6]. In the series reported by Chew et al., over half of the patients reported having multiple partners. According to Chew et al., 37 % of patients had had more than seven partners at the time of the interview. Similar observations can be made regarding the percentage of subjects who report having a stable relationship. Transsexual patients who establish a stable relationship report a high level of sexual satisfaction, which led to a significant improvement in their QoL.

Some patients have a stable relationship before SRS, but it was demonstrateded that the chance to have a stable relationship significantly increases after surgery. In particular, De Cuypere and colleagues [10] showed that the percentage of subjects who had a stable relationship increased from 34 % preoperatively to 59 % postoperatively. Moreover, 2 % of subjects decide to get married, in countries where this is allowed. In our experience many MtoF transsexual subjects with a stable relationship before the surgery change partners after the operation. This observation is shared by other authors [3]. In fact, after SRS some patients change their sexual orientation. According to a work by Lawrence on 232 MtoF subjects before surgery, 54 % were predominantly attracted to females and only 9 % to males, whereas after surgery, the ratio was reversed, with 25 % of people attracted to females and 34 % attracted to males. This trend was also confirmed by other authors [9]; therefore, we believe that some patients before surgery tend to retain heterosexual orientation according to their phenotypic sex, and after surgery they feel freer concerning their sexual orientation, choosing a male partner.

23.3 Quality of Life After Female to Male Sexual Reassignment Surgery

23.3.1 Physical Determinants of Quality of Life After Female to Male SRS

Female to male transsexuals need to address multiple surgical procedures in order to adapt their body to their mind. First of all, mastectomy and hystero-ovariectomy have to be performed. Second, several reconstructive procedures can be used to adapt the external genitalia: the World Professional Association of Transgender Health (WPATH) consider vaginectomy, phalloplasty and urethroplasty to be standard operations for genital transformation, whilst at a later stage testicular prosthesis and penile prosthesis implantation can be considered to achieve the final result. The transition path is time-consuming and challenging, both for the patient and for the medical team; thus, patient QoL can be affected by the extensive “medicalisation”. Nevertheless, usually at the end of the process, the physical aspect of the subject is very close to what he desires and the new genitalia usually have a good aspect and satisfactory functional features, depending on the surgical technique used [34]. There are some issues related to surgical treatment that directly affect patient satisfaction and thus can be considered physical determinants of his QoL.

23.3.1.1 Number of Procedures

A complete penile reconstruction is a complex surgery requiring a staged procedure. Monstrey et al. reported a single-stage procedure for genital transformation with good results [28]. Nowadays, the WPATH consensus agrees on a multiple-stage procedure consisting of phallus configuration, a join-up urethroplasty and finally prosthesis implantation. The advantage of a staged procedure is to avoid a lengthy procedure with increased intraoperative and postoperative complications.

23.3.2 The Aesthetic Appearance of the Neophallus

The main purpose of the phalloplasty procedure is to create an aesthetically acceptable neophallus. Among the different techniques the forearm free flap has the advantage of having a thin flap, which is tabularised, with excellent results in terms of aesthetic appearance. Moreover, the vascularisation of the flap permits a glanduloplasty with a skin patch to be performed safely, according to Norfolk. The aim of this procedure is to permit the patient to have a “socially accepted” phallus.

23.3.3 Functional Outcomes: Sensitivity, Penetration, Orgasmic Feelings

A purpose that has to be perceived in this procedure is not only to permit the patients to have penetrative sexual intercourse, but also to have an erogenous sensation on the neophallus and to provide the possibility of reaching an orgasm during intercourse. The fore-arm free flap permits the surgeon to create an anastomosis between the antero-brachial and ileo-inguinal nerve or the dorsal clitoridal nerve. The presence of the tactile sensation of the phallus is extremely important in order to avoid complications after penile prosthesis implantation. Different studies reported high sensitivity in the neophallus and high satisfactory penetrative intercourse achieving orgasmic sensations [15].

23.3.4 Micturition in a Standing Position

Probably the main difference in social appearance between a biological man and woman is the ability of a man to void while standing. It is well known that one of the priorities of a man undergoing phalloplasty is to have the possibility of urinating while standing. This main goal can be achieved with free flap phalloplasty and also with metoidioplasty. Unfortunately, the reconstruction of the urethra is a tricky stage of the reconstructive process with a high incidence of complications, such as fistulas and strictures [5, 27]. Considering the high risk of complications, this step should be discussed extensively with the patients.

23.3.5 Complications

The penile reconstruction is an aesthetic procedure to prevent a psychiatric disturbance from affecting the patient's life. This consideration underlines the need to minimise complications as far as possible. As with all surgical procedures, general complications such as bleeding, pulmonary embolism and wound infections have to be considered. Deaths have not been reported in the literature. Fortunately, there were very few complications related to the flap in the series reported in the scientific literature. Despite these data, early reinterventions related to ischaemia of the flap were reported in 12 % of cases. As we discussed in the previous paragraph, the main complications are related to the urethral reconstruction. The risks of the procedure have to be discussed and shared with the patients.

23.3.6 Scarring in the Donor Area

The impact of scarring at the donor site has to be extensively discussed and accepted by the patients. Metoidioplasty is the best procedure with which to address patients asking for low morbidity related to the donor area. Free flap phalloplasty is characterised by a certain degree of aesthetic impairment in the site of the donor area. Different studies have demonstrated that the scar is well accepted by transsexual patients, viewing the scarring site as a requirement to reach their aim: creation of the phallus. Nowadays, surgical techniques permit morbidity of the donor area to be reduced through the use of skin graft and tattoos [41]. Female to male transsexual patients comprise an increasing population of patients asking medical professionals to achieve satisfying aesthetic and functional outcome whilst minimising complications. Different surgical approaches can be considered to reach this goal, but every procedure has its own advantages and risks [2]. In general, good results are reported in literature with every technique, in expert hands; thus, it could be argued that is not difficult to make patients happy and satisfied [43]. In reality, it is not that simple, and patients are requested to have good compliance with the therapeutic programme: once again, we have to underline the need to share with the patients the benefits and the risks of each procedure to obtain satisfaction and thus to provide the best conditions to enjoy a good QoL. Free-flap phalloplasty with urethral reconstruction and penile prosthesis implantation, for instance, obtains good patient satisfaction, but the need for revision of the vascular anastomosis has to be considered in 12 % of cases treated using this procedure. Whatever the technique adopted, the main problems are related to the urethroplasty; Monstrey et al. reported 41 % urological complications in terms of cutaneous fistula or stricture. Moreover, scarring of the donor area has to be accepted by the patients. Penile prosthesis implantation is a tricky stage of the reconstructive path. Hoebeke et al. reported the largest series of hydraulic devices in neophallus, with an explantation rate of 44 %. Despite the high complication rate, the results in terms of patient satisfaction are extremely high, with more than 80 % of patients reporting an improvement in their sexual function [21]. In patients who do not require a functional phallus for sexual intercourse a metoidioplasty could be proposed; this procedure gives excellent results in terms of patient satisfaction [11] with minimal complications. Furthermore, this procedure does not result in adjunctive scarring.

23.3.7 Social and Relational Determinants of Quality of Life After Female to Male SRS

23.3.7.1 Social and Labor Integration After SRS

From the data available in the literature, the same aspects and critical points described for MtoF transsexuals are valid for patients undergoing FtoM sexual reassignment in all areas of daily life. The main difference between MtoF and FtoM patients, as reported in the literature, consists of a more simple process of socio-professional reintegration. The available data support that there is less difficulty in this fundamental step for FtoM transsexual individuals, because of a greater ability to adapt and to start interpersonal relationships compared with MtoF transsexuals [29]. Even for FtoM transsexuals, the available literature data on the effects of SRS on the scope of employment are conflicting, but the data support in a stronger way a real improvement (30–60 % of cases) in terms of FtoM patient satisfaction with regard to this area.

23.3.7.2 Sexual Relationships After SRS

As with MtoF patients, the main determinant of the social QoL of FtoM subjects is the possibility to of having a satisfying, active sexual life and a stable relationship. Few data on the social life of FtoM transsexuals have been reported in the scientific literature compared with MtoF subjects. A few authors report that about a third are not able to start a relationship after surgery, despite a normally active sexual desire.

Despite major difficulties in starting a relationship, FtoM transsexuals are more suitable for marriage. Parola et al. [29] reported that 30.4 % of FtoM transsexuals were married versus 2 % of MtoF transsexuals after SRS. Despite acceptable aesthetic results after SRS, some of these patients probably avoid a relationship with a potential partner because they do not feel confident about their masculinity and retain high levels of anxiety. Once this first hurdle has been crossed, they are more likely to maintain a stable relationship.

Conclusions

In conclusion, the QoL in patients undergoing SRS is a very complex subject because of the wide variety of determinants that may influence them from medical, biological and socio-relational points of view. Moreover, few and heterogeneous data are reported in the literature. According to our experience and to the data reported in the literature, after SRS the vast majority of transsexual individuals lead a life with satisfaction rates comparable with those of non-transsexuals. The duration of life of transsexual subjects who underwent SRS seems to be comparable with that of the general population [10, 19, 23, 42]. Previously, some authors reported higher mortality rates in the 10 years after SRS, but the values are gradually returning to those of the normal population, probably because of refinement of surgical techniques and protocols of hormone replacement therapy (HRT) [12]. The increased frequency of cardiovascular disease and cancer may also be increased for habits such as smoking (about 50% of MtoF and 20% of FtoM are smokers), adverse effects of hormonale replacement therapies (actually in a constant optimization process) and infectious disease such as AIDS [1, 13, 20, 30, 40, 44]. It is possible that transsexual people avoid the healthcare system because of a presumed risk of discrimination [10]. Despite these encouraging data, it is clear from several works that there is an increased rate of suicides in transsexual subjects, both before and after intervention [19, 37, 42]. The fact that transsexualism is a risk factor for suicide [12] emphasises once again the duty of the medical/surgical care team not only to undertake conversion of the sexual characteristics but also to extensively monitor parameters such as satisfaction and QoL of patients, even after surgery.

References

1. Bauer GR, Hammond R, Travers R, Kaay M, Hohenadel KM, Boyce M (2009) "I don't think this is theoretical; this is our lives": how erasure impacts health care for transgender people. J Assoc Nurses AIDS Care 20(5):348–361. doi:10.1016/j.jana.2009.07.004
2. Bettocchi C, Ralph DJ, Pryor JP (2005) Pedicled pubic phalloplasty in females with gender dysphoria. BJU Int 95(1):120–124
3. Bodlund O, Kullgren G (1996) Transsexualism–general outcome and prognostic factors: a five-year follow-up study of nineteen transsexuals in the process of changing sex. Arch Sex Behav 25(3):303–316
4. Brunocilla E, Soli M, Franceschelli A, Schiavina R, Borghesi M, Gentile G, Pultrone CV, Martorana G, Orrei MG, Colombo F (2012) Radiological evaluation by magnetic resonance of the 'new anatomy' of transsexual patients undergoing male to female sex reassignment surgery. Int J Impot Res 24(5):206–209. doi:10.1038/ijir.2012.18
5. Cavadas PC, Landin L (2005) Treatment of urethral stricture in a female-to-male transsexual with a tubulized flap from the labia minora. J Reconstr Microsurg 21(3):153–156
6. Chew S, Tham KF, Ratnam SS (1997) Sexual behaviour and prevalence of HIV antibodies in transsexuals. J Obstet Gynaecol Res 23:33–36
7. Costantino A, Cerpolini S, Alvisi S, Morselli PG, Venturoli S, Meriggiola MC (2013) A prospective study on sexual function and mood in female-to-male transsexuals during testosterone administration and after sex reassignment surgery. J Sex Marital Ther 39(4):321–335. doi:10.1080/0092623X.2012.736920
8. Cova M, Mosconi E, Liguori G, Bucci S, Trombetta C, Belgrano E, Pozzi-Mucelli R (2003) Value of magnetic resonance imaging in the evaluation of sex-reassignment surgery in male-to-female transsexuals. Abdom Imaging 28(5):728–732
9. Daskalos CT (1998) Changes in the sexual orientation of six heterosexual male-to-female transsexuals. Arch Sex Behav 27(6):605–614
10. De Cuypere G, T'Sjoen G, Beerten R, Selvaggi G, De Sutter P, Hoebeke P, Monstrey S, Vansteenwegen A, Rubens R (2005) Sexual and physical health after sex reassignment surgery. Arch Sex Behav 34(6):679–690
11. Djordjevic ML, Stanojevic D, Bizic M, Kojovic V, Majstorovic M, Vujovic S, Milosevic A, Korac G, Perovic SV (2009) Metoidioplasty as a single stage sex reassignment surgery in female transsexuals: Belgrade experience. J Sex Med 6(5):1306–1313
12. Dhejne C, Lichtenstein P, Boman M, Johansson AL, Langstrom N, Lande M (2011) Long-term follow-up of transsexual persons undergoing sex reassignment surgery: cohort study in Sweden. PLoS One 6(2):e16885
13. Elamin MB, Garcia MZ, Murad MH, Erwin PJ, Montori VM (2010) Effect of sex steroid use on cardiovascular risk in transsexual individuals: a systematic review and meta-analyses. Clin Endocrinol (Oxf) 72:1–10
14. Fisher AD, Castellini G, Bandini E, Casale H, Fanni E, Benni L, Ferruccio N, Meriggiola MC, Manieri C, Gualerzi A, Jannini E, Oppo A, Ricca V, Maggi M, Rellini AH (2014) Cross-sex hormonal treatment and body uneasiness in individuals with gender dysphoria. J Sex Med 11(3):709–719. doi:10.1111/jsm.12413, Epub 2013 Dec 16
15. Garaffa G, Christopher NA, Ralph DJ (2010) Total phallic reconstruction in female-to-male transsexuals. Eur Urol 57(4):715–722
16. Giraldo F, Esteva I, Bergero T, Cano G, González C, Salinas P, Rivada E, Lara JS, Soriguer F, Andalusia Gender Team (2004) Corona glans clitoroplasty and urethropreputial vestibuloplasty in male-to-female transsexuals: the vulval aesthetic refinement by the Andalusia Gender Team. Plast Reconstr Surg 114(6):1543–1550
17. Godano A, Maggi M, Jannini E, Meriggiola MC, Ghigo E, Todarello O, Lenzi A, Manieri CJ (2009) SIAMS-ONIG Consensus on hormonal treatment in gender identity disorders. J Endocrinol Invest 32(10):857–864
18. Goddard JC, Vickery RM, Qureshi A, Summerton DJ, Khoosal D, Terry TR (2007) Feminizing genitoplasty in adult transsexuals: early and long-term surgical results. BJU Int 100(3):607–613
19. Gooren LJ, Giltay EJ, Bunck MC (2008) Long-term treatment of transsexuals with cross-sex hormones: extensive personal experience. J Clin Endocrinol Metab 93(1):19–25
20. Gooren LJ, van Trotsenburg MA, Giltay EJ, van Diest PJ (2013) Breast cancer development in transsexual subjects receiving cross-sex hormone treatment. J Sex Med 10(12):3129–3134. doi:10.1111/jsm.12319
21. Hoebeke PB, Decaestecker K, Beysens M, Opdenakker Y, Lumen N, Monstrey SM (2010) Erectile implants in female-to-male transsexuals: our experience in 129 patients. Eur Urol 57(2):334–340
22. Imbimbo C, Verze P, Palmieri A, Longo N, Fusco F, Arcaniolo D, Mirone V (2009) A report from a single institute's 14-year experience in treatment of male-to-female transsexuals. J Sex Med 6(10):2736–2745
23. Johansson A, Sundbom E, Höjerback T, Bodlund O (2010) A five-year follow-up study of Swedish adults with gender identity disorder. Arch Sex Behav 39(6):1429–1437
24. Kirk S (1997) A survey of post-operative male to female transsexuals from health care to sexual experience and points in between. Paper presented at the XV Harry Benjamin International Gender Dysphoria Association Symposium, Vancouver
25. Kuhn A, Bodmer C, Stadlmayr W, Kuhn P, Mueller MD, Birkhauser M (2009) Quality of life 15 years

after sex reassignment surgery for transsexualism. Fertil Steril 92(5):1685–1689
26. Lawrence AA (2003) Factors associated with satisfaction or regret following male-to-female sex reassignment surgery. Arch Sex Behav 32:299–315
27. Lumen N, Monstrey S, Goessaert AS, Oosterlinck W, Hoebeke P (2011) Urethroplasty for strictures after phallic reconstruction: a single-institution experience. Eur Urol 60(1):150–158. doi:10.1016/j.eururo.2010.11.015, Epub 2010 Nov 21
28. Monstrey SJ, Ceulemans P, Hoebeke P (2011) Sex reassignment surgery in the female-to-male transsexual. Semin Plast Surg 25(3):229–244. doi:10.1055/s-0031-1281493
29. Parola N, Bonierbale M, Lemaire A, Aghababian V, Michel A, Lançon C (2010) Study of quality of life for transsexuals after hormonal and surgical reassignment. Sexologies 19(1):24–28
30. Pattison ST, McLaren BR (2013) Triple negative breast cancer in a male-to-female transsexual. Intern Med J 43(2):203–205. doi:10.1111/imj.12047
31. Rakic Z, Starcevic V, Maric J, Kellin K (1996) The outcome of sex reassignment surgery in Belgrade: 32 patients of both sexes. Arch Sex Behav 25:515–525
32. Rehman J, Lazer S, Benet AE, Schaefer LC, Melman A (1999) The reported sex and surgery satisfactions of 28 postoperative male-to-female transsexuals patients. Arch Sex Behav 28(1):71–89
33. Rolle L, Falcone M, Vighetti S, Ceruti C, Sedigh O, Timpano M, Molo MT, Castelli L, Preto M, Gontero P, Frea B (2014) Does sex reassignment surgery induce cerebral modifications in MTF transsexuals? J Sex Med 11(1):312
34. Selvaggi G, Dhejne C, Landen M, Elander A (2012) The 2011 WPATH standards of care and penile reconstruction in female-to-male transsexual individuals. Adv Urol 2012:581712
35. Sohn MH, Hatzinger M, Wirsam K (2013) Genital reassignment surgery in male-to-female transsexuals: do we have guidelines or standards? Handchir Mikrochir Plast Chir 45(4):207–210. doi:10.1055/s-0033-1343427, Epub 2013 Jul 9
36. Soli M, Brunocilla E, Bertaccini A, Palmieri F, Barbieri B, Martorana G (2008) Male to female gender reassignment: modified surgical technique for creating the neoclitoris and mons veneris. J Sex Med 5(1):210–216
37. Sørensen T, Hertoft P (1982) Male and female transsexualism: the Danish experience with 37 patients. Arch Sex Behav 11(2):133–155
38. Trombetta C, Liguori G, Bucci S, Salamè L, Garaffa G, Cova M, Belgrano E (2004) Radiological evaluation of vaginal width and depth in male-to-female transsexuals by the use of magnetic resonance imaging. World J Urol 22(5):405–408
39. Trombetta C, Liguori G, Benvenuto S, Petrovic M, Napoli R, Umari P, Rizzo M, Zordani A (2011) Neo-urethroclitoroplasty according to Petrovic. Urologia 78(4):267–273. doi:10.5301/RU.2011.8855
40. Turo R, Jallad S, Prescott S, Cross WR (2013) Metastatic prostate cancer in transsexual diagnosed after three decades of estrogen therapy. Can Urol Assoc J 7(7–8):E544–E546. doi:10.5489/cuaj.175
41. Van Caenegem E, Verhaeghe E, Taes Y, Wierckx K, Toye K, Goemaere S, Zmierczak HG, Hoebeke P, Monstrey S, T'Sjoen G (2013) Long-term evaluation of donor-site morbidity after radial forearm flap phalloplasty for transsexual men. J Sex Med 10(6): 1644–1651
42. Van Kesteren PJ, Asscheman H, Megens JA, Gooren LJ (1997) Mortality and morbidity in transsexual subjects treated with cross-sex hormones. Clin Endocrinol (Oxf) 47(3):337–342
43. Wierckx K, Van Caenegem E, Elaut E, Dedecker D, Van de Peer F, Toye K, Weyers S, Hoebeke P, Monstrey S, De Cuypere G, T'Sjoen G (2011) Quality of life and sexual health after sex reassignment surgery in transsexual men. J Sex Med 8(12):3379–3388
44. Wierckx K, Elaut E, Declercq E, Heylens G, De Cuypere G, Taes Y, Kaufman JM, T'Sjoen G (2013) Prevalence of cardiovascular disease and cancer during cross-sex hormone therapy in a large cohort of trans persons: a case-control study. Eur J Endocrinol 169(4):471–478. doi:10.1530/EJE-13-0493, Print 2013 Oct
45. Zimmermann A, Zimmer R, Kovacs L, Einodshofer S, Herschbach P, Henrich G, Tunner W, Biemer E, Papadopulos NA (2006) Transsexuals' life satisfaction after gender transformation operations. Chirurg 77:432–438

Imaging

24

Michele Bertolotto, Rosaria Perrone, Francesca Cacciato, Giovanni Liguori, and Maria A. Cova

24.1 Introduction

The goal of male to female (MtoF) sex reassignment surgery (SRS) is to provide an aesthetically attractive and functional result, which permits the new female effortless intromission, preserving the potential for orgasm. Although many of these patients would benefit from imaging investigation, either to plan SRS or to manage postoperative complications, imaging is not routinely performed in the standard clinical practice. This likely arises, at least in part, from the lack of confidence of most radiologists with the pelvic anatomy after genital reconfiguration and possible postoperative complications.

M. Bertolotto, MD (✉) • R. Perrone
F. Cacciato • M.A. Cova
Department of Radiology, University of Trieste, Ospedale di Cattinara, Strada di Fiume 447, Trieste 34149, Italy
e-mail: bertolot@units.it; ros.perrone@gmail.com; francescacacciato@gmail.com; cova@gnbts.units.it

G. Liguori
Department of Urology, University of Trieste, Ospedale di Cattinara, Strada di Fiume 447, Trieste 34149, Italy
e-mail: gioliguori@gmail.com

24.2 Magnetic Resonance Anatomy After MtoF SRS

The superior soft-tissue contrast resolution afforded by magnetic resonance (MR) imaging provides an opportunity to advance imaging evaluation of the postoperative anatomy in MtoF SRS. Full evaluation of normal postoperative changes and the presence of postoperative complications can be documented.

24.2.1 Evaluation of the Neovagina

The configuration of a neovagina of adequate depth and inclination is mandatory in achieving satisfying sexual intercourse. These parameters, as well as the straight or angulated course of the neovagina, are best estimated on T2-weighted images (Fig. 24.1) [1–3]. Neovaginal and rectal distension with gel optimises evaluation of the wall and the length. Previous investigations showed an average neovaginal length of about 9.3 cm (range: 6–11 cm) [2, 3]. Physiological inclination in the sagittal plane is from front to rear and from low to high.

A minor but relatively common complication of MtoF SRS is neovaginal prolapse (Fig. 24.2). Diagnosis is clinical, but MR imaging is indicated when associated inflammatory ischaemic changes are suspected. Abscesses are frequently localised in the labia (Fig. 24.3) [4], but can also involve the dissected rectoprostatic fascia and the tissues around the urethral stump. They are

C. Trombetta et al. (eds.), *Management of Gender Dysphoria: A Multidisciplinary Approach*, DOI 10.1007/978-88-470-5696-1_24, © Springer-Verlag Italia 2015

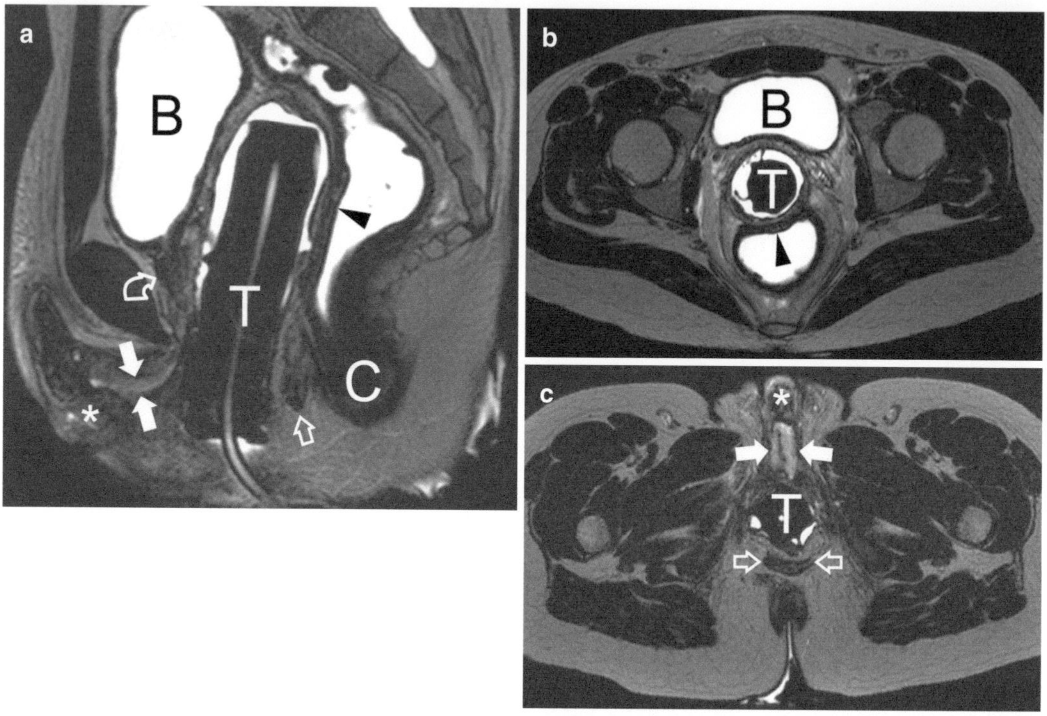

Fig. 24.1 Evaluation of the new female anatomy in a 25-year-old male to female (MtoF) transsexual investigated 8 days after sex reassignment surgery (SRS). The neovagina and the rectum are distended with gel. Imaging has been performed with the vaginal tutor (*T*) inserted. (**a**) Midsagittal T2-weighted magnetic resonance (MR) image shows the new female normal anatomy of the patient. The neovagina has an adequate length of 11 cm and inclination from front to rear. Note the prostate (*curved arrow*), rectovaginal septum (*arrowhead*), anal canal (*C*), bladder (*B*), urethral remnant (*arrows*), neoclitoris (*asterisk*), and bulbocavernous muscle (*open arrow*). (**b**, **c**) Appearance of the same anatomical features on axial T2-weighted MR images

usually treated conservatively with incision and drainage and with cephalosporin-based antibiotics until complete remission. In a minority of cases wound exploration is required.

24.2.2 Thickness of the Rectovaginal Septum

During MtoF SRS the neovagina is obtained by dissecting the space between the rectum posteriorly and the prostate anteriorly. This is the most dangerous phase of the operation because accidental rectal injuries are possible with fistula formation. The bulbocavernous muscle may be used to reinforce the distal portion of the septum and reduce the risk of fistulisation.

Introduction of gel into the rectum and neovagina eases evaluation of the rectoneovaginal septum, which is only a few millimetres thick [1–3], of the bulbocavernous muscle, and of its relationships with the distal portion of the neovagina and of the anal canal (Fig. 24.1).

24.2.3 Evaluation of the Neoclitoris

Magnetic resonance imaging allows excellent evaluation of the neoclitoris early after SRS and later during the follow-up (Fig. 24.4). Variations in the surgical technique can be identified, such as preservation of the dorsal aspect of the tunica albuginea, isolated or with a small amount of cavernosus tissue (Fig. 24.5). Bleeding of the tissues used to manufacture the neoclitoris is common in the early postoperative period (Fig. 24.6). It is usually self-limiting, but may occasionally require medical treatment, interventional procedures or surgical revision. Fat-saturated T1-weighted images obtained after gadolinium contrast medium administration are the most informative when evaluating the urethral stump, glans remnant, neurovascular bundle, blood extravasation, and ischaemic changes.

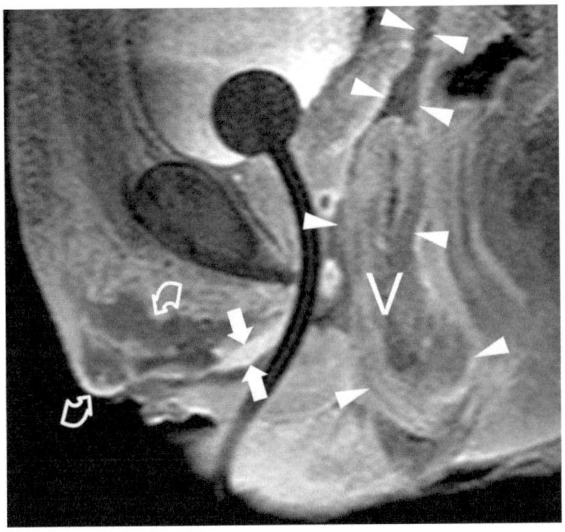

Fig. 24.2 Prolapse of the neovagina in a 35-year-old MtoF transsexual investigated 5 days after SRS. The patient was investigated because ischaemia of the neovaginal wall was clinically suspected. Midsagittal fat-suppressed T1-weighted MR image obtained after the administration of a gadolinium-based contrast agent shows a partially prolapsed, non-ischaemic neovagina (*V*) in the lower portion of the space created between the prostate and the rectum (*arrowheads*). Fluid (*curved arrows*) is also shown anterior to the urethral remnant (*arrows*)

24.2.4 Evaluation of Cavernosal and Spongiosal Remnants

In early surgical variations for MtoF SRS a neoclitoris was not created. The crura of the corpora cavernosa and the bulbus of the corpus spongiosum were preserved as they were thought to increase sensitivity and enhance sexual satisfaction. Long-term experience has demonstrated, on the contrary, that engorgement of the residual erectile tissue during sexual arousal and foreplay causes the patient discomfort and dyspareunia during penetration. MR imaging allows an excellent depiction of the remnants and of their relationship with the surrounding structures [1, 2]. T2-weighted images obtained after ultrasound-guided PGE1 injection are the most informative (Fig. 24.7).

24.3 Breast Imaging

After taking hormonal therapy in MtoF transsexuals breast tissue closely resembles that of natal women [5]. Breasts present on the

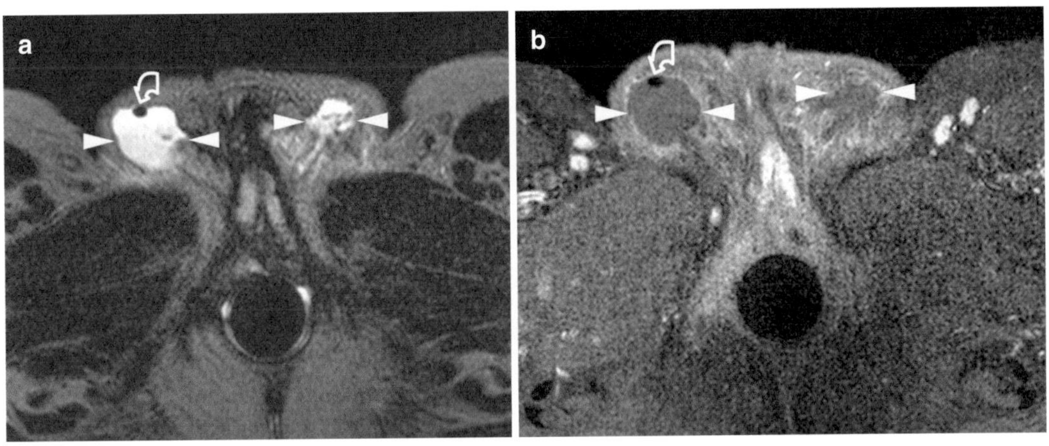

Fig. 24.3 Abscess formation in the labia of a 22-year-old MtoF transsexual investigated 9 days after SRS. Axial T2-weighted (**a**) and fat-suppressed T1-weighted MR image (**b**) obtained after the administration of a gadolinium-based contrast agent show fluid collections within the labia (*arrowheads*) with an air bubble (*curved arrow*) and a peripheral rim of enhancement consistent with abscesses. The patient was treated with systemic antibiotics and subsequently underwent successful percutaneous drainage

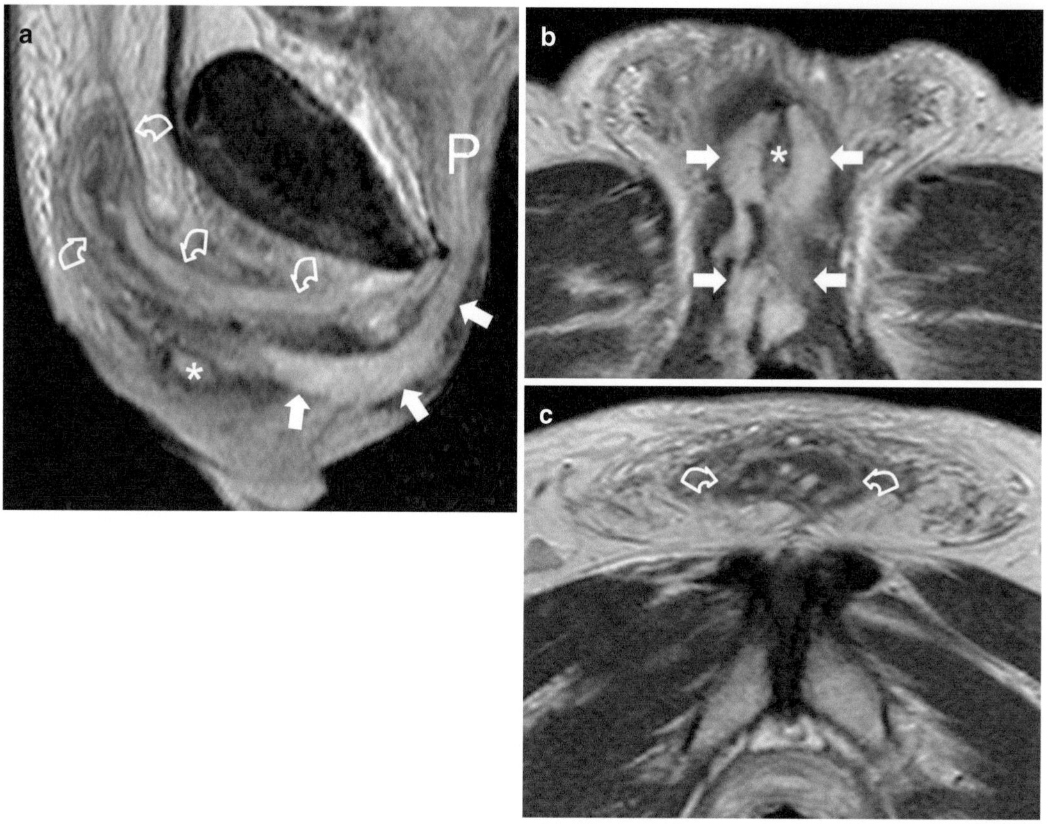

Fig. 24.4 Evaluation of the neoclitoris in a 41-year-old MtoF transsexual investigated 8 days after SRS. (**a**) Midsagittal T1-weighted MR image obtained after the administration of a gadolinium-based contrast agent shows the urethral remnant (*arrows*), the dorsal neurovascular bundle of the penis (*curved arrow*) folded up under the pubic subcutaneous fat to form the mons veneris, and the neoclitoris (*asterisk*), which is in the natural anatomical position of the female clitoris. (**b**, **c**) Axial gadolinium-enhanced T1-weighted images at the level of the neoclitoris (**a**) and of the mons veneris (**b**) show: (**b**) the urethral remnant (*arrows*) opened, incised distally in a Y shape, and sutured around the neoclitoris (*asterisk*), and (**c**) the neurovascular bundle of the penis within the pubic subcutaneous fat. *P* prostate

mammogram with a spectrum of tissue density, including heterogeneously dense and extremely dense breast tissue (Fig. 24.8). Cancer has been rarely reported [6]. Given the biological plausibility of increased risk and the lack of sufficient evidence evaluating the risk, regular monitoring is recommended. Breast self-examination, clinical breast examination at regular appointments and routine mammogram and ultrasound screening should continue in MtoF patients on cross-sex hormone therapy, the same as recommendations for screening in biological women. In MtoF transsexuals with breast augmentation imaging plays the same role as in natal women.

24.4 Voice Feminisation Surgery

Anatomical and functional assessment of the larynx is usually considered sufficient for the management of patients undergoing voice feminisation surgery [7]. Ultrasound is commonly performed in these patients by the surgeon himself to measure the anterior cricothyroid space (Fig. 24.9) [8]. No further imaging is usually carried out. Postoperative ultrasound is often technically limited because there are artefacts from the implanted miniplate. Following vocal surgery, unsatisfactory results are obtained in a not negligible percentage of patients [9–11]. In fact, movement of the cricothyroid joint during

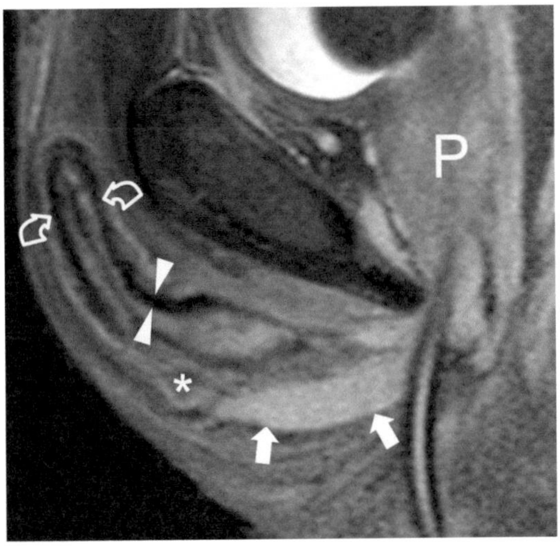

Fig. 24.5 Variation of the surgical technique for creating the neoclitoris in a 22-year-old MtoF transsexual. Midsagittal fat-suppressed T1-weighted MR image obtained after the administration of a gadolinium-based contrast agent shows the urethral remnant (*arrows*), the dorsal neurovascular bundle of the penis (*curved arrow*) and the neoclitoris (*asterisk*). A strip of the dorsal portion of the tunica albuginea has been preserved, which is visible as a hypointense line (*arrowheads*) stuck on the neurovascular bundle. *P* prostate

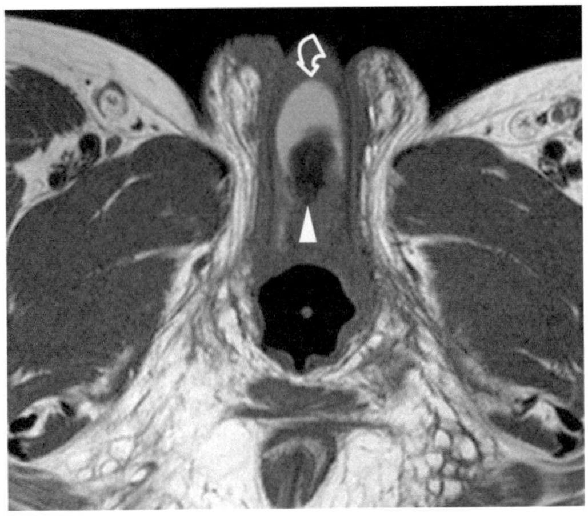

Fig. 24.6 Male to female SRS complicated by bleeding of the wedge of the glans when the neoclitoris was manufactured. MR imaging was performed 2 days after the operation. Axial T1-weighted image shows a small extravasation of blood (*curved arrow*) surrounding the neoclitoris (*arrowhead*). The haematoma was reabsorbed spontaneously within 1 week

phonation is complex [9, 12], and evidence is increasing that a detailed preoperative analysis of the laryngeal anatomy and biomechanics is needed to improve the rate of patient satisfaction. Helical CT makes it possible to demonstrate the structures of the larynx both before and after the operation, and to measure vocal cord length [10]. Preclinical studies show the potential for detailed three-dimensional evaluation of the biomechanics of the larynx in real time [13, 14].

24.5 Vaginoplasty

Vaginal strictures and loss of depth are major functional complications in MtoF SRS [4]. Use of vaginal dilatators, inflatable silicon tutors, or suitable substitutes is necessary to keep the neovagina open. Discontinued dilatation results in neovaginal stenosis to some degree and strictures of the introitus, which require stretching again, or vaginoplasty. Moreover, local infection and reduction of the local blood supply may cause severe stenosis. When the patency of the neovagina cannot be restored using non-surgical techniques, reconstruction is indicated with skin flaps or other lining materials [15], the rectosigmoid colon [16], or an ileal segment [17]. MR imaging is the modality of choice for investigating patients undergoing surgical reconstruction of the neovagina, to assess postoperative ischaemic or inflammatory complications, and to evaluate the surgical results (Fig. 24.10).

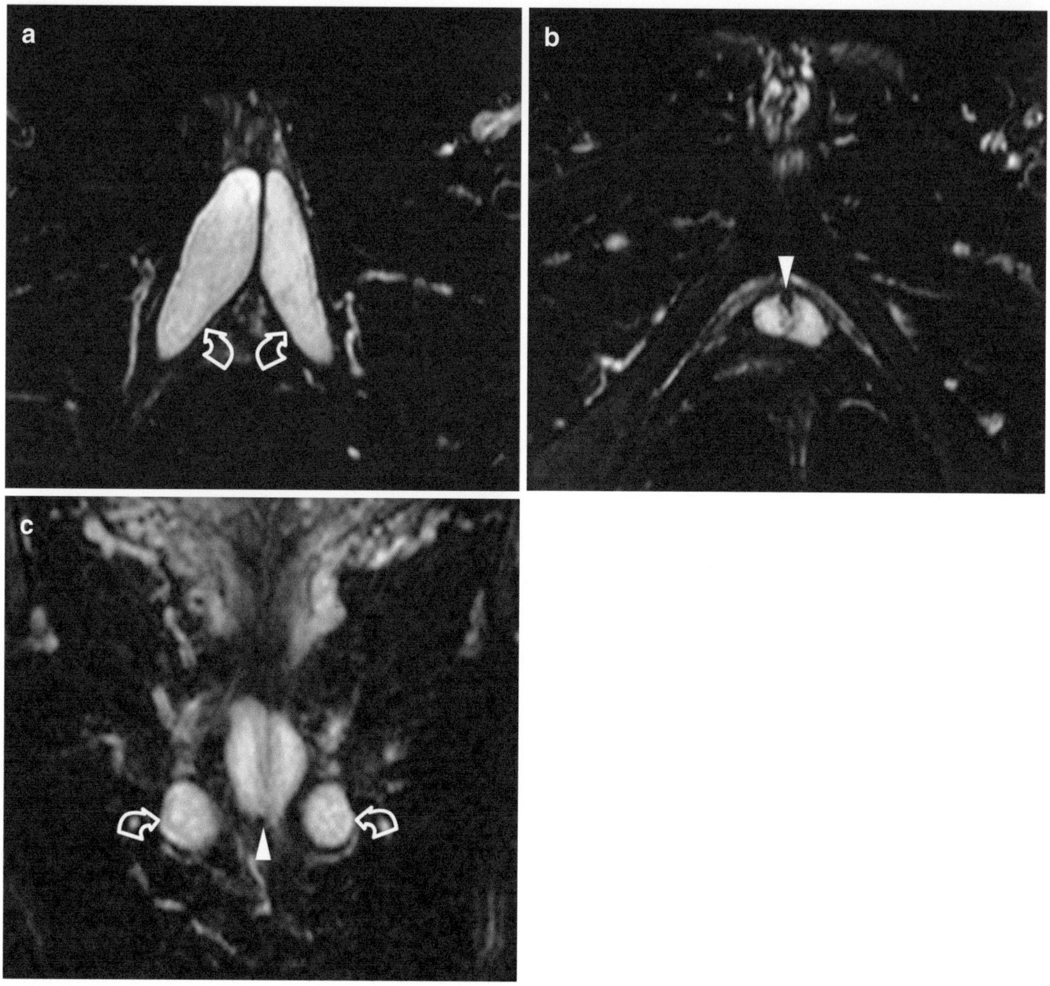

Fig. 24.7 Axial (**a**, **b**) and coronal (**c**) T2-weighted images with fat saturation obtained after ultrasound-guided intracavernosal PGE1 injection showing the remnants of the corpora cavernosa (*curved arrows*) and the bulbus of the corpus spongiosum (*arrowhead*) in a MtoF transsexual patient operated on 22 years ago

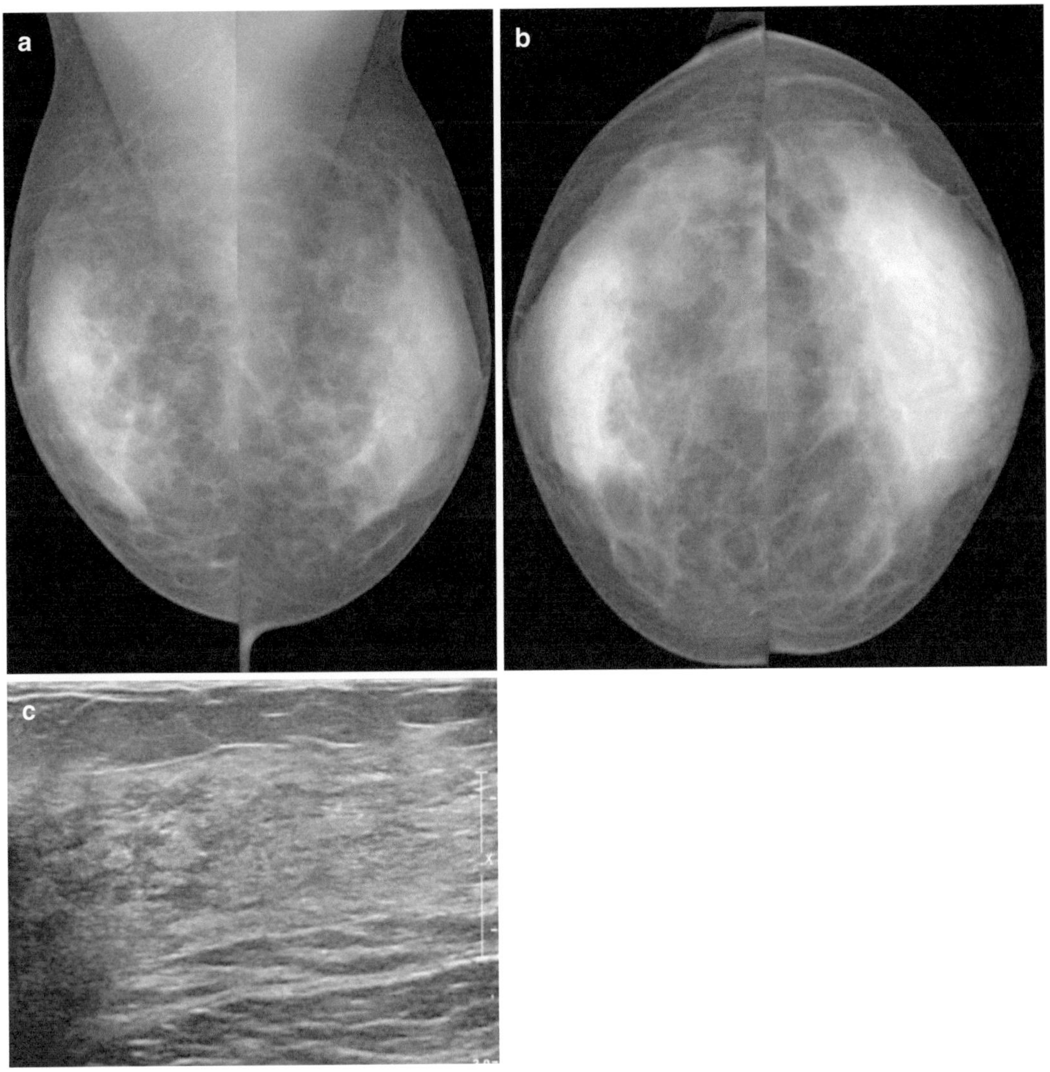

Fig. 24.8 Routine imaging screening in a 44-year-old MtoF transsexual taking hormonal therapy for 27 years. (**a**, **b**) Mammogram shows dense breast parenchyma. (**c**) Ultrasound appearance of the breasts of the same patient shows a prevalence of echogenic fibroglandular tissue

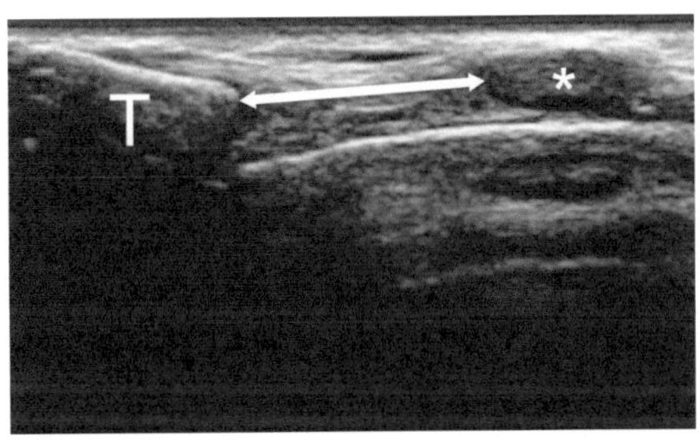

Fig. 24.9 Ultrasound evaluation of the cricothyroid space in a 28-year-old MtoF transsexual undergoing voice surgery. Longitudinal ultrasound view of the anterior aspect of the neck shows partially calcified thyroid cartilage (*T*), cricoid cartilage (*), and the cricothyroid space (*double arrow*) measuring 1.2 cm

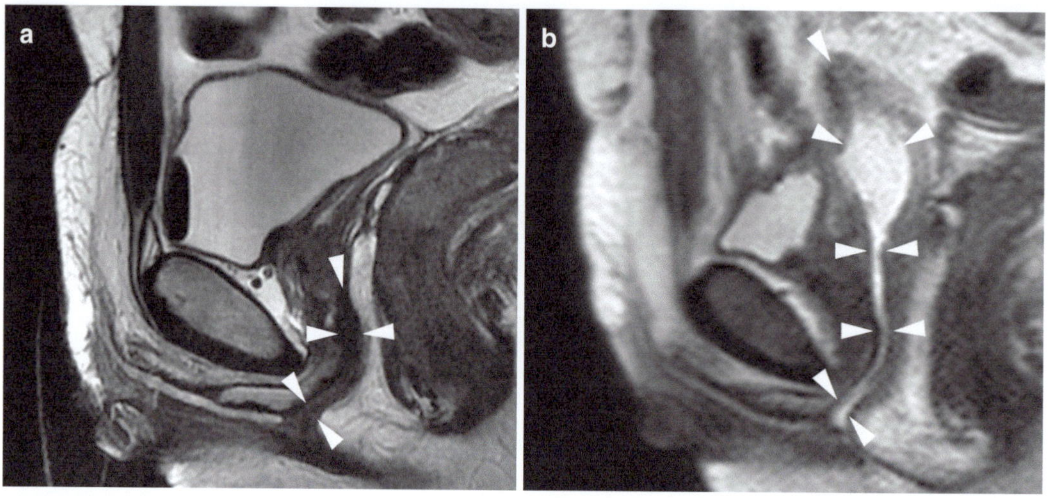

Fig. 24.10 Vaginoplasty in a 30-year-old MtoF transsexual who had undergone SRS 8 years previously and had developed stenosis of the neovagina. Midsagittal T2-weighted images. (**a**) Before the operation a non-patent neovagina measuring 5 cm in length (*arrowheads*) is present. (**b**) After ileal vaginoplasty a neovagina measuring 13 cm in length, distended with gel, is shown

Conclusions

Male to female SRS is complex and difficult surgery and is fraught with risk. Optimal treatment requires a multidisciplinary approach with a nucleus of dedicated physicians. Radiologists must be confident with the pelvic anatomy after genital reconfiguration and with possible postoperative complications. MR imaging is often the imaging modality of choice because it allows a detailed assessment of the new pelvic anatomy after sex reassignment, identifies postoperative complications, and provides information that can be useful in planning further intervention.

References

1. Cova M, Mosconi E, Liguori G et al (2003) Value of magnetic resonance imaging in the evaluation of sex-reassignment surgery in male-to-female transsexuals. Abdom Imaging 28:728–732
2. Trombetta C, Liguori G, Bucci S et al (2004) Radiological evaluation of vaginal width and depth in male-to-female transsexuals by the use of magnetic resonance imaging. World J Urol 22:405–408
3. Brunocilla E, Soli M, Franceschelli A et al (2012) Radiological evaluation by magnetic resonance of the 'new anatomy' of transsexual patients undergoing male to female sex reassignment surgery. Int J Impot Res 24:206–209
4. Rossi Neto R, Hintz F, Krege S, Rubben H, Vom Dorp F (2012) Gender reassignment surgery–a 13 year review of surgical outcomes. Int Braz J Urol 38:97–107
5. Kanhai RC, Hage JJ, van Diest PJ, Bloemena E, Mulder JW (2000) Short-term and long-term histologic effects of castration and estrogen treatment on breast tissue of 14 male-to-female transsexuals in comparison with two chemically castrated men. Am J Surg Pathol 24:74–80
6. Phillips J, Fein-Zachary VJ, Mehta TS, Littlehale N, Venkataraman S, Slanetz PJ (2014) Breast imaging in the transgender patient. AJR Am J Roentgenol 202:1149–1156
7. Pickuth D, Brandt S, Neumann K, Berghaus A, Spielmann RP, Heywang-Kobrunner SH (2000) Value of spiral CT in patients with cricothyroid approximation. Br J Radiol 73:840–842
8. Gugatschka M, Kiesler K, Chibidziura-Priesching J, Schokler B, Friedrich G (2009) Pitch synchronous changes of the anterior cricothyroid gap by using ultrasonography. J Voice 23:610–613
9. Storck C, Gehrer R, Fischer C et al (2011) The role of the cricothyroid joint anatomy in cricothyroid approximation surgery. J Voice 25:632–637
10. Neumann K, Welzel C (2004) The importance of the voice in male to female transsexualism. J Voice 18. 153–167
11. Yang CY, Palmer AD, Murray KD, Meltzer TR, Cohen JI (2002) Cricothyroid approximation to elevate vocal pitch in male-to-female transsexuals:

results of surgery. Ann Otol Rhinol Laryngol 111:477–485
12. Hammer GP, Windisch G, Prodinger PM, Anderhuber F, Friedrich G (2010) The cricothyroid joint–functional aspects with regard to different types of its structure. J Voice 24:140–145
13. Storck C, Juergens P, Fischer C et al (2011) Biomechanics of the cricoarytenoid joint: three-dimensional imaging and vector analysis. J Voice 25:406–410
14. Storck C, Juergens P, Fischer C et al (2010) Three-dimensional imaging of the larynx for pre-operative planning of laryngeal framework surgery. Eur Arch Otorhinolaryngol 267:557–563
15. Panici PB, Ruscito I, Gasparri ML, Maffucci D, Marchese C, Bellati F (2011) Vaginal reconstruction with the Abbe-McIndoe technique: from dermal grafts to autologous in vitro cultured vaginal tissue transplant. Semin Reprod Med 29:45–54
16. Djordjevic ML, Stanojevic DS, Bizic MR (2011) Rectosigmoid vaginoplasty: clinical experience and outcomes in 86 cases. J Sex Med 8:3487–3494
17. Trombetta C, Liguori G, Siracusano S, Bortul M, Belgrano E (2005) Transverse retubularized ileal vaginoplasty: a new application of the Monti principle–preliminary report. Eur Urol 48:1018–1023; discussion 1023–1014

Part III

Management of Female to Male

The Hot Questions of Prepubertal Gender Dysphoria in Girls

25

Alessandra Graziottin

The Ego is first of all a "body-ego". S. Freud, Das Ich und das Es, 1923 [1]

"I woke up one morning, years ago, and suddenly I saw my road in life: I thought there must have been a mistake, but my cards have already been played. I could not get back and choose what I would have liked to be. I could not go back. I wonder why nature does not give any other chances. I'm only a mistake!". Carla 13 years, quoted in J. Baldaro Verde and A. Graziottin, L'enigma dell'identità, 1991 [2]

25.1 Introduction

Gender identity disorders (DID) and, namely, gender dysphoria (GD) are multifaceted [2–7]. The change of sex from female to male (F to M) is a challenge of the highest complexity [2–7]. Key issues involve all the three dimensions of human sexuality: *sexual identity, sexual function, and sexual relationship* (Table 25.1) [2]. *Gender identity, gender role, and gender orientation* were considered major contributors of sexual identity [2]. Encompassing the concept of sexuality, a major focus is currently devoted to the gender issues, with three readings: gender identity (which overlaps with the concept of sexual identity), gender role (a subspecification of the sexual identity), and sexual orientation, considered as three key aspects of human psychosexual differentiation in sex-dimorphic differences [3].

Satisfaction with the gender identity outcome depends on a number of variables that deserve the highest multidisciplinary consideration [2–6].

The most accurate evaluation of physical, emotional, psychoaffective, relational, and contextual difficulties should be taken into account to evaluate the best options. The goal is to offer the girl/patient (and her family) real expectations about the potential outcomes prior to starting a long treatment path. The chapter will briefly consider the most important issues in prepubertal GD girls, with a focus on the biological/medical sexological perspective, integrated with psychosexual implications.

25.2 The "Body-Ego"

As Freud stated back in 1923 [1], the sense of personal identity and gender identity are rooted first in the physical appearance: this is why the body issue of gender appearance is so vital for each of us in the lifespan, and, even more so, for children/adolescents with gender dysphoria. Early on, in 1912, he wrote "anatomy is destiny" [8]: the aspect of the external genitalia at birth is the first social cornerstone of gender identity leading to the attribution of the "anagraphic sex." The description as "male" or "female" usually triggers comprehensive and pervasive family and social interactions oriented first to appreciate and reinforce the self-perception of the child as either a boy or a girl and, second, his/her adherence to the gender norms of that family and cultural belonging [2, 9]. In girls, a rewarding identification with the mother (or another affectively persistent/constant significant female caregiver, such as the grandmother in many families) and a satisfying complementation with the father (or another affectively persistent/constant respectful male figure) further contribute to

A. Graziottin, MD
Center of Gynecology and Medical Sexology, H. San Raffaele Resnati, Via Santa Croce 10/a, 20123 Milan, Italy
e-mail: a.graziottin@studiograziottin.it; segreteria@studiograziottin.it

C. Trombetta et al. (eds.), *Management of Gender Dysphoria: A Multidisciplinary Approach*, DOI 10.1007/978-88-470-5696-1_25, © Springer-Verlag Italia 2015

Table 25.1 Key dimensions of human sexuality

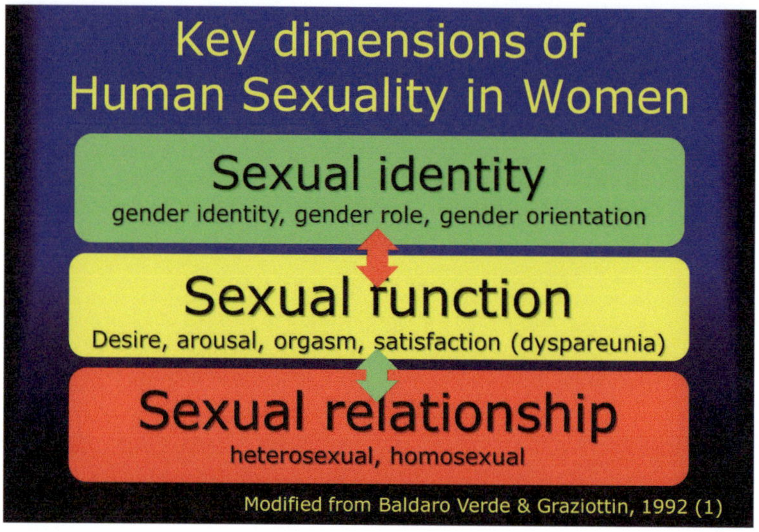

Modified from Baldaro Verde and Graziottin [2]

developing a solid and consistent female gender identity [2]. This positive self-perception is well expressed in the statement "I'm happy to be a girl": feminine, active, pretty, joyful, tender, vital, energetic, and smiling to life.

25.2.1 The Biological Priming of Brain and Body

The female genital organs (and the brain) differentiate in the feminine phenotype during the embryonic period without particular hormonal influences. Indeed, the "female" *is the* "default" *program* [10] exemplified in XO subjects (Turner syndrome): they are infertile, but the external genitalia are female and behavior is female. Not one case of gender dysphoria in Turner syndrome women is reported in the literature, in this author's knowledge. Indeed, internal and external genitalia can be differentiated into the "male" organs and functions only in presence of androgens at male physiologic levels for the gestational age [10].

This *biological asymmetry* is key for the reading of the biological contributors of gender dysphoria. In boys, a reduced androgenic priming of the brain may lead to the emergence of the original basic female brain, with coherent feelings and behaviors. Inadequate androgen priming may contribute to inadequate development of the external genitalia to frank intersex ambiguous appearance.

The key directors of male gonad differentiation are substantially three:

1. The sex-determining region Y protein (SRY) also known as testis-determining factor (TDF) [11]. It is a protein that in humans is encoded by the SRY gene located in the Y chromosome. Its expression causes the development of primary sex cords, which later develop to seminiferous tubules. These cords form in the central part of the yet-undifferentiated gonad, turning it into a testis. The now induced Leydig cells of the testis then start secreting testosterone, while the Sertoli cells produce anti-Mullerian hormone.
2. Androgens, secreted by the Leydig cells, further "force" the basic program into the progressively male phenotype.
3. Anti-Mullerian hormone (AMH) produced by Sertoli cells in men, by the granulosa cells of the ovary in women.

In summary, the gonadal differentiation takes place in the second month of the fetal life: the female phenotype depends therefore on the *absence* of sexual SRY protein, androgens, and anti-Mullerian hormone (AMH), leading to gonads composed of an inner medulla (ovarian stroma) and an outer cortex (parenchyma).

Table 25.2 "I wanted to wear *only* trousers": motivations to behave as male in prepubertal girls

Defensive against a female condition perceived as submissive, limiting, and restrictive
Expressive of desire, interests, talents, and vocations typical of male children

The biological asymmetry in the process of gender differentiation may explain why gender identity disorders are more prevalent in the male gender, although reliable epidemiological data are still lacking [12]. In terms of probability, in chromosomic XY boys, it is more likely that a biologically complex process (the androgenization of the basic female body and brain) undergoes mistakes and inadequacies leading to a self-perception and "hardwired" inner body image more adherent to the basic female gender program than vice versa. In a chromosomic girl, androgens are necessary to partially masculinize the brain, body, and genitals. Androgens can be of fetal origin, such as in the adrenogenital syndrome, maternal, or, rarely, exogenous. In girls, this author's working hypothesis is that psychodynamic, affective, and contextual factors may contribute to a mild GD of "defensive" motivational origin, while more severe GD up to a frank "expressive" transexualism requires an androgenic priming at least of the brain, if not of the genitals.

25.3 "I Want To Be a Boy"

In children and adolescent girls, this sentence is the alerting "tip of the iceberg" of a very heterogeneous set of psychodynamic and biological conditions that require the highest empathic clinical attention [13–16].

Indeed gender identity disorders encompass a spectrum of very different motivations, perceived first at the emotional level and then progressively at the cognitive one (Table 25.2).

25.3.1 The Defensive Motivation

At one extreme, clinicians recognize girls *in flight from femininity*: when the female gender is perceived as "the losing one." This is the *defensive* motivation against a female condition recognized as submissive, limiting, restrictive, and abused in all the cultures and family contexts that still stress women's inferiority. Predisposing, precipitating, and maintaining factors can be considered.

25.3.1.1 Predisposing Factors

Four leading, and often overlapping, factors can interact:

- The *disappointment/delusion* at perceiving continuously restrictive messages *killing* the personal talents ("stereotypically" considered appropriate for boys) and thirst for life with an obsessive refrain "girls must not behave as such" even when a simple extroverted joyful personality is in play or when the girl expresses a talent for autonomy and vital curiosity of the outer world: "Why boys can do what they want and I can do nothing?"
- The *early recruitment* in all kinds *of homework* while boys can still play: caring of younger sibling, cleaning the house and dresses, ironing, cooking, and in many cultures still serving the family men. The oppression of being a girl, humiliated and crushed by all-day pervading gender role female duties, may lead to sadness and depression. It is well exemplified in the photo of boys and girl of the Italian countryside (in 1952) at the end of 5 years of primary school, where sadness and joy show a dramatic gender polarization (Fig. 25.1). Girls who do not surrender to this kind of female role identity may gradually shift to desire a male gender role if not a full male gender identity. The full shift in a frank gender dysphoria may progress *with the contribution of: (1) not yet detected endocrine factors acting on the brain, during pregnancy – such as high level of maternal stress with increase of adrenal androgens* – (2) *subclinical level of adrenal congenital hyperplasia both in fetal life and early childhood, and (3) iatrogenic drugs administered in pregnancy* [2].
- *Inadequate identification with the mother* and lack of a meaningful female significant other. A mother perceived as neglecting, refusing, and abusing may be a cofactor in a girl's progressive

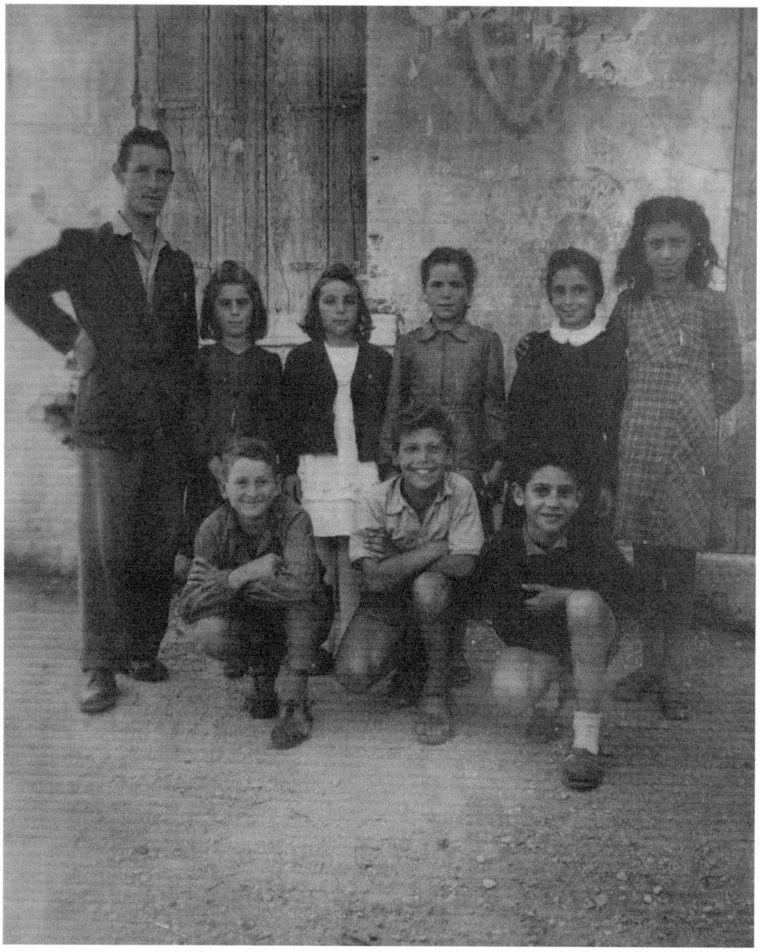

Fig. 25.1 Photo of boys and girls of the Italian countryside (in 1952) at the end of 5 years of primary school. The picture highlights the contrast between the sad (except one), concerned, and serious expression of girls and the happy, vital, energetic, and confident expression of boys. It clearly shows how gender differences in breeding styles and behavioral codes may prime the attitudes not only toward life but toward one's gender identity as well. In the 1950s, in the Italian countryside, the gender identity issue was nonexistent. Dissatisfied girls could just have thought that being a girl was a reason for sadness as it was a lesser gender. It is very likely that – were those girls living today – at least one or two would have expressed concerns and uneasiness with their gender of birth (Photo: Courtesy of Mrs Elena Bordin, Rist. Bosco del Falco, Treviso (Italy))

refusal of the female gender identity. A parallel, stronger identification with the father, or a significant other positive male in the family, including a loved brother or grandfather, may facilitate the desire/choice of becoming a boy. In girls, when the process of identifying with the same gender parent (the mother) and complementing with the parent of the opposite gender (the father) is disrupted, a psychodynamic contributor to a gender dysphoria is in play. A detached, rigid mother, emotionally distant or frankly dismissing, who does not encourage a positive identification with her, contributes to redirect the identification process on the father. "*Too much father, too little mother*" well describes the parental scenario contributing to a stronger identification with the father or his stable male surrogate. An androgenic priming during the fetal life may predispose to and potentiate such a shift.

- *Having being sexually harassed or abused, within and/or outside the family*: for this unfortunate children, being a girl equals being a prey. The escalation may move from "I want to wear only trousers" (still a symbol of male gender role in many cultures) perceived as an armor, a defense, and a key for freedom [17] to "I want myself to become a boy."

25.3.1.2 Precipitating Factors

Four other key events may precipitate a kind of "collapse of awareness" of GD.

The defensive motivations may lead to a diagnosis of gender dysphoria: this label should be kept on hold (or expressed as a very mild disorder). Colette Chiland [18], a psychiatrist with an extensive experience with children and adolescents gender disorders, warns against an early use of "diagnostic etiquettes" as such, given the high plasticity of gender identity in the lifespan and maximum at adolescence. Indeed she warns about a "mediagenic transexualism" induced by the media attitude to oversimplify the extremely demanding path of changing/reassigning sex. Such an etiquette, given to children with more simple gender dysphorias, could become a "self-fulfilling prophecy" in children with a weak sexual identity, or with nontransexual gender dysphorias, when they are desperately looking for a clearer, more solid identity, whatever it could be. Instead of following a surgical, behavioral, and social change, she suggests that psychotherapeutic support should be offered to the child/girl and to the family, to improve the psychological well-being within the gender of birth. An empathic, skilled, and experienced female psychotherapist may do a good job for and with the child. She could work for a good mediation for a well-perceived male gender *role*, when desired, preventing a likely self-damaging acting out in the search of a male *gender* identity. Clinical wisdom suggests as well to avoid a premature jump on a label of frank transexualism (sometimes "diagnosed" as such by unexperienced health-care providers). A premature diagnosis of transexualism would be harmful per se as it may be perceived as a life buoy in a sea of unhappiness by the confused child and her helpless family. Changing sex is not the magic end of a cultivated dream, but a very difficult and painful process, of uncertain outcome. In prepubertal girl, *temporal suppression of puberty* (see the paragraph XYZ) may offer a *therapeutic critical window* to appreciate with the child all the unbiased pros and cons of changing sex in the real life. Concrete alternatives of physical satisfactions should be offered in sport, music, and dance to experience joy from and with the body she has. The enormous psychoplasticity of young brains may ease the goal of a satisfactory mediation in a loving and respectful female therapeutic setting.

Precipitating factors include [2]:

- The onset of puberty, with the appearance of breast and periods, forcing the girl to move from a "totipotent, partially undifferentiated identity" to a definite female gender: a shocking discovery for many GD girls [19]
- The loss of a very significant relative, often the father or a surrogate male parent (usually the grandfather)
- The perception of an unaccepted homosexual drive
- An escape from an unacceptable masturbatory activity, as pleasure derives from the stimulation of the "hated" and somehow "untouchable" female genitalia

Maintaining factors include on one side the unaddressed persistence of predisposing and precipitating factors and on the other the lack of professional support with a careful evaluation of defensive vs expressive GD conscious and unconscious motivations.

25.3.2 The Expressive Motivation

At the opposite end of the spectrum of gender dysphoria (with all the mixed motivations in between), clinicians recognize "a boy really trapped in a girl's body." The want to *become a boy expresses lifelong desire, vocation, interests, and talents, more typical of a male child* (Table 25.3). It is not a denial of or a flight from femininity, but the real feeling of belonging to the male gender, with a male "body image" hardwired in the brain [20]. Dreams and goals of girls with severe gender dysphoria are summarized in Table 25.3. Usually these girls are recognized as

Table 25.3 Desires and goals of a girl with severe gender dysphoria up to transexualism

To live (and be accepted) in roles typical of the male sex
To have a male body
To become a member of the male gender
To acquire the social and anagraphic status coherent with the former goals

"boys" from age-mate companions since the first 2–3 years of life. Motivations and emotions to become a boy can be variably enhanced and supported by biological contributors. One of the most powerful biological contributor is brain-derived neurotrophic factors (BDNF) (with current more evidence, however, in male to female GD) [21, 22].

25.3.3 Emotions, Neurovegetative Pathways, and Motor and Hormonal Correlates

Physical appearance is shaped by the emotions that live and express themselves in the neurovegetative physical domain. Four basic emotions command systems: desire, anger, fear and panic with separation distress dominate the emotional life [23]. They pervade the body, in terms of neurovegetative correlates that activate pertinent behaviours. Emotions are the first experience we all have of our being alive, loved, disregarded/neglected or hated.

Emotions are not a cloud of feelings over the head. They have very solid somatic correlates, mediated by the *neurovegetative system* (that appears to be upregulated in persons with GD). They have an immediate *motor expression*: moving toward for desire; fight, or flight for fear; moving against for anger; and looking for a comforting presence/attachment/hug for panic with separation distress [23]. Emotions indeed reshape continuously the perception of human body image, further modulated by affective dynamics and mood (so critical to set the emotional "color" of self-perception, as we all know also in our personal life). Cognitive issues further contribute to the inner self perception of gender identity. Emotions are continuously modulated by *hormones* and by sexual hormones in the fetus and then from puberty onward. This is why endocrine medical issues are critical in this field. To reach and maintain a new, positive F to M identity requires more than a number of successful operations (but the quality of surgical outcome is certainly a powerful prerequisite though).

Body image, coherence of internal self-represented body perception with the objective body shape; the struggle to tune two divergent identities in a meaningful unified, hopefully harmonious, vision; and the identity mirroring from significant others, first, and then from the society later in life all together modulate sexual/gender identity.

25.4 Time: When to Operate

Time is a critical factor: a right treatment in the wrong moment for that individual patient is wrong. Two concepts of time are of relevance in the F to M surgery: *when to operate* in terms of:

1. Patient's age.
2. Optimal moment of the evolutive psychoemotional pathway, possibly tuned with optimal social acceptance and respect. To simplify the reasoning on time, the case of a lifelong F to M, with an early GD diagnosis, will be considered.

Why is the patient's age so critical? The age at puberty determines a basic gender-related somatic fact: *height*. In women, the progressive estrogens' uprise leading to menarche coincides with the end of the height growth, with very few centimeters obtained afterward in a minority of girls (the taller ones). Estrogens close the long bone cartilages that in childhood allow and modulate the lengthening of long bones. Within the large variety linked to race, family genes, food, and light availability, males are usually taller than females. Puberty can be delayed for a few years with GnRH analog (GnRHa): a kind of "puberty on hold," a "sleeping puberty" as it can be explained to young patients and parents, totally reversible when the final decision – to change sex or not – is finally and more serenely taken. Blocking pubertal development at Tanner stage 2 for prepubertal, gender-nonconforming children is a relatively new but reversible and highly beneficial strategy to delay puberty, giving patients and families time to come up with a transition plan – a real lifesaving choice [24].

Growth hormone (GH) administered in parallel to GnRHa seems to promote height growth more than the analogues alone in prepubertal girls with central precocious puberty [25].

GH and GnRHa combined have been used in children with idiopathic short stature, obtaining a height increase of 1.0–1.3 SD [26].

No controlled studies with GH have been carried out so far in GD girls, in this author's knowledge. The issue needs to be explored prospectically to evaluate if the advantages theoretically considered here can be substantiated in GD patients.

A delay, say from 12 up to 14–16 years of age, would offer a number of potential *advantages* to girls with *lifelong gender dysphoria* (F to M).

25.4.1 Biological Advantages

The delay of puberty/menarche may offer the possibility to reach a *height* 10–15 cm or more higher than in normal puberty: a strong basic advantage in terms of body image and self-perception. If combined with *regular physical exercise*, this delay would allow a *stronger muscle growth*, with a more solid body shape and a better bone [27].

Meanwhile, exercise will promote a *better mood*, through the physiologic motor discharge of negative emotions (so high in patients with gender dysphoria), increase endorphins, dopamine, and serotonin, thus contributing to a better psychotherapeutic emotional approach to the disturbing gender issues. Indeed physical exercise improves brain plasticity, behaving as a kind of "endogenous pharmacotherapy" [28].

It improves the perception of well-being: its usefulness should be explored in controlled studies in girls with GD.

Periodic plasmatic *check of vitamin D level* and its *supplementation* when appropriate is to be recommended also in prepubertal girls with GD. A prospective study indicate a very significant correlation between hypovitaminosis D and precocious puberty [29, 30], a problem that would be even more relevant in girls with GD, as all their psychosexual problems would be exasperated. Calcium intake should be adequate (at least 1,000 mg/day) [31].

Calcium supplementation should be considered when the daily intake is inadequate and in lactase-deficient girls to contribute to maintaining an optimal bone mass, even if prolonging the prepubertal amenorrhea with GnRHa and GH. Dehydroepiandrosterone (DHEA) supplementation could be considered to further support the height and muscle growth. Unfortunately no controlled studies are available on these issues in this author's knowledge. The overall feeling is that these important biological aspects are still underconsidered in the management of lifelong or early onset GD in girls.

25.4.2 Psychosexual Advantages

A pharmacologic (reversible) delay of puberty emphasizes the opportunity to work on the many psychosexual issues involved while the girl is still in a "neutral" physical state, not yet overdetermined by the appearance of secondary sex characteristics. GnRHa are used to give adolescents time to make balanced decisions on any further treatment steps and to obtain improved results in the physical appearance of those who opt to continue with sex reassignment. Proponents of puberty suppression emphasize the beneficial effects of GnRHa on the adolescents' mental health and quality of life and of having a physical appearance that makes it possible for the patients to live unobtrusively in their desired gender role. In the Netherlands, gender dysphoric adolescents may be eligible for puberty suppression at age 12, subsequent cross-sex hormone treatment at age 16, and gender reassignment surgery at age 18. Initially, a thorough assessment is made of the gender dysphoria and vulnerabilities in functioning or circumstances. Psychological interventions and/or gender reassignment may be offered, with increased well-being in GD adolescent patients [32]. Currently, withholding physical medical interventions in these cases seems more harmful to the well-being of both adolescents and adults when compared to cases where physical medical interventions were provided [33].

The Japanese guidelines revised in 2012 suggest delaying puberty with GnRHa until the age of 15, after which cross-sex hormones may be given [34]. However the paper does not mention the physical implications of delaying puberty mentioned above.

Ongoing studies have demonstrated that in adolescents treated with GnRHa from 12 to up to 16 years of age, behavioral and emotional problems and depressive symptoms decreased, while general functioning improved significantly during puberty suppression. The authors conclude that puberty suppression may be considered a valuable contribution in the clinical management of GD in adolescents [35].

There is a growing consensus that treatment with gonadotropin-releasing hormone analog and/or cross-sex hormones, in collaboration with transgender-competent mental health professionals, is an intervention that appears to be appropriate in carefully selected youth with gender dysphoria [36].

The attitude of working with psychosexual support and medical cross-hormonal treatment, while postponing surgery after the age of 18, is well defined in the GD M to F scientific literature [37].

Postponing puberty seems to be the most reasonable approach. From the studies that have been published so far, it seems that the benefits outweigh the risks. However, more systematic research in this area is needed to determine the safety of this approach [38].

Indeed, the appearance of breast and periods and the development of female body shape are a major physical and emotional shock for a girl with lifelong GD. Breast growth elicits negative feelings (girls with GD usually detest it) and triggers the social comments on her in fear of becoming "a real woman." All girls with GD use any type of constrictive and covering garments and attitudes (tight breast fasciae, posture with bent shoulders, oversize pullovers, and jackets) to minimize the social perception/appreciation of the breast growth. Why not prevent/delay this growth? Menarche appearance causes a major waste of emotional and physical energy that would be better utilized on the psychosexual work and real life issues. Menarche is even more disturbing if it is associated with heavy periods, dysmenorrhea, which increases significantly with increasing biological and/or psychosexual stress [39, 40], and premenstrual symptoms (depression, irritability, aggressivity outbursts, headache, food cravings, mastodynia, abdominal bloating) [41] contributing to her perception that menstruation is a curse in such a detested gender of birth. Since the appearance/diagnosis of a GD, sport, music, dancing, and all the activities that improve the girl's personal skills should be encouraged with the girl and the family: they may offer a natural positive experience of the body reality, increase self-esteem and age-mates' respect, and favor social connections while reducing the tendency to pursue the monomanic obsession of gender concerns and the tendency to isolate in a kind of virtual life. Given the complexity of factors and the importance of the therapeutic decisions, hormone treatment for pubertal suppression and subsequent gender transition needs to be always individualized within stringent protocols in multidisciplinary specialist units [42].

25.5 Relational Factors in Prepubertal Girls with GD

Relational factors play a lifelong major dynamic role in reshaping human sexual identity. They maintain such a role in GD girls as well. Family dynamics can be major contributors in the modulation of gender dysphoria, in the timing of the search for professional help, and in supporting the child in her desperate pursuit of a comforting and comfortable sexual identity [2]. It is a search of identity often dreamed of, caressed, and cultivated as an endless promise of happiness, which unfortunately is not the case in the majority of GD individuals.

25.6 Professional Issues in Prepubertal Girls with GD

In prepubertal girls with GD, the professional support should have at least five major goals:

- To establish a deep, meaningful, warm, and empathic relationship, based on nonjudgmental trust, but at the same time solid in having a concrete perspective on real life issues [43, 44]
- To understand, share, and evaluate the conscious and unconscious motivations to sex reassignment, when dreamed of and requested [45]
- To consider and discuss with the girl her expectations (real and delusional, mainly on the cosmetic and sexually functional outcome)
- Critically important, to consider a well-tailored pharmacological intervention
  - To delay puberty and optimize growth (with GnRH analogues and possibly GH)
  - To integrate vitamins and oligoelements when indicated
  - To ease the suffering with antidepressants, anxiolytics, or antipsychotics, when specifically indicated and when "giving words to the emotional pain," with psychotherapeutic support, is not enough to facilitate their search for a more satisfying identity [14]
- To support the family with a psychodynamic intervention

25.6.1 Legal Aspects

At 16 years of age, when many countries recognize the maturity to get a driving license and vote, a comprehensively diagnosed and supported GD F to M girl, maintained in a prepubertal status by a well-tailored pharmacologic treatment, is more likely to be able to make her final choice: start the appropriate hormonal treatment and then be operated of hysteroannessiectomy or to remain in her gender of birth, with a variable modulation of her final goals. When the diagnosis of severe gender dysphoria is accurate, all the examined and followed-up adolescents with a pharmacologically delayed puberty have far better psychological, emotional, and general life adjustments, a smoother transition to hormone treatment and sex reassignment [35, 46, 47].

25.7 Surgical Aspects of Delaying Puberty in Severe GD

By avoiding the breast growth, the girl will be spared the view, touch, proprioception, and perception of an organ she detests and the surgical trauma of a mastectomy later on in life. By preventing the appearance of periods, the girl will be spared the perception of a disturbing organ and function that could later on be removed with likely far less emotional (and physical?) costs. By preventing the development of a female body shape, often with cellulitis and stretch marks, a number of cosmetic interventions may be prevented later on in life. The overall result would be a significant reduction in the number of surgeries and potential side effects, an optimal timing of surgery, and a far better general cosmetic outcome and psychosexual achievement. Delaying puberty is a choice and a process more likely to be closer to a well-assisted pursuit of the best personal sexual identity than leaving the "natural" pubertal process to go on with enormous distress and more physical consequences.

Conclusion

Gender dysphoria is certainly a complex and challenging issue first for the patient, a human being that bears a tremendous need and drive to find out and determine once for all who she/he really is. It is challenging for the family, often unaware of the intense suffering of the child and as well of the intrinsically complex tasks of gender reassignment pathways. It is difficult for the health-care providers who are required to have and offer a well-balanced human touch and professional skill in an extremely complex area.

The early diagnosis of severe GD in girls and the serious consideration of the many aspects it involves should induce the health-care providers to pharmacologically *delay* the onset of puberty while appropriately supporting the growth by healthy lifestyle, with optimal diet, vitamins (especially vitamin D), and oligoelements such as calcium, magnesium, and iron when indicated, regular daily exercises and respect of the sleep hours (at least seven, better eight), and avoidance of alcohol, smoke, or drugs: all aspects frequently neglected, in this author's knowledge. Antidepressants, anxiolytics, and antipsychotics should as well be considered in selected cases.

The goal is to get quality years of personal and physical growth to optimize a more matured and "digested" choice whatever it would be: either remaining in the gender of birth with appropriate, more satisfying inner adjustments or move to a final male gender identity with real expectations and a higher probability of having them fulfilled.

References

1. Freud S (1923) Das Ich und das Es. Internationaler Psychoanalytischer Verlag, Wien
2. Baldaro Verde J, Graziottin A (1991) L'enigma dell'identità – Il transessualismo. Edizioni Gruppo Abele, Torino
3. Zucker KJ, Bradley SJ, Oliver G et al (1996) Psychosexual development of women with congenital adrenal hyperplasia. Horm Behav 30(4):300–318
4. Ercan O, Kutlug S, Uysal O et al (2013) Gender identity and gender role in DSD patients raised as females: a preliminary outcome study. Front Endocrinol (Lausanne) 4:86–93
5. Sandberg DE, Gardner M, Cohen-Kettenis PT (2012) Psychological aspects of the treatment of patients with disorders of sex development. Semin Reprod Med 30(5):443–452
6. Martin CL, DiDonato MD, Clary L et al (2012) Preschool children with gender normative and gender non-normative peer preferences: psychosocial and environmental correlates. Arch Sex Behav 41(4): 831–847
7. Mattila AK, Fagerholm R, Santtila P et al (2012) Gender identity and gender role orientation in female assigned patients with disorders of sex development. J Urol 188:1930–1937
8. Freud S (1912) Über die allgemeinste Erniedrigung des Liebeslebens (Beiträge zur Psychologie des Liebeslebens, Bd. 2). Jahrbuch für psychoanalytische und psychopathologische Forschungen 4(1):40–50
9. Money JW, Ehrhardt AA (1996) Man & woman, boy & girl: gender Identity from conception to maturity. Jason Aronson, Northvale
10. Graziottin A, Gambini D (2015) Anatomy and physiology of genital organs. Women: what is relevant for the clinical practice. In: Vodusek D, Boller F (eds) Neurology of sexual and bladder disorders, Handbook of clinical neurology. Elsevier BV, Amsterdam
11. Harley VR, Clarkson MJ, Argentaro A (2003) The molecular action and regulation of the testis-determining factors, SRY (sex-determining region on the Y chromosome) and SOX9 [SRY-related high-mobility group (HMG) box 9]. Endocr Rev 24(4):466–487
12. Shields JP, Cohen R, Glassman JR et al (2013) Estimating population size and demographic characteristics of lesbian, gay, bisexual, and transgender youth in middle school. Adolesc Health 52(2):248–250
13. Levine DA, Committee on Adolescence (2013) Office-based care for lesbian, gay, bisexual, transgender, and questioning youth. Pediatrics 132(1):e297–e313
14. Leibowitz SF, Telingator C (2012) Assessing gender identity concerns in children and adolescents: evaluation, treatments, and outcomes. Curr Psychiatry Rep 14(2):111–120
15. Wallien MS, Cohen-Kettenis PT (2008) Psychosexual outcome of gender-dysphoric children. J Am Acad Child Adolesc Psychiatry 47(12):1413–1423
16. Drummond KD, Bradley SJ, Peterson-Badali M, Zucker KJ (2008) A follow-up study of girls with gender identity disorder. Dev Psychol 44(1):34–45
17. Cardella L (1989) Volevo i pantaloni. Mondadori, Milano
18. Chiland C (1988) Enfance et transsexualisme. Psychiatr Enfant 31(2):313–373
19. Steensma TD, Kreukels BP, de Vries AL, Cohen-Kettenis PT (2013) Gender identity development in adolescence. Horm Behav 64(2):288–297
20. Ramachandran VS, McGeoch PD (2007) Occurrence of phantom genitalia after gender reassignment surgery. Med Hypotheses 69(5):1001–1003
21. Fuss J, Biedermann SV, Stalla GK, Auer MK (2013) On the quest for a biomechanism of transsexualism: is there a role for BDNF? J Psychiatr Res 47(12): 2015–2017
22. Fontanari AM, Andreazza T, Costa ÂB et al (2013) Serum concentrations of brain-derived neurotrophic factor in patients with gender identity disorder. J Psychiatr Res 47(10):1546–1548
23. Panksepp J (1998) Affective neuroscience: the foundations of human and animal emotions. Oxford University Press, New York
24. Forcier MM, Haddad E (2013) Health care for gender variant or gender non-conforming children. R I Med J 96(4):17–21
25. Pasquino AM, Pucarelli I, Segni M et al (1999) Adult height in girls with central precocious puberty treated

with gonadotropin-releasing hormone analogues and growth hormone. J Clin Endocrinol Metab 84(2): 449–452
26. Wit JM, Balen HV, Kamp GA, Oostdijk W (2004) Benefit of postponing normal puberty for improving final height. Eur J Endocrinol 151(Suppl 1):S41–S45
27. Scerpella TA, Dowthwaite JN, Gero NM et al (2010) Skeletal benefits of pre-menarcheal gymnastics are retained after activity cessation. Pediatr Exerc Sci 22(1):21–33
28. Sale A, Berardi N, Maffei L (2014) Environment and brain plasticity: towards an endogenous pharmacotherapy. Physiol Rev 94(1):189–234
29. Villamor E, Marin C, Mora-Plazas M, Baylin A (2011) Vitamin D deficiency and age at menarche: a prospective study. Am J Clin Nutr 94(4):1020–1025
30. Chew A, Harris SS (2013) Does vitamin D affect timing of menarche? Nutr Rev 71(3):189–193
31. Esterle L, Nguyen M, Walrant-Debray O (2010) Adverse interaction of low-calcium diet and low 25(OH)D levels on lumbar spine mineralization in late-pubertal girls. J Bone Miner Res 25(11):2392–2398
32. Cohen-Kettenis PT, Steensma TD, de Vries AL (2011) Treatment of adolescents with gender dysphoria in the Netherlands. Child Adolesc Psychiatr Clin N Am 20(4):689–700
33. de Vries AL, Cohen-Kettenis PT (2012) Clinical management of gender dysphoria in children and adolescents: the Dutch approach. J Homosex 59(3):301–320
34. Nakatsuka M (2013) Puberty-delaying hormone therapy in adolescents with gender identity disorder] [Article in Japanese. Seishin Shinkeigaku Zasshi 115(3):316–322
35. de Vries AL, Steensma TD, Doreleijers TA, Cohen-Kettenis PT (2011) Puberty suppression in adolescents with gender identity disorder: a prospective follow-up study. J Sex Med 8(8):2276–2283
36. Khatchadourian K, Amed S, Metzger DL (2014) Clinical management of youth with gender dysphoria in Vancouver. J Pediatr 164(4):906–911
37. Milrod C (2014) How young is too young: ethical concerns in genital surgery of the transgender MTF adolescent. J Sex Med 11(2):338–346
38. Kreukels BP, Cohen-Kettenis PT (2011) Puberty suppression in gender identity disorder: the Amsterdam experience. Nat Rev Endocrinol 7(8):466–472
39. Ju H, Jones M, Mishra G (2014) The prevalence and risk factors of dysmenorrhea. Epidemiol Rev 36(1): 104–113
40. Iacovides S, Avidon I, Bentley A, Baker FC (2014) Reduced quality of life when experiencing menstrual pain in women with primary dysmenorrhea. Acta Obstet Gynecol Scand 93(2):213–217
41. Craner J, Sigmon S, Martinson A, McGillicuddy M (2013) Perceptions of health and somatic sensations in women reporting premenstrual syndrome and premenstrual dysphoric disorder. J Nerv Ment Dis 201(9):780–785
42. Hewitt JK, Paul C, Kasiannan P et al (2012) Hormone treatment of gender identity disorder in a cohort of children and adolescents. Med J Aust 196(9): 578–581
43. Schwartz D (2012) Listening to children imagining gender: observing the inflation of an idea. J Homosex 59(3):460–479
44. Zucker KJ, Wood H, Singh D, Bradley SJ (2012) A developmental, biopsychosocial model for the treatment of children with gender identity disorder. J Homosex 59(3):369–397
45. Ehrensaft D (2012) From gender identity disorder to gender identity creativity: true gender self child therapy. J Homosex 59(3):337–356
46. Hembree WC (2011) Guidelines for pubertal suspension and gender reassignment for transgender adolescents. Child Adolesc Psychiatr Clin N Am 20(4):725–732
47. Shumer DE, Spack NP (2013) Current management of gender identity disorder in childhood and adolescence: guidelines, barriers and areas of controversy. Curr Opin Endocrinol Diabetes Obes 20(1):69–73

The Female-to-Male Medical Treatment

26

Bruno Fabris and Stella Bernardi

26.1 On the Way to Medical Treatment

Transsexualism refers to a condition where an individual identifies with a gender that differs from the assigned sex [1]. Transsexual subjects may suffer from gender dysphoria, which is the distress caused by the feeling of being born to the wrong biologic sex. Gender dysphoria is undoubtedly a complex and multifaceted problem that requires a multidisciplinary approach for its diagnosis and treatment [2]. It goes without saying that the goal of the therapy is to harmonize physical appearance with gender identity [3]. In order to do so, treatments need to be customized, as some individuals need cross-sex hormone therapy and surgery to alleviate their gender dysphoria, others need only one of these treatment options, and some need neither [2].

Having said that before starting any medical or surgical treatment, the diagnosis of gender dysphoria should be established by a mental health professional [3]. The World Professional Association for Transgender Health (WPATH), formerly known as the Harry Benjamin International Gender Dysphoria Association [4], has drafted Standards of Care for the diagnosis and treatment of transsexual individuals [2]. The WPATH Standards of Care indicate that, beside gender dysphoria, the other criteria for cross-sex hormone therapy prescription to adult transsexuals include: (i) capacity to make a fully informed decision and to consent for treatment, (ii) age of majority, and (iii) prior management of coexisting medical or mental health concerns.

Gender dysphoria is not always a straight forward diagnosis. As a result, the prescription of cross-sex hormone therapy is accompanied by a period of time during which the patient lives as a person of the desired sex. This real-life experience is essential for providing insight into the new sex status, confirming the diagnosis, considering surgery [5]. Before starting the therapy, patients should be educated on its risks and adverse effects as well as on what could be their realistic and unrealistic expectations about outcomes. Moreover, patients should be counselled about the available options for fertility. Lastly, an informed consent should be obtained.

26.2 The Female-to-Male Medical Treatment

26.2.1 Androgens

In female-to-male (FtM) transsexuals, cross-sex hormone therapy aims at reducing female secondary sex characteristics and at inducing male secondary characteristics. This therapy is based on the use of testosterone. Testosterone is

B. Fabris (✉) • S. Bernardi
Department of Medicine, Surgery and Health Sciences, U.C.O. Medicina Clinica, University of Trieste, Trieste, Italy
e-mail: b.fabris@fmc.units.it

C. Trombetta et al. (eds.), *Management of Gender Dysphoria: A Multidisciplinary Approach*,
DOI 10.1007/978-88-470-5696-1_26,

available in different forms, including intramuscular (i.m.) injections, topical gels, patches, buccal tablets, and implantable pellets (Table 26.1). The dose of testosterone required to virilize biological females is generally slightly higher than that used as replacement therapy in hypogonadic men [6]. Common dosage ranges are reported in Table 26.1. Finding the right type of hormone therapy is a challenging task, given that there are no prospective or retrospective studies indicating what is the optimal formulation and dose of hormones. As a result, any prescription of cross-sex hormone therapy is primarily based on expert opinions [3]. In the second place, hormone therapy should be continued after sex-reassignment surgery to maintain virilization and prevent osteoporosis. Nevertheless, there are no recommendations as to what age cross-sex hormone administration must be continued, and there is presently no evidenced-based recommendation on risks/benefits of continuing/stopping hormones. Often, cross-sex hormone treatment is maintained for lifetime, for FtM themselves are usually reluctant to stop administration of hormones worrying that the secondary sex characteristics of the acquired sex will diminish [7]. Moreover, testosterone treatment does not require any interruption before sex-reassignment surgery or any other surgical procedure [6]. Although there have been no reports that the long-term administration of testosterone increases mortality and morbidity [8], FtM subjects seem to have a higher risk of cardiovascular diseases (CVD) [9]. Therefore, before starting any FtM cross-sex hormone therapy, it is recommended to ensure that patients do not have comorbid conditions that could be exacerbated by hormonal treatments (Table 26.2) [3, 10]. In addition, before starting such therapy, FtM people should be strongly advised to give up smoking and to lose weight as a measure to reduce their cardiovascular risk [3, 9, 11].

26.2.2 Intramuscular Injections

The i.m. administration of testosterone esters, such as testosterone enanthate and testosterone

Table 26.1 Hormones used in female to male treatment and potential disadvantages

Testosterone	Dosage range	Disadvantages
Oral		
Testosterone undecanoate	160–240 mg/day	Variable clinical response
Transbuccal		
Buccal tablets	30 mg twice daily	Gum-related adverse effect
Transdermal		
Testosterone gel 1 %	2.5–10 g/day	Potential transfer to a female partner or child
Testosterone patch	2.5–7.5 mg/day	Skin irritation, musky odor
Parenteral		
Testosterone esters (enanthate or cypionate)	100–200 mg i.m. every 2 weeks or 50–100 mg i.m. every wk	Requires i.m. injections, peaks and valleys in serum T levels
Mixture of testosterone esters	1 ampoule i.m. every two wks	
Testosterone undecanoate	1,000 mg every 12 weeks	Requires i.m. injections of a large volume
Subcutaneous		
Testosterone pellets	3–6 pellets; dose and regimen vary with formulation	Requires surgical incision for insertion; pellets may extrude spontaneously

Table 26.2 Contraindications to cross-sex hormone therapy in female-to-male transsexual patients

Absolute (very high risk of serious adverse outcomes)
Pregnancy
Unstable coronary artery disease
Active substance abuse
Breast or uterine cancer
Erythrocytosis (hematocrit >50 %)
Severe liver dysfunction
Relative (moderate to high risk of adverse outcomes)
Coronary artery disease
Hyperlipidemia
Severe obstructive sleep apnea
Refractory migraine headaches
Uncontrolled hypertension
Heavy tobacco use
Obesity
Advanced age

cypionate, is the preferred and most widely used treatment modality for providing testosterone replacement in FtM subjects [3, 12]. Injectable testosterone esters do not undergo first-pass metabolism and thus do not cause hepatotoxicity. Moreover, esterization allows for a sustained release of testosterone from the site of injection to the blood. Consistent with it, i.m. injectable testosterone esters have been recommended due to their lipophilicity, resulting in the storage and gradual release from the oil-based vehicle in which they are administered and limiting the need for frequent injections [13]. Testosterone enanthate and testosterone cypionate are almost interchangeable, apart from the fact that they may be mixed with different oils, so some individuals may tolerate one better than the other. Other i.m. injectable formulations of testosterone esters include a mixture of short- and long-acting testosterone esters and testosterone undecanoate. The testosterone mixture, also known as *Sustanon*, is an oil-based blend of testosterone propionate, testosterone phenylpropionate, testosterone isocaproate, and testosterone decanoate [14]. On the other hand, testosterone undecanoate is a newly marketed formulation of i.m. injectable testosterone in oil, which allows for only four yearly injections [15]. Nevertheless, each dose of testosterone undecanoate consists of 4 ml which may require multiple simultaneous injections, without considering that it is much more expensive and currently unavailable in the United States. Limitations of i.m. injectable testosterone esters include high peak levels of androgens in the first few days after an injection (except for testosterone undecanoate), which can be ameliorated by reducing the dosing interval while maintaining the same total dose [12]. Moreover, due to the variability in absorption between users, some subjects may experience fluctuations in energy [16]. In the third place, injection site reactions are frequent side effects [16]. In addition to this, due to the viscous nature of the vehicle in which testosterone is delivered and the muscularity of the injection site, a long, large-gauge needle is required to administer the drug, which can be a barrier to someone [12].

26.2.3 Topical and Transdermal Preparations

Transdermal testosterone is available in either patches or gels, and both reproduce normal testosterone levels better than injectable preparations. Both are absorbed quickly when applied and produce a temporary drug depot in the skin, whereby testosterone diffuses into the circulation, peaking at 4 h and decreasing slowly over the rest of the day. Clinical studies have demonstrated that gels allow for longer-lasting serum testosterone levels as compared to transdermal patches [17]. Notwithstanding these clear advantages, transdermal testosterone preparations are often poorly effective to induce rapid and complete amenorrhea and may translate to a lessened change in physical appearance and virilization [12]. In addition to this, patches cause skin irritation in 2 patients out of 3 [16], while gels put patients at risk of testosterone transmission with skin contact. This is particularly worrisome if the transfer occurs in children, where it may cause penile or clitoral enlargement, premature development, and aggressive behavior [16, 18]. Lastly, all transdermal formulations of testosterone can be quite costly for patients who cannot apply prescription insurance benefits for this elective therapy.

26.2.4 Oral Preparations

Oral testosterone is occasionally used in Europe while it is not available in the United States due to its risk of hepatotoxicity [16, 19]. The safest oral formulation is testosterone undecanoate, but it is still less effective than intramuscular or transdermal testosterone and much more expensive than testosterone enanthate and testosterone cypionate. Moreover, testosterone undecanoate bioavailability seem to be affected by food and dietary fat content.

26.2.5 Transbuccal System

Testosterone may also be taken by buccal tablets, which release it as excipients are slowly hydrated in the mouth [16]. These buccal systems release testosterone in a pulsatile manner, which is similar to endogenous testosterone secretion. Peak testosterone levels are reached rapidly, and the steady state is achieved by the second dose. The advantages of this route of administration include avoidance of first-pass hepatic metabolism and patient compliance, since it is well tolerated. On the other hand, though, transient mouth and gum reactions, as well as a bitter taste or other forms of dysgeusia, are the chief complaints. At the moment, its use in FtM transsexuals is limited.

26.2.6 Subcutaneous Testosterone Implants

Implants of crystalline testosterone can be inserted into the subcutaneous tissue to maintain adequate serum testosterone levels for up to 6 months [16]. The chief adverse events with testosterone pellets include pellet extrusion, minor bleeding, and infection, which are not frequent and may also result in pellet extrusion.

26.2.7 Progestins

Progestins may be used with testosterone if menses do not cease [20]. At the beginning of FtM cross-sex hormone therapy, medroxyprogesterone can be given by i.m. injection at a dose of 150 mg every 3 months in addition to testosterone, and it is usually discontinued once the patient has had 3–6 months of testosterone therapy [12]. Progestins may be also indicated in order to avoid endometrial hyperplasia in those rare patients who take testosterone for more than 3 years and are not willing to undergo hysterectomy [6].

26.3 Effects of Female-to-Male Medical Treatment

26.3.1 Physical Changes

The degree of changes that are induced by hormone therapy is highly variable for fully mature adult genetic females, and outcome predictive criteria are scarce. Physical changes depend on medication, as well as on their dose and route of administration, and on individual sensitivity [6]. Androgen effects are in fact primarily mediated by their specific receptors, whose polymorphism can be responsible for different responses to steroid hormones in different subjects [21]. Treatment duration is also an important variable to consider when evaluating physical changes, given that at least 2 years of therapy are necessary to get the full effect of the treatment [22]. The first physical changes appear after 3–6 months of testosterone therapy, and they include menses cessation, facial and body hair increase, oiliness of skin, libido increase, clitoral enlargement, and muscle and fat mass redistribution [3]. Then over a long period of time, ovaries undergo polycystic transformation [23, 24], and endometrium may become either hyperplastic or atrophic [24]. Endocrinologists should closely monitor the physical signs of masculinization for judging the efficacy of the treatment. It has also to be noted that the physical changes induced by sex hormone transition are usually accompanied by an improvement in mental well-being and a better quality of life [25]. Unrealistic expectations include skeletal changes and male distribution of body fat changes.

26.3.2 Menses Cessation

Menses arrest is a very important goal of the FtM cross-sex hormone therapy. In the vast majority of recipients, testosterone therapy interrupts the menses after 3–6 months from the start, especially if it is administered i.m. [26]. If this is not achieved, as in the cases of transdermal testosterone administration, progesterone therapy can be added to the therapy in order to stop menstrual flow [12, 20].

26.3.3 Hair Growth and Skin Sebum Production

It is well known that sex steroids regulate the skin pilosebaceous unit, as both the sebaceous gland epithelial cells and the hair follicle mesenchymal cells contain androgen receptors [27]. Here, androgens promote hair growth and skin oiliness, and, in case of an excess of androgenic activity, hirsutism and acne usually develop [28, 29]. So androgen treatment in FtM transsexuals results in the induction of facial hair growth and the increase in sebum production, which can be usually seen after 4 months and continue to develop beyond 1 year [30]. Acne occurs in approximately 40 % of the subjects, and it is usually most pronounced on the back and shoulders rather than in the face [30]. The degree of hirsutism can be generally predicted from the degree and pattern of hair distribution in male members of the same family. Likewise, androgenic alopecia, which affects approximately 50 % of the patients [31], is influenced by genetic background.

26.3.4 Clitoral Enlargement

Clitoral enlargement occurs in all the recipients but its degree varies. The younger the patient is at the start of androgen administration, the more it is encountered [32]. In approximately 5–8 % of people, the clitoral length may reach up to 6 cm and become sufficient for vaginal intercourse [20].

26.3.5 Libido Increase

Most FtM subjects report an increase in the frequency of masturbation, sexual desire, arousal, and sexual fantasies after testosterone administration [33]. Solitary or dyadic sexual desires have been found to correlate positively with testosterone levels [34], while they are inversely associated with LH levels [33]. Unfortunately, there has been little focus so far on the sexual health of transsexuals after sex-reassignment surgery. In one of the very few papers on this issue, Costantino and colleagues reported that sexual parameters such as kissing, arousal, and sexual fantasies returned to baseline levels after surgery. This can be probably ascribed to the fact that in Italy phalloplasty or metoidoplasty are not routinely performed in every center, which may have generated dissatisfaction, failed expectations, and ultimately contributed to the decrease of some aspects of sexual function after surgery [34].

26.3.6 Breast

Androgen effects on breast differ widely from one subject to the other. In most FtM transsexuals, long-term testosterone administration markedly reduces the glandular tissue while promoting connective tissue formation [35]. These changes are similar to the mammary involution that is observed at the end stage of the menopause [35]. The effects on breast are likely to reflect the simultaneous action of androgens and estrogens, which are generated by androgen peripheral aromatization. Sometimes, FtM people utilize the breast-binding technique to flatten their breast and create a male chest contour before sex-reassignment surgery.

26.3.7 Ovaries

Exogenous androgens in FtM transsexuals induce the morphological feature characteristic of the polycystic ovary disease, often encountered in polycystic ovarian syndrome (PCOS) [36]. In these cases the ovaries are enlarged probably in relation to the high number of antral follicles as well as to the hyperplasia of both theca interna and connective tissue.

26.3.8 Endometrium

It is not entirely clear what are the effects that androgen have on the uterus. Having said that androgen receptors are detected in the epithelial cells and connective tissue of the endometrium, during all the phases of the menstrual cycle [37]. Here, the effect of long-term androgen administration is quite variable ranging from endometrial hyperplasia to atrophy [24]. The pathophysiological mechanisms leading to endometrial hyperplasia during androgen therapy remain debated. Nevertheless, one possible explanation is that the chronic lack of progesterone accompanying hyperandrogenemia and anovulation might stimulate endometrial proliferation and hyperplasia [37].

26.3.9 Body Composition

It is well known that men, on average, have less fat mass and that its distribution is more central or intra-abdominal than that of women [38]. On the other hand, premenopausal women have more fat, whose distribution is more gluteal/femoral. In addition, women generally have more subcutaneous fat [38, 39], while men carry more visceral fat [40]. Consistent with this, it has been demonstrated that FtM cross-sex hormone therapy causes a reduction in subcutaneous fat and an increase in thigh muscle area as well as visceral fat [41]. Moreover, testosterone treatment would also lead to an increase in BMI and in lean mass. The increase in lean body mass is on average 4 kg, and the increase in body weight is usually above 7 kg [20].

26.3.10 Voice

Voice deepening occurs after 6–10 weeks of androgen administration and is irreversible [32].

26.4 Side Effects of Female-to-Male Medical Treatment

26.4.1 Cardiovascular Events

There are no adequate data yet to assess the long-term cardiovascular risks of testosterone therapy in the general population [42]. The same could obviously be said for the risks of such a therapy in FtM transsexuals [43]. On one hand, there is some evidence that patients with testosterone deficiency have a higher risk of CVD [44], as treatment with testosterone has been shown to improve lipid profiles [45, 46] and insulin resistance [45, 46] and to increase the time to ST depression during stress testing [47]. On the other hand, though, other studies have demonstrated that there is a clear association between testosterone therapy and risk of serious, adverse cardiovascular-related events, including nonfatal myocardial infarction, which could be ascribed to the induction of an atherogenic lipid profile [3, 43], to the increase in plasma total homocystein [48] and C-reactive protein levels [7]. This discordance can only be partly explained by the notion that the effects of endogenous and exogenous testosterone may differ [49]. Going back to FtM transsexuals, in a recent meta-analysis of 16 studies that included 651 FtM subjects, testosterone treatment was associated with a significant decrease in high-density lipoprotein levels and a modest increase in systolic blood pressure. However, testosterone did not have any significant effect on cardiovascular outcomes such as death, stroke, myocardial infarction, or venous thromboembolism [43]. This is consistent with long-term studies from the Netherlands that did not find any increase in the risk for cardiovascular mortality in patients taking cross-sex hormone therapy [8]. In conclusion, in spite of current limitations, the most important issue raised by all these apparently conflicting findings is that testosterone effects may partly depend on the population that is being treated with it. Therefore, since cardiovascular risk increases with aging, in both FtM transsexuals and hypogonadic males treated with testosterone, glucose, lipid profile, and blood pressure should be monitored regularly and managed according to established guidelines [2, 3].

26.4.2 Cancer

Malignancies related to cross-sex hormone treatment of transsexuals have so far, fortunately, been a rare occurrence. Nevertheless, they are a concern in FtM subjects treated with long-term testosterone therapy [50], given that androgens are converted to estrogens [51], which could then increase the risk of breast or ovarian cancer. FtM transsexuals receiving androgen treatment have in fact high circulating 17β-estradiol levels, coming from the peripheral aromatization of testosterone [50]. A direct effect of testosterone on the tissues expressing the androgen receptors cannot be excluded [51]. The vast majority of FtM subjects undergo mastectomy as part of their sex-reassignment therapy. In those who have not undergone mastectomy, clinicians should be aware of the potential development of breast carcinoma. In addition, Endocrine Society guidelines suggest that total hysterectomy and oophorectomy should also be considered as a part of the sex-reassignment surgery in FtM transsexuals [3].

26.4.2.1 Breast Cancer

Although some authors have reported an association between circulating testosterone levels and the risk of developing breast cancer in postmenopausal women [52], according to the North American Menopause Society, there are no randomized controlled trials of sufficient size and duration to conclusively assess if testosterone has an effect on breast cancer risk in postmenopausal women [53]. Accordingly, almost all long-term follow-up studies of women with hyperandrogenism from PCOS, which is characterized by the simultaneous presence of high circulating androgen and estradiol levels, do not provide evidence of a higher breast cancer risk in these women [54, 55]. In FtM transsexuals, three cases of breast cancer have been reported so far. These were all cases where supraphysiologic doses of testosterone were used [51, 56].

26.4.2.2 Ovarian Cancer

Thus far, three cases of ovarian carcinoma have been reported in testosterone-treated FtM transsexuals who had not undergone sex-reassignment surgery [57, 58]. Having too much high androgen levels, as it may have happened in these subjects, is one of the putative mechanisms underlying the development of ovarian cancer, given that ovarian epithelial cells express androgen receptors [59] and experimental data show that testosterone may increase ovarian tumor growth [60]. In addition to this, exogenous testosterone would in any case promote the development of polycystic ovaries [23], which are more likely to develop malignancies. Therefore, although there are no epidemiological studies showing a higher incidence of ovarian cancer in FtM transsexual as compared to the general population, it seems reasonable to suggest that androgen-treated FtM people should undergo laparoscopic oophorectomy after a successful transition to the male role [20].

26.4.2.3 Endometrial Cancer

Prolonged testosterone exposure can lead to an increase in endogenous estrogen levels and the risk of endometrial hyperplasia [24], but whether this condition could represent a premalignant lesion is unknown [61]. Although there has been no report of cases of endometrial cancer in FtM transsexuals, bleeding should not be neglected [3].

26.4.2.4 Tumors of Other Organs

Rare cases of hormone-dependent tumors in organs such as the lung, colon, bladder and brain (in particular meningiomas) have also been reported in transsexuals, but not in numbers that could suggest a causative link between their development and cross-sex hormone therapy [46].

26.4.3 Osteoporosis

Sex steroids are important regulators of bone metabolism and bone mineral density. Since postmenopausal women and hypogonadal men have an increased risk of fractures, long-term bone health is a matter of concern in the treatment of transsexual persons especially after gonadectomy. In FtM transsexuals, it is well documented that androgens protect the bone from estrogen deprivation [62]. This positive effect on bone turnover can be ascribed to both a direct effect of testosterone on bone mass and an indirect effect that is due to the aromatization of testosterone to estradiol [7]. A bone histomorphometric study carried out in 15 FtM transsexuals, who had undergone hysterectomy with bilateral ovariectomy and had been treated with 250 mg testosterone i.m. every fortnight for an average of 39 months, showed intact trabecular bone structure, increased cortical thickness, and low bone turnover indices as compared to 11 healthy men and 8 postmenopausal women [62]. Consistent with it, it has been found an inverse relationship between serum LH concentrations and bone mineral density, so that serum LH could be used as an indicator of the adequacy of sex steroid administration [63]. At the moment, it is not known whether and when cross-sex hormone therapy can be discontinued, without inducing an unacceptable risk of osteoporosis and bone fractures. Unfortunately, fracture data in transsexual men and women are not available. Otherwise, vitamin D and calcium supplementation should be initiated according to standard guidelines for the general population.

26.4.4 Mortality

In FtM transsexuals, the use of testosterone at doses similar to those used for hypogonadal men seems to be safe, and deaths are not significantly different from those expected [8]. In contrast to male-to-female, in FtM, transsexuals, the external causes of death (suicide, illicit drugs, and AIDS) are extremely rare [8].

26.5 Monitoring and Safety of Female-to Male Medical Therapy

During cross-sex hormone therapy, a continuous medical supervision by a trained endocrinologist is strongly recommended, as androgens may produce serious adverse effects. In the vast majority of cases, risks come from and are worsened by the intentional or unintentional use of either too elevated or inadequate doses of sex hormones to maintain normal physiology [3]. Transsexual subjects tend to self-administer higher hormonal doses in order to achieve more rapid physical changes and therefore to obtain better results. Therefore, once the treatment has been started, the most important rule is avoiding supraphysiological doses of androgens, which may sensibly increase the risk of cardiovascular diseases, including thromboembolic events as well as of other adverse effects. In the second place, total testosterone and estradiol levels should be monitored regularly in order to maintain total testosterone plasma concentrations within the normal range for men (320–1,000 ng/dl) [3], and this goal should be shared with patients [64].

Regular clinical and laboratory monitoring of androgen administration should be scheduled at baseline and every 3 months during the first year and then once or twice yearly. Patient history, drug history, current complaints, and patient ideas, concerns, and expectations should always be evaluated. The physical examination should focus on secondary sex characteristics as well as on the monitoring of body weight and blood pressure. Laboratory tests that include complete blood count, renal and liver function, and lipid and glucose metabolism should be performed. Other exams such as ECG or DEXA should be considered in selected patients. ECG should be performed in smokers or hypertensive patients during the first year of follow-up, whereas DEXA should be taken into account at baseline if there are other risk factors for fracture or in patients older than 60 years, especially if they have stopped cross-sex hormone therapy and have had gonadectomy [3]. An ultrasound scan of the abdomen should be periodically performed in patients who have not undergone ovarian removal. If breast and cervical tissue are present, FtM people should be followed according to screening guidelines as recommended by the American Cancer Society and by the American College of Obstetricians and Gynecologists, respectively [3]. A standard monitoring plan for FtM transsexuals on testosterone therapy is found in Table 26.3.

Lifestyle changes, such as eating healthy food, giving up smoking, and taking regular exercise, should be strongly encouraged in FtM transsexual persons to avoid cardiovascular complications.

Table 26.3 Clinical assessment and follow-up of MtF transsexuals during cross-hormone therapy

Assessments	Timing of clinical and laboratory assessment
Routine health questions focused on risk factors and medications Karyotype in case of a surgical reassignment or according to clinical indication HBsAg, HBsAb, HCV, HIV, TPHA	Baseline
Complete physical examination including: Blood pressure, body weight Extent of masculinization Palpation of breast for masses Examinations of genitalia	Baseline, every 3 months after starting treatment for the first year Every 6–12 months after the first year
Laboratory investigation including: Creatinine, blood urea Liver function tests Fasting glucose and lipid profile CBC, hemoglobin LH, total testosterone, estradiol	Baseline, every 3 months after starting treatment for the first year Every 6–12 months after the first year
ECG	Within the first year of hormone treatment
Bone mineral density	At baseline if risk factors are present and at age 60 in low-risk people
Lower abdomen ultrasound	After 2–3 years of testosterone therapy waiting hystero-adnexectomy
Cervical PAP test	In case of prolonged androgen treatment
Mammography	Annually after age 50

CBC complete blood count, *HBsAg* hepatitis B surface antigen, *HBsAb* hepatitis B surface antibody, *HCV* hepatitis C virus, *HIV* human immunodeficiency virus, *TPHA* treponema pallidum hemagglutination, *LH* luteinizing hormone, *ECG* electrocardiogram, *PAP* papanicolaou

Conclusion

Transsexualism is a rare condition of unknown cause that is accompained by gender dysphoria, whose diagnosis should be first assessed by an experienced mental health professional [3].

Although hormonal treatment with androgens is an indispensable tool to alleviate gender dysphoria in FtM people, by inducing and mantaining male characteristics [3], cross-sex hormone therapy can be associated with many potentially serious long-term complications [33].

Comparative and long-term multicenter follow-up studies are necessary to test the efficacy of different regimens and dosing of cross-sex hormones and its potential risks and benefits.

References

1. Knudson G, De Cuypere G, Bockting W (2010) Process toward consensus on recommendations for revision of the DSM diagnoses of gender identity disorders by the World Professional Association for Transgender Health. Int J Transgenderism 12(2):54–59
2. Coleman E, Bockting W, Botzer M, Cohen-Kettenis P, DeCuypere G et al (2011) Standards of care for the health of transsexual, transgender and gender-nonconforming people, Version 7. Int J Transgenderism 13:165–232
3. Hembree WC, Cohen-Kettenis P, de Delemarre-van Waal HA, Gooren LJ, Meyer WJ 3rd et al (2009) Endocrine treatment of transsexual persons: an Endocrine Society clinical practice guideline. J Clin Endocrinol Metab 94(9):3132–3154
4. Meyer WJ III, Bockting W, Cohen-Kettenis P et al (2001) The Harry Benjamin International Gender Dysphoria Association's standards of care for gender identity disorders, 6th version. Int J Transgenderism 5:1–22. Available from http://www.wpath.org/Documents2/socv6.pdf
5. Gooren LJ (2011) Care of transsexual persons. N Engl J Med 364(13):1251–1257
6. Godano A, Maggi M, Jannini E, Meriggiola MC, Ghigo E, Todarello O, Lenzi A, Manieri C (2009) SIAMS-ONIG consensus on hormonal treatment in gender identity disorders. J Endocrinol Invest 32(10):857–864
7. Gooren LJ, Giltay EJ, Bunck MC (2008) Long-term treatment of transsexuals with cross-sex hormones: extensive personal experience. J Clin Endocrinol Metab 93(1):19–25
8. van Kesteren PJ, Asscheman H, Megens JA, Gooren LJ (1997) Mortality and morbidity in transsexual subjects treated with cross-sex hormones. Clin Endocrinol (Oxf) 47(3):337–342
9. Wierckx K, Mueller S, Weyers S, Van Caenegem E, Roef G et al (2012) Long-term evaluation of cross-sex hormone treatment in transsexual persons. J Sex Med 9:2641–2651

10. Tangpricha V, Ducharme SH, Barber TW, Chipkin SR (2003) Endocrinologic treatment of gender identity disorders. Endocr Pract 9(1):12–21
11. Wylie KR, Fung R Jr, Boshier C, Rotchell M (2009) Recommendations of endocrine treatment for patients with gender dysphoria. Sex Relationsh Ther 24(2):175–187
12. Knezevich EL, Viereck LK, Drincic AT (2012) Medical management of adult transsexual persons. Pharmacotherapy 32(1):54–66
13. Beg S, Al-Khoury L, Cunningham GR (2008) Testosterone replacement in men. Curr Opin Endocrinol Diabetes Obes 15(4):364–370
14. Kalra S, Agrawal N, Kumar S, Sharma A (2010) Testosterone replacement in male hypogonadism. Clin Pharmacol 2:149–153
15. Harle L, Basaria S, Dobs AS (2005) Nebido: a long-acting injectable testosterone for the treatment of male hypogonadism. Expert Opin Pharmacother 6:1751–1759
16. Seftel A (2007) Testosterone replacement therapy for male hypogonadism: Part III. Pharmacologic and clinical profiles, monitoring, safety issues, and potential future agents. Int J Impot Res 19:2–24
17. Swerdloff RS, Wang C, Cunningham G, Dobs A, Iranmanesh A, Matsumoto AM et al (2000) Long-term pharmacokinetics of transdermal testosterone gel in hypogonadal men. J Clin Endocrinol Metab 85:4500–4510
18. Bhowmick SK, Ricke T, Retting KR (2007) Sexual precocity in a 16-month-old boy induced by indirect topical exposure to testosterone. Clin Pediatr 46:540–543
19. Bird DR, Vowles KD (1977) Liver damage from long-term methyl-testosterone. Lancet 2:400–401
20. Gooren L (2005) Hormone treatment of the adult transsexual patient. Horm Res 64(Suppl 2):31–36
21. Zitzmann M, Nieschlag E (2007) Androgen receptor gene CAG repeat length and body mass index modulate the safety and long-term intramuscular testosterone undecanoate therapy in hypogonadal men. J Clin Endocrinol Metab 92:3844–3853
22. Dahl M, Feldman JL, Goldberg JM, Jaberi A (2006) Physical aspects of transgender endocrine therapy. Int J Transgenderism 9:111–134
23. Amirikia H, Savoy-Moore RT, Sundareson AS, Moghissi KF (1986) The effects of long-term androgen treatment on the ovary. Fertil Steril 45:202–208
24. Futterweit W, Deligdish L (1986) Histopathological effects of exogenously administered testosterone in 19 female to male transsexuals. J Clin Endocrinol Metab 62:16–21
25. Gorin-Lazard A, Baumstarck K, Boyer L, Maquigneau A, Gebleux S et al (2012) Is hormonal therapy associated with better quality of life in transsexuals? A cross-sectional study. J Sex Med 9(2):531–541
26. Moore E, Wisniewski A, Dobs A (2003) Endocrine treatment of transsexual people: a review of treatment regimens, outcomes, and adverse effects. J Clin Endocrinol Metab 88(8):3467–3473
27. Choudhry R, Hodgins MB, Van der Kwast TH, Brinkmann AO, Boersma WJ (1992) Localisation of androgen receptor in human skin by immunohistochemistry: implications for the hormonal regulation of hair growth, sebaceous glands and sweat glands. J Endocrinol 133(3):467–475
28. Marynick SP, Chakmakjian ZH, McCaffree DL, Herndon JH Jr (1983) Androgen excess in cystic acne. N Engl J Med 308(17):981–986
29. Lai JJ, Chang P, Lai KP, Chen L, Chang C (2012) The role of androgen and androgen receptor in skin-related disorders. Arch Dermatol Res 304(7):499–510
30. Giltay EJ, Gooren LJ (2000) Effects of sex steroid deprivation/administration on hair growth and skin sebum production in transsexual males and females. J Clin Endocrinol Metab 85(8):2913–2921
31. Giltay EJ, Toorians AW, Sarabdjitsingh AR, De Vries NA, Gooren LJ (2004) Established risk factors for coronary heart disease are unrelated to androgen-induced baldness in female-to-male transsexuals. J Endocrinol 180(1):107–112
32. Gooren LJ, Giltay EJ (2008) Review of studies of androgen treatment of female-to-male transsexuals: effects and risks of administration of androgens to females. J Sex Med 5(4):765–776
33. Wierckx K, Elaut E, Van Caenegem E, Van De Peer F, Dedecker D et al (2011) Sexual desire in female-to-male transsexual persons: exploration of the role of testosterone administration. Eur J Endocrinol 165(2): 331–337
34. Costantino A, Cerpolini S, Alvisi S (2013) A prospective study on sexual function and mood in female-to-male transsexuals during testosterone administration and after sex reassignment surgery. J Sex Marital Ther 39(4):321–335
35. Slagter MH, Gooren LJ, Scorilas A, Petraki CD, Diamandis EP (2006) Effects of long-term androgen administration on breast tissue of female-to-male transsexuals. J Histochem Cytochem 54(8):905–910
36. Baba T, Endo T, Honnma H, Kitajima Y, Hayashi T et al (2007) Association between polycystic ovary syndrome and female-to-female transsexuality. Hum Reprod 22(4):1011–1016
37. Grynberg M, Fanchin R, Dubost G, Colau JC, Bremont-Weil C et al (2010) Histology of genital tract and breast tissue after long-term testosterone administration in a female-to-male transsexual population. Reprod Biomed Online 20(4):553–558
38. Shi H, Seeley RJ, Clegg DJ (2009) Sexual differences in the control of energy homeostasis. Front Neuroendocrinol 30(3):396–404
39. Kotani K, Tokunaga K, Fujioka S, Kobatake T, Keno Y et al (1994) Sexual dimorphism of age-related changes in whole-body fat distribution in the obese. Int J Obes Relat Metab Disord 18(4):207–212

40. Wajchenberg BL (2000) Subcutaneous and visceral adipose tissue: their relation to the metabolic syndrome. Endocr Rev 21(6):697–738
41. Elbers JM, Asscheman H, Seidell JC, Gooren LJ (1999) Effects of sex steroid hormones on regional fat depots as assessed by magnetic resonance imaging in transsexuals. Am J Pathol 276(2 Pt 1):E317–E325
42. Vigen R, O'Donnel CI, Baron A, Grunwald GK, Maddox TM et al (2013) Association of testosterone therapy with mortality, myocardial infarction, and stroke in men with low testosterone levels. JAMA 310(17):1829–1836
43. Elamin MB, Garcia MZ, Murad MH, Erwin PJ, Montori VM (2010) Effect of sex steroid use on cardiovascular risk in transsexual individuals: a systematic review and meta-analyses. Clin Endocrinol (Oxf) 72(1):1–10
44. Tirabassi G, Gioia A, Giovannini L, Boscaro M, Corona G et al (2013) Testosterone and cardiovascular risk. Intern Emerg Med 8(Suppl 1):S65–S69
45. Jones TH, Arver S, Behre HM, Buvat J, Meuleman E et al; TIMES2 Investigators (2011) Testosterone replacement in hypogonadal men with type 2 diabetes and/or metabolic syndrome (the TIMES study). Diabetes Care 34(4):828–837
46. Jones TH, Saad F (2009) The effects of testosterone on risk factors for, and the mediators of, the atherosclerotic process. Atherosclerosis 207(2):318–327
47. Mathur A, Malkin C, Saeed B, Muthusamy R, Jones TH, Channer K (2009) Long-term benefits of testosterone replacement therapy on angina threshold and atheroma in men. Eur J Endocrinol 161(3):443–449
48. Giltay EJ, Hoogeveen EK, Elbers JM, Gooren LJ, Asscheman H, Stehouwer CD (1998) Effects of sex steroids on plasma total homocysteine levels: a study in transsexual males and females. J Clin Endocrinol Metab 83(2):550–553
49. Xu L, Freeman G, Cowling BJ, Schooling CM (2013) Testosterone therapy and cardiovascular events among men: a systematic review and meta-analysis of placebo-controlled randomized trials. BMC Med 11:108
50. Mueller A, Gooren L (2008) Hormone-related tumors in transsexuals receiving treatment with cross-sex hormones. Eur J Endocrinol 159(3):197–202
51. Shao T, Grossbard ML, Klein P (2011) Breast cancer in female-to male transsexuals: two cases with a review of physiology and management. Clin Breast Cancer 11(6):417–419
52. Key T, Appleby P, Barnes I, Reeves G, Endogenous hormones and breast cancer collaborative group (2002) Endogenous sex hormones and breast cancer in postmenopausal women: reanalysis of nine prospective studies. J Natl Cancer Inst 94(8):606–616
53. North American Menopause Society (2005) The role of testosterone therapy in postmenopausal women: position statement of The North American Menopause Society. Menopause 12(5):496–511
54. Anderson KE, Sellers TA, Chen PL, Rich SS, Hong CP, Folsom AR (1997) Association of Stein-Leventhal syndrome with the incidence of postmenopausal breast carcinoma in a large prospective study of women in Iowa. Cancer 79(3):494–499
55. Balen A (2001) Polycystic ovary syndrome and cancer. Hum Reprod Update 7(6):522–525
56. Burcobe RJ, Makris A, Pittam M, Finer N (2003) Breast cancer after bilateral subcutaneous mastectomy in a female-to-male transsexuals. Breast 12(4):290–293
57. Hage JJ, Dekker ML, Karim RB, Verheijen RHM, Bloemena E (2000) Ovarian cancer in female-to-male transsexuals: report of two cases. Gynecol Oncol 76(3):413–415
58. Dizon DS, Tejada-Berges T, Koelliker S, Steinhoff M, Granai OC (2006) Ovarian cancer associated with testosterone supplementation in a female-to-male transsexual patient. Gynecol Obstet Invest 62(4):226–228
59. Chadha S, Pache TD, Huikeshoven JM, Brinkmann AO, van der Kwast TH (1994) Androgen receptor expression in human ovarian and uterine tissue of long-term androgen-treated transsexual women. Hum Pathol 25(12):1198–1204
60. Hillier SG, Ross GT (1979) Effects of exogenous testosterone on ovarian weight, follicular morphology and intraovarian progesterone concentration in estrogen-primed hypophysectomized immature female rats. Biol Reprod 20(2):261–268
61. Futterweit W (1998) Endocrine therapy of transsexualism and potential complications of long-term treatment. Arch Sex Behav 27(2):209–2266
62. Lips P, van Kesteren PJ, Asscheman H, Gooren LJ (1996) The effect of androgen treatment on bone metabolism in female-to-male transsexuals. J Bone Miner Res 11(11):1769–1773
63. van Kesteren P, Lips P, Gooren LJ, Asscheman H, Megens J (1998) Long-term follow-up of bone mineral density and bone metabolism in transsexuals treated with cross-sex hormones. Clin Endocrinol (Oxf) 48(3):347–354
64. Meriggiola MC, Jannini EA, Lenzi A, Maggi M, Manieri C (2010) Endocrine treatment of transsexual persons: an Endocrine Society Clinical Practice Guideline: commentary from a European perspective. Eur J Endocrinol 162(5):831–833

Total Phallic Reconstruction in Female-to-Male Transsexuals by the Pedicle Anterolateral (ALT) Flap

27

Zoran Marij Arnež, Vittorio Ramella, and Giovanni Papa

27.1 Introduction and History

Total phallic construction is an important step in surgical treatment of female-to-male transsexuals (FTMT) for gender reassignment.

Female-to-male gender reassignment consists of subcutaneous mastectomy, hysterectomy, salpingo-oophorectomy, and vaginectomy which are performed typically prior to phallic construction and insertion of penile and testicular prostheses which can be done simultaneously or at a later stage.

The ideal total phallic reconstruction should create an aesthetically acceptable, sensate phallus with the neourethra permitting voiding in a urinal and enough tissue to allow for insertion of a penile prosthesis permitting sexual intercourse [1].

However, selection of the reconstructive method depends largely on patients' desires: some of the patients prefer a reconstruction without the neourethra; others may refuse insertion of a penile prosthesis.

Z.M. Arnež, MD, PhD (✉)
Department of Medicine, Surgery and Health
University of Studies of Trieste,
Strada di Fiume 447, Trieste 34149, Italy
e-mail: zoran.arnez@aots.sanita.fvg.it

V. Ramella • G. Papa
Department of Plastic and Reconstructive Surgery,
Cattinara Hospital, University Hospital of Trieste,
Strada di Fiume 447, Trieste 34149, Italy
e-mail: vittorio.ramella@aots.sanita.fvg.it;
giovanni.papa@aots.sanita.fvg.it

Historically, the first penile reconstructions started in the late 1930s with random pedicled oblique abdominal tube flaps with no neourethra and optional insertion of costal cartilage to obtain rigidity [2].

Later, in the 1940s, in order to reconstruct the neourethra, the "tube-within-a-tube" concept was added to the original Borgas' technique [3, 4].

With the advent of axial pattern flaps, the groin flap was introduced into phallic reconstruction. Because it was wedge shaped and insensate, it never gained popularity [5–7].

Pedicle musculocutaneous flaps from the thigh (gracilis) led to poor results and were abandoned [8, 9].

In 1984 Chang and Hwang published a series of 7 total phallic reconstructions by the free radial forearm flap which revolutionized phallic reconstruction. This flap offered the possibility of reconstructing a well-vascularized, sensate penile shaft of generous dimensions and neourethra using the "tube-within-a-tube" principle from the non-hirsute skin in one stage, making possible an insertion of a penile prosthesis [10].

Later, the design of this flap has been modified to improve the aesthetic results and to reduce the complication rate (mainly connected to meatal stenosis and urethral fistulae) and the donor site morbidity.

Other microvascular reconstructions include the island lateral arm flap [11, 12], deltoid flap [13], pedicled TFL [14] flap, SCIP flap [15],

C. Trombetta et al. (eds.), *Management of Gender Dysphoria: A Multidisciplinary Approach*,
DOI 10.1007/978-88-470-5696-1_27, © Springer-Verlag Italia 2015

sensate fibula OC flap [16], radial forearm OC flap [17], pedicled and free anterolateral thigh flaps [18, 19], and latissimus dorsi myocutaneous flap [20].

However, total phallic reconstruction by the free microvascular radial forearm flap remains also nowadays the "gold standard" to which all new methods need to be compared. The main disadvantage of this flap remains necessity of donor site skin grafting around at least two thirds of the forearm circumference in the distal and middle third. Because of this stigma of the operative procedure, the surgeons are constantly exploring other donor sites for flaps convenient for total phallic reconstruction.

In 1984 Song introduced the free septocutaneous anterolateral thigh (ALT) flap [21]. In the era of perforator flaps, the ALT flap, because of its numerous advantages, became the most popular flap in practically all fields of reconstructive microsurgery [22].

In fact, in 2005 Felici introduced the free ALT flap into total phallic reconstruction [18].

Microsurgery is neither performed in all centers where FTMT are treated for gender reassignment nor all patients are suitable for microsurgical procedures.

Pedicle flaps have been used at the beginnings of total phallic reconstruction before the advent of microsurgery [2–9] and are still a valid arm in the armamentarium of reconstructive procedures aimed at total phallic reconstruction.

Their main advantage is their reliability.

Free flaps work on "all or none" principle: they can fail totally but partial failures are rare. The average failure rate in free flap surgery today remains somewhere between 1 and 5 % which is considered acceptable. However, for the patient a total flap failure represents a 100 % loss because the aim of the operation was not achieved and the problem remains the same in spite of the additional price that has been paid (scars, pain, and discomfort) in the donor area.

Total failure of pedicle flaps in total phallic reconstruction is extremely rare. Partial failures (loss of a part of the flap) happen more often depending on the type and the design of the pedicle flap.

Pedicle flaps from the infraumbilical portion of the abdomen (Pryor and Gill [23]) based on superficial pudendal vessels became popular in the 1990s.

In 2000 two other pedicle flaps were introduced: the island tensor fascia lata flap (Santanelli and Scuderi [14]) and the "Istanbul" flap (Mutaf [24]).

In 2006 Mutaf [25] described the use of a pedicle ALT flap for total phallic reconstruction. Rubino et al. [19] innervated the pedicle ALT by anastomosing the lateral cutaneous femoral nerve to the dorsal clitoris branch of the pudendal nerve.

27.2 Flap Dimensions

The anterolateral thigh offers a large donor site for harvesting of a (pedicle or free) flap called the anterolateral thigh (ALT) flap composed of skin, subcutaneous fat, fascia, and a vascularized nerve (lateral cutaneous nerve of the thigh) based on the descending branch of the lateral circumflex femoral artery (LCFA).

The flap can be as long as 35 cm and as wide as 25 cm, but when large like that, the donor area requires split-thickness skin grafting. Only donor defects of less than 8 cm width can be closed primarily and wider defects should be closed by an STSG (usually over a dermal substitute to reduce the steplike deformity at skin borders) (Figs. 27.1 and 27.2).

Total phallic reconstruction requires flaps at least 15 cm or more wide and 12–15 cm long, and therefore patients have to be informed about the donor site closure. When the patient requires phallic reconstruction without the urethra by the pedicle ALT flap and the patient is thin, a flap width of 8–10 cm only is necessary which (sometimes) makes direct donor closure possible (see Fig. 27.1).

A tube within a tube for neourethral reconstruction is possible only in extremely thin patients with little/no subcutaneous tissues; the outer tube is impossible to close without split-thickness skin grafts (Fig. 27.3). Generally, all patients with subcutaneous fat tissue thicker than 2 cm are discouraged from phallic reconstruction by this flap.

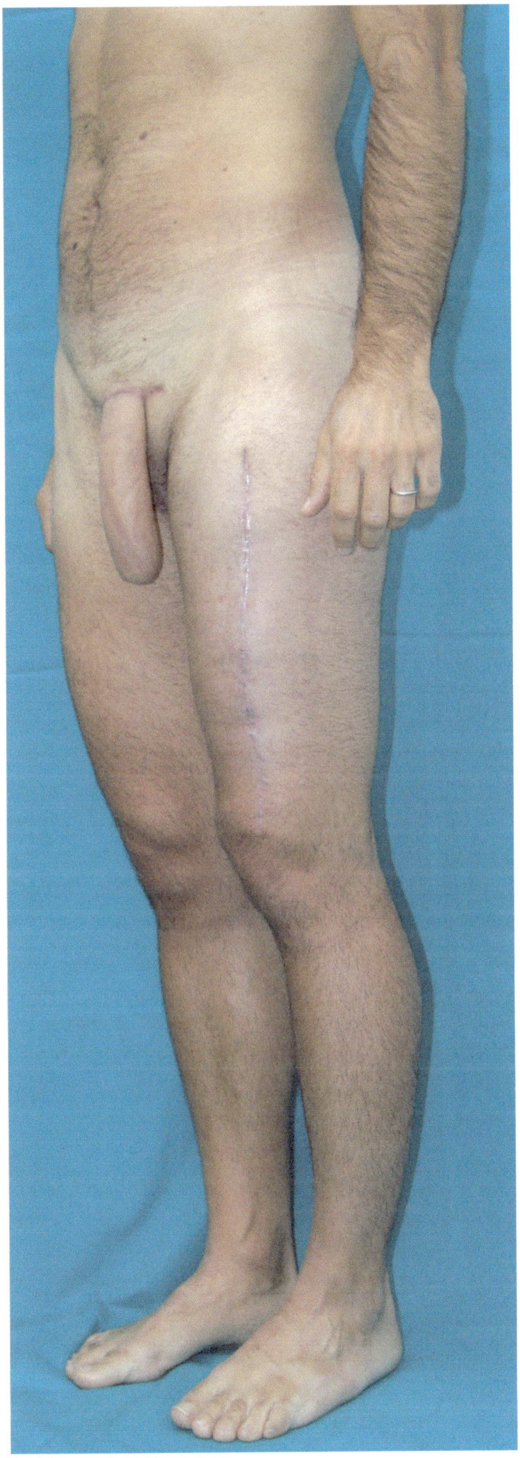

Fig. 27.1 Reconstruction of the phallus without the urethra by the pedicle ALT flap – direct donor site closure. In thin patients, when the donor defect is less than 8–10 cm large, direct donor closure is possible

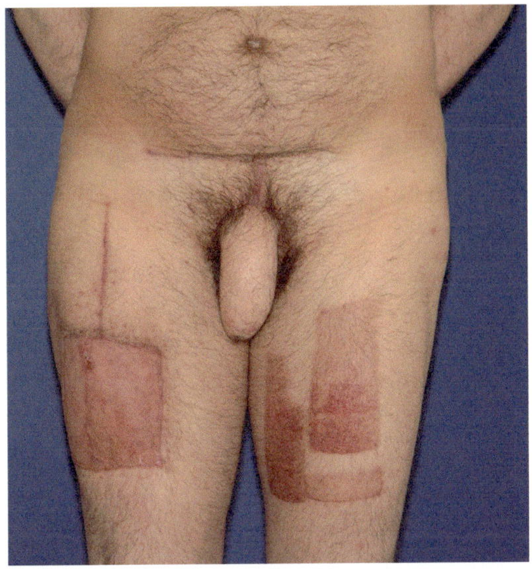

Fig. 27.2 Reconstruction of the phallus without the urethra by the pedicle ALT flap – donor closure by dermal substitute (Integra) and split-thickness skin graft. When subdermal fat on the thigh is thicker, to avoid a steplike deformity, the donor site is closed first by the dermal substitute covered by a silicone sheath and 2–3 weeks later by a split-thickness skin graft

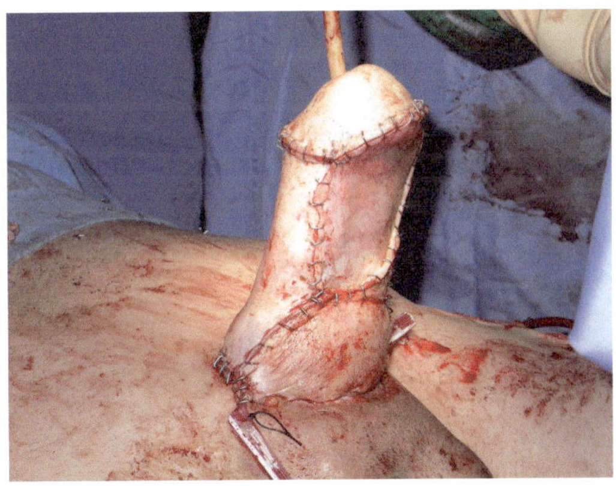

Fig. 27.3 Total phallic reconstruction ("tube within a tube") in a patient with subdermal fat thicker than 2 cm (result at the end of reconstruction). Since, because of the thickness of the flap, it was impossible to close primarily the "outer tube," split-thickness skin grafting was necessary on the ventral side of the penile shaft

27.3 Preoperative Diagnostics

The simplest way of finding the most constant perforator (within a circle of 3 cm of midpoint of the line drawn between the anterior superior iliac

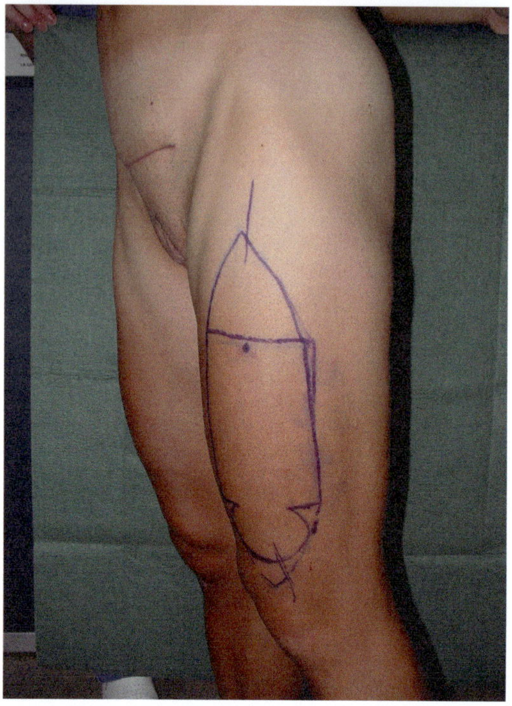

Fig. 27.4 Preoperative flap design. The design is incorporated in an ellipse to facilitate donor site closure. Note the location of the perforator (*dot*) 1–2 cm distal to the base of the future shaft

spine and the superolateral corner of the patella [26]) is by handheld Doppler device (see Fig. 27.4). Color flow Doppler and CT angiography have greater sensitivity and specificity in localizing perforators, but they are time consuming and expensive.

27.4 Designing and Harvesting of the Pedicle ALT Flap

Once the perforator has been identified, the design of the flap has to be transferred to the skin of the thigh. The flap base starts 1–2 cm proximal to the point where the perforator enters into the flap, and the flap is centered over the intermuscular septum between the rectus femoris and the vastus lateralis muscles (see Fig. 27.4). The design of the flap is different when the neo-phallus will have no urethra from the design of total phallic reconstruction.

The flap design is incorporated into an elliptical form for easier wound closure (see Fig. 27.4). First, the anterior incision of the flap is made along the anterior part of the predesigned ellipse through skin, subcutaneous fat, and fascia. Care is taken to preserve some 5 cm of the lateral femoral cutaneous nerve which will be later used to provide sensitivity.

The fascia is elevated by the single hooks, and the dissection proceeds in the posterior direction toward the intermuscular septum between the rectus femoris and the vastus lateralis muscles. The more the septum is being approached, the more care must be taken about any perforators piercing the rectus muscle which are preserved. Then the posterior incision is made, again through skin, fat, and fascia, and the septum is being approached taking care to preserve any perforator through the vastus lateralis muscle. The septum is opened, and the descending branch of the lateral circumflex femoral artery (LCFA) is identified lying on the vastus intermedius muscle between the rectus femoris and vastus lateralis muscles. As soon as it becomes evident that the major perforator from the LCFA is either septocutaneous or musculocutaneous perforating the vastus lateralis muscle, all anterior perforators perforating the rectus muscle are safely divided. The selected perforator is then dissected to the source vessel (LCFA). When the perforator pierces the vastus lateralis muscle, the pedicle dissection may be time consuming since multiple muscle branches have to be carefully identified and divided by bipolar coagulation or micro-clips to preserve the muscle.

Then the descending branch of LCF vessels (artery and vein) is divided from the motor nerve (preserving it) starting distal to the entrance of the perforator. Distal to that point, the vessels are ligated and divided and the dissection proceeds proximally. To be able to liberate the descending branch, multiple artery and vein branches are clipped or ligated.

The dissection stops at the level where the perforator through the tensor fasciae latae muscle to the skin takes off. At that point the flap is passed posterior to the rectus femoris and sartorius muscles from the lateral to the medial part of the thigh (Fig. 27.5).

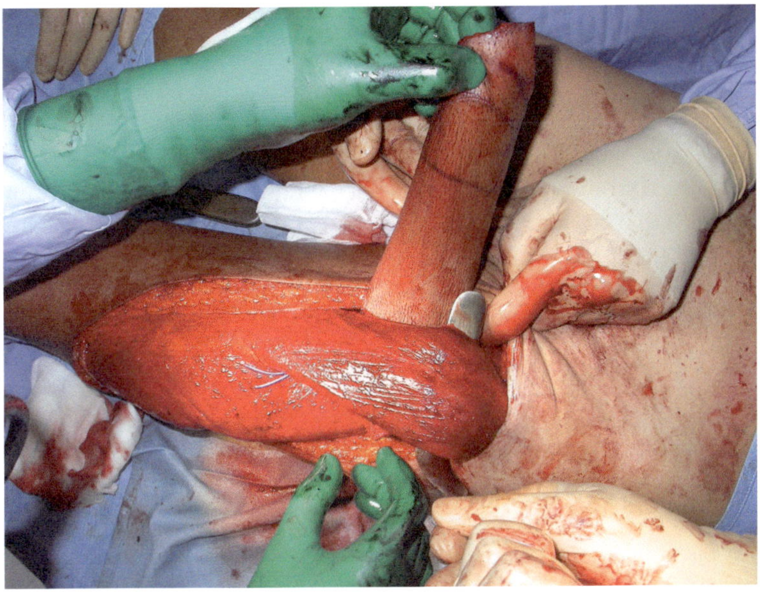

Fig. 27.5 Intraoperative view. Passing the pedicle ALT flap ventral to the rectus femoris and sartorius muscles from the anterolateral to the medial side of the thigh

The pedicle length should be such to permit tension-free reaching of the midline just cranial to the clitoris where the neo-phallus should be positioned. If the pedicle is too short, further pedicle dissection is necessary which can reach as far as to the profunda femoris vessels. To be able to do that, first the TFL perforator and later the ascending branch of the LCFA have to be ligated and divided.

After the optimal pedicle length is ascertained, the elliptical flap is trimmed to the preoperative design discarding all unnecessary tissue. This is followed by tubulization: the flap is sutured into a tube (or a "tube within a tube" in case the urethra is being reconstructed), passed under the rectus muscle, and delivered to the recipient site.

There the lateral cutaneous nerve of the thigh is trimmed to the necessary length and coapted by microsutures to the dorsal clitoris branch of the pudendal nerve to provide sensation. The neourethral tube is sutured to the urethral prolongation made from vascularized labial flaps over a Foley catheter. The cranial portion of subcutis at 12 h is fixed to pubic symphysis and the wounds are closed.

It is our experience to leave scrotal sac reconstruction, insertion of testicular prostheses, and penile prosthesis insertion for the second phase of the operation.

Donor defect is closed after generous undermining of the anterior and posterior skin and the subcutaneous fat dorsal to the fascia, and when possible, direct wound closure is carried out. Otherwise, positioning of the dermal substitute (Integra) and split-thickness skin grafting after 2–3 weeks are required.

27.5 Indications

The primary indication for an innervated pedicle LTF flap in our hands is reconstruction of a neophallus without the urethra in thin patients where direct donor site closure is expected (Fig. 27.1).

When the patient wishes a total phallic reconstruction, our first choice is the radial forearm free flap.

However, if the patient would like to avoid its stigma on the forearm, we would harvest a pedicle ALT flap to reconstruct the "outer tube" and an ulnar forearm (UF) free flap to reconstruct the urethra and glans. In this way one can close the donor site on the thigh directly and transfer the scar on the forearm to the ulnar side where it is less obvious. However, such a reconstruction requires microsurgery not only to coapt nerves but also the UF vessels and can take longer.

27.6 Advantages

The pedicle-innervated ALT flap phallic reconstruction offers several advantages.

The first one is that it remains reliable. The procedure is safe. We never encountered any problems with total or partial flap necrosis.

The only possible problem can be a short vascular pedicle resulting in suboptimal – out of midline – positioning of the flap (Fig. 27.1).

When this is the case, the flap can easily be transformed into a free flap.

The second advantage, being a pedicle flap, is that the procedure is much quicker than the radial forearm free flap. By avoiding microvascular anastomoses and (possibly) split-thickness skin grafting, at least 1 h and a half can be spared.

The third advantage is the color match which is even more important in patients with dark pigmented skin where a "whitish" radial forearm flap has a patchy appearance, whereas the color of thigh skin resembles that of the perineum much better.

A further advantage of the pedicle ALT flap transfer is that it does not require any postoperative anticoagulant/antiaggregation therapy.

27.7 Disadvantages

With total phallic reconstructions, a large soft tissue defect remains on the anterolateral aspect of the thigh and requires split-thickness skin grafting. In overweight or obese patients, a "steplike" deformity is created. This can be partially overcome by placing the dermal substitute Integra on the exposed rectus and vastus lateralis muscles and grafting it after 2–3 weeks (see Fig. 27.2).

Contrary to the donor site of the radial forearm flap where skin grafts are placed on the tendons of the wrist, harvesting of pedicle ALT flap does not leave any functional disability.

However, harvesting of skin grafts leaves hypo-/hyperpigmentation on the donor site. Although color match between the skin from the thigh and perineum is better compared to the forearm, it is not exactly the same.

27.8 Personal Experience

The Trieste Plastic Surgery Department started to use the pedicle ALT flap in 2007 and presented it at the SICPRE meeting in Bari in 2007.

From 2007 to 2013 we performed 3 pedicle ALT flaps, 2 total reconstructions, and 1 penile reconstruction without the urethra. During the same period we performed 7 free ALT penile reconstructions, one total and 6 "outer circle" (tube) only.

References

1. Hage JJ, Bloem JJ, Suliman HM (1993) Review of the literature on techniques for the phalloplasty with emphasis on the applicability in female-to-male transsexuals. J Urol 150:1093–1098
2. Bogoras N (1936) Uber die volle plastische Wiederherstellung eines zum Koitus fahigen Penis (Penisplastica totalis). Zentralbl Chir 22:1271–1276
3. Maltz M (1946) Maltz reparative technique for the penis. In: Maltz M (ed) Evolution of plastic surgery. Froben Press, New York, pp 278–279
4. Gillies HD, Harrison RJ (1948) Congenital absence of the penis with embryological consideration. Br J Plast Surg 1:8–28
5. McGregor IA, Jackson IT (1972) The groin flap. Br J Plast Surg 25:3–16
6. Puckett CL, Montie JE (1978) Construction of male genitalia in the transsexual, using a tubed groin flap for the penis and a hydraulic inflation device. Plast Reconstr Surg 61:523–530
7. Perović S (1995) Phalloplasty in children and adolescent using the extended pedicle island groin flap. J Urol 154:848–853
8. Orticochea M (1972) A new method of total reconstruction of the penis. Br J Plast Surg 25:347–366
9. Persky L, Resnick M, Desprez J (1983) Penile reconstruction with gracilis pedicled flaps. J Urol 129: 603–605

10. Chang TS, Hwang WY (1984) Forearm flap in one stage reconstruction of the penis. Plast Reconstr Surg 129:603–605
11. Upton J, Mortimer KL, Loughlin K et al (1987) Penile reconstruction using the lateral arm flap. J R Coll Surg Edinb 32:97
12. Hage JJ, de Graaf FH, van den Hoek J et al (1993) Phallic construction in female-to-male transsexuals using a lateral upper arm sensate free flap and a bladder mucosa graft. Ann Plast Surg 31:275–280
13. Harashina T, Inoue T, Tanaka I et al (1990) Reconstruction of the penis with a free deltoid flap. Br J Plast Surg 43:217
14. Santanelli F, Scuderi N (2000) Neophalloplasty in female-to-male transsexuals with the island tensor fasciae latae flap. Plast Reconstr Surg 105: 1990–1996
15. Koshima I, Nanba Y, Nagai A et al (2006) Penile reconstruction with bilateral superficial circumflex iliac artery perforator (SCIP) flaps. J Reconstr Microsurg 22:137–142
16. Sengezer M, Ozturk S, Deveci M et al (2004) Long-term follow-up of total penile reconstruction with sensate osteocutaneous free fibula flap in 18 biologically male patients. Plast Reconstr Surg 114: 439–450
17. Fang RH, Kao YS, Ma S et al (1999) Phalloplasty in female-to-male transsexuals using free radial osteocutaneous flap: a series of 22 cases. Br J Plast Surg 52:217–222
18. Felici N, Felici A (2006) A new phalloplasty technique: the free anterolateral thigh flap phalloplasty. J Plast Reconstr Aesthet Surg 59:153–157
19. Rubino C, Figus A, Dessy LA et al (2009) Innervated island pedicled anterolateral thigh flap for neo-phallic reconstruction in female-to –male transsexuals. J Plast Reconstr Aesthet Surg 62:e45–e49
20. Vesely J, Hyza P, Ranno R et al (2007) New technique in total phalloplasty with reinnervated latissimus dorsi myocutaneous free flap in female-to-male transsexuals. Ann Plast Surg 58:544–550
21. Song YG, Chen GZ, Song YL (1984) The free thigh flap: a new free flap concept based on septocutaneous artery. Br J Plast Surg 37:149–159
22. Wei FC, Jam V, Celik N et al (2002) Have we found an ideal soft-tissue flap? An experience with 672 anterolateral thigh flaps. Plast Reconstr Surg 109:2219–2226; discussion 2227–2230
23. Pryor JP, Gill H (1991) Surgical considerations in 29 female to male transsexual patients. Gend Dysphoria 1:44–47
24. Mutaf M (2000) A new surgical procedure for phallic reconstruction: Istanbul flap. Plast Reconstr Surg 105:1361–1370
25. Mutaf M (2006) A true one-stage nonmicrosurgical technique for total phallic reconstruction. Ann Plast Surg 57(1):100–106
26. Xu DC, Zhong SZ, Kong JM et al (1988) Applied anatomy of the anterolateral femoral flap. Plast Reconstr Surg 82:305–310

Surgical Therapy: Forearm Free Flap Phalloplasty

28

Carlo Trombetta, Giorgio Mazzon, Vittorio Ramella, and Zoran Marij Arnež

Phalloplasty plays a pivotal role in the management of female-to-male transsexuals and is considered to be one of the most challenging procedures in reconstructive surgery. The development of techniques of phalloplasty has paralleled the evolution of flap development in reconstructive surgery itself. In fact, with the development of microsurgery, free flaps also were introduced.

This procedure requires a neophallus cosmetically acceptable to both patient and partner, a sufficient rigidity for vaginal penetration, and tactile sensitivity maintained. Furthermore, scarring in the donor area should be minimized, and a neo-urethra should be constructed, to allow voiding while standing.

Although many patients would like to be able to use the phallus sexually and/or to void in standing position, others only express a desire for a good cosmetic appearance in order to be accepted in the society. The highest priority of most patients is the ability to urinate in public while standing, but this objective is the hardest to reach due to the high complications rate. Unfortunately, sex reassignment surgery usually requires multiple operations, which are very invasive and time consuming.

C. Trombetta • G. Mazzon (✉) • V. Ramella
Z.M. Arnež
Department of Urology, Cattinara Hospital,
Strada di Fiume 447, Trieste 34100, Italy
e-mail: trombcar@units.it;
Giorgio_mazzon@libero.it; Vittorio.ramella@gmail.com;
zoran.arnez@aots.sanita.fvg.it

Hysterectomy and ovariectomy may be performed as a preliminary procedure to reconstructive genital reassignment in female-to-male transsexuals or become an integrated part of it. 'All in one' procedure may be more cost- and time-effective, but may expose the patient to an extended trauma, blood loss and anaesthesia time [1, 2].

As the vaginal skin is no more incorporated into the reconstructive steps of genital reassignment, vaginal length should be reduced as much as possible during hysterectomy in order to facilitate later colpocleisis. Furthermore, the gynaecologist performing this procedure should be eager to prevent damage to the abdominal wall vasculature during hysterectomy, which may be important as future recipient vessels during free flap transposition for penile reconstruction (e.g., inferior epigastric artery and vein).

In this chapter, we describe the use of microsurgical forearm free flap, with or without the creation of a neo-urethra. The radial forearm flap (RFF) was initially developed for the release of cervical skin contracture in burn patients and is today a frequently used flap in head and neck reconstruction as well as limb and penile reconstructive surgery [3].

Free flaps from nearly all parts of the body were described for penile reconstruction [4, 5], but after an initial and euphoric phase, more recent publications of larger series of patients revealed a restriction to only two favourite donor sites: forearm flaps and fibula flaps.

C. Trombetta et al. (eds.), *Management of Gender Dysphoria: A Multidisciplinary Approach*,
DOI 10.1007/978-88-470-5696-1_28, © Springer-Verlag Italia 2015

First reports on the use of forearm free flap phalloplasty was in 1984 and opened the way for microsurgery in genital reconstruction [6, 7]. Biemer (1988) reported a modification of the forearm flap, which was also based on the radial artery [8]; and in 1990, Farrow and associates reported their 'cricket bat' modification of the radial forearm flap [9]. The various modifications of the forearm flap do not represent changes in the technique of flap elevation; rather, they are modifications in the design of the skin island and the relative position of the urethral paddle in relation to the skin that will eventually become the shaft coverage. Each of these modifications has advantages in different situations.

Initial results of this technique were not good. Matti et al. in 1988 reported the results in five transsexuals cases. They had partial success in two cases, both complicated by a fistula, and complete failure in three cases due to a vascular thrombosis [10]; however, in experienced hands this procedure has gained increasing acceptance over the last 23 years since its first description.

Actually, in high-volume centres, on which urologists and plastic surgeons cooperate in common teams, forearm free flap with or without urethral prelamination and without inclusion of osseosegments has become the first choice for penile reconstruction [1, 2, 11–14]. Although no phalloplasty technique is accepted as the standard, there is clear evidence to suggest that the radial artery-based forearm free flap (RAFFF) phalloplasty will give the best cosmetic and functional results, with 99 % of patients able to void from the tip of the phallus while standing and 97 % fully satisfied with cosmesis and size [15, 16].

Details of the operation may differ between different centres, as timing of hysterectomy and ovariectomy, which may well be performed in a previous session in order to reduce blood loss and operative trauma.

Herein we report how we perform phalloplasty according to Chang's technique [6]. The forearm flap is usually harvested from the non-dominant forearm. Preoperatively, the Allen test is used to screen patients carefully for arterial insufficiency. In Fig. 28.1, we report the scheme of incision.

The forearm flap can be elevated and transferred on the superficial fascia. The lateral and medial antebrachial cutaneous nerves appear proximally beneath the fascia. The cephalic, basilic and medial antebrachial veins are also included in the flap and constitute a portion of the venous drainage (Fig. 28.2).

The shaft is covered with the radial aspect of the skin paddle. A deepithelialized strip is made, and a second skin island, on the ulnar aspect of the skin paddle, is tubed to form the urethra. The urethral tube is then rolled within the tube of skin to form a tube-within-tube design, around a 16-F catheter (Fig. 28.3).

T-shaped radial forearm free flap that retains the lateral antebrachial nerve is raised and transferred. The reconstructed penile vascular pedicle is divided and the transplantation is completed by vascular anastomosis by serrated sutures. The vascular pedicle of the reconstructed penis is tunnelled into the inguinal region subcutaneously. The vascular anastomosis of the cephalic vein or its branches and the radial artery to the superficial epigastric artery or the femoral artery (previously prepared and tunnelled into the inguinal region) is carried out under operating microscopes (Fig. 28.4). The anastomosis may be either end to end or end to side as the case necessitates. Cutaneous nerves in the proximal shaft aspect of the flap are coapted to the clitoral nerves.

If the neo-urethra is created, the construction of the fixed part of the urethra up to the level of the clitoris is accomplished using an anterior vaginal flap. The vaginal mucosa is initially separated posteriorly; the anterior wall of the vagina is preserved while the rest of vaginal mucosa is removed. This mucosa is rolled up to provide extension of urethra to the base of the clitoris. The labia minora are then sutured in the midline and the urethra is closed over for healing phalloplasty. Extension of the urethra to the base of the clitoris with the anterior vaginal mucosa has greatly reduced fistula formation. Colpocleisis also better supports the vascularity of this area, providing a well-vascularized anastomosis site for neo-urethra creation. Subsequently, a neo-glans is modelled, as shown in Fig. 28.5. In the final step, urethral anastomosis is completed. A urethral

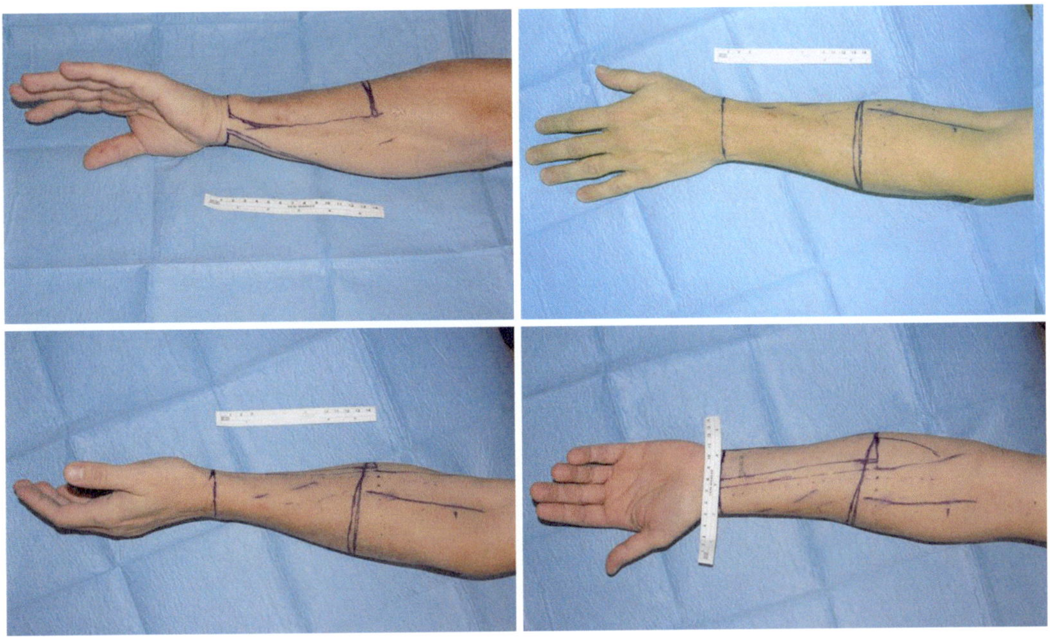

Fig. 28.1 Scheme of incision (Courtesy of Prof. Zoran Marij Arnež)

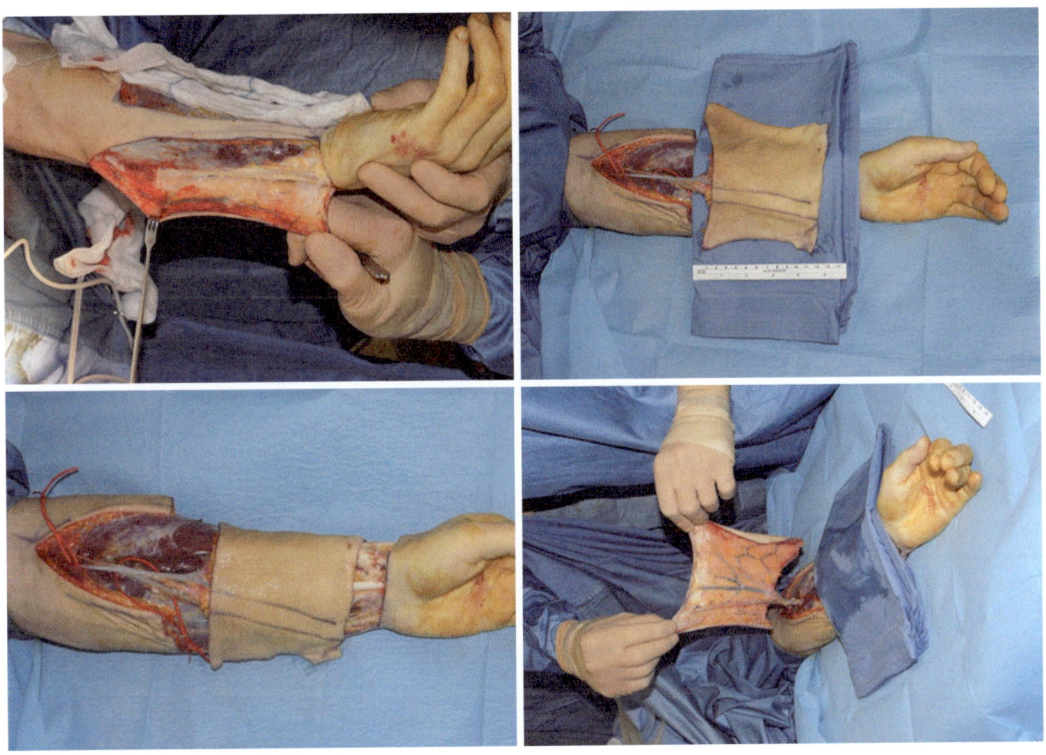

Fig. 28.2 The flap is isolated and mobilized; the neuro-vascular pedicle is well evident (Courtesy of Prof. Zoran Marij Arnež)

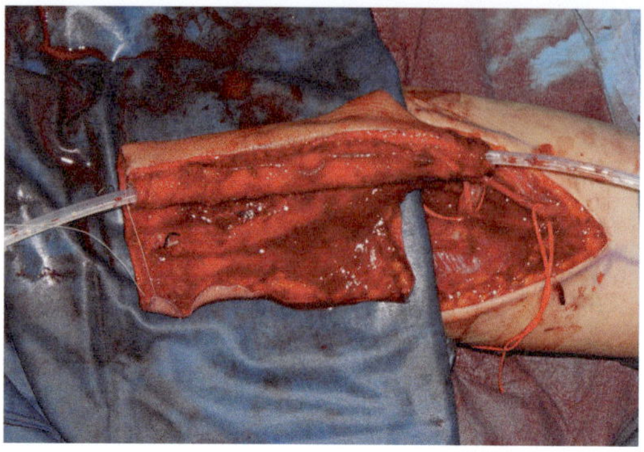

Fig. 28.3 Neo-urethra is created around a 16-French catheter; the flap is then rolled to create a neophallus (Courtesy of Prof. Zoran Marij Arnež)

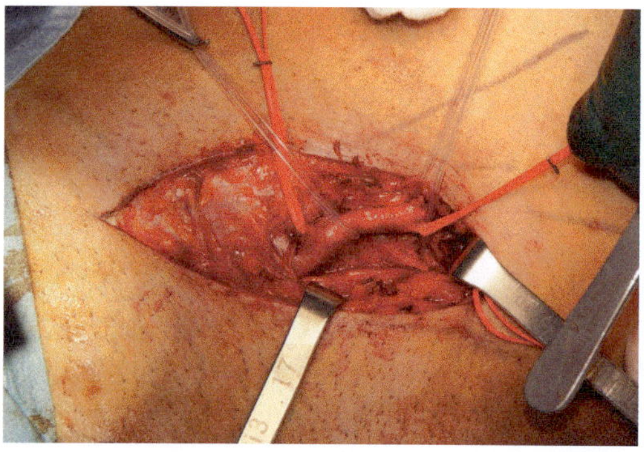

Fig. 28.4 Femoral artery and its branches are isolated and subsequently prepared for anastomosis (Courtesy of Prof. Zoran Marij Arnež)

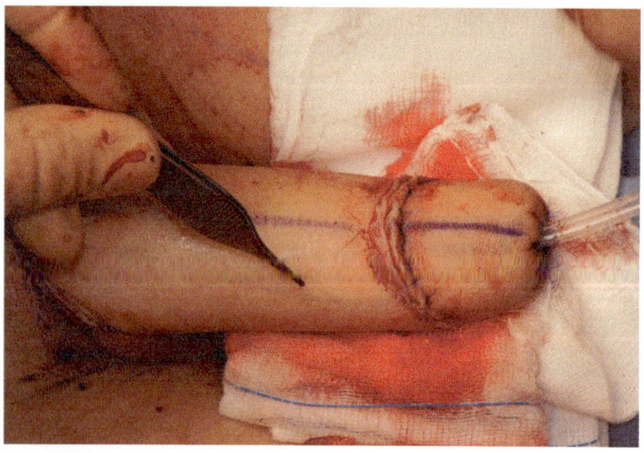

Fig. 28.5 Glanduloplasty (Courtesy of Prof. Zoran Marij Arnež)

catheter is inserted during this procedure (Fig. 28.6). That will be removed 3 weeks after surgery and the defect on the donor arm site is covered with a full-thickness skin graft harvested

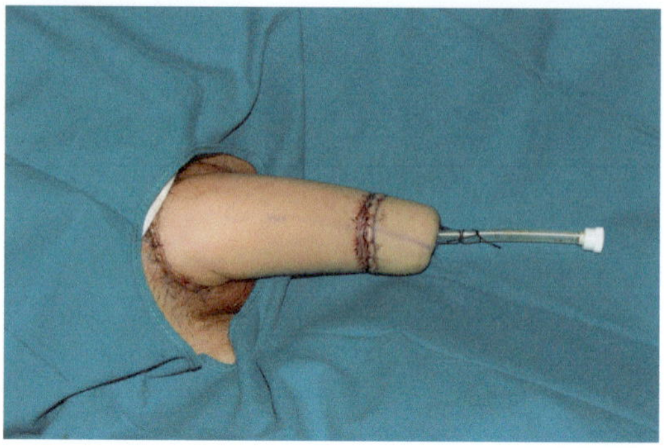

Fig. 28.6 Final results (Courtesy of Prof. Zoran Marij Arnež)

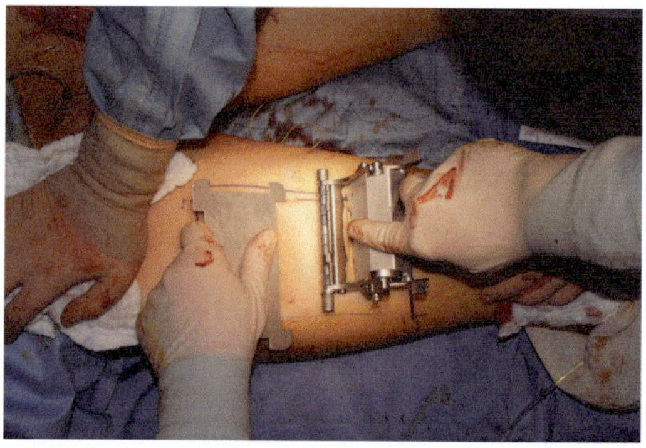

Fig. 28.7 Harvesting of the skin graft from the upper thigh (Courtesy of Prof. Zoran Marij Arnež)

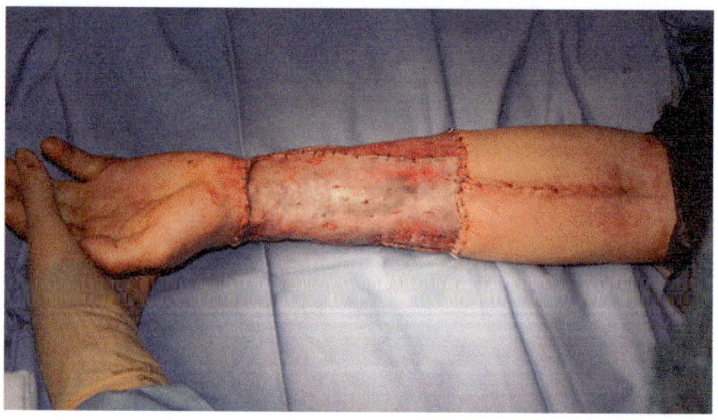

Fig. 28.8 Forearm is covered with a full-thickness skin graft (Courtesy of Prof. Zoran Marij Arnež)

from the upper thigh (Figs. 28.7 and 28.8); harvest from the buttock or the abdomen is described. A compressive dressing is applied to the graft and the arm kept elevated for 1 week. The arm is then inspected every week thereafter. Figure 28.9 shows the final results after a 3-month follow-up.

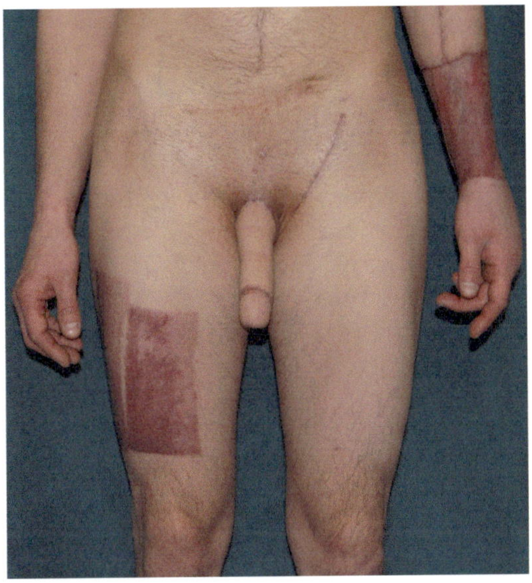

Fig. 28.9 Results after 3-month follow-up (Courtesy of Prof. Zoran Marij Arnež)

In literature, the use of an osteocutaneous free flap is reported [17]. In these cases, a piece of radial bone, based on the diaphyseal periosteal branches of the radial artery, approximately 10 cm in length and not more than one-third of the thickness of the radius, was harvested with the flap.

Due to the complex nature of the operation, complications are numerous and should be explained in detail to the patient: in experienced hands, partial or total flap loss should be expected in less than 5 % of the cases, and nerve compression or compartment syndromes due to the prolonged lithotomy position in less than 2 %. Urethral complications such as fistula and/or stenosis formation still are the leading reasons for reinterventions in around 50–60 % of all patients.

Traditionally local flaps without the need for microsurgical vascular anastomoses were seen to be less prone for complications than free flaps. From recent publications of experienced high-volume centres, it becomes obvious that the more complex the primary procedure is designed, the more possible complications are implicated independently from the surgical technique [18, 19]. In 2005, Monstrey et al. demonstrated on 81 patients with phalloplasty derived from forearm free flaps a 3.6 % rate of partial or total flap loss, 22 % of wound healing problems and 42 % of urinary fistulas or stenosis.

Another recent paper from Leriche et al. dealt with the follow-up of 56 patients after forearm free flap phalloplasty. A 5 % flap loss rate was reported, 37 % had urethral complications, and 29 % had prostatic complications [19].

Even if reinterventions for urethral problems may be successful, nearly half of the patients report urinary problems as reduced urinary stream, dribbling or recidivant urinary infections [20].

Possible complications after free flap phalloplasty comprise early and late anastomotic revisions due to venous, arterial or combined thromboses, partial or total flap loss and urological complications such as fistulas and strictures, which frequently require multiple urological revisions.

Urethral fistulas and strictures are the two main problems arising in patients with total phallic reconstruction; in particular, one-stage procedure seems to be associated with a higher risk of urinary complications. Reasons may be the insufficient vascular supply of the local flaps and the inappropriate width of the phallic urethra, the latter being responsible for relative obstruction of the urinary stream and increased force on the 'bulbar urethra' and anastomotic sites.

In the series of Biemer [8], the neo-urethra was constructed from a 3-cm-wide skin strip. In 9 of 10 patients evaluated after an average of 30 months, urethral fistulas were observed. In 7 of these patients, 3–4 reoperations did not solve the problem; moreover, in 4 patients urethral strictures were present as well. Rohrman et al. reported a casistic with 25 cases with primary female transsexualism underwent phalloplasty with a radial forearm free flap, vaginectomy and urethroplasty in a one-stage procedure. In 16 of these patients, the fixed part of the neo-urethra ('bulbar urethra') was constructed from a vaginal flap. In 9 patients, flaps of the labia minora (5 patients) or the 'urethral plate' (4 patients) were used. In 14 (58 %) patients, fistulas and/or strictures in the newly constructed urethra occurred. Eleven (69 %) of 16 patients in whom the 'bulbar urethra' was constructed from a vaginal flap experienced fistulas and/or stricture formation.

Fistulas and/or strictures occurred in 3 of 5 patients with labia minora flaps and none of 4 patients with the urethral plate procedure. Repair of fistula and strictures was performed by primary closure of fistulas, staged urethroplasty with local pedicled flaps or distant tissue grafts using buccal mucosa (2–6 procedures) [21].

Partial flap necrosis is reported to occur in 7–11 % of phalloplasty cases [22, 23]. The largest series published by Doornaert et al. showed a rate of 7.2 % (23 out of 316 cases) with a higher incidence in smokers, in patients who insisted on large-sized neo-phalluses and after anastomotic revision. In 15 out of these 23 patients (63 %), debridement and secondary closure or skin grafting was necessary. 2 Partial flap necrosis frequently affects the radial and ulnar flap borders, which are both directly involved in the formation of the neo-urethra in the Chang design. This may lead to a necrotic or exposed neo-urethra and consequently to urethral dysfunction. Possible contributing factors to partial flap necrosis in a tube-within-tube setting are the flap width and the need for double bending of the flap. Additionally, postoperative flap swelling may cause venous congestion.

Baumeister et al. reported a series with 135 radial forearm flaps, in which 10 flaps had a thrombosis (3 arterial, 4 venous, 3 combined) on postoperative day 0, 1 ($n=5$), 4, 4, 5 and 24. Six revisions were successful; 4 flaps failed (3 %). Twelve flaps (9 %) showed a partial or superficial necrosis which required an operative revision [22].

In case of partial flap necrosis with involvement of neo-urethra in toto, some authors suggested a salvage procedure with a second RFF from the contralateral side providing well-vascularized tissue. No flap-related complications were observed [24].

In case of thrombosis of arterial pedicle which results in ischemia of neophallus, some authors reported the perfusion of the flap with streptokinase which restored venous return. Flap perfusion was thereafter confirmed by intraoperative direct angiography of the neophallus [25].

Another important issue is morbidity on donor site after forearm free flap phalloplasty. In fact, despite continuous improvements in the technique of preparing the donor site for grafting that have allowed a significant improvement of the final cosmetic result, the residual scar on the donor arm still represents a 'stigma'. Unaesthetic scarring, reduced bone density, limited range of motion, decreased pinch and grip strength or graft loss, delayed healing and sensory changes have all been reported after a radial forearm flap [26–30].

However, large series describing long-term results are scarce in literature. Van Caenegem et al. reported a 7-year follow-up on 44 F-to-M transsexuals treated with forearm free flap phalloplasty [31].

They observed no functional limitations on daily life activities, a pain-free and rather aesthetic scar and unaffected bone health a median of 7 years after radial forearm flap phalloplasty. Over 75 % of transsexual men were either satisfied or neutral with the appearance of the scar.

In other and older series, morbidity of the donor site arm after forearm free flap phalloplasty has been reported to be higher, including poor wound healing [29, 32], bone fracture [17, 27, 32], persisting pain [33] or varying degrees of functional loss [28, 34, 35].

This difference may be explained by the use of supra- or subfascial flap. A suprafascial dissection may lead to a lower morbidity.

At the time, it is relatively difficult to give reliable data or long-term follow-up of FM-TS patients due to the plethora of operative techniques used in the last 20 years. Follow-up studies published before 1991 are not helpful due to the lack of modern phalloplasty techniques at that time.

Wirsaw et al. reported data from 29 patients undergoing subjective and objective follow-up showed that 70 % were able to have vaginal sexual intercourse, 72 % were able to reach orgasm by neopenis stimulation, 90 % were able to void in a standing position and 90 % would do the procedure again if necessary . The measurement of sensory evoked potentials (SEP) showed normal to slightly prolonged latency times in 27 patients. In all these patients, at least one clitoral nerve was adapted to the forearm flap nerves under microsurgical conditions, which may prove the possible efficiency of this technique to give erotic sensitivity to a neopenis [36].

Another technique using a free flap is fibula flap phalloplasty which will be herein shortly described because it is not covered in this chapter. This procedure was first published in 1993 by Sadove et al. [37] as free sensate osteocutaneous fibula flap. Part of the fibula is included as a substitute for penile stiffening. The lateral sural cutaneous nerve can be coapted to adequate nerves deriving from ilioinguinal nerve or iliohypogastric nerve. One dorsal clitoral nerve can be used as a recipient nerve. The recipient vessels are the femoral artery and branches of the long saphenous vein. The size of the flap, whose blood supply relies on the peroneal artery, is about 20 cm long and 12 wide. The inclusion of part of the fibula into the flap is still a point of debate: in long-term follow-up studies, some authors proved that such bone transplants remain vital and stable in contrast to free transplanted cartilage or bone fragments [38]. Nevertheless, a permanently rigid structure in the neopenis has to be considered an impediment at best. Furthermore, proximal bone fixation remains problematic resulting in insufficient penile stability during intercourse. The most important shortcoming is donor site morbidity with need for wearing a lower leg splint for at least 6 weeks and the potential for long-term problems with decreased power, suboptimal gait, coordination and ankle instability after loss of the fibula. In 2006, a successful penile reconstruction using a septocutaneous fibula free flap without fibula bone had been reported; it can help decrease morbidity and will be a welcome alternative for patients who refuse forearm scar or are not suited for forearm surgery because of other reasons [39].

References

1. Monstrey S et al (2001) Surgical therapy in transsexual patients: a multi-disciplinary approach. Acta Chir Belg 101(5):200–209
2. Jarolim L (2000) Surgical conversion of genitalia in transsexual patients. BJU Int 85(7):851–856
3. Yang GF et al (1981) Forearm free skin flap transplantation: a report of 56 cases. Br J Plast Surg 50(3): 162–165
4. Vesely J, Haage J (1999) From the history of penis reconstruction. Acta Chir Plast 41(2):43–45
5. Hage JJ, Bloem JJ, Suliman HM (1993) Review of the literature on techniques for phalloplasty with emphasis on the applicability in female-to-male transsexuals. J Urol 150(4):1093–1098
6. Chang TS, Hwang WY (1984) Forearm flap in one-stage reconstruction of the penis. Plast Reconstr Surg 74(2):251–258
7. Kao XS et al (1984) One-stage reconstruction of the penis with free skin flap: report of three cases. J Reconstr Microsurg 1(2):149–153
8. Biemer E (1988) Penile construction by the radial arm flap. Clin Plast Surg 15(3):425–430
9. Semple JL et al (1991) The "cricket bat" flap: a one-stage free forearm flap phalloplasty. Plast Reconstr Surg 88(3):514–519
10. Matti BA, Matthews RN, Davies DM (1988) Phalloplasty using the free radial forearm flap. Br J Plast Surg 41(2):160–164
11. Vesely J et al (1999) Our standard method of reconstruction of the penis and urethra in female to male transsexuals. Acta Chir Plast 41(2):39–42
12. Hu ZQ et al (2005) Penis reconstruction using three different operative methods. Br J Plast Surg 58(4): 487–492
13. Hage JJ et al (1993) Construction of the neophallus in female-to-male transsexuals: the Amsterdam experience. J Urol 149(6):1463–1468
14. Meyer R, Daverio P (1987) One-stage sensible phalloplasty in the transsexual female. Helv Chir Acta 54(1–2):175–176
15. Garaffa G, Christopher NA, Ralph DJ (2010) Total phallic reconstruction in female-to-male transsexuals. Eur Urol 57(4):715–722
16. Monstrey S et al (2009) Penile reconstruction: is the radial forearm flap really the standard technique? Plast Reconstr Surg 124(2):510–518
17. Fang RH et al (1999) Phalloplasty in female-to-male transsexuals using free radial osteocutaneous flap: a series of 22 cases. Br J Plast Surg 52(3):217–222
18. Sohn M, Bosinski HA (2007) Gender identity disorders: diagnostic and surgical aspects. J Sex Med 4(5):1193–1207; quiz 1208
19. Leriche A et al (2008) Long-term outcome of forearm flee-flap phalloplasty in the treatment of transsexualism. BJU Int 101(10):1297–1300
20. Hoebeke P et al (2005) Impact of sex reassignment surgery on lower urinary tract function. Eur Urol 47(3):398–402
21. Rohrmann D, Jakse G (2003) Urethroplasty in female-to-male transsexuals. Eur Urol 44(5):611–614
22. Baumeister S et al (2011) Phalloplasty in female-to-male transsexuals: experience from 259 cases. Handchir Mikrochir Plast Chir 43(4):215–221

23. Doornaert M et al (2011) Penile reconstruction with the radial forearm flap: an update. Handchir Mikrochir Plast Chir 43(4):208–214
24. Tchang LA et al (2014) Second free radial forearm flap for urethral reconstruction after partial flap necrosis of tube-in-tube phalloplasty with radial forearm flap: a report of two cases. Microsurgery 34:58–63
25. Noordanus RP, Hage JJ (1993) Late salvage of a "free flap" phalloplasty: a case report. Microsurgery 14(9): 599–600
26. Bardsley AF et al (1990) Reducing morbidity in the radial forearm flap donor site. Plast Reconstr Surg 86(2):287–292; discussion 293–294
27. Boorman JG, Brown JA, Sykes PJ (1987) Morbidity in the forearm flap donor arm. Br J Plast Surg 40(2):207–212
28. Jaquet Y et al (2012) Radial forearm free flap donor site morbidity: ulnar-based transposition flap vs split-thickness skin graft. Arch Otolaryngol Head Neck Surg 138(1):38–43
29. Loeffelbein DJ et al (2012) Reduction of donor site morbidity of free radial forearm flaps: what level of evidence is available? Eplasty 12:e9
30. Lutz BS et al (1999) Donor site morbidity after suprafascial elevation of the radial forearm flap: a prospective study in 95 consecutive cases. Plast Reconstr Surg 103(1):132–137
31. Van Caenegem E et al (2013) Long-term evaluation of donor-site morbidity after radial forearm flap phalloplasty for transsexual men. J Sex Med 10(6): 1644–1651
32. Richardson D et al (1997) Radial forearm flap donor-site complications and morbidity: a prospective study. Plast Reconstr Surg 99(1):109–115
33. Sardesai MG et al (2008) Donor-site morbidity following radial forearm free tissue transfer in head and neck surgery. J Otolaryngol Head Neck Surg 37(3):411–416
34. Ma S et al (1991) Clinical application of Chinese forearm flap: 5-year review. Zhonghua Yi Xue Za Zhi (Taipei) 47(1):45–49
35. Song C et al (2011) Modifications of the radial forearm flap phalloplasty for female-to-male gender reassignment. J Reconstr Microsurg 27(2): 115–120
36. Wirsam K, Sohn M, Exner K, Horbach C (2006) Pudendus-reinnervation after penile reconstruction: sensory-evoked potentials (SEP) in correlation to subjective questionnaire results. J sex Med 3(5):391
37. Sadove RC et al (1993) One-stage total penile reconstruction with a free sensate osteocutaneous fibula flap. Plast Reconstr Surg 92(7):1314–1323; discussion 1324–1325
38. Papadopulos NA, Schaff J, Biemer E (2002) Long-term fate of the bony component in neophallus construction with free osteofasciocutaneous forearm or fibula flap in 18 female-to-male transsexuals. Plast Reconstr Surg 109(3):1025–1030; discussion 1031–1032
39. Dabernig J, Chan LK, Schaff J (2006) Phalloplasty with free (septocutaneous) fibular flap sine fibula. J Urol 176(5):2085–2088

Surgical Therapy: Metoidioplasty Technique and Results

29

Rados P. Djinovic

29.1 Introduction

Despite a long time having passed since its inception, female to male sex reassignment surgery (SRS) remains very challenging and demanding. The principal objective of medical treatment is to conform the body to the self-perception of the gender. Surgical gender conversion is the last step of a fairly lengthy process that involves psychological, endocrinological, aesthetic, and legal procedures. There is no general consensus in the literature with regard to the length of time spent living as a female-to-male transsexual before gender reassignment surgery is undertaken. Gender reassignment surgery for the female to male transsexual involves breast surgery, hysterectomy, salpingo-oophorectomy, vaginectomy, metoidioplasty or total phalloplasty and placement of a testicular prosthesis. Despite a variety of surgical techniques for total phalloplasty, none fulfills all the criteria and none has been accepted as being the best method.

Metoidioplasty is the only procedure that enables the creation of small neophallus – a "penoid" – with completely preserved tactile and erogenous sensitivity. Simultaneously, a scrotum is created from the labia majora with two implanted testicular prostheses. The goal of metoidioplasty is to form a small penis and to enable voiding in a standing position. It consists of the elongation and displacement of an overdeveloped clitoris after hormonal therapy to construct a microphallus. This is possible because of the similar embryological development of male and female external genitalia. Although a neophallus created in this way is not large enough to enable sexual intercourse with vaginal penetration, a certain number of transgender patients are satisfied with this solution; this is very important for better socialization of these patients because it enables them to use male public toilets. Also, some of them are not willing to undergo major surgery with the consequent big scars that are connected with total phalloplasties. In any case, we noted that 1 % of these patients change their mind after surgery and require total phalloplasty later. We previously published our variant of metoidioplasty with functional and cosmetic outcome that generated further improvements [1]. Experience in the repair of perineal hypospadias with penoscrotal transposition was very important in helping us to improve the technique because of its great similarity to female external genitalia [2].

29.2 Patients and Methods

In the period between October 2004 and May 2014 a total of 93 patients with a mean age of 27 years (range, 18–54 years) underwent metoidioplasty as a part of SRS. It was done simultaneously

R.P. Djinovic
Sava Perovic Foundation,
Center for Genito-Urinary Reconstructive Surgery,
Borisavljeviceva 58, Belgrade 11000, Serbia
e-mail: djinovic@gmail.com

C. Trombetta et al. (eds.), *Management of Gender Dysphoria: A Multidisciplinary Approach*,
DOI 10.1007/978-88-470-5696-1_29, © Springer-Verlag Italia 2015

with removal of female genitalia and sometimes mastectomy. Thirty-six of these patients (39 %) had undergone previous hysterectomy with bilateral salpingo-oophorectomy (13 laparoscopic, 8 transvaginal, and 15 open surgeries) in other centers and required only vaginectomy, whereas the remaining 57 (61 %) had no previous genital surgery. Uterus and ovaries are removed using a transvaginal (52 patients; 56 %) or laparoscopic approach (5 patients; 5 %). In 9 patients (7 %) breasts were removed simultaneously. All patients were treated hormonally from 6 months to 16 years preoperatively (mean, 4 years). Also, all patients are advised to use dihydrotestosterone gel (ANDRACTIM®) topically twice per day and to use a vacuum device to stretch the clitoris for at least 3 months before surgery to maximally increase its size.

29.2.1 Indications

The procedure is used in female transsexuals who wish to undergo one-stage SRS without having a complex, multistage total phalloplasty or in those who want this procedure later. The clitoris has to be large enough, i.e., measuring over 2 cm in a stretched position, and the patient should be without severe obesity, to enable creation of a sufficiently long "penoid" to satisfy the patient's wish to void in a standing position (Fig. 29.1). Labia minora and clitoral skin should be normally developed to use as an onlay flap or for

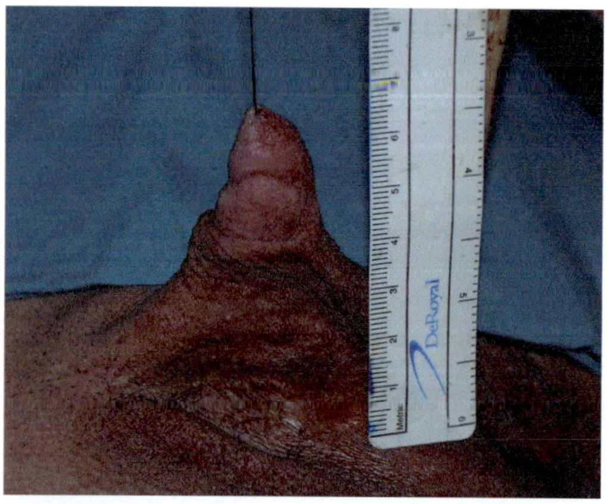

Fig. 29.1 Clitoral length in a stretched position should be at least 2 cm

tubularized urethroplasty. If the mons pubis is prominent, simultaneous lipectomy or liposuction should be performed to allow better neophallic exposure, depending on the amount of fat and overstretched skin.

29.2.2 Operative Technique

The procedure starts with removal of the internal genitalia, usually via a vaginal approach. Conversion was performed only in one patient who had a large myoma of the uterus that had not been diagnosed preoperatively. The vaginal fornix is opened circumferentially, the sacrouterine ligaments detached, and after ligation of the uterine vessels, the uterus with the tubes and ovaries are removed. In some patients a laparoscopic approach was used, but we found no advantage and longer operative times. The vaginal epithelium is completely removed starting with a circumferential superficial incision with cautery at the level of the introitus and carefully continued toward vaginal end (Fig. 29.2). The

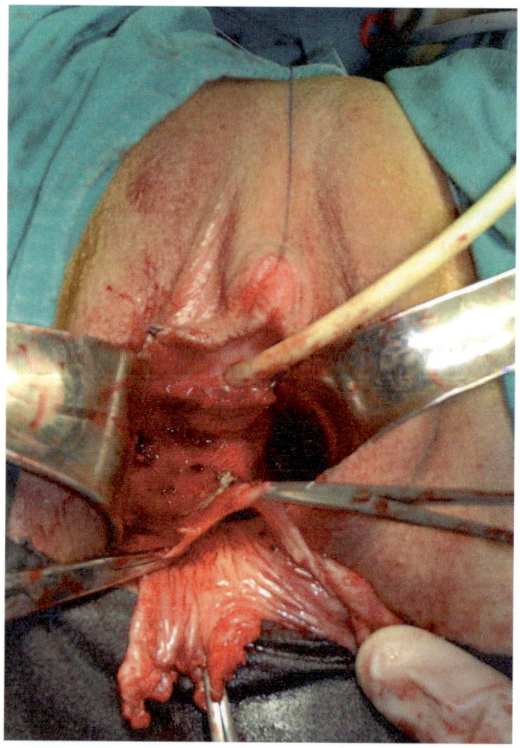

Fig. 29.2 Vaginal mucosa is excised by careful cauterization

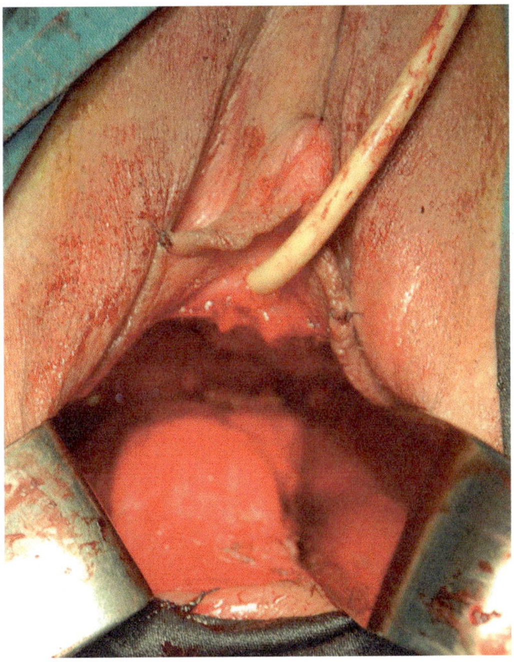

Fig. 29.3 De-epithelialized vaginal cavity

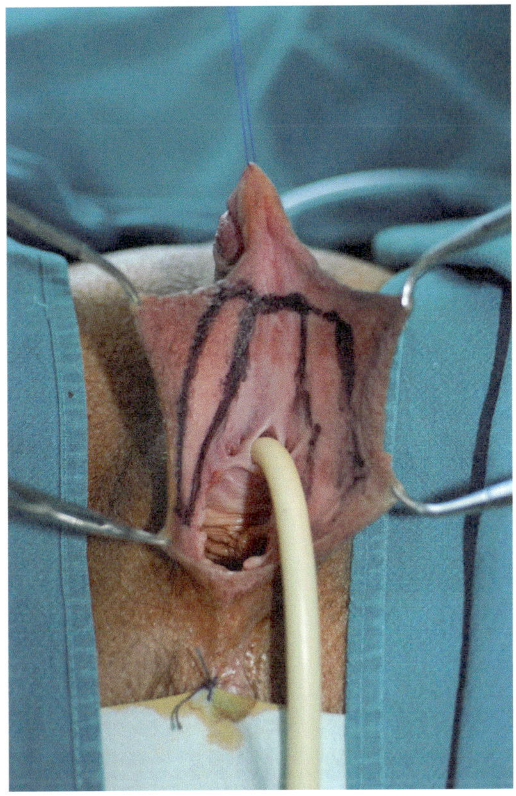

Fig. 29.4 Lines of incision show the design of the urethral plate (UPF) and labia minora flaps (LMF)

peritoneum is closed a using continuous suture, and the vaginal vault completely obliterated using a spiral suture up to the perineum (Fig. 29.3). Two longitudinal parallel incisions about 2.5 cm apart are made along the "urethral plate," starting from the native urethral meatus up to the subcoronal level of the clitoris (Fig. 29.4). The urethral plate in females is short, pulling the clitoris down o the pubis; thus, it is transacted at a subcoronal level and carefully dissected off the ventral side of the clitoral bodies up to the urethral meatus, together with its thick spongiosum. This maneuver significantly lengthens the clitoris, forming a gap between the divided edges of the urethral plate, usually 4–7 cm long (Fig. 29.5). Mobilization of the clitoral skin off the corporal bodies follows without a subcoronal incision, to provide wide exposure of the suspensory ligament; it differs from that in males because it is much bigger, starting from mid-pubis proximally and spreading from the clitoral base up to the subcoronal level distally, in this way strongly pulling the whole clitoris toward the symphysis. The skin is fully released from the clitoral body and excised, leaving only its most proximal part intact to avoid the clitoris falling downward (Fig. 29.6). This procedure enables additional clitoral lengthening. Clitoral skin is tacked to the remaining proximal part of the suspensory ligament at its base using a mattress suture, which helps its distribution over the maximal clitoral length dorsally. The urethra is reconstructed after placement of a Ch12 siliconized Foley catheter – the proximal part is mobilized by tubularizing and transecting the urethral plate, which is carefully fixed to the base of the cavernosal bodies (Fig. 29.5). The distal part of the neourethra at the level of the gap between the transected urethral edges is created in two different ways, depending on the size of the labia minor; if it is not well developed, a combination of a dorsal inlay buccal mucosa graft and a ventral flap created from the labia minora or clitoral skin is used (63 patients – 68 %). The buccal mucosa graft is fixed to the corporal body by quilting (Fig. 29.7). Graft length ranged from 4 to 7 cm and width from 1 to 1.5 cm. The ventral

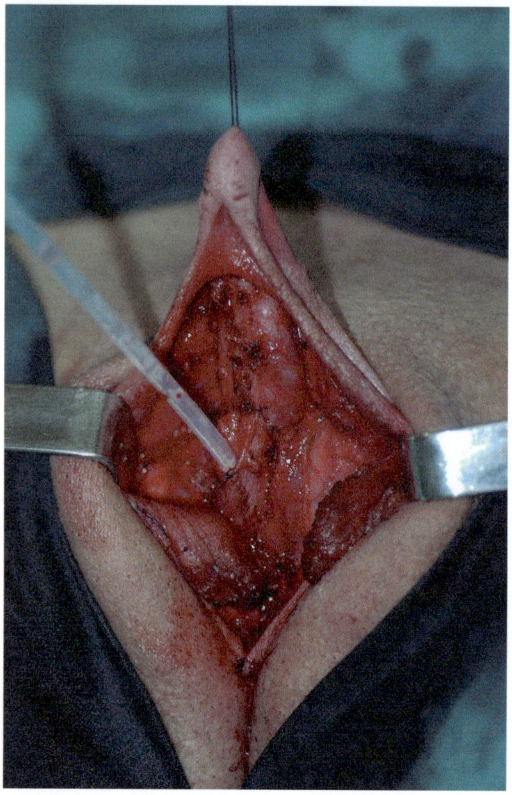

Fig. 29.5 Clitoral lengthening after division of the urethral plate. The proximal part of the urethra is created from a mobilized urethral plate and fixed to the corporal body. The area for de-epithelialization of the outer surface of the labia minora is marked

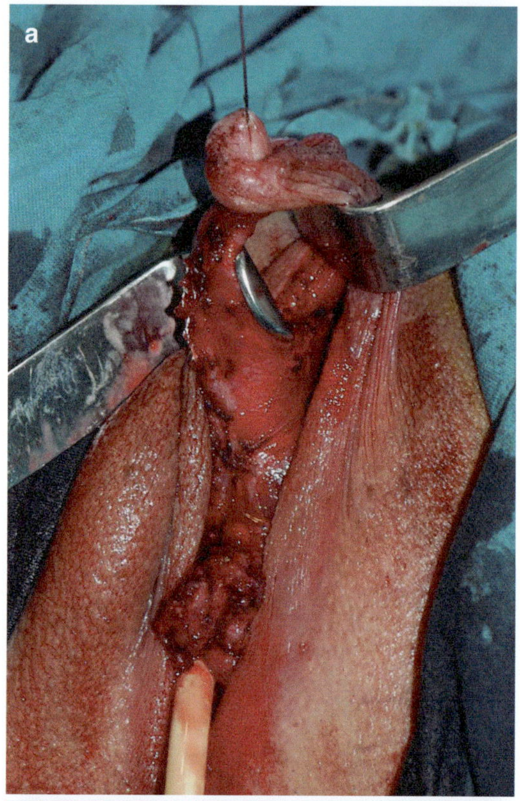

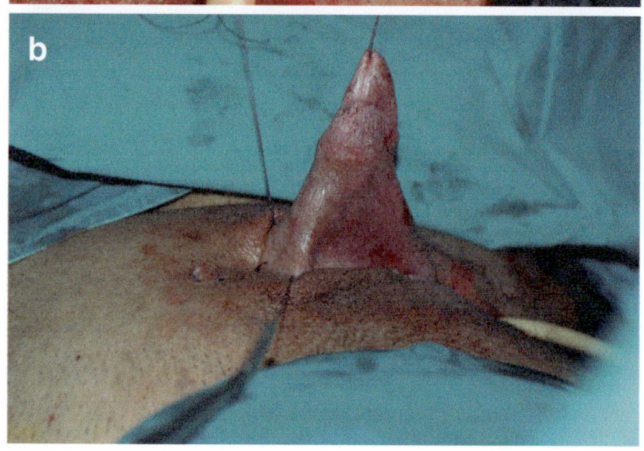

Fig. 29.6 (**a**) Subtotal division of the suspensory clitoral ligament with preservation of the clitoral skin. (**b**) Fixation of the clitoral base skin to the albuginea to prevent retraction

part of the distal neourethra was created using a labia minora flap (Fig. 29.8). The lower parts of the labia minora are detached from their base and mobilized upward; flap vascularity is based solely on deep and superficial external pudendal vessels. The lateral side, together with the edge of one of the labia minora is de-epithelialized and its medial epithelial surface sutured over the quilted buccal/vaginal mucosa graft as an onlay (Fig. 29.9); its proximal part is anastomosed with the vaginal mucosa graft. The edges of the subglandular parts of the prepuce are de-epithelialized and sutured in two layers, creating a wide neourethral meatus at the coronal level (Fig. 29.10). In this way the neourethra is formed. In the remaining 30 patients (32 %) the urethra was created from combined labia minor flaps bilaterally, which are detached proximally, preserving their ventral vascularity from the pudenda externa superficialis and profunda

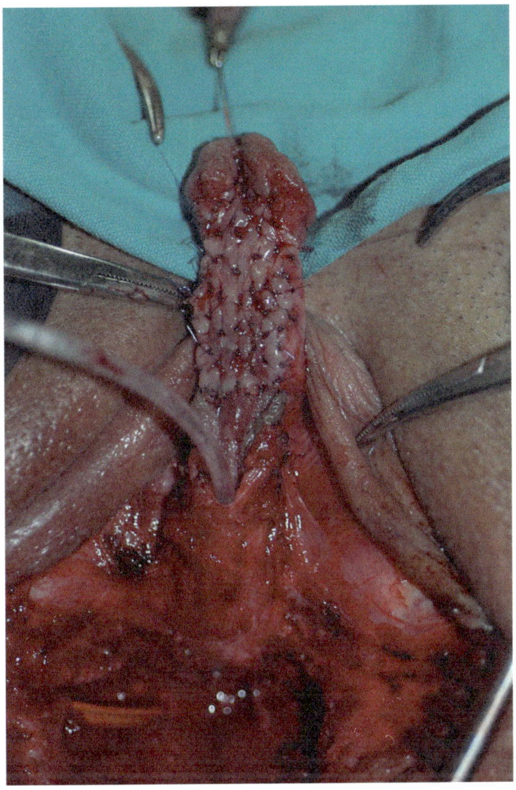

Fig. 29.7 Gap created after division of the urethral plate is covered with a buccal mucosa graft

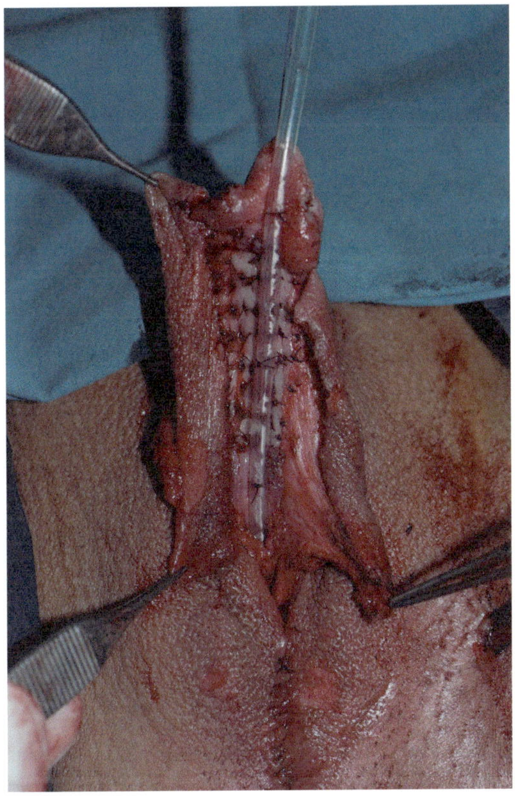

Fig. 29.8 Labia minora flap is pulled distally and fixed to the buccal mucosa laterally

(Fig. 29.11). The flaps are pulled-up distally and one of them fixed to the ventral part of the albuginea, creating the dorsal part of the urethra (Fig. 29.12). On the other side the flap is tubularized ventrally over the contralateral one and a tube is created that is fixed to the urethra proximally and to the glans distally (Fig. 29.13).

The pelvic gap is obliterated by the approaching levators and the perineum is reconstructed in several layers continuing over a proximal neourethral part; the labia majora are mobilized posteriorly as V-shaped flaps and joined in the midline to form the scrotum (Fig. 29.14). Ventral neophallic skin is reconstructed by de-epithelialization of the edge and medial side of the remaining labia minora, and overlapping the pendular neourethra. The two raw surfaces of the labia minora are tucked with several sutures and the skin sutured laterally; in this way, a well-vascularized protective layer for prevention of fistulas is formed and the neophallus is thickened. Testicular prostheses are implanted through oblique lateral incisions above the labia majora to decrease tension on the suture line. In patients with a prominent pubic area, liposuction or lipectomy is carried out to better expose the neophallus. The urethra is stented with a Foley silicone catheter Ch12 for 2–3 weeks and suprapubic urinary drainage is placed for approximately 3 weeks. Broad spectrum antibiotics are administered postoperatively for 7 days. A specially designed vacuum device is advised for at least 6 months, starting 4 weeks postoperatively, to lengthen the neophallus during the healing process.

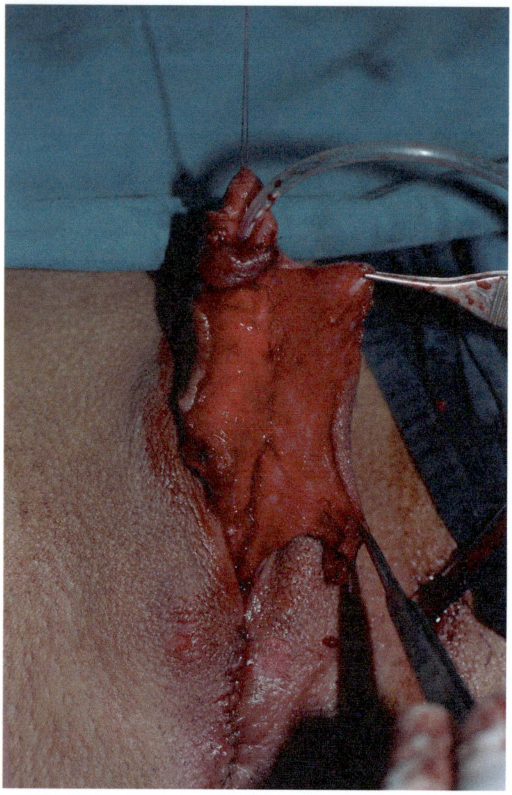

Fig. 29.9 Labia minora flap (LMF) over a buccal mucosa graft onlay (BMG) for pendular urethra reconstruction. The de-epithelialized outer surface of the other LMF is visible

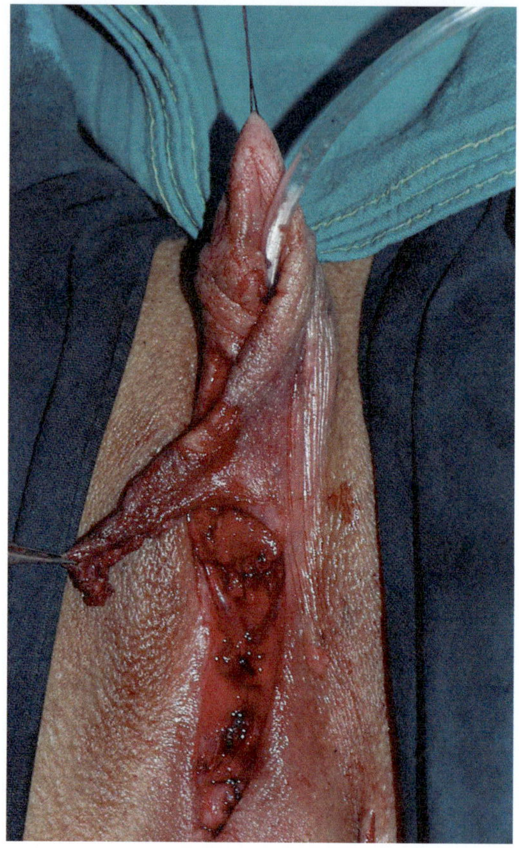

Fig. 29.10 The de-epithelialized flap is used to cover the urethra to prevent fistulas

29.3 Results

Follow-up ranged from 1 to 114 months (mean 47). Neophallus length ranged from 2.5 to 7 cm (mean 4 cm) in a stretched position (Fig. 29.15). Voiding in a standing position was reported in all but 12 patients (13 %). Protective and orgasmic sensitivity was unchanged in all patients. Temporary spraying of urine during voiding was reported by 18 patients and resolved spontaneously in all by 3–6 months after surgery. Twelve patients (13 %) developed fistulas after infection and 9 (10 %) short strictures on anastomosis between the vaginal and labial flaps, probably because of impaired vascularity. They were treated by minor additional surgery and normal voiding was re-established in all. Voiding uroflowmetry was within the normal range (14–28 mL/s) in all patients, including patients with complications after repair (controlled in 37 patients). Six patients (6 %) had testicular prosthesis protrusion, which required removal and later reimplantation (Fig. 29.16).

29.4 Discussion

Despite many advances in the understanding and treatment of transgender patients, one-stage female to male SRS remains a very challenging and demanding task. One of the alternative operative techniques for these patients is metoidioplasty with simultaneous removal of internal genitalia. In some cases, breast removal is performed in the same stage. This procedure provides creation of small male-like external genitalia and voiding in a standing position.

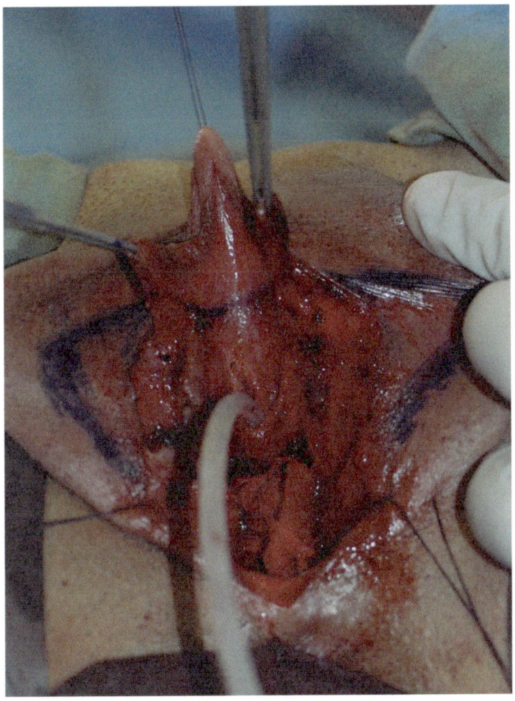

Fig. 29.11 The labia minora flaps are marked bilaterally

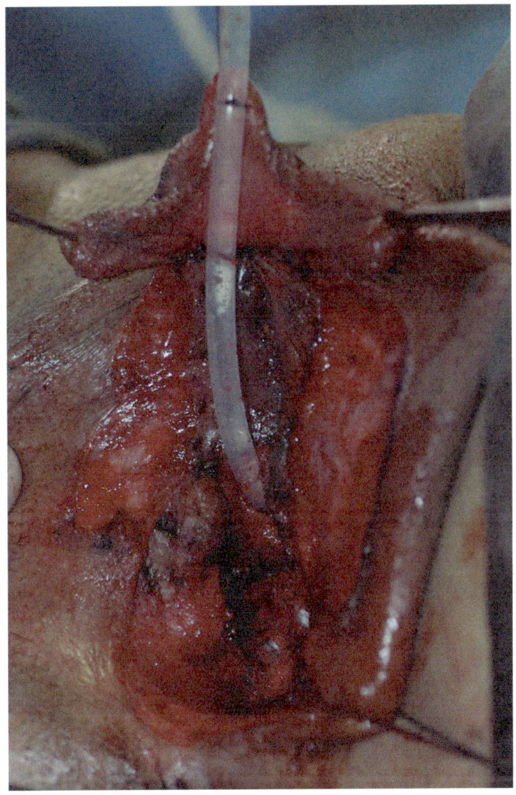

Fig. 29.13 The other flap is used as an onlay

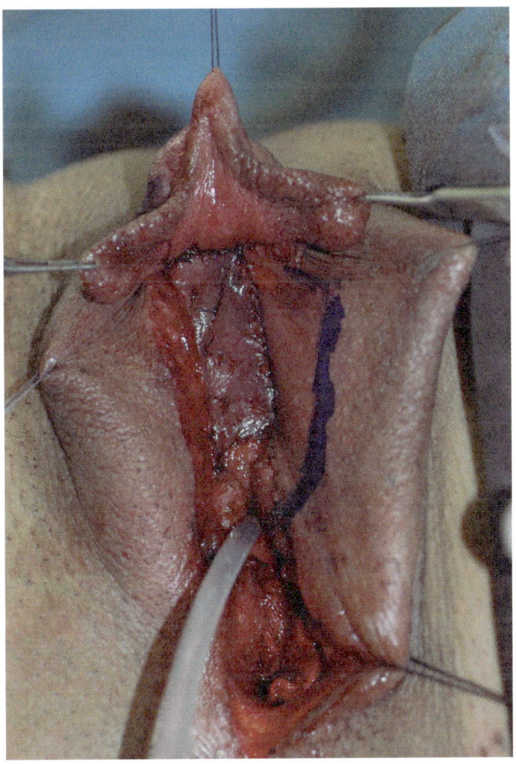

Fig. 29.12 The right flap is fixed to the clitoral body

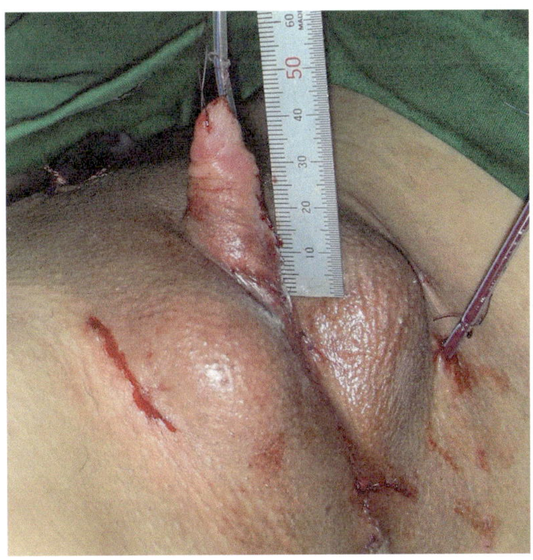

Fig. 29.14 Appearance at the end of surgery

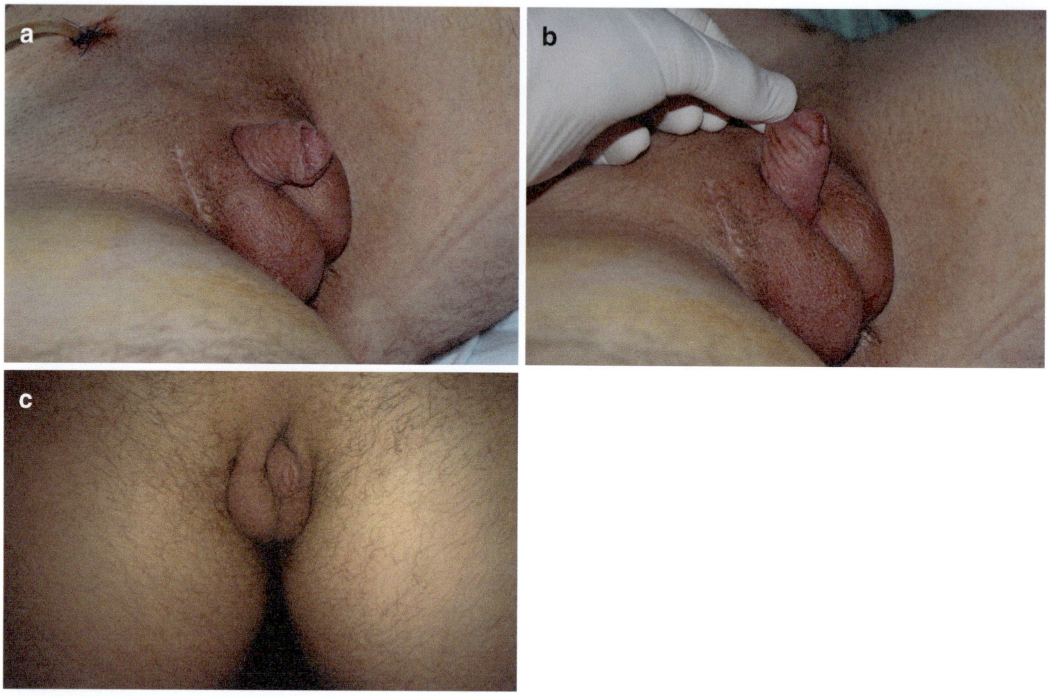

Fig. 29.15 (**a**–**c**) Late outcome after metoidioplasty

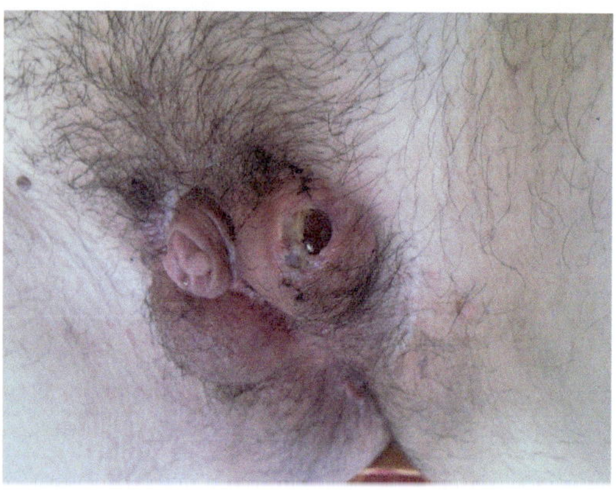

Fig. 29.16 Testicular implant protrusion

There are very few published data on this technique. Lebovic and Laub first introduced the main principles of the procedure and named it metoidioplasty [3]. Later, Hage and Turnhout published their modification with long-term outcome [4]. We also developed our variant of metoidioplasty, but outcomes led us to search for new improvements, mainly based on our experience in the repair of perineal hypospadias with penoscrotal transposition [1, 2].

The goal of reconstruction is to create as large a neophallus as possible with satisfactory cosmesis and a competent neourethra. To achieve this, it is important to understand some of the anatomical particularities of the clitoris that are different from the penis and try to correct them [5]. During our work, we noticed two features that strongly attach the clitoris to the pubic symphysis and shorten its length: the "urethral plate," which bends and pulls the clitoris down, and the suspensory ligament, which differs from the analogous structure in males because it inserts over the dorsal side of the clitoris – up to the subcoronal level. Thus, the clitoris is stretched between these two structures and pulled toward the symphysis; their release is the mean rationale for its straightening and lengthening. We also noticed that releasing the most proximal part of the ligament causes descent of the clitoris because of its already low position under the symphysis and decreases the possibility of voiding in a standing position; for this reason we always preserve it. Also, female transgender patients often have more prominent pubis and buttocks, which makes neophallic exposure more difficult.

Creation of a neourethra after urethral plate division is a much more demanding task owing to the formed gap and the need to make the distal, pendular part of the urethra. Previously, we used a tubularized longitudinal dorsal penile skin flap transposed ventrally by a button-hole maneuver. A common drawback of this technique was the lack of remaining skin for neophallic coverage and the complications of tubularized urethroplasty [1]. This is why we started to create a "composite" pendular neourethra, i.e., a dorsal graft/ventral flap urethroplasty to preserve more skin. In the beginning, we used solely an inlay buccal mucosa graft, which is the most popular and proven technique for urethral replacement [6]. The inner side of the labia minora flap is used as an onlay over the mucosal inlay. It is hairless, elastic and well-vascularized, receiving blood from three sources: the superficial and deep external pudendal as well as perineal arteries. During flap mobilization, its lower part with perineal vessels is cut from the base, but its vascularity is always excellent because of abundant collaterals.

The other advantage of this approach is decreased invasiveness, since we perform complete degloving and suspensory ligament release via the lateral approach, without circumferential clitoral skin incision. In this way, the problem with neophallic shaft coverage is avoided. A peno-pubic angle is created by fixing the clitoral base skin to the remaining deep part of the suspensory ligament using a mattress suture; this maneuver stretches the skin over the entire pendular part of the neophallus, which enhances its exposure, i.e., visible length. Reconstruction of the ventral skin is easily performed by overlapping the pendular neourethra with the opposite labia minora, which is medially de-epithelialized; in the same way, it provides coverage of the neourethra with thick, well-vascularized tissue, at the same time thickening the penis.

Creation of a scrotum from the labia majora and implantation of testicular prostheses is another important issue for the formation of male-like external genitalia. The lower parts of the labia major are mobilized and medially rotated to create a saccular scrotum. Implants should be positioned in the upper part of the labia, just under the neophallic base to avoid a too low position – if implants are positioned further down they are subject to increased external pressure and the risk of wound dehiscence and protrusion through the suture line. To avoid this, an oblique incision for their implantation is made well above their position and they are placed through the subcutaneous channel of the labia majora. Regarding the final outcome of this technique, the majority of patients were satisfied with the male-like appearance of their genitalia and with voiding in a standing position.

Metoidioplasty, compared with other phalloplasty techniques, involves a shorter hospital stay, minimal donor site morbidity, and entirely retains erogenous sensitivity; however, it creates a very short phallus that is barely capable of sexual penetration, if at all.

Conclusions

Metoidioplasty with simultaneous removal of internal genitalia is a one-stage, time-saving procedure. Preconditions are a large enough clitoris for the creation of a male-like neophallus and a scrotum, and normally developed labia minora. The technique is demanding and meticulous with many details, but it can provide a outcome that can satisfy the majority of patients if performed properly. We recommend it as a good choice for female transgenders whose only requirements are male-like external genitalia and voiding in a standing position.

References

1. Perovic SV, Djordjevic M (2003) Metoidioplasty: a variant of phalloplasty in female transsexuals. BJU Int 92(9):981–985
2. Perovic S, Vukadinovic V (1992) Penoscrotal transposition with hypospadias: 1-stage repair. J Urol 148:1510–1513
3. Lebovic GS, Laub DR (1999) Metoidioplasty. In: Ehrlich RM, Alter GJ (eds) Reconstructive and plastic surgery of the external genitalia. WB Saunders Co., Philadelphia, pp 355–360
4. Hage JJ, Turnhout WM (2006) Long-term outcome of metoidioplasty in 70 female to male transsexuals. Ann Plast Surg 57(3):312–316
5. Patterson JM, Chapple CR (2008) Surgical techniques in substitution urethroplasty using buccal mucosa for the treatment of anterior urethral strictures. Eur Urol 53(6):1162–1171. Review
6. Baskin LS, Erol A, Wu Li Y, Hui Liu W, Kurzrock E, Cunha GR (1999) Anatomical studies of the human clitoris. J Urol 162:1015–1020

Surgical Therapy: Phalloplasty with Suprapubic Flap, Pryor's Technique

30

Carlo Bettocchi and Marco Spilotros

Several surgical techniques are available to fashion a neophallus in female-to-male patients. The majority of studies on this topic report satisfactory outcomes with few complications for each of the individual procedures rating mainly the aesthetical appearance, the ability to void while standing, and the capacity to perform penetrative sexual intercourse.

The ideal surgical technique should be a one-stage procedure allowing cosmetically and functionally acceptable results to both patient and partner. Furthermore the fulfillment of a competent neourethra represents a challenging procedure in sex reassignment surgery (SRS) for those patients who require to void while standing [1]. The scar in the donor area is one of the main issues related to phalloplasty, and according to the technique performed, the defect can be more evident.

The surgical procedure available can be classified as (1) metoidioplasty, (2) pedicled flap, and (3) free flaps (radial artery forearm flap, anterolateral thigh flap, and latissimus dorsi flap). Metodioplasty [2] is a simple procedure but leads to less satisfactory results. With this technique the clitoris, hypertrophic after the hormonal treatment, is tailored to create a microphallus. The advantage of this technique, when compared to the others, is that it does not leave any scars outside the genital area and makes the patient possible to void in standing position; the main disadvantage is that it does not allow the creation of a neophallus of satisfactory dimension.

The radial artery phalloplasty (RAP) and the anterolateral thigh (ALT) flap phalloplasty are procedures characterized by a remarkable aesthetic results of the phallus, but patients end up with an evident scar on the arm and thigh, respectively. During RAP and ALT, a neourethra can be fashioned at the same time and generally is joined up to the native one during the following stage. The abdominal flap is a pedicled flap and represents an ideal procedure for patients with an adequate amount of abdominal fat: it is a straightforward operation characterized by reasonable results and an acceptable scar in the lower aspect of the abdomen. Compared to the creation of a free flap, it has a reduced complication rate considering that, keeping its own blood supply, microanastomosis is not performed. Another advantage lies in the possibility of performing the hysterectomy with bilateral salpingo-oophorectomy during the same procedure through the abdominal incision. Despite that few considerations are mandatory, with this approach the neourethra cannot be created at the same time and, if needed, a free-flap urethroplasty can be performed in a second stage [3, 4]. Furthermore abdominal scars resulting from previous surgery can cause

C. Bettocchi (✉) • M. Spilotros
Department of Urology, Policlinico,
University of Bari, Bari, Italy
e-mail: carlo.bettocchi@uniba.it

C. Trombetta et al. (eds.), *Management of Gender Dysphoria: A Multidisciplinary Approach*,
DOI 10.1007/978-88-470-5696-1_30, © Springer-Verlag Italia 2015

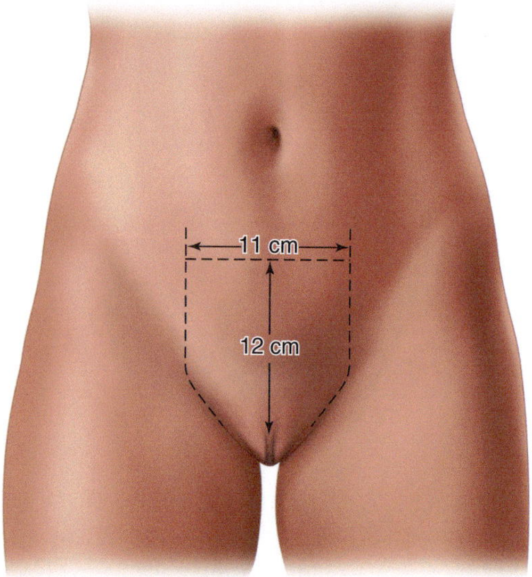

Fig. 30.1 Schematic representation of the abdominal flap prior to its rise [4]

a reduced blood supply with partial necrosis of the flap.

30.1 Pryor's Technique

The patient can be placed in a modified lithotomy or supine position. The flap is drawn on the anterior abdominal wall measuring 12 cm in length from the base of the clitoris and 11 cm in girth as shown in Fig. 30.1.

The flap is then mobilized from the distal edge to the base: during this phase it is important to lift up the skin and the subcutaneous tissue down to the fascia of the rectus abdominis muscle in order to keep a satisfactory blood supply for the whole surface of the flap. In order to achieve a reasonable girth at the base of the phallus without tension in this area it is mandatory to fully mobilize this portion trying to preserve and include the superficial external pudendal vessels into the base of the phallus (Fig. 30.2).

Once the flap is lifted up, it is tubularized to fashion the neophallus. The success of this procedure is related to the blood supply coming from the base of the flap and to the pressure inside the phallus: for this reason the redundant

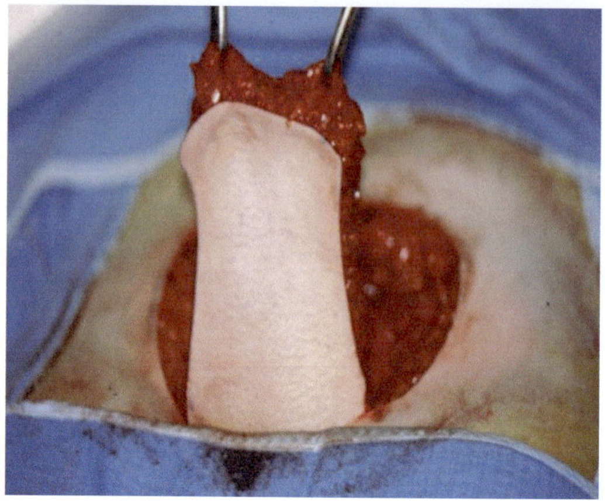

Fig. 30.2 Abdominal flap before tubularization

fat should be removed to reduce the tension before suturing the edges.

The complete exposure of the fascia of the rectus abdominis muscle at this stage of the procedure allows performing a hysterectomy with salpingo-oophorectomy through a U-shaped incision of the fascia that allows having a good exposure of the uterus.

The abdominal incision can be closed mobilizing an advancement flap from the upper abdomen that is pulled till the base of the phallus, but in thin patients the available tissue could not be enough. For this reason, in order to close the incision with minimal tension, two lateral abdominal flaps can be rotated medially in addition to the above mentioned advancement flap. In the postoperative period the complete rest with both legs bent toward the abdomen for 48 h is mandatory to decrease the tension along the abdominal suture line, while the sutures are removed 2 weeks after surgery.

The Pryor technique is a reliable approach to create a phallus with satisfactory cosmetic results and reduce morbidity of the donor area. The positive aspect of this treatment is represented by a relative ease compared to a free flap: performing this technique the possible risks related to the complication of the microanastomosis are avoided. Furthermore the absence of scars on the arm or on the thigh (evident instead when a free flap is raised from these donor areas) represents another reason why patients choose this treatment.

The negative aspect is represented by a less enthusiastic appearance of the neophallus compared to the RAP and ALT and by the need of an additional procedure to incorporate a neourethra into the phallus if the patient requires voiding while standing. To reach this purpose several techniques have been adopted and, according to the author's experience, the radial artery urethroplasty can be a valid option [5]. With this technique the phallic urethra is reconstructed in its total length and is joined to the native urethra during the following procedure. During this procedure the skin of one side of the clitoris and an omolateral strip of skin of the major labia are mobilized and tubularized around a Foley catheter connecting the native urethra and the phallic urethra. The suture line is then covered with a Martius flap to reduce the risk of fistula formation. Garaffa et al. [5] performing this technique reported an overall satisfaction rate of 92 % with the ability to void from the tip of the phallus in all patients and minimal morbidity of the donor site. At the same time, for patients that do not want any female part left behind, the clitoris can be buried into the base of the phallus to maintain erogenous sensation and the vagina can be completely removed.

In order to improve the cosmesis and the functional outcomes of the phalloplasty, glans sculpting can be performed and, as the last step of the SRS, a penile implant can be inserted into the neophallus.

Glanuloplasty can be performed during the following stage. There are several techniques with controversial results in terms of cosmetic outcome and complications. At the moment, the most commonly used procedure is the Norfolk modification of the Munawar technique [6]: with this approach the tip of the phallus is incised circumferentially and a skin flap is lifted up and folded to recreate the shape of a glans. The incision on the neophallus is then covered with a split-thickness skin graft raised from the abdomen (Fig. 30.3).

The insertion of a penile implant can provide an adequate rigidity for sexual intercourse: inflatable implant is generally preferred rather than semirigid one due to the increased risk of erosion with the latter [7]. The bottom of each cylinder is covered with a Dacron sock which is sutured to the pubic bone with nonabsorbable suture to fix the prosthesis. The same material can be used to cover the tips of the cylinder to decrease the risk of erosion. Despite the technical improvement of the procedure of the prosthesis, the risk of malfunctioning and infection of the device is about 10 times higher than in normal patients [7].

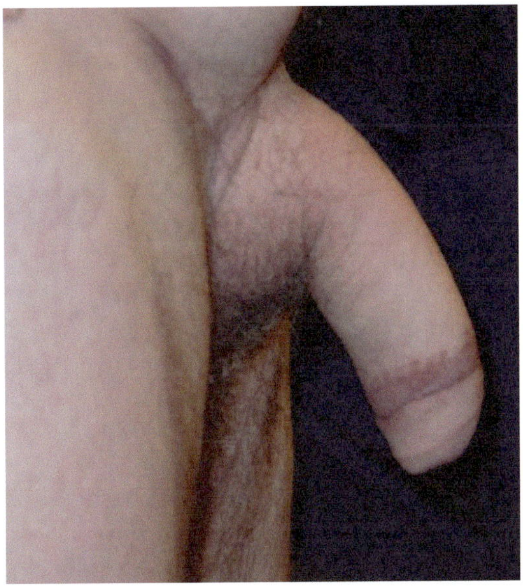

Fig. 30.3 Final result after glans sculpture

30.2 Outcomes and Complications

The cosmetic appearance of the phallus is satisfactory in 95 % of the patients [8]. The abdominal scar is generally minimal; it can be easily concealed with clothes and it is less evident than the scar on the arm and thigh after RAP and ALT, respectively. The survival of the pedicled flap relies on the blood supply from the base of the phallus and on the absence of scars from previous procedures. In this case it is suggested to mobilize the flap without lifting it up in order to check the survival of the flap; 3 months after this procedure, in case of absence of complications, the flap is tubularized to create the phallus.

Tactile sensation on the phallus is preserved while the erogenous sensation is based on the stimulation of the clitoris. The urinary function is satisfactory, and in previous series all patients undergoing urethral reconstruction could void while standing with 92 % satisfaction rate [5]. The main risk of the urethral reconstruction is fistula and stricture formation: in case of total phalloplasty and urethroplasty at the same stage, the incidence rate can reach 58 % [9].

In the two-stage technique these complications are slightly less common: stricture has been reported in 44 % of patients (meatus 25 %, distal urethra 17 %, perineal urethra 4 %) and fistula in 42 % of patients [10]. The incidence of perineal fistula can be further decreased by using the Martius flap or performing a vaginectomy [4].

References

1. Hage JJ, de Graff FG (1993) Adressing the ideal requirements by free flap phalloplasty. Some reflections on refinements of technique. Microsurgery 14:592–598
2. Hage JJ (1996) Metaidoioplasty: an alternative phalloplasty technique in transsexuals. Plast Reconstr Surg 97(1):161–167
3. Bogoras N (1936) Plastic construction of penis capable of accomplishing coitus. Zentralbl Chir 14:1271–1276
4. Bettocchi C, Ralph DJ, Pryor JP (2004) Pedicled pubic phalloplasty in females with gender dysphoria. BJU Int 95:120–124
5. Garaffa G, Christopher AN, Ralph DJ (2010) Total urethral construction with the radial artery-based forearm free flap in the transsexual. BJU Int 106(8):1206–1210
6. Rong-Hwang F, Yi-Sheng K, Shiuh M, Jin-The L (1998) Glans sculpting in phalloplasty: experience in female to male transsexuals. Br J Plast Surg 51(5):376–379
7. Hage JJ, Bouman FG, De Graaf FH, Bloem JJA (1993) Construction of the neophallus in female-to-male transsexuals: the Amsterdam experience. J Urol 149:1463–1468
8. Terrier JE, Courtois F, Ruffion A et al (2014) Surgical outcomes and patients' satisfaction with suprapubic phalloplasty. J Sex Med 11(1):288–298
9. Rohrmann D, Jakse G (2003) Urethroplasty in female-to-male transsexuals. Eur Urol 44:611–614
10. Hage JJ, Bloem JJ (1993) Review of the literature on construction of the a neourethra in female-to-male transsexuals. Ann Plast Surg 30:278–286

Surgical Therapy: Total Phalloplasty Using Latissimus Dorsi Flap

31

Rados P. Djinovic

31.1 Introduction

Sex reassignment surgery in female-to-male transgender patients presents the most demanding tasks in genitalia reconstruction. It includes removal of female and creation of male external genitalia. Male genitalia has unique characteristics with complex anatomy, and creation of their substitute using present surgical techniques is still far from ideal. Despite achievement of satisfactory esthetic and functional result (regarding voiding and sexual function), we cannot really say that we can create "normal" penis with both flaccid and erect state and good erogenous sensation. Russian surgeon Borgoras has done the first described total phalloplasty using abdominal pedicle flap in 1936 [1]. This event stimulated other surgeons to search for better solution, describing many techniques that use different free or local flaps [2–6]; however, none of them was able to fulfill all goals of total phalloplasty, i.e., creation of normal-size penis that enables safe prosthesis insertion with good aesthetic appearance with hairless and normal skin color, good tactile and erogenous sensation, and competent neourethra with meatus at the top of the glans, all of this together with acceptable donor site morbidity.

The most widely used flap for total phalloplasty nowadays is the radial forearm flap [2, 4], but it has many weaknesses, such as unsightly donor site scar, very frequent urethral complications, small size that does not allow safe prosthesis insertion in many patients, and too soft consistency, often with pale skin. Those were the main reasons why we, searching for better solution, started to use musculocutaneous latissimus dorsi free transfer flap, which can satisfy most of the abovementioned requirements. Latissimus dorsi is a very reliable flap, often used in plastic reconstructive surgery for different indications (ref.). In urology it was used in atonic bladder for its overlapping flap, which provides better bladder emptying [7–9]. The flap has suitable anatomy (i.e., good size, volume, and length of neurovascular pedicle) to meet esthetical and functional needs for phallic reconstruction. It can be also used successfully in pediatric population [10].

31.2 Patients and Methods

In the period between February 2005 and January 2014, total phalloplasty using musculocutaneous latissimus dorsi flap was performed in 216 transgender patients aged between 18 and 58 years (mean 26 years). Patients with other indications are excluded from this number. All patients were

R.P. Djinovic
School of Medicine, Belgrade University,
Belgrade, Serbia

"Sava Perovic Foundation" – Center for Genito-Urinary Reconstructive Surgery,
Borisavljeviceva 58, Belgrade 11000, Serbia
e-mail: djinovic@gmail.com

C. Trombetta et al. (eds.), *Management of Gender Dysphoria: A Multidisciplinary Approach*,
DOI 10.1007/978-88-470-5696-1_31, © Springer-Verlag Italia 2015

previously diagnosed by qualified psychologist/psychiatrist and were on hormonal treatment at least 6 months before surgery. The necessary precondition for this technique is a normal BMI (body mass index) in order to avoid creation of too thick neophallus and difficult urethroplasty.

Donor site was prepared preoperatively in all patients by skin massage with the use of antiscarring ointment at least 1 month before surgery in order to improve skin elasticity and enable direct donor site closure. In six obese patients who failed to lose weight, donor site liposuction was performed at least 3 months before surgery in order to decrease flap thickness and enable its safe tubularization without compromising its blood supply.

Table 31.1 Surgical stages of total phalloplasty using musculocutaneous latissimus dorsi flap

Stages	Surgeries	Time between stages
1st stage	Transvaginal hysterectomy, adnexectomy colpocleisis, proximal urethroplasty, perineoplasty, and scrotoplasty. Neophallus creation using musculocutaneous latissimus dorsi free flap with one-stage urethroplasty	
2nd stage	Two-stage urethroplasty: neourethral plate tubularization. Implantation of testicular implants	3–6 months
3rd stage	Penile prosthesis implantation	3–6 months

31.2.1 Surgical Anatomy

Musculocutaneous latissimus dorsi flap, first described by Baudet et al. [11], is dependable and versatile for free tissue transfer: it is easily elevated with a large surface area, with thoracodorsal artery that provides large, long, and reliable pedicle [12–14]. The subscapular artery divides after 3–5 cm from its origin into two branches, circumflex scapular and thoracodorsal artery, which continue downward, and it is the dominant vessel supplying the flap. There are usually two venae comitantes which join to form a single large thoracodorsal vein prior to entering the subscapular vein. The latissimus dorsi muscle is innervated by the thoracodorsal nerve, a branch of the posterior cervical cord. The neurovascular hilum is positioned 8–9 cm from the axillary artery and enters the deep surface of muscle 1.5–3.0 cm medially from its anterior border. The vessels and nerve usually bifurcate and then run together on the deep surface of the muscle: one main branch runs parallel to anterior while the other one parallel to superior border of the muscle. A large musculocutaneous flap, up to 18 cm wide and 28 cm long, can be raised on a 3–4 cm narrow strip of muscle after dividing several reliable perforators over the anterior intramuscular branch. Also, only the skin flap can be raised by careful mobilization of the pedicle from the muscle.

31.2.2 Surgical Technique

Total phalloplasty using a latissimus dorsi flap is standardly performed in three stages (Table 31.1). The first stage includes also removal of the female genitalia (transvaginal hysterectomy with bilateral adnexectomy, colpocleisis) and urethral advancement till the pubis, perineoplasty, and scrotoplasty in the last 6 years. Previously we did total vaginectomy with removal of full-thickness vaginal muscle, but we gave up on this due to bladder and rectal fall into the perineum because of loosing vaginal muscle support. After this, the patient is repositioned in lateral decubitus using beanbags, with the upper torso placed in a full lateral position at 90° and pelvis tilted at 20–30° to provide access to groins, allowing simultaneous flap harvesting and recipient site preparation. Care is taken that there is neither excessive nor prolonged abduction of the upper shoulder during dissection. Flap planning begins with marking of the anterior and superior muscle border (Fig. 31.1). Projection of thoracodorsal artery is defined and flap design is marked with base positioned over its hilum and extending 6–7.5 cm on either side of the artery. Flap dimensions were created according to normal penile size in adults – 12–15 cm in width and 13–18 cm in length – depending on the patient's wish on one side and fat and muscle thickness on the other.

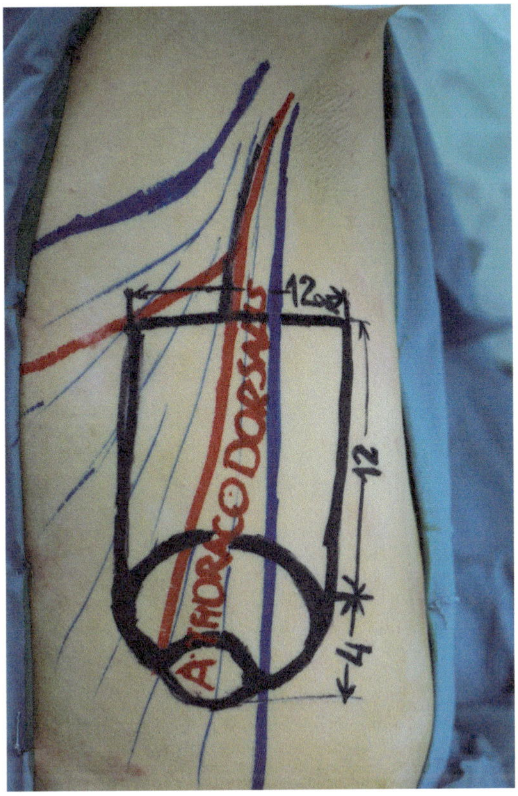

Fig. 31.1 Musculocutaneous latissimus dorsi flap design

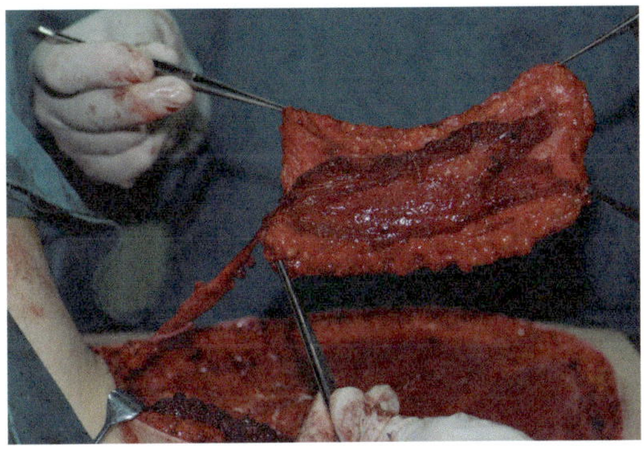

Fig. 31.2 Flap elevation on a long neurovascular pedicle

Flap elevation is started with incision of anterior skin margin down to the deep fascia over the serratus anterior muscle; plane is developed between latissimus dorsi and serratus anterior muscle, using combined sharp and blunt dissection. The flap is divided inferiorly and medially, cauterizing large posterior perforators of the intercostal vessels, and then slowly lifted proximally to expose neurovascular pedicle. The amount of the harvested muscle tissue around the blood vessels depends on fat thickness – in slim patients more muscle is harvested and vice versa. The pedicle surrounded by fatty tissue is identified and dissected proximally up to the axillary vessels (Fig. 31.2). All major branches are identified and carefully ligated using monofilament ligatures, while smaller ones are cauterized. The thoracodorsal nerve is identified and isolated proximally from vessels for the length of 5–6 cm, taking care to preserve its vascularization. During dissection, care is taken to avoid injury of the long thoracic nerve which can cause winging of the scapula. A neophallus is created while the flap is still perfusing on its vascular pedicle: the flap is tubularized fully, leaving 3–4 cm-wide muscle surface exposed ventrally, which is grafted with split-thickness skin graft (STSG) taken from some available skin, most often from the labia minora (Fig. 31.3a, b) but, sometimes, from the long skin flap from clitoral and labia minora skin (Fig. 31.3c). Heparin is administered intravenously, and few minutes later neophallus is detached from the axilla after clamping and dividing the subscapular artery, vein, and thoracodorsal nerve at its origin, in order to achieve maximal pedicle length and wider blood vessel diameter. Donor site defect is closed directly using one or two local rotational flaps (Fig. 31.4a, b). Previously, we used STSG for donor site closure when it was not possible to close it directly, but due to non-satisfactory esthetic result, we started to use rotational flaps instead. In the second stage, the surgical team prepares the recipient site simultaneously – superficial femoral artery, saphenous (or some other local) vein, and ilioinguinal nerve are dissected and mobilized through the oblique inguinal incision. Another, a Y incision is made on the pubis for neophallus attachment, and a wide tunnel is created between two incisions for pedicle placement. After neophallus transfer and its fixation to the recipient area, microsurgical anastomoses are done between the subscapular and femoral artery (latero-terminal) and between

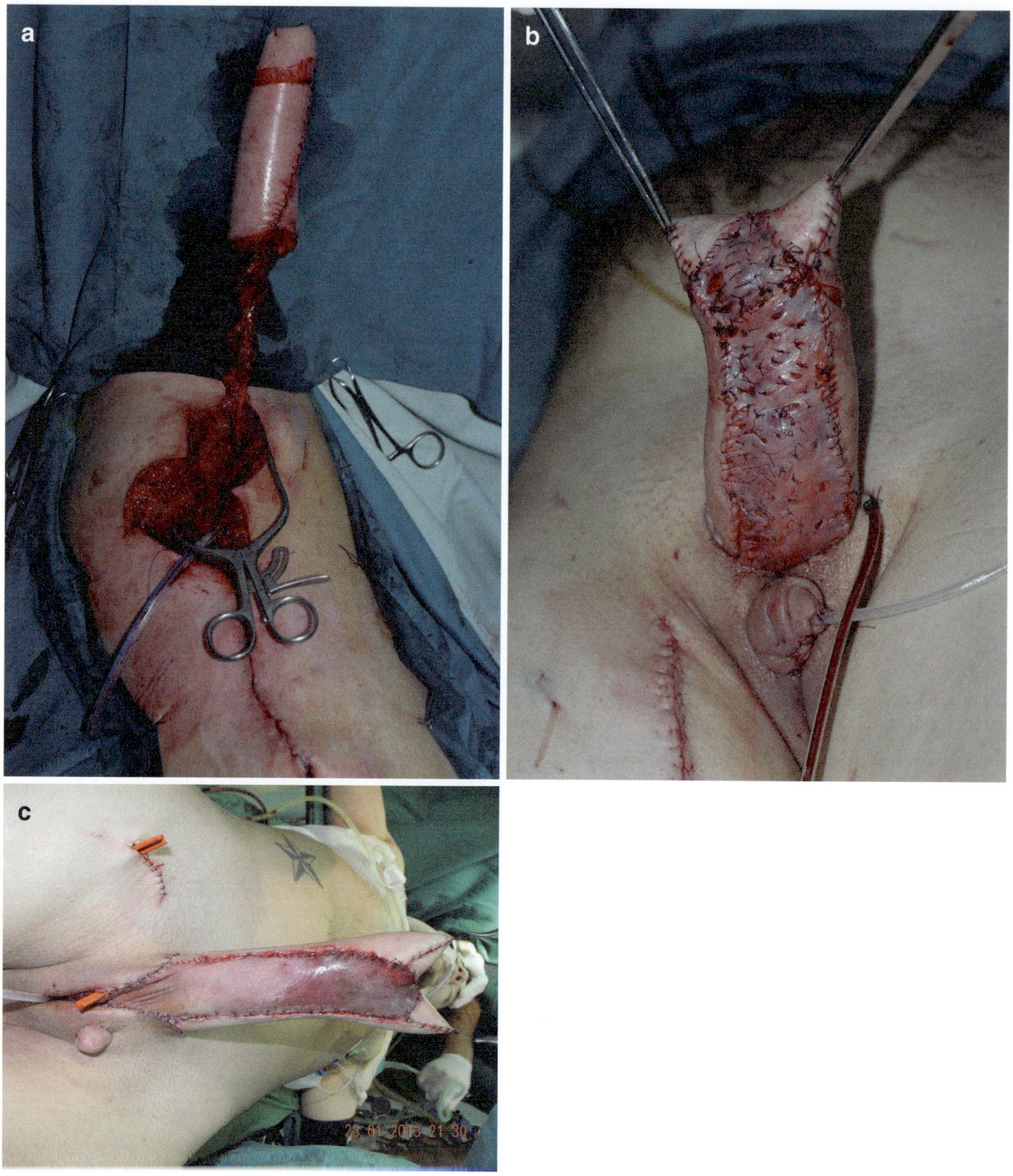

Fig. 31.3 (**a**) On-site neophallus creation, including the glans. (**b**) Ventral flap grafting using STSG. (**c**) Ventral flap covering with long labia minora/clitoral skin flap

the subscapular and saphenous vein (terminoterminal) using operative loops (Fig. 31.5). The epineural microneurorrhaphy is then completed between the ilioinguinal and thoracodorsal nerve (Fig. 31.6). Previously extended proximal urethra is joined to the neourethral plate on the ventral side of the flap. The clitoris with preserved neurovascular bundle is mobilized and fixed at the base of the neophallus for its better stimulation during sexual intercourse. A Foley catheter is inserted for one 2–3 weeks. The neophallus is fixed in an elevated position for 7–10 days to the specially constructed dressing, which is important to prevent pedicle kinking. Flap viability is assessed by clinical examination (i.e., skin color, turgor, and capillary refill).

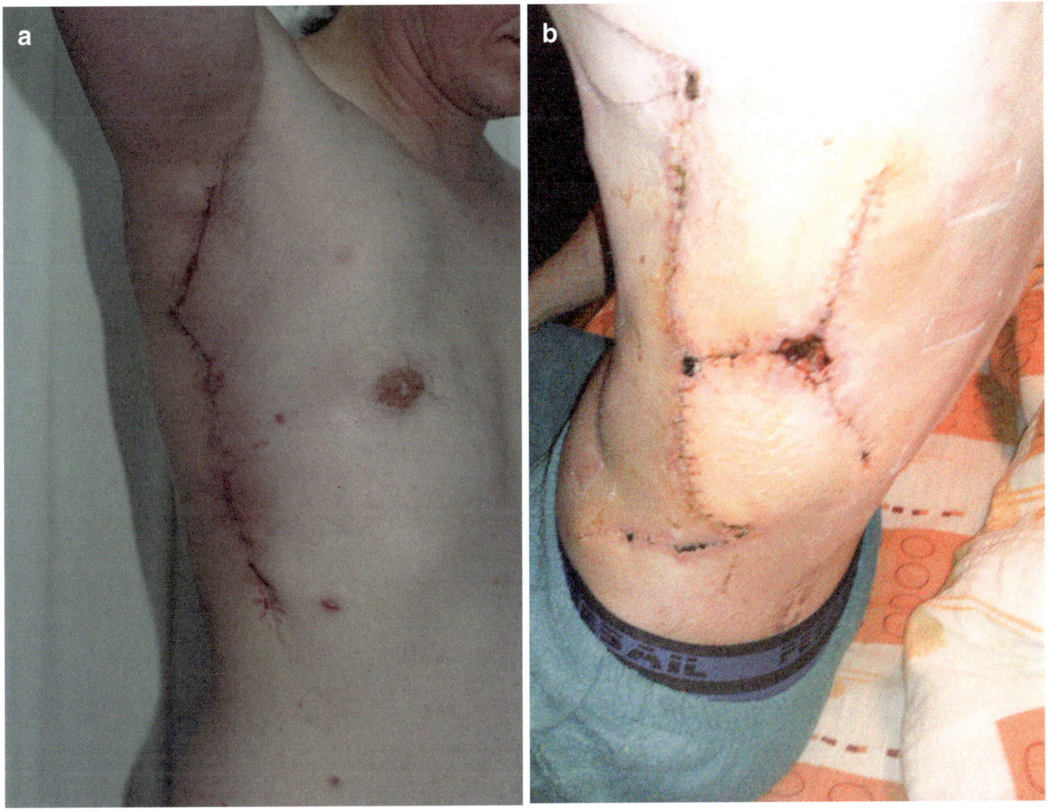

Fig. 31.4 (**a**) Direct donor-site closure. (**b**) Donor-site closure using 2 rotational flaps

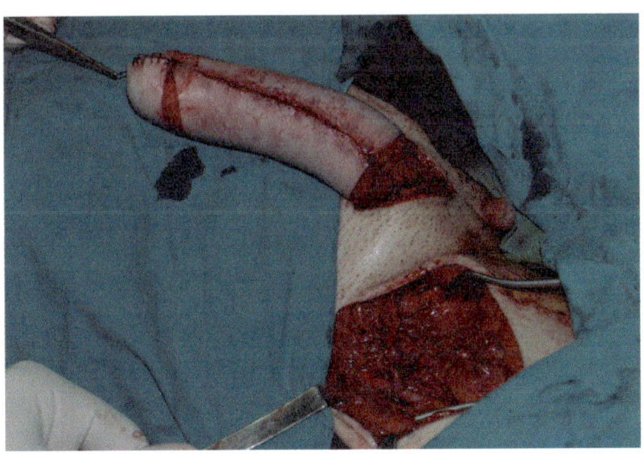

Fig. 31.5 Flap transfer to the pubic region

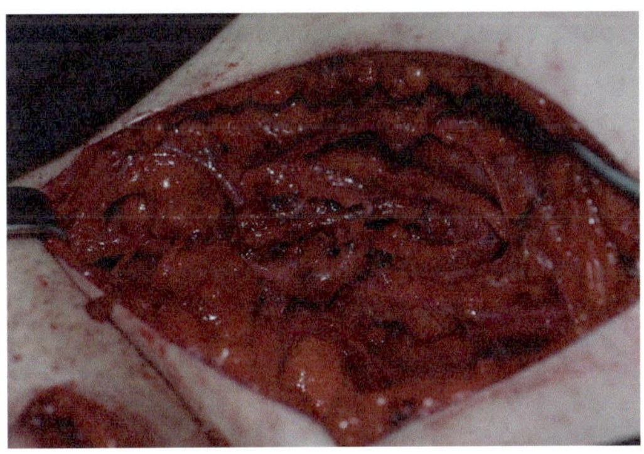

Fig. 31.6 Microsurgical anastomoses

The second stage includes tubularizing urethroplasty over 14 Ch silicone Foley catheter and is performed at least 6 months after first surgery; in the majority of patients penile urethra was joined with proximal part of the neourethra, but in some, which were on the risk for urethral stricture, small fistula was leaved for voiding at their junction, while penile part is dilated for few months and then joined in the next stage (Fig. 31.7). Care is taken to avoid overlapping of urethral and skin suture lines. The neophallus is created by tubularization, with glans designed and created over the distal 4–6 cm of the flap by tangential skin cutting and joined subdermally

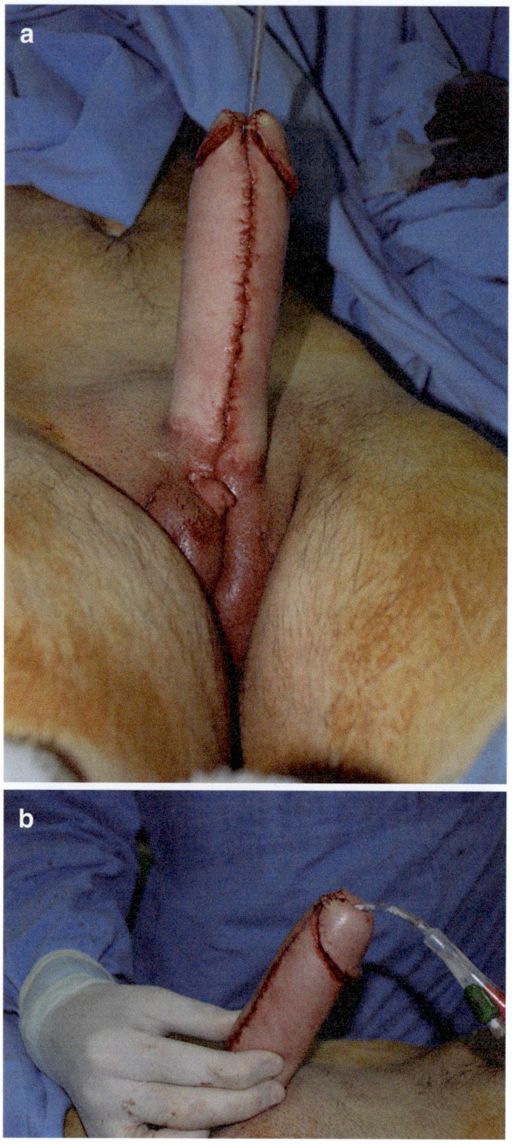

Fig. 31.7 (**a**, **b**) Tubularized flap after the second stage

with the proximal part (Fig. 31.7b). In this stage, testicular implants are usually implanted. Suprapubic catheter is placed for 3–4 weeks. Patients start to void 3–4 weeks after completion of urethroplasty. After healing is finished, neophallus already will have its definitive shape (Fig. 31.8a–c).

In the third stage, implantation of penile prosthesis is performed through infrapubic approach. In majority of patients, a 3-piece inflatable prosthesis with two cylinders is implanted. The flap is detached partially from the pubis and contralaterally from the pedicle, and tunnels are created in the phallus on both sides using Hegar dilators at the border between the muscle and fatty tissue, taking care to avoid urethral damage and not to go too distally. Spaces are also created close to pubic rami for prosthesis base fixation. Reservoir is placed paravesically. The proximal and distal neotunica sleeves are created by enveloping cylinders/rods with hernia mesh, which are then fixed to the periosteum of the inferior pubic rami (Fig. 31.9a, b).

Some patients did not want to have urethroplasty due to concern of complications that were the most common. In some of them, perineostomy was created, while some wanted to have both metoidioplasty and phalloplasty at the same time – this way complications bonded with long urethra through the neophallus are avoided, and they are able to void in standing position (Fig. 31.10a, b).

31.3 Results

Follow-up was 4–99 months (mean 58 months). All stages are performed in 167 patients; additional 15 patients underwent also urethroplasty, 5 patients wanted only perineostomy, 8 wanted metoidioplasty with phalloplasty, while the remaining 21 were waiting for the prosthesis implant. Urethral stricture developed in 32 patients – in the majority in the penile part, but in 5 also at the junction between the proximal and penile urethra. Nine patients developed consequent urethral diverticulum at the pubic part. All but 4 of them are treated surgically. Urethral fistula developed in 8 patients – in 2, it healed spontaneously, while in the remaining 6, it was closed surgically. Penile prosthesis is implanted in 172 patients – in 117, inflatable three-component; in 12, two-component; and in the remaining 43, malleable. Two cylinders are implanted in all patients. Nine patients did not want penile prosthesis implantation. Penile size varies from 12 to 26 cm in length and from 11 to 17 cm in circumference. Five partial and 4 total flap losses occurred. Donor site healed satisfactorily in 194 patients, while in

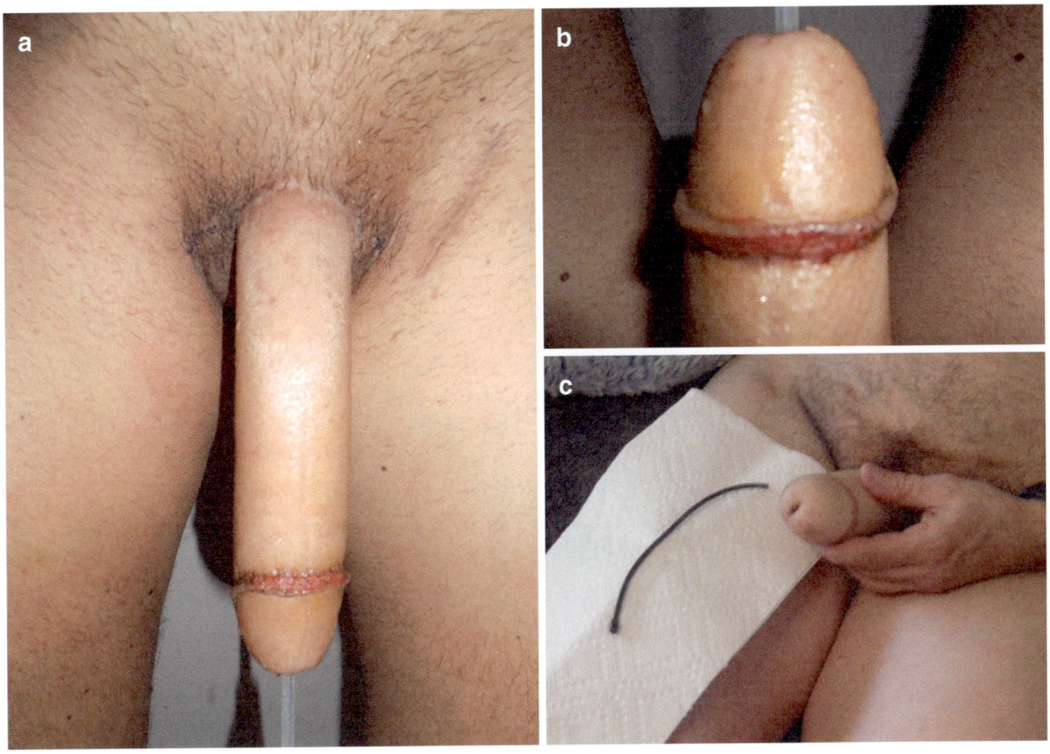

Fig. 31.8 (**a**–**c**) Appearance after the second stage healing

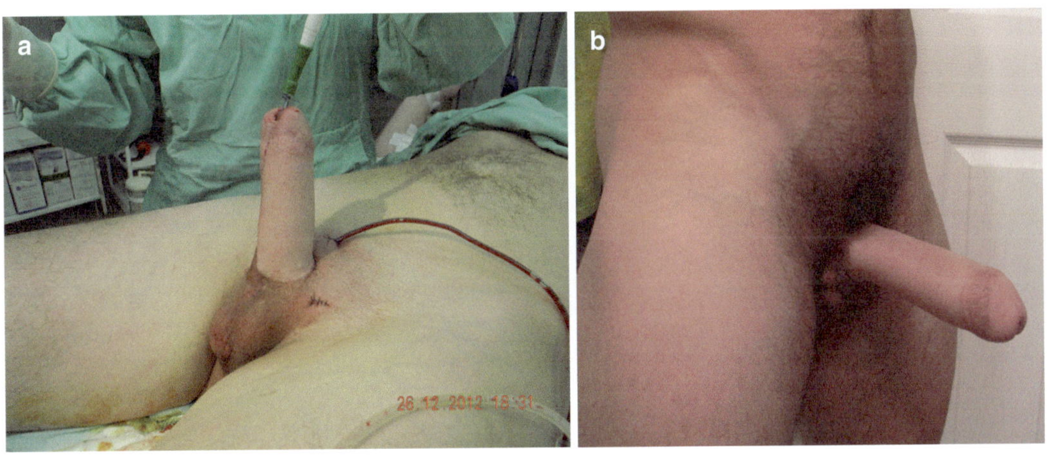

Fig. 31.9 (**a**, **b**) End surgical and final outcome after the third stage

the remaining, mild to moderate scarring occurred. 59 patients required additional scar correction in the second or third stage. Infection with prosthesis removal was present in 11 patients, prosthesis protrusion in 7, malleable prosthesis braking in 6, inflatable prosthesis dysfunction in 4, and misplacement that needed revision in 8.

31.4 Discussion

Penile reconstruction in transsexual patients presents great task and challenge for the surgeon who deals with genital reconstruction. Indications for phallic construction are growing; initially, they were limited to posttrauma victims who required

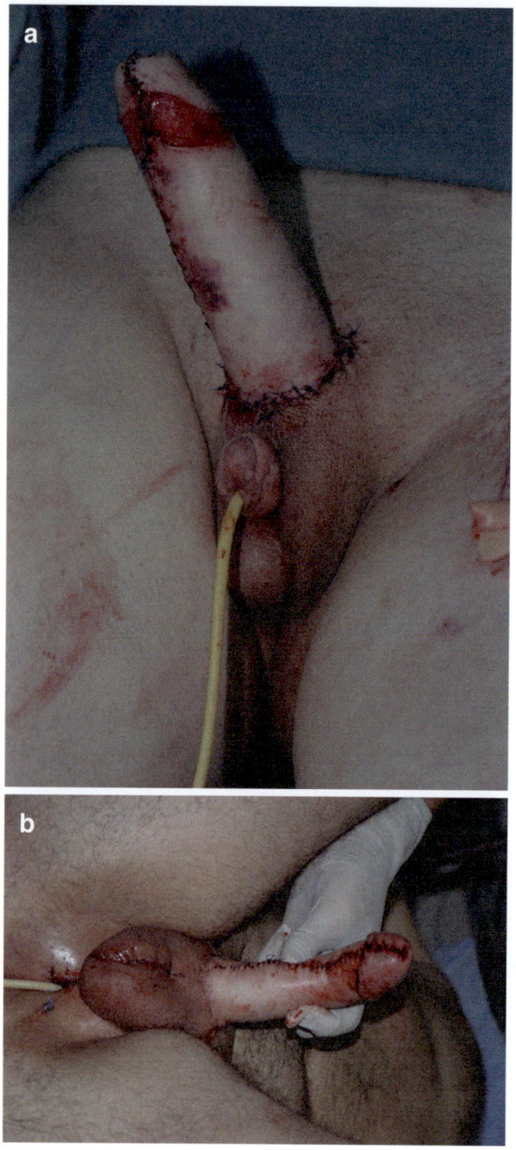

Fig. 31.10 (**a**) Combined total phalloplasty and metoidioplasty. (**b**) Total phalloplasty with perineostomy

surgery to retain their male anatomy. Today, indications are expanded to many other disorders such as penile agenesis, micropenis, intersex conditions, epispadias or hypospadias, and transsexualism. The penis is a unique organ of the male body characterized by the presence of a vascularized urinary conduit surrounded by erectile tissue and capacity to achieve erogenous sensibility, making completely successful phallic construction elusive at present. An ideal phalloplasty would include one surgical stage, protective and erogenous sensibility, esthetic resemblance, volume enough to place a protected prosthesis, sufficient rigidity to allow sexual intercourse, patency of the neourethra, and low donor-site morbidity. However, many different surgical techniques are reported using available local vascularized tissues or microvascular tissue transfer [15]. After initial experience with local [16] and free flaps [17], we developed technique for total phalloplasty using the musculocutaneous latissimus dorsi free transfer flap that, in our opinion, gives the most satisfactory phalluses. The main advantage of this flap is its large surface area that gives excellent penile size – large enough to allow urethroplasty as well as penile prosthesis implantation. Moreover, penile size can be made according to the patient's wish.

Musculocutaneous latissimus dorsi flap is easily elevated on a very long and reliable pedicle that allows creation of direct anastomosis with femoral artery without interposition of venous graft. Removal of the muscle is associated with minimal weakness which is rarely of functional significance [14], especially when only thin muscle strip is harvested as in our technique. Creation of the neoglans gives satisfactory esthetic appearance. Neophallus retraction and discoloration of the musculocutaneous flap are less likely than of the fasciocutaneous one.

Donor site can be closed directly in most of the patients with satisfactory outcome if it is prepared appropriately by superficial skin massage using some skin-softening cream to improve skin elasticity. We also perform liposuction of the donor area in obese patients several weeks before flap harvesting in order to decrease flap bulkiness and allow its tubularization.

Penile prosthesis implantation is technically easier and better tolerated in a neophallus which contain muscle inside [18]. Disadvantage could be mild protective sensitivity of the neophallus that presents a risk for prosthesis protrusion, but we solved this problem by enveloping of the proximal and distal part of cylinders/rods with hernia mesh and their fixation to the pubic bones. The issue of sexual function in the neophallus remains problematic since the flap lacks orgasmic sensitivity; it is restricted to the clitoris with preserved dorsal nerve bundle incorporated at the base of the neophallus. Strong motivation as well as good partner's cooperation is mandatory for successful sexual intercourse.

Functional repair, patient satisfaction, and quality of life are main goals in total phalloplasty. The musculocutaneous latissimus dorsi flap provides excellent neophallic size with good esthetic appearance. It allows easy implantation of penile prosthesis as well as sexual intercourse in all cases, which is very often the main patient's request. Urethroplasty using buccal mucosa graft is the most appropriate choice.

Conclusions

The use of musculocutaneous latissimus dorsi flap is a reliable technique that allows creation of neophalluses of normal size with good esthetic appearance and functional outcome.

Function of implanted penile prosthesis is satisfactory in all patients, and a great majority of them report successful sexual intercourse. Although neural anastomosis is made between the sensory and motor nerves, slow development of protective sensibility is present in all patients, first felt inside the muscle on pressure and progressing toward the skin. Erogenous sensitivity and orgasm is based on clitoris incorporated at the penile base.

References

1. Borgoras NA (1936) Plastic Reconstruction of penis capable of accomplishing coitus. Zentralbl Chir 63:1271
2. Chang TS, Hwang WY (1984) Forearm flap in one-stage reconstruction of the penis. Plast Reconstr Surg 74:251–258
3. Biemer E (1988) Penile construction by the radial arm flap. Clin Plast Surg 15:425–430
4. Sadove RC, Sengezer M, McRoberts JW, Wells MD (1993) One-stage total penile reconstruction with a free sensate osteocutaneous fibula flap. Plast Reconstr Surg 92:1314–1323
5. Khouri RK, Young VL, Casoli VM (1998) Long-term results of total penile reconstruction with a prefabricated lateral arm free flap. J Urol 160: 383–388
6. Felici N, Felici A (2006) A new phalloplasty technique: the free anterolateral thigh flap phalloplasty. J Plast Reconstr Aesthet Surg 59:153–157
7. Stenzl A, Ninkovic M, Willeit J, Hess M, Feichtinger H, Schwabegger A (1997) Free neurovascular transfer of latissimus dorsi muscle to the bladder acontractility. I. Experimental studies. J Urol 157:1103–1108
8. Stenzl A, Ninkovic M, Kolle D, Knapp R, Anderl H, Bartsch G (1998) Restoration of voluntary emptying of the bladder by transplantation of innervated free skeletal muscle. Lancet 351:1483–1485
9. Stenzl A, Schwabegger A, Bartsch G, Prosser R, Ninkovic M (2003) Free neurovascular transfer of latissimus dorsi muscle for the treatment of bladder acontractility: II. Clinical results. J Urol 169: 1379–1383
10. Djordjevic ML, Bumbasirevic MZ, Vukovic PM, Sansalone S, Perovic SV (2006) Musculocutaneous latissimus dorsi free transfer flap for total phalloplasty in children. J Pediatr Urol 2:333–339
11. Baudet J, Guimberteau J, Nascimento E (1976) Successful clinical transfer of two free thoraco dorsal axillary flaps. Plast Reconstr Surg 58:680–688
12. Lassen M, Krag C, Nielsen I (1985) The latissimus dorsi flap. An overview. Scand J Plast Reconstr Surg 19:41–51
13. Manktelow RT (1986) Microvascular reconstruction. Springer, Berlin/Heidelbergh
14. Cormack GC, Lamberty BG (1994) The arterial anatomy of skin flaps, 2nd edn, revised. Churchill Livingstone, Edinburgh
15. Perovic S (1995) Phalloplasty in children and adolescent using the extended pedicle island groin flap. J Urol 154:848–853
16. Gilbert DA, Jordan GH, Devine CJ Jr, Winslow BH, Schlossberg SM (1993) Phallic construction in prepubertal and adolescent boys. J Urol 149:1521–1526
17. Gilbert DA, Jordan GH, Schlossberg SM, Winslow BH (1999) Forearm free flap for pediatric phallic reconstruction. In: Erlich RM, Alter GJ (eds) Reconstructive and plastic surgery of the external genitalia. W.B. Saunders Company, Philadelphia, pp 327–334
18. Hoebeke P, de Cuypere G, Ceulemans P, Monstrey S (2003) Obtaining rigidity in total phalloplasty: experience with 35 patients. J Urol 169:221–223

Surgical Therapy: Chest Wall Contouring for Female-to-Male Transsexuals

32

Vittorio Ramella, Giovanni Papa, and Zoran Marij Arnež

32.1 Introduction

The contouring of the *chest wall* is usually the first surgical step in female-to-male transsexuals. Its aim is to transform the female chest in one with a male appearance. It is usually the most sought after procedure in female-to-male transsexuals and the one that is performed almost on every patient with this gender disorder, as it provides the most visible result and has major implications in daily social interactions.

Sometimes, it is the only surgical procedure desired and required by the patient, and it has a high postoperative satisfaction rate [1].

A multidisciplinary approach leads to better results in transsexual patients [2]: in our practice, we often combined it with hysterectomy and bilateral salpingo-oophorectomy performed by the gynaecologist to minimize the total number of surgical procedures.

V. Ramella (✉) • G. Papa, PhD • Z.M. Arnež, PhD
Plastic and Reconstructive Surgery, Ospedale di Cattinara, Strada di Fiume 447, Trieste 34149, Italy
e-mail: vittorio.ramella@aots.sanita.fvg.it; giovanni.papa@aots.sanita.fvg.it; zoran.arnez@aots.sanita.fvg.it

32.2 Preoperative Planning

The goals of the ideal chest wall contouring have been established by Hage et al. in the 1990s [3, 4]:

- Removal of breast tissue and excessive skin
- Repositioning and remodelling of the *nipple-areola complex* (NAC)
- Minimization of chest wall scars

These goals can be achieved by careful patient evaluation:

- Breast volume (small, medium or large)
- Breast ptosis and excess skin
- NAC size and position
- Skin elasticity (can be reduced by previous breast binding) [5]
- Inframammary fold (usually lower than in a male chest)
- Patient body mass index (BMI)

In patients with large breasts, the technique that gives the best result is the mastectomy with free nipple-areola complex grafting [5]. The resulting scar is positioned lower or higher on the chest, based on the breast size/ptosis and the initial position of the *inframammary fold.*

For medium- and small-sized breasts, there are two options, based on breast volume and NAC position relative to the inframammary fold (depending on previous breast binding). In young patients with elastic skin and a NAC positioned cranially to the inframammary fold, we use a semicircular technique: after the removal of the mammary gland, the skin adapts to the contour of

C. Trombetta et al. (eds.), *Management of Gender Dysphoria: A Multidisciplinary Approach*,
DOI 10.1007/978-88-470-5696-1_32, © Springer-Verlag Italia 2015

the underlying pectoral muscle. If the NAC is positioned caudally to the inframammary fold, even in young patients with elastic skin, the semicircular technique should not be used. In this case the skin will not adapt, and there will be an excess with a poor aesthetic result. If the breast ptosis is moderate, the skin excess can be reduced with a concentric circular technique and the NAC lifted and repositioned.

32.2.1 Nipple-Areola Complex Positioning and Size

The NAC position in a normal male chest wall has been described by many authors [6–10]. In our experience, the best way to determinate the right spot is to follow the anatomical structures of the thorax. The sternocostal head of the pectoralis major muscle arises from the anterior part of the sternum, the superior six costal cartilages and the abdominal aponeurosis, and it converges with the clavicular head into a common insertion on the bicipital groove of the humerus. Its inferior-lateral border starts horizontally from the sternum and then shifts obliquely towards the shoulder. The NAC should be positioned where this border shifts from horizontal to oblique.

To ensure the correct position, the preoperative markings should be drawn prior to surgery with the patient in erect position and with the upper limbs at sides. In this position, the patient contracts the pectoralis major muscle to aid locating the angle between the horizontal and oblique vector of the inferior-lateral border of the muscle.

In patients with larger breasts and higher BMI, the mammary gland displaces upwards the overlying adipose tissue and skin. If the position is marked preoperatively on a standing patient, the final position will be lower.

Usually, also the NAC morphology is different: in the female, both the nipple and the areola are bigger. The female areola is circular, while the male one is oval, about 3×2 cm in size and with the main axis oriented in a latero-medial way [7].

If the original areola is very big (6 or more centimetres) and the nipple is about 1–2 cm, the grafting can be very challenging, as the defatted nipple alone would be big enough to reach the size of a male NAC. In these cases, an alternative option would be to graft a lateral part of the areola and position a cartilage graft or a cutaneous bud under the dermis to reconstruct the nipple.

32.3 Surgical Techniques

With every surgical technique, it is important to remove the whole mammary gland but preserve the subcutaneous fat to avoid depression/retraction of the skin [5]. The thickness of the skin flaps should be consistent with the other body parts and thus with the patient's BMI. The patients should be informed that scars in the sternal and thoracic region have an increased risk of becoming hypertrophic or even keloidal.

32.3.1 Mastectomy with Free Nipple-Areola Complex Grafting

Mastectomy with free NAC grafting (Fig. 32.1) was the first technique described for chest wall contouring in female-to-male transsexuals [11–13]. During the preoperative planning and marking, the position of the upper limbs of the patient is very important. As we can see in Fig. 32.2, the NAC position changes when the upper limbs are positioned at 90° as during the operation. Due to this fact, the preoperative markings should always be done in an orthostatic position with the upper limbs completely adducted. In this position, both the lower and upper limits of the amputation are marked.

To achieve an aesthetically pleasing result, the scar is more important than the survival of the grafted NAC. The scar should be positioned on the border between two aesthetic units of the male chest, on the lower border of the pectoralis major muscle, and it should follow its profile also laterally, where it will go obliquely towards the anterior pillar of the axilla.

In patients with high BMI and breasts with a large base, the markings should extend laterally to avoid the creation of lateral dog-ears.

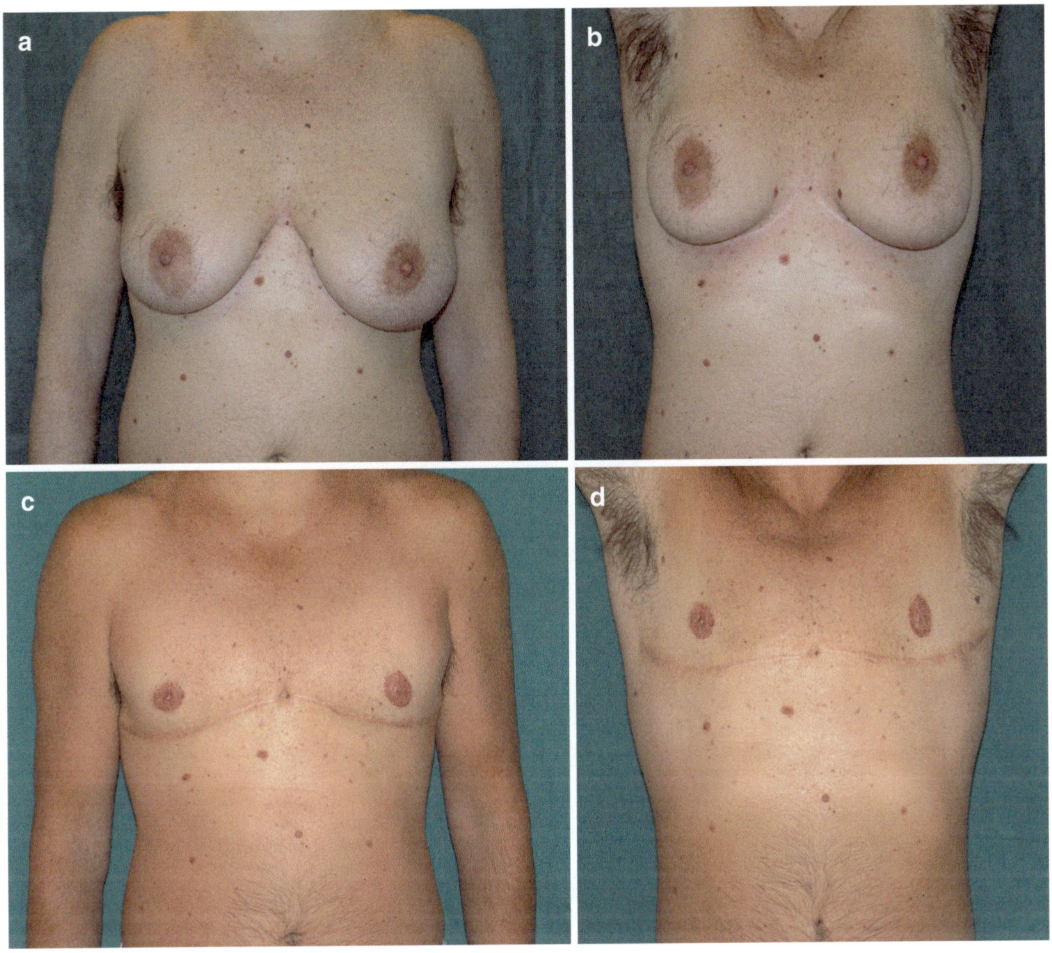

Fig. 32.1 Mastectomy with free nipple-areola complex grafting: (**a**, **b**) preoperative view; (**c**, **d**) postoperative view

Even with careful preoperative planning, they can still occur, but they are easy to correct in a secondary outpatient procedure. In these patients, care must be taken to avoid the joining of the median portion of the resulting scars, as this will make them even more visible. Even if small dog-ears arise intraoperatively, they can be left in place as they will usually disappear in the following months with a good morphologic result.

The tension between the two adipocutaneous flaps is evaluated with the patient's forearms positioned horizontally on his head by trying to join the upper and lower markings. If the tension is excessive, the upper limit of the excised skin must be lowered until it is reduced or almost eliminated.

The operation starts with the incision and elevation of the planned NAC grafts that are placed in saline-soaked gauzes. The next step is the surgical incision of the lower preoperative marking. Both incisions can be oblique to preserve as much derma as possible and reduce the tension on the skin. The dissection continues caudally until the plane between the pectoralis major fascia and the *mammary gland* is reached, which is followed upwards to the upper pole of the mammary gland. The mastectomy is then completed with the upper incision, which should get to the same plane as the lower one. The axillary tail of the breast is a part of the gland that should not be left in place. That would be wrong from an oncological point of view, and it will cause a very

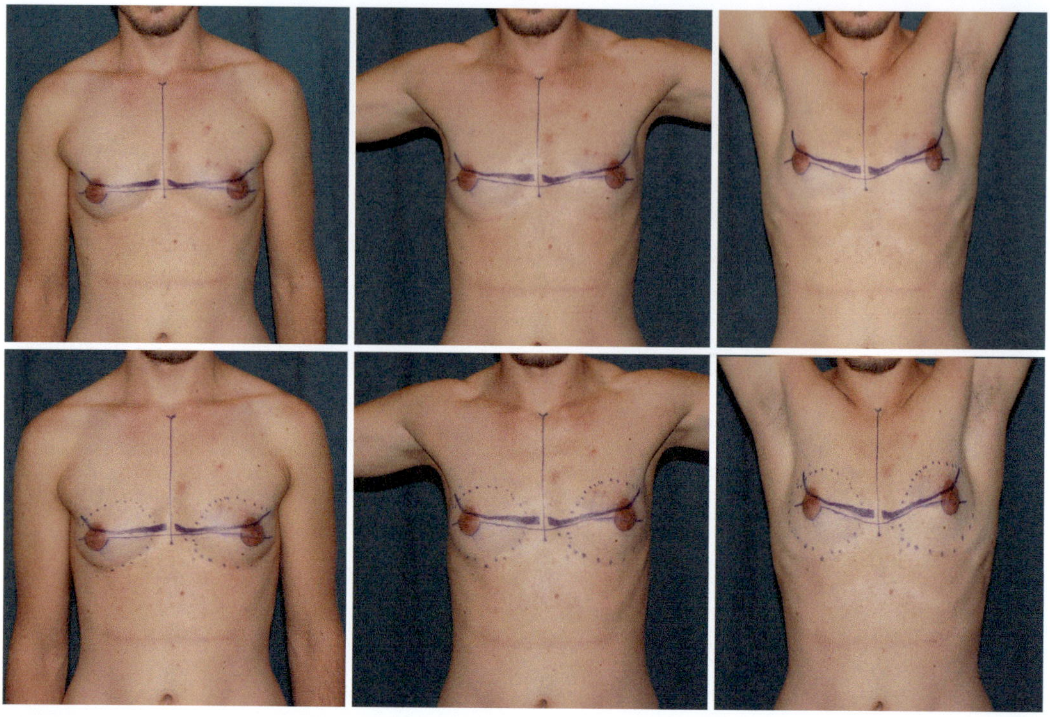

Fig. 32.2 NAC position and mammary tissue distribution changes with different positions of the upper limbs

visible, aesthetically unappealing result. After the mastectomy, the correct new position of the NAC can be double-checked, as the underlying structures are clearly visible, even in patients with higher BMI and less developed muscles.

The flaps on both sides are undermined to allow a tension-free closure. In some patients, the mammary fold has to be released without removing the overlying skin to position the scar and the NAC in the correct anatomic position [5]. After an accurate haemostasis, a drain is placed and the flaps are sutured. If the preoperative markings were correct, the suture should be on the lower border of the pectoralis major muscle. The NAC is defatted, as a thinner graft has a better chance of taking. The receiving bed is deepithelialized and the NAC positioned and secured in place with a tie-over suture over a paraffin gauze, which will stay in place for 5 days to allow the process of graft taking to complete. An *elastic bandage* is applied at the end of the operation that should be kept continuously by the patient for at least a month [5].

The drains are removed as soon as the amount of drainage is 30 cc or lower in 24 h. The sutures (usually intradermal) are removed 14 days postoperatively.

32.3.2 Semicircular Technique

The *semicircular* mastectomy technique (Fig. 32.3) was first described by Webster [14] for gynecomastia and is the best choice in small to medium breasts with good elasticity and without excessive ptosis. A well-distributed medium-sized mammary has a NAC that is central to the breast mound and thus just 2–3 cm from the male position. The skin elasticity will allow the surgeon to create a male-looking chest without additional scars on the skin.

In this surgical technique, the only incision is done on the lower border of the areola between the skin and the areola. In very small areolas, the incision can be extended laterally to form an inverted omega.

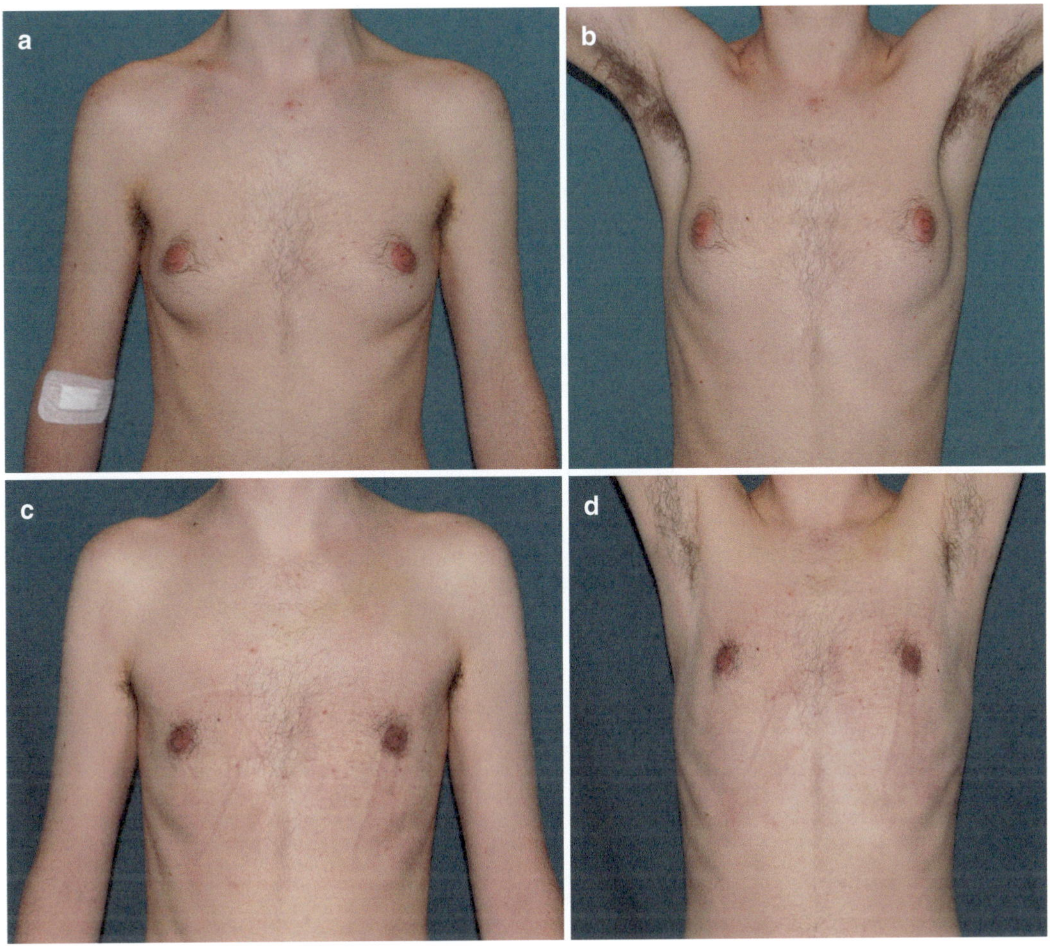

Fig. 32.3 Semicircular technique: (**a**, **b**) preoperative view; (**c**, **d**) postoperative view

With this access, it is possible to get to the inframammary fold and severe the breast gland insertions inferiorly. After doing so, the avascular plane of lax areolar tissue between the fascia of the pectoralis major muscle and the mammary gland should be found. By following this plane, the whole mammary gland can be raised from the underlying structures without significant bleeding. The mastectomy is then completed by dissection on the superficial plane between the gland and the overlying adipose tissue.

Due to the small surgical access, care must be taken to avoid traumas to the perforators of the mammary artery on the sternal side of the mastectomy, as they will be very difficult to locate and coagulate or ligate.

Lighted retractor blades are very useful in this procedure and should be used, if available, both during and after the mastectomy to double check the haemostasis. This is very important to avoid excessive postoperative bleeding that can potentially cause haematomas. To reduce the visibility of the final scar, we usually remove about 1 mm of skin and areola along the incision, as it has been traumatized during the surgical procedure. The skin is closed with simple interrupted sutures that will be removed 2 weeks later. An elastic bandage is applied at the end of the procedure, but there is less compression, compared to mastectomy with free NAC grafting. To avoid excessive pressure that could lead to partial or total necrosis, no additional gauzes are positioned on the NAC.

32.3.3 Round Block: Concentric Circular Technique

The *concentric circular technique* (Fig. 32.4) used in female-to-male transsexuals is very similar to the technique described for gynecomastia [15]. In our experience, it is usually associated with the semicircular and can be seen as a variation of this technique. It aims to reduce both the mammary gland and the overlying skin without doing a full mastectomy. It can be used in patients that have small- to medium-sized breasts with a minimal amount of ptosis that the semicircular technique alone cannot correct. In patients with asymmetrical breasts, both techniques can be used together to achieve a better result. The round block can be used also as a secondary corrective procedure.

With the concentric circular technique, the skin in excess and areolar tissue is reduced by deepithelialization with a pattern, made of concentric circles or ovals to reposition the NAC in the correct male position (which is usually higher compared to a female breast).

Due to the different diameter of the neo-areola and the skin that should be sutured together, the scar will not be uniform with the skin profile – festoons will form to compensate the difference.

As the areola is very elastic compared to the skin, it will usually enlarge in the following months. This should be kept in mind during the preoperative planning and marking. Both the festoons and the areola stretching can be corrected with a secondary procedure, but even that cannot always provide a perfect morphologic result.

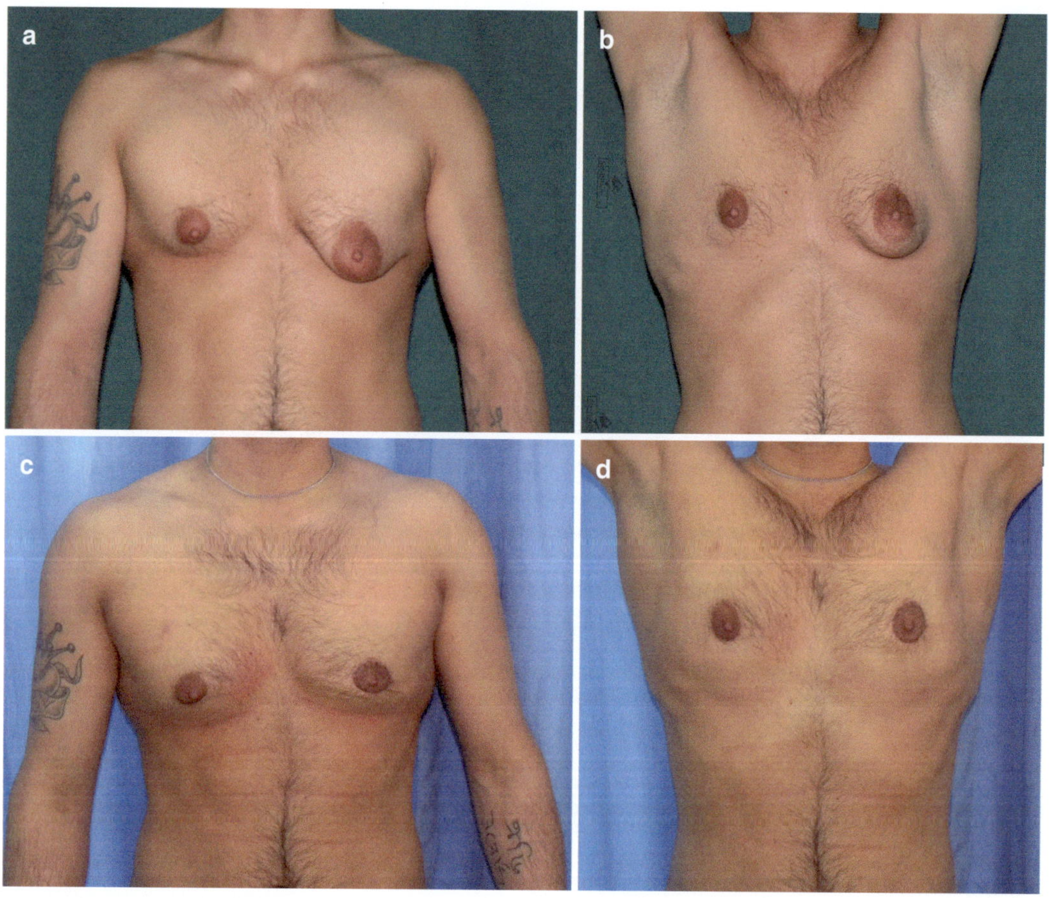

Fig. 32.4 Concentric circular technique: (**a**, **b**) preoperative view; (**c**, **d**) postoperative view

32.3.4 Complications and Their Management

Postoperative bleeding that causes a *haematoma* can arise as a life-threatening complication that should be treated with an immediate reoperation, removal of the clotted blood, coagulation or ligation of the bleeding vessels. Seromas can also occur but are usually treated conservatively.

Small wound dehiscences are treated conservatively with dressings, while bigger ones can be treated with a small revision in an outpatient setting. Partial or total loss of the NAC is treated conservatively in the immediate postoperative period. After the stabilization of the scar (6 months to 1 year after the operation), the dyschromic area (usually hypopigmented) is corrected with a tattoo.

If the nipple is too big after the primary procedure, it can be reduced by removal of the distal part and/or part of the nipple [5].

References

1. Nelson L, Whallett EJ, McGregor JC (2009) Transgender patient satisfaction following reduction mammaplasty. J Plast Reconstr Aesthet Surg 62(3): 331–334
2. Monstrey S, Hoebeke P, Dhont M, De Cuypere G, Rubens R, Moerman M, Hamdi M, Van Landuyt K, Blondeel P (2001) Surgical therapy in transsexual patients: a multi-disciplinary approach. Acta Chir Belg 101(5):200–209
3. Hage JJ, Bloem JJ (1995) Chest wall contouring for female-to-male transsexuals: amsterdam experience. Ann Plast Surg 34:59
4. Hage JJ, Kesteren PJM (1995) Chest-wall contouring in female-to-male transsexuals: basic considerations and review of the literature. Plast Reconstr Surg 96:386
5. Monstrey S, Selvaggi G, Ceulemans P, Van Landuyt K, Bowman C, Blondeel P, Hamdi M, De Cuypere G (2008) Chest-wall contouring surgery in female-to-male transsexuals: a new algorithm. Plast Reconstr Surg 121(3):849–859
6. Atiyeh BS, Dibo SA, El Chafic AH (2009) Vertical and horizontal coordinates of the nipple-areola complex position in males. Ann Plast Surg 63(5):499–502
7. Beer GM, Budi S, Seifert B, Morgenthaler W, Infanger M, Meyer VE (2001) Configuration and localization of the nipple-areola complex in men. Plast Reconstr Surg 108(7):1947–1952; discussion 1953
8. Shulman O, Badani E, Wolf Y, Hauben DJ (2001) Appropriate location of the nipple-areola complex in males. Plast Reconstr Surg 108(2):348–351
9. Beckenstein MS, Windle BH, Stroup RT Jr (1996) Anatomical parameters for nipple position and areolar diameter in males. Ann Plast Surg 36(1):33–36
10. Murphy TP, Ehrlichman RJ, Seckel BR (1994) Nipple placement in simple mastectomy with free nipple grafting for severe gynecomastia. Plast Reconstr Surg 94(6):818–823
11. Kluzak R (1968) Sex conversion operation in female transsexualism. Acta Chir Plast 10:188
12. Hoopes JE (1974) Surgical construction of the male external genitalia. Clin Plast Surg 1:325
13. Lindsay WRN (1979) Creation of a male chest in female transsexuals. Ann Plast Surg 3:39
14. Webster JP (1946) Mastectomy for gynecomastia through a semicircular intra-areolar incision. Ann Surg 124:557
15. Davidson BA (1979) Concentric circle operation for massive gynecomastia to excise the redundant skin. Plast Reconstr Surg 63:350

Surgical Therapy: Possible One-Step Solutions

33

Nicola Pavan, Francesca Vedovo, Giovanni Liguori, and Carlo Trombetta

33.1 Surgical Therapy

33.1.1 Possible One-Step Solutions

Gender reassignment, which is a comprehensive treatment aiming to alter the phenotype with hormonal therapy and/or surgery, has been demonstrated to be the best solution available for persons affected by gender dysphoria in order to ease their condition, facilitating a person's gender role and altering sex characteristics [1].

Gender reassignment surgery (GRS) is a complex process of surgical procedures, including both genital and nongenital surgery, performed to alter the phenotypic expression of the biological sex in order to alleviate gender dysphoria.

For the female-to-male patient, surgical procedures may include the following:

1. Breast/chest surgery: subcutaneous mastectomy and creation of male chest
2. Genital surgery: hysterectomy/salpingo-oophorectomy; reconstruction of the fixed part of the urethra, which can be combined with a metoidioplasty or with a phalloplasty (employing a pedicled or free vascularized flap); vaginectomy; scrotoplasty; and implantation of erection and/or testicular prostheses (Table 33.1)
3. Nongenital, nonbreast surgical interventions: voice surgery, liposuction, lipofilling, pectoral implants and various aesthetic procedures

Most recent reviews [1, 2] in penile reconstruction for female-to-male patients confirm the difficulty of this peculiar surgery in terms of possible complications and limits of the final achievable outcomes, with surgery necessitating several steps and high number of revision.

Currently, there are several different operative techniques for penile reconstruction. Choices for a specific technique may be restricted by anatomical and surgical considerations [1, 3]. If the patient's goal is a neophallus of good appearance, standing micturition, sexual sensation, and/or coital ability, patients should be clearly informed that surgery would require several separate stages, with technical difficulties and high likelihood of additional operations [1, 3].

Phalloplasty, using a pedicled or a free vascularized flap, is a lengthy, multistage procedure with significant morbidity that includes frequent urinary complications (urinary tract stenoses and fistulas (can be as high as to 20–40 %)), unavoidable donor site scarring, and occasionally necrosis (partial or total) of the neophallus (1–2 %) [1, 2, 4].

Even *metoidioplasty* (clitoris enlargement), which in theory is a one-stage procedure for construction of a microphallus, often requires more than one operation, and standing micturition cannot be guaranteed. Furthermore, metoidioplasty results in a micropenis, without the capacity for

N. Pavan (✉) • F. Vedovo • G. Liguori
C. Trombetta
Urological Department, University of Trieste, Strada di Fiume 447, Trieste 34149, Italy
e-mail: nicpavan@gmail.com; superfv@libero.it; gioliguori@libero.it; trombcar@units.it

C. Trombetta et al. (eds.), *Management of Gender Dysphoria: A Multidisciplinary Approach*, DOI 10.1007/978-88-470-5696-1_33, © Springer-Verlag Italia 2015

Table 33.1 Surgical techniques for female-to-male dysphoria

Surgical technique	Limitations	Benefits
One-step technique	Long operatory time Stiffener required	One surgical solution Ability for sexual intercourse Good cosmetic result
Radial forearm flap	Possible urinary tract complication Multiple stages Stiffener required Microsurgical ability required	Ability for sexual intercourse Good cosmetic result
Anterolateral thigh flap	Similar limitation of radial forearm flap	Easier to hide the donor site disfigurement
Fibula flap	Permanent erection Similar limitation of radial forearm flap Extrusion risk increased Infection risk increased	No need of prosthesis
Suprapubic flap/groin flap	Cosmetic appearance unsatisfactory	
Latissimus dorsi flap	Urinary tract not reconstructed Erection function based on muscle contraction? Donor site morbidity Sexual and tactile sensitivity not reported No long-term follow-up available Microsurgical skills required	No need of prosthesis?

standing urination or sexual intercourse [1, 2]. Finally, erectile function is difficult to achieve. The radial forearm flap requires an inflatable penile prosthesis, with a considerable failure/revision rate. When a latissimus dorsi myocutaneous free flap is used, sexual intercourse is possible by contraction of the muscle, which stiffens, but shortens, the penis, with no need of an inflatable implant. Flaps harvested with bone (e.g. fibula and osteocutaneous radial forearm flap) do not need stiffeners, but this flap type results in a permanent erection [1].

For these reasons, many female-to-male transsexuals never undergo genital surgery other than hysterectomy and salpingo-oophorectomy [5].

Theoretically, the ideal female-to-male sex reassignment surgery should be a *one-stage procedure*. The resulting neophallus should be cosmetically acceptable to both patient and partner, should have sufficient rigidity for vaginal penetration, and should maintain tactile sensitivity. Furthermore, scarring in the donor area should be minimized, and a neourethra constructed to allow voiding while standing [6]. Although many patients would like to be able to use the phallus sexually and/or to void while standing, others only express a desire for a good cosmetic appearance to be accepted as males in society. Unfortunately, sex reassignment surgery usually requires several operations, which are very invasive and time-consuming. Herein we present our recent experience with single-stage sex reassignment surgery in female-to-male transsexuals, where *mastectomy* and chest contouring are carried out with oophorectomy and hysterectomy at the same time as the pedicled pubic phalloplasty.

Since 2000 we offered one-stage sex reassignment surgery in our departments. Before surgery each underwent a complete psycho-sexological evaluation, and hormonal therapy was discontinued 1 month before the intervention for anaesthetic reason.

Two operative teams are necessary: while the first team performs subcutaneous adenomammectomy and mastopexy using the round-block technique, hystero-oophorectomy, phalloplasty and testicular prosthesis implantation are carried out by the second team (Fig. 33.1).

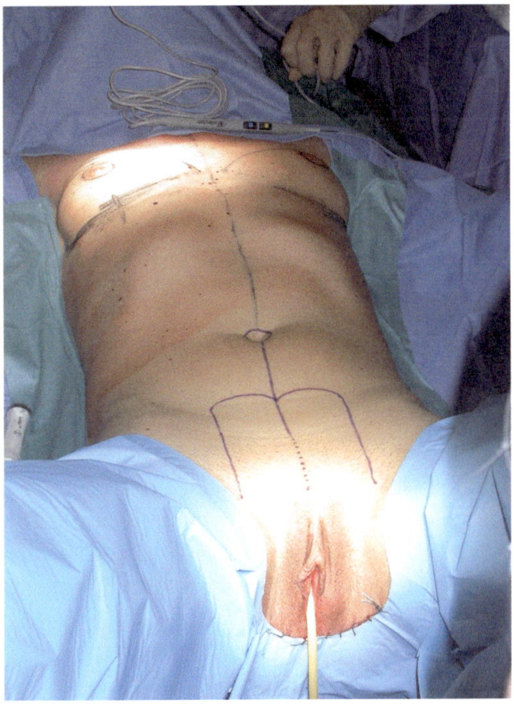

Fig. 33.1 Preoperative management

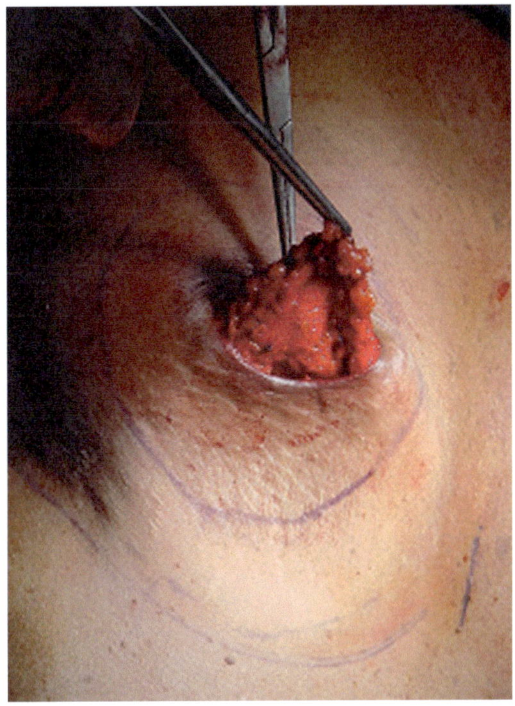

Fig. 33.2 Round-block technique

The mastoplasty technique used in the one-stage procedure in these patients consists of subcutaneous adenomammectomy and mastopexy using the *round-block technique* (Fig. 33.2). Cutaneous excision depends upon the size and volume of the breast skin. A second round-block excision for a better aesthetic result is optional, but it is always undertaken when the breast is particularly big and a large amount of skin removed. In some cases, a high degree of ptosis may require an inferior pedicle mastopexy technique, leaving only periareolar and inframammary fold scars [7].

The phallus is fashioned from a flap of the anterior abdominal wall skin, 10×10 cm, measured from the base of the clitoris. Skin, subcutaneous fat and Scarpa's fascia are incised superiorly and laterally. Superficial inferior epigastric and external pudendal vessels are incorporated into the flap pedicle. After mobilization of the flap, any excess subcutaneous tissue is excised to give better cosmesis. The abdominal design is then completed through skin excision. Through the same incision, hysterectomy and bilateral salpingo-oophorectomy are easy. The

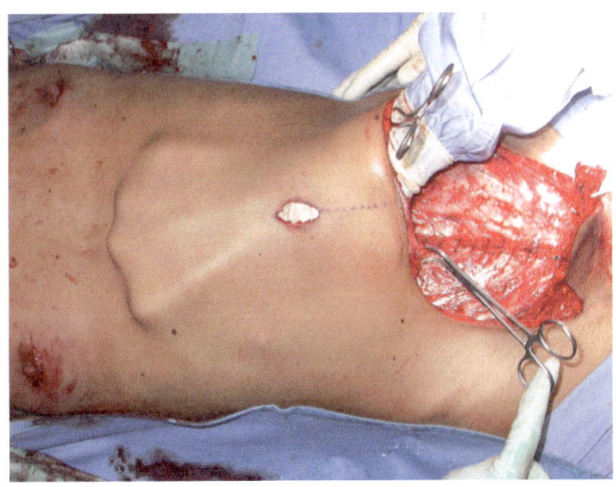

Fig. 33.3 Dissection of the abdominal skin and subcutaneous fat

abdominal fascia is closed, and the umbilicus is incised and separated from the abdominal skin (Fig. 33.3). The abdominal skin and subcutaneous fat are widely dissected from the abdominal wall up to the costal edge. The incision of the former umbilicus is closed and the neo-umbilicus repositioned 5 cm above the old one. The donor area of the phalloplasty flap may be closed

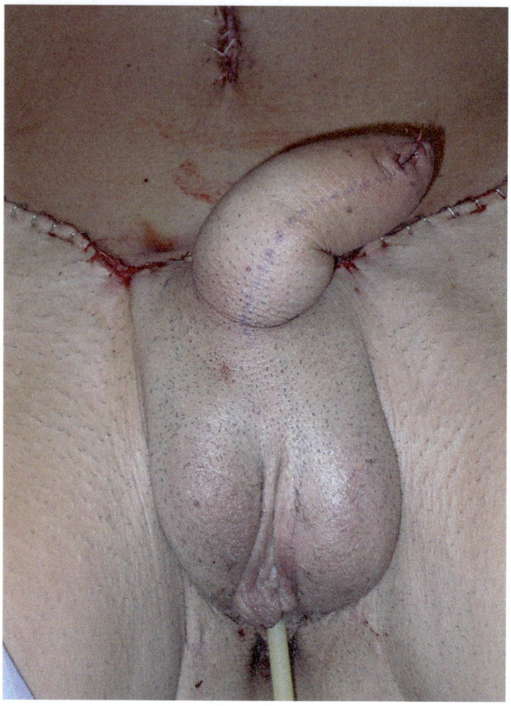

Fig. 33.4 Postoperative result

in a tension-free manner. Suction drainage is applied bilaterally. The flap is then tubularized on its dorsal side. A neourethra was not constructed because the patients did not wish to have one when they were informed of the possible complications. Testicular prostheses were inserted easily into the labia majora through the abdomen to avoid exterior skin incisions.

The mean duration of the procedure was 6 h, after which a moderately compressive abdominal dressing was positioned from the costal margin to the iliac crests, which was substituted after 15 days with an elastic bandage. The phallus is left in a semierect position to facilitate venous outflow. Patients were discharged home 12 days after surgery; there were no complications except for a partial dehiscence of the dorsal suture of the neophallus in one patient and that healed spontaneously in 4 weeks. The cosmetic outcome was considered excellent by both the surgeons and patients (Fig. 33.4). Although erogenous sensitivity should not be expected with this technique, sensitivity to pressure stimuli and vibratory sense recurred in the neophallus of two patients.

The aim of mastoplasty in female-to-male sex reassignment surgery is to give a more masculine appearance to the patient's thorax. To obtain satisfactory results, five different problems must be solved concurrently, i.e. reduction of gland tissue, reduction of excessive skin, reduction and rearrangement of the areola-nipple complex, revision of the inframammary fold, and minimization of resulting scars [8].

The creation of a neophallus is usually associated with different surgical problems, and several efforts are underway to improve function and appearance. In our opinion *pubic phalloplasty* is a simple and relatively quick procedure, leads to minimal scarring or disfigurement in the donor area, and is well accepted by the patients [9, 10]. Because of the high neourethral complication rate, we prefer to use urethroplasty only if patients wish to have a functional phallus and thus to void while standing.

Pedicled pubic flap phalloplasty offers an acceptable neophallus with minimal disfigurement in the donor area. Although erogenous sensitivity should not be expected with this technique, tactile and vibratory sensitivity can recur in the neophallus.

To our knowledge another case of complete one-stage procedure for sex reassignment surgery in female-to-male transsexuals has not yet been described. The major surgical problem is the creation of a functional and cosmetically acceptable neophallus. Many techniques have been reported, and results are more or less aesthetically acceptable. All surgical options should be discussed with the patient, together with the most frequent complications [11]. The use of a pedicled myocutaneous flap has some advantages because a skin-lined urethra may be preconstructed, but obvious scarring of the donor site is inevitable and cicatricial retraction of the migrated muscle is frequent [12]. Furthermore no erogenous sensitivity is obtained in the neophallus [13]. Metoidioplasty [14] can be a method of choice when the clitoris is large enough after prolonged hormonal therapy. The advantage of this technique is the optimal erogenous sensitivity obtained, but the length of the penis is generally insufficient for intercourse, and possible complications such as necrosis of the corpora cavernosa are severe.

Functionally and cosmetically, the microsurgical free flap phalloplasty techniques give the best results [15].

These flaps can offer the advantages of better sensitivity, if a neural microsurgical anastomosis is used, and can include a vascularized urethra. Vaginal penetration is possible only after implantation of a penile prosthesis [16]. However, it is very invasive and time-consuming. The complication rate is relatively high, especially for urethral stenosis and formation of fistula [17]. Moreover, there is always a large scar in the donor area, with possible functional loss [18]. Minimal disfigurement with no functional loss in the donor area should be possible in cooperation with a plastic surgeon. Abdominoplasty allows a tension-free closure of the flap donor site with minimal scar retraction and a neophallus of sufficient length positioned in the pubic area.

In conclusion, a one-stage sex reassignment procedure for female-to-male transsexuals is feasible, with acceptable cosmetic and functional results. The advantage is a significant reduction in morbidity, pain, scarring and convalescence. Our results show the importance of a multidisciplinary approach to such patients; we have a team of psychologists, psychiatrists, endocrinologists, and plastic, urological, and gynaecological surgeons to care for these patients.

The *quality of surgical results* has been demonstrated to be one of the best predictors of the overall outcome of sex reassignment [19, 20].

References

1. Selvaggi G, Bellringer J (2011) Gender reassignment surgery: an overview. Nat Rev Urol 8(5):274–282
2. Selvaggi G, Elander A (2008) Penile reconstruction/formation. Curr Opin Urol 18(6):589–597
3. The World Professional Association for Transgender Health (2011) Standards of care for the health of transsexual, transgender, and gender nonconforming people. 7th version http://www.wpath.org
4. Monstrey S, Hoebeke P, Selvaggi G et al (2009) Penile reconstruction: is the radial forearm flap really the standard technique? Plast Reconstr Surg 124(2): 510–518
5. Hage JJ, De Graaf FH (1993) Addressing the ideal requirements by free flap phalloplasty: some reflections on refinements of technique. Microsurgery 14(9):592–598
6. Chesson RR, Gilbert DA, Jordan GH et al (1996) The role of colpocleisis with urethral lengthening in transsexual phalloplasty. Am J Obstet Gynecol 175:1443–1449
7. Pascone M (1999) Il transessualismo gino-androide – la mastoplastica. In: Belgrano E, Fabris B, Trombetta C (eds) Il transessualismo – identificazione di un percorso diagnostico e terapeutico milano. Kurtis Editrice, Milano, pp 223–240
8. Lindsay WR (1979) Creation of a male chest in female transsexual. Ann Plast Surg 3:39–46
9. Pryor JP, Gill H (1991) Surgical considerations in 29 female to male transsexual patients. Gend Dysphoria 1:44–46
10. Snyder CC, Browne EZ (1977) Chapter 100. Intersex problems and hermaphroditism. In: Converse JM (ed) Reconstructive plastic surgery: principles and procedures in correction, reconstruction and transplantation, 2nd edn. WB Saunders, Philadelphia, pp 3941–3949
11. Hage JJ, Bout CA, Bloem JJ, Megens JA (1993) Phalloplasty in female-to-male transsexuals. What do our patients ask for? Ann Plast Surg 30:323–326
12. Hage JJ, Bloem JJ, Suliman HM (1993) Review of the literature on techniques for phalloplasty with emphasis on the applicability in female-to-male transsexuals. J Urol 150:1093–1098
13. Davies DM, Matti BA (1988) A method of phalloplasty using the deep inferior epigastric flap. Br J Plast Surg 41:165–168
14. Gilbert DA, Winslow BH, Gilbert DM, Jordan GH, Horton CE (1988) Transsexual surgery in the genetic female. Clin Plast Surg 15:471–487
15. Chang TS (1992) Priority in the use of the forearm free flap in one-stage phalloplasty. J Reconstr Microsurg 8:335–336
16. Jordan GH, Alter GJ, Gilbert DA, Horton CE, Devine CJ Jr (1994) Penile prosthesis implantation in total phalloplasty. J Urol 152:410–414
17. Young VL, Khouri RK, Lee GW, Nemecek JA (1992) Advances in total phalloplasty and urethroplasty with microvascular free flaps. Clin Plast Surg 19:927–938
18. Fang RH, Lin JT, Ma S (1994) Phalloplasty for female transsexuals with sensate free forearm flap. Microsurgery 15:349–352
19. Lawrence AA (2006) Patient-reported complications and functional outcomes of male-to-female sex reassignment surgery. Arch Sex Behav 35(6):717–727
20. Wierckx K, Van Caenegem E, Elaut E et al (2011) Quality of life and sexual health after sex reassignment surgery in transsexual men. J Sex Med 8(12): 3379–3388

34 Surgical Therapy: Scrotal Reconstruction in Female-to-Male Transsexuals

Gennaro Selvaggi

Since surgeons started to perform sex reassignment surgery in FTM, attention was mainly focused to phalloplasty, while the scrotum received less attention.

In the last 20 years, transsexuals became more demanding, and surgeons started to focus on scrotoplasty as well.

Currently, the creation of an aesthetically acceptable result, both for the phallus and the scrotum, is one of the goals of genital construction in female-to-male (FTM) transsexuals [1].

Traditional flaps for scrotal reconstruction as usually performed in biological male are not really applicable in the group of transsexual patients.

Older techniques for scrotal reconstruction in transsexuals consist of leaving the labia in situ with midline closure and prosthetic implant filling. These techniques are aesthetically unappealing and remind the patients their female past.

More elaborate techniques applying pedicled thigh, groin, and pubic flaps are too elaborate for scrotal reconstruction in transsexuals; require longer operating time; cause extra donor site morbidity, eventually with unsatisfactory scars in the donor area; and place additional risk for complications which may require extra surgical step(s); finally, aesthetic results are often not pleasing enough for patients and surgeons.

G. Selvaggi, MD, PhD
Department of Plastic and Reconstructive Surgery, Sahlgrenska University Hospital, Gröna Stråket 8, Gothenburg SE-413 45, Sweden
e-mail: selvaggigennaro@yahoo.it

Myocutaneous flaps are also too complex and unnecessary, with final unnatural feeling and absence of erogenous sensation; finally, the palpation of the testicular implants under the myocutaneous flap might be difficult [1, 2].

Further to these, scrotoplasty should not interfere with the reconstruction of the proximal part of the urethra (pars fixa), not increasing risk of urinary problems, neither with the vaginectomy [3–23].

Expansion of the labia majora has widely been performed and even with good results [23]. However, tissue expansion of the labia majora is adding extra surgical procedures and clinic visits to these patients, and, further, cannot reach a scrotum located completely in front of the legs but mainly in between [2].

Figure 34.1 is showing the result of tissue expansion on the labia.

Today, most of the surgeons performing scrotoplasty in transsexual patients prefer techniques involving the use of labia majora flaps; since labia majora flaps are not bulky enough, testicular implants are usually needed and inserted in a later stage.

The labia majora, in fact, are the embryologic counterpart of the scrotum: these are both, in fact, matching for color and texture and hair bearing, and these have the same tactile and erogenous innervations.

Furthermore, the labia majora presents with fat tissue which can give adequate protection to the testicular implants [2].

C. Trombetta et al. (eds.), *Management of Gender Dysphoria: A Multidisciplinary Approach*, DOI 10.1007/978-88-470-5696-1_34, © Springer-Verlag Italia 2015

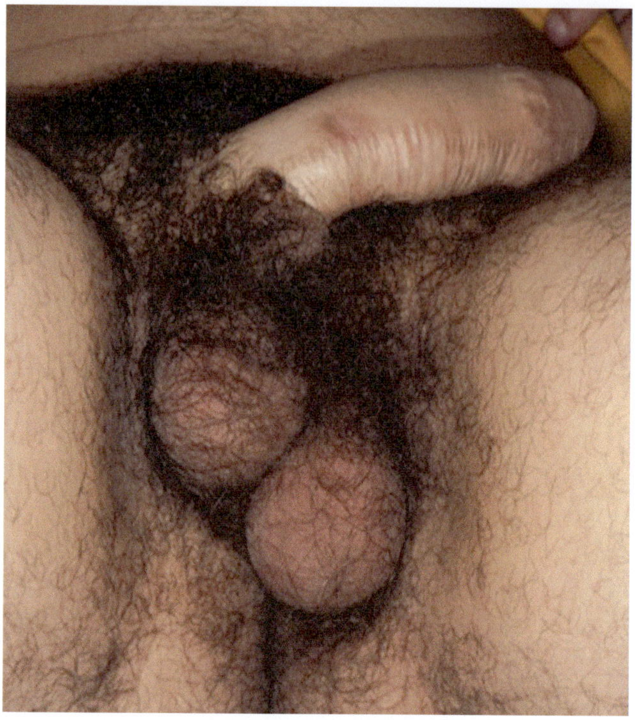

Fig. 34.1 Scrotoplasty performed with direct skin expansion in the labia majora, with no flap surgery: the scrotum is located completely in between the legs

For these reasons, labia majora flaps are overcoming many disadvantages posed by older techniques, such as the procedure results technically easier less additional donor site morbidity and better sensitivity [2].

With the introduction of labia majora V-Y plasties [1–3, 5–19], surgeons aimed to bring the scrotum in front of the legs and at the same time obtaining a natural sack-looking scrotum [2].

Figure 34.2 is showing a scrotoplasty performed with inferiorly based labia majora flaps, at the same time of a metoidioplasty. These flaps are simply harvested with subcutaneous fat, lifted downward, and sutured together. This ends into a scrotum in between the legs.

According to the Hoebecke's novel technique for scrotoplasty [2], a V-Y 90° rotation labial plasty can bring the scrotum more in front of the legs. Today, their series constitute the largest and longest follow-up, with more than 240 operated patients with successful results.

This method is always performed at the same time of the phalloplasty, with no extra expansion needed.

Table 34.1 (modified from Selvaggi et al. [2]) is summarizing the most representative techniques described in the literature.

34.1 Hoebecke's Surgical Technique

This surgical approach is for scrotoplasty, vaginectomy, and reconstruction of the pars fixa in one stage, at the same time of a penile reconstruction, which is mostly performed with a free radial forearm flap by the authors of the technique. The same scrotoplasty technique can be used also in combination with other phalloplasty methods.

We hereby limit our description to the scrotoplasty step only.

The incision lines are marked on the borders of the labia majora and on top of the clitoris (Fig. 34.3). A total submucosal vaginectomy is performed.

A traction suture is placed on the tip of the clitoris, and the lengthening of the urethra is started incising and suturing together two vertical lines made on the internal side of the labia

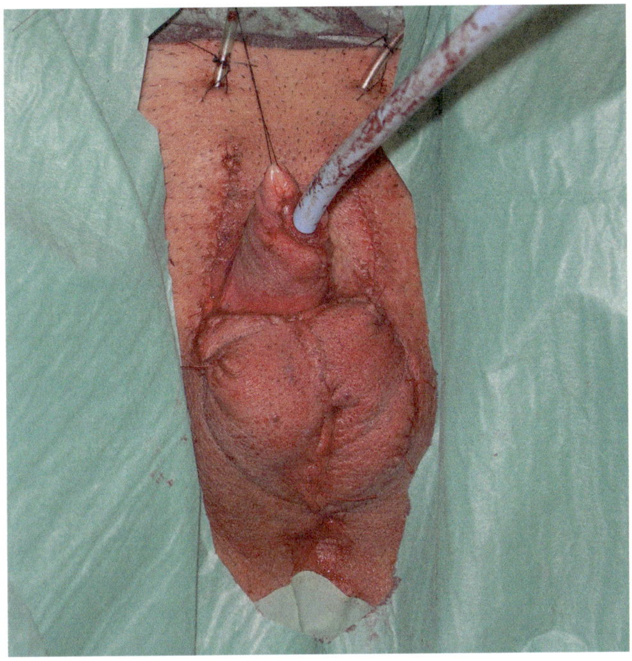

Fig. 34.2 Scrotoplasty performed with inferiorly based labia majora flaps, at the same time of a metoidioplasty

Table 34.1 Surgical techniques using labia majora flaps for scrotal reconstruction in transsexual patients

Authors	Flap' s description	Advantages	Disadvantages
Gonzalez-Ulloa [5]	Bilateral advancement of M-like-incised skin flaps		Not aesthetically pleasing results: scrotum results in between legs
Snyder and Browne [8]	Bilateral skin flaps from perineum and medial aspect of the thighs (skin in the midline is deepithelialized, and closure is started laterally, incorporating a V-Y advancement)		Not aesthetically pleasing results: scrotum results more anteriorly than Gonzalez-Ulloa' s technique, but still not in front of the legs
Hage et al. [1]	Labia majora incised in a reversed V-like manner; the skin of the dorsally based skin flaps is undermined; testicular prostheses are immediately inserted; skin is closed in a Y-like fashion		Not aesthetically pleasing results: scrotum results in between legs
Others (Millard [6]; Puckett and Montie [9]; Reid and Wright [13]; Meyer and Daverio [16]; Still and Goodman [20]; Exner [19]; Stark [21]; Hage et al. [1]; Small and Becker [22]; Sengezer and Sadove [23])	Different kinds of labial rotation and V-Y closure, with or without implants		Similar to previous techniques Few cases performed, or numbers not mentioned Some do not reconstruct urethra

(continued)

Table 34.1 (continued)

Authors	Flap' s description	Advantages	Disadvantages
Hoebeke's technique (Selvaggi et al. [2])	Superiorly based bilateral V-Y flaps, rotated medially and bent on themselves	Increased possibility for local erogenous sensation (preserving the dorsal skin of the clitoris to create the anterior part of the scrotum) Possibility for orgasm during displacement of the clitoris at the base of the phallus (allowing for orgasm during masturbation or penetration) Better cosmetic result and positioning of the scrotum "in front of the legs" Better coverage for the reconstruction of the "pars fixa" of the urethra reducing urinary fistulas	

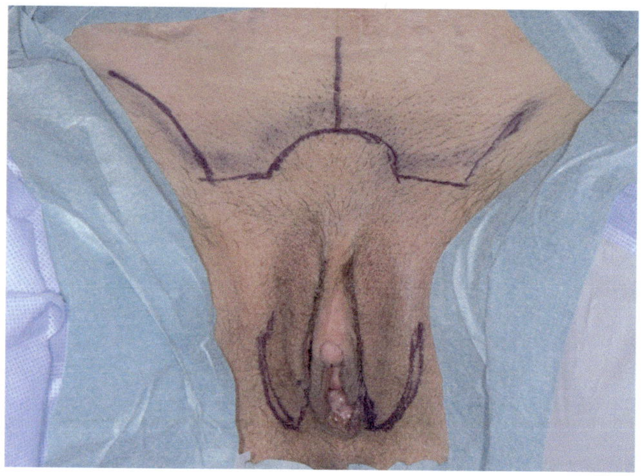

Fig. 34.3 Drowning of the incision on the labia majora

minora, approximately 2 mm laterally to the original urethral end.

The upper parts of the labia minora, often excessive, are resected. A labia minora-clitoral hood flap is created; the mucosa of the glans of the clitoris is completely resected, and the clitoris is rotated ventrally and buried at the base of the flap.

The V-shaped labia majora flaps are harvested based on a superior pedicle. These are never defatted, and all the tissue included between the lateral and the medial borders of each labium majus is included in the flaps. Once elevated, labial flaps are rotated 90° medially and bent on themselves superiorly, then joined to the midline.

The tips of the two triangular labia majora flaps are medially approximated, sutured to each other, and lifted upward, while labia minora-clitoral hood flap is pulled down [2].

The effect of the 90° rotation, bending of the flaps superiorly, and lowering the dorsal skin of the clitoris is creating wrinkles to the lateral and anterior part of the scrotum, increasing the natural appearance, while the two flaps joined together on the midline are resembling the scrotum bifidity.

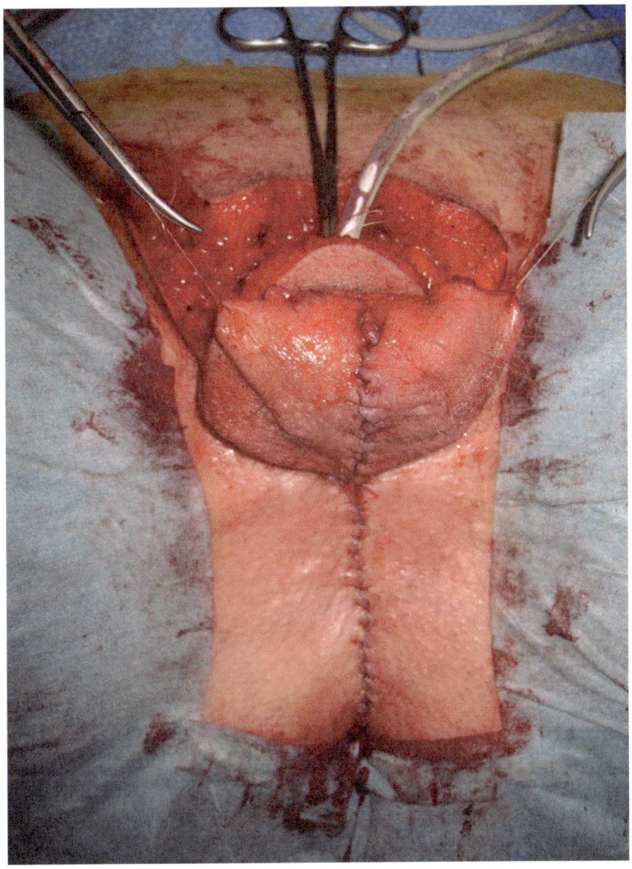

Fig. 34.4 Final result of Hoebecke's scrotoplasty just after surgery: the scrotum is lifted ventrally and detached from the thighs

Figure 34.4 is showing a final result just after surgery. The scrotum, lifted ventrally, is detached from the thighs and moved forward in front of the legs. Figure 34.5 is showing a final result after surgery with the scrotum hanging down from its attachment.

It must be said that in a normal biological male, scrotal volume and shape present a large number of variations among different people, ages, and temperature conditions. This variation is not possible with any of the techniques available. However, the Hoebecke's scrotoplasty achieves a standard result that is within the wide range of normal scrotal variations [2].

34.2 Testicle Implants

Following scrotoplasty, most of the patients are requesting testicle implants.

The reason for the testicle implants is to give consistency and firmness to the empty scrotal bag and to let palpation of two different testicular structures in order to resemble normal male anatomy.

Testicle implants are usually inserted 6–12 months after the original scroto-phalloplasty procedure.

If a hydraulic erection device is chosen, one testicle implant and one pumping valve (to act as a second testicle implant) are positioned in the scrotal sack.

If a malleable erection device is chosen, then 2 testicle implants are inserted in the scrotal sack usually at the same time the malleable erection implant is inserted into the reconstructed penis.

The combination of the labial flaps (with the labial fat tissue included within the flaps) with the silicon testicle implants is providing a natural feeling on palpating the scrotum.

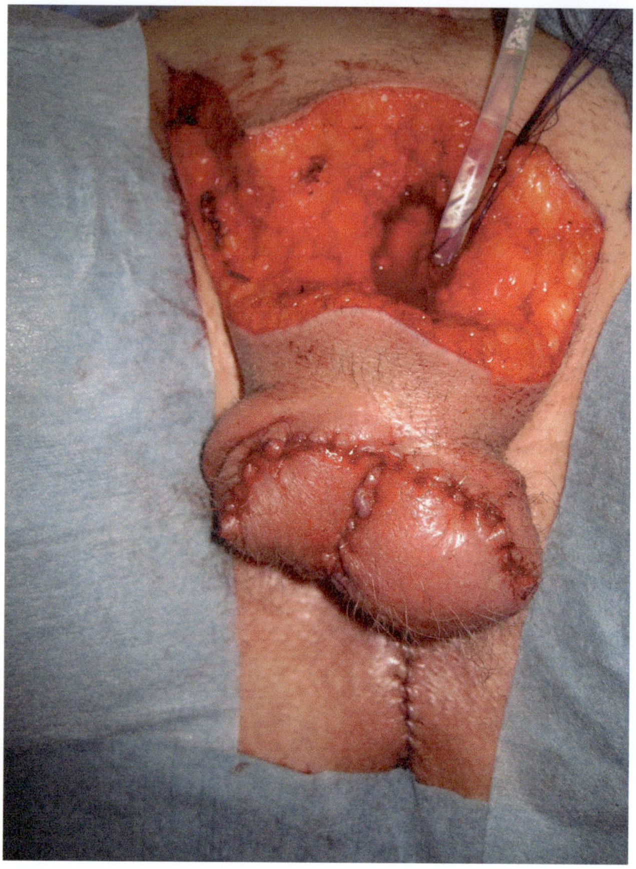

Fig. 34.5 Final result of Hoebecke's scrotoplasty just after surgery: the scrotum is hanging down from its attachment

34.3 Results and Complications

Literature is poor in providing specific results of scrotoplasty techniques.

No major complications, related to the scrotoplasty, are reported.

Hematoma of the scrotum is in the range of 0–2 %. Wound dehiscence is up to 5 % [2]. Nevertheless, revision surgery following scrotoplasty is very rare, and most of the complications are solved conservatively.

It is reported in literature that tactile and erogenous sensitivity of the genital area is preserved [24, 25].

34.4 The Future

Few has to be ameliorated on scrotoplasty itself for female-to-male transsexuals. Mostly, research should be aimed in finding surgical refinements for improving the contemporary reconstruction of the pars fixa of the urethra, in order to prevent urinary fistulas.

References

1. Hage JJ, Bouman FG, Bloem JJ (1993) Constructing a scrotum in female-to-male transsexuals. Plast Reconstr Surg 91(5):914–921
2. Selvaggi G, Hoebecke P, Ceulemans P et al (2009) Scrotal reconstruction in Female-to-Male Transsexuals: the novel scrotoplasty. Plast Reconstr Surg 123(6):1710–1719
3. Millard DR Jr (1966) Scrotal construction and reconstruction. Plast Reconstr Surg 38:10
4. Pfeiffer DB, Miller DB (1950) Traumatic avulsion of skin of penis and scrotum: a simplified method of reconstruction. Plast Reconstr Surg 5:520
5. Gonzalez-Ulloa M (1963) Severe avulsion of the scrotum in a bullfighter: reconstruction procedure. Br J Plast Surg 16:154
6. Noe JM, Birdsell D (1973) A surgical program for female-to-male transsexuals. In: Laub DR, Gandy P (eds) Proceedings of the second interdisciplinary

symposium on gender dysphoria syndrome. Stanford University Press, Palo Alto, pp 152–162
7. Noe JM, Sato R, Coleman C et al (1974) The surgical construction of the male genitalia for the female-to-male transsexual. Plast Reconstr Surg 53:511
8. Snyder CG, Browne EZ Jr (1977) Intersex problems and hermafroditism. In: Converse JM (ed) Reconstructive plastic surgery. Saunders, Philadelphia, pp 3941–3949
9. Puckett CL, Montie JE (1978) Construction of male genitalia in the transsexuals, using a tubed groin flap for penis and a hydraulic inflation device. Plast Reconstr Surg 61:523–530
10. Biemer E (1982) Transsexualismus: geschlechtsumwandelnde Operationen. Med Klin 77:16
11. Foerster DW (1983) Female-to-male transsexual conversion: a 15-year follow-up. Plast Reconstr Surg 72:237
12. Eicher W (1984) Transsexualismus: moglichkeiten und grenzen der geschtsumwandlung. Gustuv Fischer Verlag, Stuttgart
13. Reid CF, Wright JH Jr (1985) Scrotal reconstruction following an avulsion injury. J Urol 133:881
14. Lim SM (1986) Surgery in transsexuals. Ann Acad Med Singapore 15:22
15. Meyer R, Daverio PJ, Dequesne J (1986) One-stage phalloplasty in transsexuals. Ann Plast Surg 16:472
16. Meyer R, Daverio PJ (1987) One-stage phalloplasty without sensory deprivation in female transsexuals. World J Urol 5:9
17. Gilbert DA, Winslow BH, Gilbert DM et al (1988) Trassexual surgery in the genetic female. Clin Plast Surg 15:471
18. Laub DR, Eicher W, Laub DR II et al (1989) Penis construction in female-to-male transsexuals. In: Eicher W (ed) Plastic surgery in sexually handicapped. Springer, Berlin
19. Exner K (1991) Der plastichen chirurgie bei geslechtsanpassenden operationen in fer femin-zu-mzsculinen transsexualitat. In: Das phanomen der frau-zu-mann transsexualitat von anita. Transidentitas, Offenbach
20. Still EF II, Goodman RC (1990) Total reconstruction of a two-compartment scrotum by tissue expansion. Plast Reconstr Surg 85:805
21. Stark GB (1991) Total reconstruction of scrotum by tissue expansion. Plast Reconstr Surg 87:192
22. Small MP, Becker H (1989) Use of tissue expanders in genitourinaryreconstructive surgery for transsexuals. In: Proceedings of the eleventh Harry Benjamin International Gender Dsphoria Association Symposium, Cleveland
23. Sengezer M, Sadove RC (1993) Scrotal construction by expansion of labia majora in biological female transsexuals. Ann Plast Surg 31(4):372–376
24. De Cuypere G, T'Sjoen G, Beerten R et al (2005) Sexual and physical health after sex reassignment surgery. Arch Sex Behav 34(6):679–690
25. Selvaggi G, Monstrey S, Ceulemans P et al (2007) Genital sensitivity in sex reassignment surgery. Ann Plast Surg 58(4):427–433

Complications 35

Michael Sohn

In comparison to male-to-female sex reassignment surgery, female-to-male (F-t-M) transsexuals need more operative sessions and interdisciplinary cooperation for complete reassignment to a male body in appearance and function. Generally speaking, surgery is more complicated and less standardized. As a result of a recent international consensus meeting on transsexual surgery, the following recommendation (Grade B) following the rules of evidence-based medicine could be published:

> Breast reduction, oophorectomy, hysterectomy and vaginectomy should be offered to all patients. There are many phalloplasty techniques involving local or free flaps and microsurgery. Patients should be warned that multiple stages are often needed with high urethral and prosthetic complication rates. However, a universal satisfaction rate of 80 % should be expected. Metoidioplasty can be offered to those who wish to stand to void but do not want sexual intercourse. [1]

These recommendations do not differ essentially from the recommendations of the 7th version of the "Standards of Care" (SOC) published recently by the World Professional Association for Transgender Health (WPATH) in 2011 [2]. The SOC further demands that physicians performing surgical treatment should be urologists, gynecologists, plastic surgeons, or general surgeons, board-certified as such by the relevant national associations. They should have specialized competence in genital reconstructive techniques and have documented supervised training with a more experienced surgeon. Furthermore, surgeons on this field should be knowledgeable about more than one surgical technique for genital reconstruction so that they can choose the ideal technique for the individual patient [2].

Currently no literature reporting percentages of patients' preference of one or another technique or reporting on goal priority is available [3].

In the following, typical complications of several surgical procedures will be explained with actual data, compiled from the literature and personal experience of the author's interdisciplinary team.

35.1 One-Stage, Two-Stage, or Multiple-Stage Sex Reassignment Surgery?

Essentially surgical sex reassignment in F-t-M transsexuals can be separated into breast reduction, hysterectomy with ovariectomy, and genital reconstruction. All three steps can be performed in one session or as a two-stage procedure. Only one study of an experienced team compared the risks and benefits of both approaches in a peer-reviewed publication [4]. The authors concluded that one-stage reassignment was associated with more blood loss but no difference in operative and

M. Sohn
Urology Department, Agaplesion Markus-Krankenhaus, Wilhelm-Epstein-Straße 4, Frankfurt am Main 60431, Germany
e-mail: Michael.Sohn@fdk.info

C. Trombetta et al. (eds.), *Management of Gender Dysphoria: A Multidisciplinary Approach*, DOI 10.1007/978-88-470-5696-1_35, © Springer-Verlag Italia 2015

postoperative complications. As a consequence after finalization of the study, the team followed the two-stage strategy in the future: the first session included laparoscopic hysterectomy and ovariectomy as well as breast reduction, and the second session included vaginectomy and genital reconstruction always followed by a separate session for prosthetic implantation [3]. In our own experience also, a two-stage procedure is clearly preferred, as vaginectomy during genital reconstruction is easier to perform several months after hysterectomy and ovariectomy.

35.2 Breast Reduction

With very few exceptions, all F-t-M transsexual patients need surgical breast reduction as the first step of surgical sex reassignment. There exists general consensus that this type of breast surgery should only be performed by surgeons with broad experience in F-t-M surgery [3]. An algorithm of several surgical techniques has recently been proposed for chest wall contouring surgery in these patients [5]. In small breasts, satisfactory results may be expected by subcutaneous mastectomy via a circumareolar incision [3]. The majority of patients need more extensive surgery as breast amputation with free or pedicled nipple-areola grafting. Furthermore, the nipple itself and the areola diameter often have to be reduced [3, 6]. Minor revisions to ameliorate the final cosmetic result are frequently necessary. In a recent study, 23 % of patients needed at least one further correction after applying an elaborated algorithm of several surgical techniques [6]. The application of poor techniques without experience in F-t-M patients may lead to unacceptable cosmetic results with high risks of nipple or areola necrosis and abundant scar formation.

35.3 Hysterectomy and Ovariectomy

Hysterectomy and bilateral ovariectomy can be performed by open abdominal, laparoscopic, or transvaginal access routes. This part of surgery is necessary in all patients, because lifelong exposure to exogenous testosterone risks the development of endometrial or ovarian carcinoma [3, 7]. Leading centers prefer a simultaneous laparoscopic approach for hysterectomy combined with chest wall contouring surgery [4]. It seems prudent to reduce as much as possible the vaginal length during hysterectomy in order to simplify later vaginectomy during genital reconstruction [3, 8]. Pure transvaginal hysterectomy and ovariectomy may be tedious and challenging after long-term testosterone application due to bulky musculature and reduced tissue elasticity, especially in case of virgo intacta. If transvaginal hysterectomy is preferred, it may also be performed under laparoscopic assistance. The risks of intra- or postoperative complications after hysterectomy have been extensively published in the relevant gynecological literature and should not be further detailed in this review.

35.4 Genital Surgery

The ideal goals in performing genital reconstruction in F-t-M patients have been repeatedly described: they include the construction of an aesthetically appealing penis and scrotum (if possible in a one-stage procedure), the preservation or reconstruction of erogenous and tactile sensation, the ability of micturition in a standing position, and the possibility of regaining erectile function enabling the patient to have penetrative intercourse [3, 9, 10].

A multitude of free and pedicled flaps have been described for penile reconstruction, but still the radial free forearm flap has emerged as the most widely used flap, being considered nearly as a gold standard in F-t-M genital surgery [11].

A minor invasive solution for patients who restrain from the risks of phalloplasty represents the so-called metoidioplasty which in most cases enables the patient to void in a standing position but which does not permit sexual intercourse. The limitations and benefits of the most frequently used techniques in genital reconstruction of F-t-M transsexuals are shown in Table 35.1 [3].

Table 35.1 Techniques for female-to-male sex reassignment surgery

Surgical technique	Limitations	Benefits
Metoidioplasty	Short phallus, not capable of sexual penetration, does not always enable voiding while standing	Easy technique, reduced risk of complication, quick recovery time
Radial forearm flap	Urinary tract problems, multiple stages, stiffener or permanent erection if bone is used, donor site morbidity	Possible ability for sexual intercourse; possibly, best cosmetic result in penile reconstruction?
Anterolateral thigh flap	No long-term follow-up available: possibly similar limits to radial forearm flap	Easy to hide the donor site disfigurement
Fibula flap	No long-term follow-up available in the past few years, possibly similar limits to radial forearm flap	Easy to hide the donor site disfigurement, no need for an inflatable erection device
Latissimus dorsi flap	No long-term follow-up available, urinary tract not reconstructed, muscle or erection function questionable, donor site morbidity, sexual and tactile sensitivity not reported	No need for an inflatable erection device
Suprapubic flap	Cosmetic appearance unsatisfactory, donor site morbidity possible, urinary tract problems, fully or only partially sensate, stiffener or erection possible? Multiple stages	Easy technique

From Selvaggi and Bellringer [3]

35.5 Complications of Phalloplasty and Genital Reconstruction

As a simple rule, it may be concluded from the actual literature that the more sophisticated genital sex reassignment is planned, the more complications can be expected.

In the following, typical complications of single steps of the procedure will be explained.

35.6 Complications of Vaginectomy and Colpocleisis

In most centers, vaginectomy is performed during phalloplasty or metoidioplasty at least 6 weeks after breast reduction and hysterectomy. A recent study from London revealed that most complications intra- and postoperatively concerned bleeding, which appeared to be related to vaginal length [8]. The median intraoperative blood loss was 700 ml (range 100–3,000 ml), mean postoperative blood loss was 200 ml (range 20–1,490 ml), and 22 % of all patients needed blood transfusions. Postoperative complications included wound infection (12.3 %), wound bleeding (14.6 %), and vaginal hematoma/abscess formation (6.7 %). In 5 %, bladder or urethral perforations occurred during the procedure, which could all be closed primarily without further consequences. Four percent needed prolonged catheterization due to the development of temporary hypotonic bladder. While most authors prefer only a mucosal vaginectomy, in our hands a radical vaginectomy including the vaginal muscle wall is preferred. The risk of leaving mucosal islands behind with later abscess or fistula formation seems to be reduced by this more radical approach. On the other hand, care has to be taken to close properly the peritoneal cavity in case it has been opened inadvertently. During 270 radical vaginectomies, we observed three cases of severe intra-abdominal bleeding postoperatively which demanded transabdominal revision.

In general, it is helpful to resect as much as possible of the vagina during previous hysterectomy and ovariectomy in order to reduce the risk of bleeding complications during vaginectomy [8].

35.7 Complications of Metoidioplasty

Modern metoidioplasty is intended to be a one-stage procedure with simultaneous lengthening and straightening of the hypertrophied clitoris, combined with urethroplasty to the tip of the clitoris, vaginectomy, and neoscrotum formation by implantation of two testicular prostheses. Urethral reconstruction seems to be the most difficult part of the procedure and is responsible for most of the possible complications. Hage et al. described a high rate of urethral fistula (37 %) and stenosis formation (35 %) in a large series of 70 patients [12]. Loss or dislocation of testicular prostheses also frequently occurred (80 %). Overall patients needed an average of 2.6 operations to complete genital reconstruction; 25 % of all patients later demanded phallic reconstruction by radial forearm flaps.

A recent publication on two different methods of metoidioplasty utilizing buccal mucosa and labia minora flaps for urethral formation in 207 patients reported significantly less urethral complications (8–20 %). Minor complications were noted in nearly 30 %. Nearly 90 % of patients were able to void in a standing position after completing the procedure. Twelve percent later demanded for complete phallic reconstruction [13].

In conclusion, metoidioplasty may be suited for F-t-M transsexuals who have no interest in penetrative sexual intercourse and who have developed significant clitoral hypertrophy after long-term testosterone application. Genital sensation is generally well preserved [3].

35.8 Complications of Phalloplasty and Urethroplasty

As previously mentioned, the most widely used free flap for penile and urethral reconstruction actually is the radial free forearm flap with more than 800 cases published until 2013. Even if modifications and flap designs differ between several author groups, complication rates seem to be quite similar in large centers [3, 9, 14]. Monstrey and coworkers reported a rate of 226 operative revisions due to complications after 316 phalloplasties by radial free forearm flaps, mostly due to urethral and prosthetic complications [9]. Ralph and coworkers reported a 34 % revision rate only for urethral complications after 115 free forearm phalloplasties, even if phalloplasty was performed as a multistage procedure [15]. In our personal experience after 270 phalloplasties using a free forearm flap, more than 60 % needed urethral revision surgery, and 37 % had to be reoperated due to prosthetic complications. Following a suggestion from Monstrey, the numerous complications after microsurgical phalloplasty can be divided in several subgroups:

(a) *Flap-related complications:*

In large centers with extensive microvascular experience, the total flap loss rate due to microvascular perfusion complications should be less than 5 % [9, 14–16]. Partial flap loss occurred in 7–9 % and can be limited by close flap perfusion control and early re-intervention [9, 14]. Smokers and adipose patients are at higher risk to suffer from these complications. Patients who do not quit their smoking habits or who are not willing to reduce their body mass index should be excluded from the waiting list for the operation.

(b) *Donor site-related complications*

The major drawback of the radial forearm flap is donor site morbidity, consisting mostly of a permanent and visible scar on the forearm [3]. This is the dominant reason for searching alternative flaps from less exposed areas of the body as, for example, pedicled anterolateral thigh (ALT) flaps or latissimus dorsi flaps or fibula free flaps [17, 18].

Recently a long-term follow-up study on donor site morbidity after radial forearm flap phalloplasty revealed that over 75 % of transsexual patients were either satisfied or neutral with the appearance of the scar [19]. No functional limitation on daily life activities was noted. Regrafting for various reasons was necessary in 2.8 % [9]. Up to now no consensus exists about the ideal material for primary coverage of the donor area: in our hands full-thickness skin grafts from the groin area give better results; other authors prefer split-thickness skin grafts of intermediate thickness [14, 19].

(c) *Urethral complications*

Fistula or stenosis rates have to be expected in a range of 20–40 % [3, 20]. There are several reasons responsible for such high complication rates: in radial forearm flaps the penis and urethra are formed following the tube-in-a-tube principle. Arterial perfusion and venous runoff of the inner neourethral tube may be compromised by pressure from the surrounding tissue, especially in obese patients. Perfusion of the inner tube cannot be controlled after penile formation, and consequent malnutrition of this tissue remains undetected. Most stenoses occur at the junction of the mucosal prolongation of the original urethra with the forearm skin part of the distal urethra, an area prone to minor perfusion and vascular malnutrition.

Some surgeons, especially plastic surgeons, who perform the procedure without urological assistance prefer to "prefabricate" the distal urethra several months before phallic reconstruction: a subcutaneous channel in the forearm area is covered by split skin grafts and held open by leaving a large-sized catheter for several months. Due to the lack of data on long-term function of these neourethras, no recommendation can be given concerning this approach, but significant shrinkage and development of stenoses can be suspected from extended urological experience with free skin grafts in conventional urethral surgery. Recently a combination of radial forearm flaps for neourethral formation with ALT flaps for reconstruction of the penile shaft has been proposed in order to reduce the development of urethral complications in phalloplasties [17].

Many small fistulas will close spontaneously after prolonged catheterization, but in our hands most cases of fistula and/or stenoses demand a surgical correction [12, 14]. There is a broad-spectrum of surgical techniques in urethral repair, as well known from urological publications and textbooks. Nevertheless, conditions are different after total phalloplasty and urethroplasty in F-t-M transsexual patients. Buccal mucosa grafts which have a dominant role in conventional urethral surgery are less suited in these patients, as no spongiosal tissue is present for graft nutrition and coverage. Two-stage repairs following the Johansson technique are sometimes necessary, especially in case of long strictures. Short strictures of less than 3 cm length developing after a long-term interval to phalloplasty are best suited for endoscopic urethrotomy with success rates of over 40 % [21]. In desperate cases a second radial free forearm flap of smaller dimensions only for urethral reconstruction may be considered, as well as return to the original female meatus position (perineal urethrotomy).

Intraurethral stone formation may occur due to extensive hair growth inside the urethra. If stone formation recurs after endoscopic extraction, opening the hair-bearing urethra may be considered, followed by depilation and secondary closure.

In general F-t-M patients should be warned before phalloplasty that urinary habits change after the operation, with 79 % complaining of postmicturition dribble and prolonged micturition time [3, 20].

(d) *Prosthetic complications*

If no urologists are involved in phalloplasty, plastic surgeons tend to use osteocutaneous flaps including radial or fibular bone strips as a permanent stiffener [18]. Apart from possible complications as less stability in the donor area, bone-bearing flaps result in a permanent erection without proximal stability [3].

The implantation of semirigid prostheses is dangerous, as no tunica albuginea exists and protrusion of these devices is impending.

Most high-volume centers in phalloplasty actually prefer to implant two- or three-piece hydraulic prosthetic devices within a sleeve of polyethylene terephthalate or other synthetic materials [14, 15, 22]. Complication rates as infections, erosion, or malfunction are significantly higher than in impotent biologic males. In order to reduce infection rates due to prolonged OR times, we prefer at our institution to perform prosthetic surgery in a two-stage session rather than in one extended session (see Figs. 35.1, 35.2, and 35.3).

In a recent report on 129 F-t-M patients after prosthetic implantation, a 41 % revision-rate was noted [22]. The infection-rate was 12 %. In our own experience after two-staged

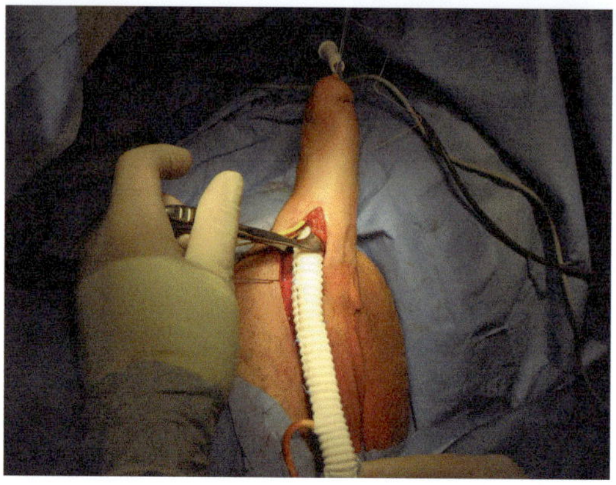

Fig. 35.1 Implantation of one hydraulic prosthesis cylinder in a complete Dacron® sheet into the neopenis (session one)

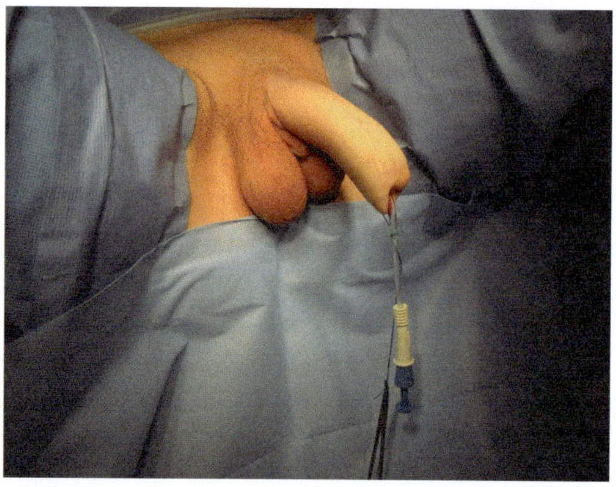

Fig. 35.2 Neopenis and neoscrotum 3 months after session one with additional implantation of two testicular prostheses into neoscrotum

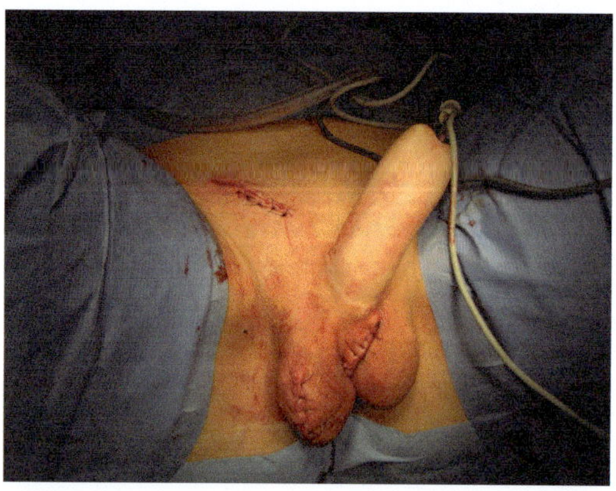

Fig. 35.3 Final result after implantation of hydraulic pump and reservoir and explantation of one testicular prosthesis (session two)

prosthetic implantation in 175 patients a revision-rate of 37 % had to be observed, mostly due to infection and malfunction.

Nearly all types of hydraulic prostheses have been used after phalloplasty but the actual data do not permit a recommendation for a certain ideal device in this patient-group. Furthermore, it remains open to debate whether one or two cylinders should be implanted into the neopenis and to which extent they should be covered with synthetic material. From the actual data it can be assumed that after 4–5 years still 50–60 % of all prostheses are still in place and well functioning. Whether this rate will drop with more long-term follow-up has to be awaited. Anyhow, about 80 % of all patients report to have satisfying sexual intercourse after completing penile prosthetic implantation [9, 16].

Conclusions

Recent reports demonstrate that penile and urethral reconstruction in F-t-M patients is feasible with reproducible satisfying results. Free radial forearm flaps are preferred by most high-volume centers and nearly emerge as a "gold standard" for phalloplasty. Best results may be achieved in multidisciplinary cooperation, involving plastic surgeons, urologists, and gynecologists. Complication rates in total phalloplasty still are remarkably high and represent a challenge to all involved specialists in the near future.

Hydraulic penile prosthesis implantation should be considered for all patients who wish to participate in penetrative sexual intercourse. These procedures should be performed after return of tactile and erotic sensation to the neopenis, before time-related slight volume loss of the neopenis occurs [9].

Urethral and prosthetic complications may occur many years after phalloplasty and demand a close long-term urologic follow-up of these patients, as long-term data on the urodynamic consequences of urethroplasty in originally female urinary tracts are still lacking [9, 20, 23, 24].

References

1. Ralph D, Gonzalez-Cadavid N, Mirone V et al (2010) Trauma, gender reassignment and penile augmentation. J Sex Med 7:1657–1667
2. Coleman E, Bockting W, Botzer M et al (2011) Standards of Care for the health of transsexual, transgender and gender-non-conforming people. J Transgend 13:165–232
3. Selvaggi G, Bellringer J (2011) Gender reassignment surgery: an overview. Nat Rev Urol 8:275–281
4. Weyers S, Selvaggi G, Monstrey S et al (2006) Two-stage versus one-stage sex reassignment surgery in female-to-male transsexual individuals. Gynecol Surg 3:190–194
5. Monstrey S (2008) Chest wall contouring surgery in female-to-male (FtM) transsexuals: a new algorithm. Plast Reconstr Surg 121:849–859
6. Morath S, Papadopulos N, Schaff J (2011) Operative management and techniques of mastectomy in female-to-male transsexuals. Handchir Mikrochir Plast Chir 43:232–239
7. Kaiser C, Stoll J, Ataseven B et al (2011) Vaginal hysterectomy and bilateral adnexectomy for female-to-male transsexuals in an interdisciplinary concept. Handchir Mikrochir Plast Chir 43:240–245
8. Spilotras M, Ralph DJ, Christopher AN et al (2012) Outcome and risk factors for vaginectomy in female-to-male transsexuals. J Sex Med 9(Suppl 4):184
9. Doornaert M, Hoebeke P, Ceulemans P et al (2011) Penile reconstruction with the radial forearm flap: an update. Handchir Mikrochir Plast Chir 43:208–214
10. Gilbert DA, Horten CE, Tercis JK et al (1987) New concept in phallic reconstruction. Ann Plast Surg 18:128–136
11. Monstrey S, Hoebeke P, Selvaggi G et al (2009) Penile reconstruction: is the radial forearm flap really the standard technique? Plast Reconstr Surg 124:510–518
12. Hage JJ, Arjen AWM, van Turnhout M (2006) Long-term outcome of metoidioplasty in 70 female-to-male transsexuals. Ann Plast Surg 57:312–316
13. Djordjevic ML, Biziz MR (2013) Comparison of two different methods for urethral lengthening in female-to-male (Metoidioplasty) surgery. J Sex Med 10:1431–1438
14. Baumeister S, Sohn M, Domke C et al (2011) Phalloplasty in female-to-male transsexuals: experience from 259 cases. Handchir Mikrochir Plast Chir 43:215–221
15. Garaffa G, Christopher A, Ralph DJ (2010) Total phallic reconstruction in female-to-male transsexuals. Eur Urol 57:715–722
16. Sohn M (2010) Complications in transgender genital surgery. In: Austoni E (ed) Atlas of reconstructive penile surgery. Pacini, Pisa, pp 455–459
17. Sinove Y, Kyriopoulos E, Ceulemans P et al (2013) Preoperative planning of a pedicled anterolateral thigh (ALT) flap for penile reconstruction with the multidetector scan. Handchir Mikrochir Plast Chir 45:217–222
18. Dabernig J, Chan LKW, Schaff J (2006) Phalloplasty with free (septocutaneous) fibular flap sine fibula. J Urol 176:2085–2088
19. Van Caenegem E, Verhaeghe E, Taes Y et al (2013) Long-term evaluation of donor-site morbidity after radial forearm flap phalloplasty for transsexual men. J Sex Med 10:1644–1651
20. Hoebeke P, Selvaggi G, Ceulemans P et al (2005) Impact of sex reassignment surgery on lower urinary tract function. Eur Urol 47:398–402
21. Lumen N, Oosterlinck W, Decaestecker K et al (2009) Endoscopic incision of short urethral strictures after phallic reconstruction. J Endourol 23:1–4
22. Hoebeke PB, Decaestecker K, Beysens M et al (2010) Erectile implants in female-to-male transsexuals: our experience in 129 patients. Eur Urol 57:334–341
23. Lumen N, Monstrey S, Goessaert AS et al (2011) Urethroplasty for strictures after phallic reconstruction: a single institution experience. Eur Urol 60: 150–158
24. Rohrmann D, Jakse G (2003) Urethroplasty in female-to-male transsexuals. Eur Urol 44:611–614

36 Penile Prosthesis Implantation in Phalloplasty in Female-to-Male Transsexuals

Giulio Garaffa and David J. Ralph

36.1 Introduction

The ideal goal of total phallic construction is the creation in few surgical stages of a cosmetically acceptable sensate phallus with incorporated neourethra, to allow the patient to void in the standing position in a male urinal, and enough bulk to house a stiffener, to guarantee the adequate rigidity for penetrative sexual intercourse [1, 2].

Achieving the rigidity necessary for sexual penetration has always been a challenge as no tissue available for phallic construction represents an adequate substitute for the unique cavernosal tissue.

Autologous bone and cartilage transplants have been initially advocated as the solution for obtaining rigidity as they are usually not extruded, but resorption, fracture and poor concealment were major drawbacks, and therefore these methods have been progressively abandoned [3, 4].

Initially described in 1977, implantation of an inflatable penile prosthesis now represents the solution of choice for the achievement of rigidity in a phalloplasty [5–7].

Although various case reports have described implantation of an erectile device in phalloplasty in a single patient, only three series report of a larger number of cases and deserve mention [4, 8, 9–13].

G. Garaffa, MD, FRCS (✉) • D.J. Ralph
St Peter's Andrology and The Institute of Urology, The London Clinic, University College London Hospitals, 145 Harley Street, London W1G 6BJ, UK
e-mail: giuliogaraffa@gmail.com

This chapter describes the various surgical steps, intra- and postoperative complications and long-term outcome of penile prosthesis implantation in female-to-male transsexuals who had previously undergone total phallic construction.

36.2 Penile Prosthesis Implantation

The main challenge surgeons have to face when implanting a penile prosthesis in a phallus is the lack of the tunica albuginea, which naturally houses and protects the cylinders and minimizes the risk of extrusion. Implantation of semirigid devices was associated with ischaemia in the distal aspect of the phallus as the device was producing constant compression on the surrounding tissues. As this process led to the formation of pressure sores and ultimately to the erosion of the device through the skin, at present, malleable implants are not routinely implanted in a phallus.

Superior results can be achieved with hydraulic devices, as they can be inflated, when rigidity is required, and in flaccidity they relieve the pressure on the surrounding phallic tissues, and therefore the chance of pressure sores are minimized.

Due to the lack of the tunica albuginea in the neophallus, the cylinders need to be wrapped in a synthetic sheath to anchor them to the pubic bone and minimize distal erosion, as described in detail in the following sections of this chapter.

C. Trombetta et al. (eds.), *Management of Gender Dysphoria: A Multidisciplinary Approach*, DOI 10.1007/978-88-470-5696-1_36, © Springer-Verlag Italia 2015

36.3 Patient Choice and Preparation

Ideally penile prosthesis implantation should be carried out at least 1 year after the initial phallic construction, once cutaneous sensation is likely to have developed and all urethral complications have been successfully corrected. This is because the presence of cutaneous sensation reduces the chance of pressure sores and ultimately of erosion of the device, while the surgical correction of urethral complications with a penile implant in situ is quite challenging and the risk of inadvertently damaging or exposing the cylinders has to be taken into consideration [1, 2, 6, 7].

Due to the higher risk of complications and the shorter life expectancy of penile prosthesis in a phallus, only highly motivated patients with good hand dexterity, who have a partner and who are otherwise ready to engage in penetrative sexual intercourse should be offered penile prosthesis implantation. The choice of the type of implant (three pieces AMS 700 CX/CXR® [American Medical Systems, Minnetonka, Minnesota, USA] or Titan Coloplast® [Coloplast Corporation, Copenhagen, Denmark] versus two pieces AMS Ambicor® [American Medical Systems, Minnetonka, Minnesota, USA]) and of the number of cylinders (one or two) should be discussed with the patient during the preoperative visit, and the decision should be made according to the size and shape of the phallus and patients' preference. The insertion of two cylinders should be offered only in patients with wider phalluses and if the surgeon suspects that one cylinder would not guarantee enough rigidity for penetrative intercourse.

To minimize the chance of infection, implantation of the device should be carried out after intravenous administration of broad-spectrum antibiotic and 10 min scrub of the surgical field with povidone-iodine (Betadine®, Meda, Sweden).

36.4 Surgical Technique

Typically, implantation of three-piece inflatable penile prostheses (3P-IPP) should be performed either in one or two stages. In patients who undergo the procedure in two stages, a testis prosthesis is inserted in the labia ipsilateral to the dominant hand, and the reservoir is implanted under direct vision in the extraperitoneal space at the time of the glans sculpture with the use of a full-thickness skin graft according to the Norfolk technique. The reservoir is inflated, and its tubing capped off with a deactivation plug and left in proximity of the testicular prosthesis, in a position easily identifiable by the surgeon during the following stage. The rationale of inserting the reservoir at this stage lies on the fact that an incision in the inguinal fossa has to be carried out anyway at this stage to allow the harvesting of the skin graft, and therefore it is easy to deepen the incision to create the space for the reservoir just below the transversus abdominis muscle, in the preperitoneal space. The second stage, which is performed at least 3 months afterwards, consists in the implantation of 1 or 2 cylinder(s) and of the pump of an inflatable penile prosthesis, which are then connected with the pre-existing reservoir. The pump is fitted in the space previously occupied by the testicular prosthesis, which is transferred to the contralateral labia, to form a neo-scrotum. The aim of splitting the procedure in two stages is to allow the formation of a mature capsule around the full reservoir and the testis prosthesis, in order to minimize the chance of autoinflation of the device when the reservoir is connected to the rest of the device and to form an adequate space where to fit the pump [1].

Two 2-piece inflatable penile prostheses (2P-IPP) are instead implanted in only one stage, as they have no separate reservoir.

As the implantation of the reservoir in the female-to-male transsexual is performed with the same technique used in male patients, this chapter focuses only on the implantation of the cylinders and pump.

Preparation for the implantation of the cylinder(s) and pump involves hair shave in the operative theatre, 10' min scrub with antiseptic solution and administration of broad-spectrum antibiotics. A 14 French catheter is usually inserted at the beginning of the procedure to allow the identification of the urethra intraoperatively, as in case of urethral injury the procedure has to be abandoned. The implantation of the cylinder(s) is carried out through a groin incision in the skin crease on the side of the testis and reservoir; if the simultaneous insertion of a second cylinder is planned, an additional incision in the contralateral groin crease is necessary. The incision is deepened to the pubic bone, and all tissues are retracted medially to expose the central aspect of the pubic symphysis. Once the periosteum is fully exposed, 4 J-needle 0 polyester sutures (Ethibond®, Ethicon, Somerville, New Jersey, USA) are inserted into the pubic bone in two parallel rows approximately 2 cm apart for prosthesis anchorage; in case of insertion of two cylinders, the procedure is repeated on the contralateral side.

The neophallus is then sequentially dilated with Hegars up to size 17, to create enough space to house the cylinder and the polyethylene terephthalate tip (Dacron®, Invista, Kansas, USA), making sure that the cavity is away from the skin and neourethral surface in order to minimize the risk of extrusion of the implant at a later date.

The phallus length is then measured from its tip to the pubic symphysis, and the size of the cylinder(s) is chosen accordingly. A polyethylene terephthalate sock is then fashioned to house the rear of the cylinder(s) with incorporation of the exit tubing. This is used for anchorage to the pubic bone. In order to decrease the risk of infection of the implant, the polyethylene terephthalate can be soaked in an antibiotic solution, usually gentamicin (Gentamicin®, Sandoz, Holzkirchen, Germany) and rifampicin (Rifadin®, Aventis, Paris, France). The use of silver impregnated polyethylene terephthalate seems to be associated with a significant reduction in infection rates. A similar polyethylene terephthalate cap is fashioned to incorporate the tip of the cylinder to prevent hypermobility and erosion.

After the cylinder is implanted by the use of the Furlow introducer, the polyethylene terephthalate sock is anchored to the pubic bone using the 4 polyester sutures that had been previously inserted.

The testicular prosthesis is then removed, and the pump placed into its capsule in order to allow for extra mobility and ease of access by the patient; all the cylinders', pumps' and reservoirs' tubings are then connected. A 10 French suction drain can be left in situ, the skin incision closed in layers with desorbable sutures, and the cylinder(s) left semi-inflated to minimize the chance of haematoma formation.

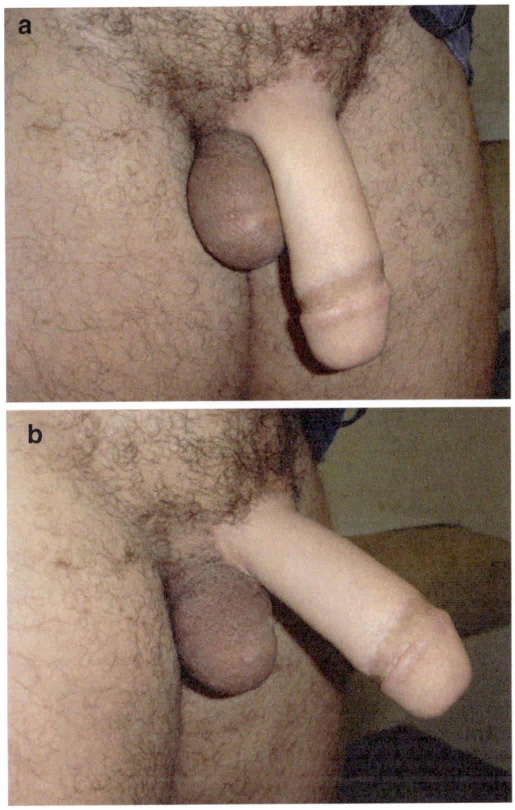

Fig. 36.1a, b The final result after implantation of a three-piece inflatable penile prosthesis in the flaccid and in the erect state

Finally, the original testicular prosthesis is inserted into the contralateral labia through a separate incision so that the neo-scrotum contains the pump on the side of the dominant hand and one testis on the contralateral side.

The catheter and drain are usually removed on postoperative day one, and the patient is discharged on oral amoxicillin/clavulanic acid for 5 days; the penile prosthesis is usually deflated 1 week postoperatively in the clinic and the patient taught how to cycle the prosthesis 3 weeks later, when the postoperative swelling had settled, and encouraged to have penetrative sexual intercourse as soon as the wounds are completely healed (Fig. 36.1a, b; the final result after implantation of a three-piece inflatable penile prosthesis in the flaccid and in the erect state).

36.5 Intraoperative Complications

Intraoperative complications include inadvertent injury to the vascular pedicle of the phallus and urethral perforation. Although the role of the vascular pedicle is uncertain, as 1 year after the phallic construction it is likely that the phallus has grown a new, independent blood supply arising from the pubic area, preservation of the pedicle is always advisable.

In order to minimize the chance of inadvertent injury to the vascular pedicle and the neourethra, it is paramount to create the space for the insertion of the cylinders with blunt dissection with Metzenbaum scissors and Hegar dilators. Performing the dissection laterally should reduce the chance of hitting the vascular pedicle, which runs on the dorsal aspect at the base of the phallus before moving towards its ventral aspect in an anticlockwise fashion towards the tip, if the radial artery flap has been harvested from the left forearm. In patients who had their phallus harvested from the right forearm, the pedicle instead runs in a clockwise fashion.

In order to minimize the risk of urethral injury, the catheter should be squeezed between the thumb and index finger of the nondominant hand in order to keep the neourethra away from the tip of the scissors and of the dilators. The presence of a urethral injury should be ruled out before proceeding with the insertion of the cylinder(s), and to do so the phallus should be irrigated with antibiotic solution. In case of fluid at the neomeatus, the presence of a neourethral injury should be suspected, and the procedure should be therefore abandoned. The catheter should be left in situ for 2 weeks to allow the urethra to heal, and a new attempt of penile prosthesis implantation should be deferred for 6 months to allow for the healing process to be complete and to rule out the presence of urethral strictures and fistulas.

36.6 Postoperative Complications

Immediate postoperative complications include ischaemic necrosis of the phallus and penile prosthesis infection.

Ischaemic necrosis of the phallus is extremely rare and is either secondary to injury to the vascular pedicle or to excessive compression by the cylinders on the surrounding tissues. If phallic ischaemia is suspected, the only advisable procedure is to deflate the prosthesis, to reduce the pressure exerted by the cylinders on the phallus.

Penile prosthesis infection rate can be as high as 15 % [12–16], significantly higher than in virgin implants in the male. This is mainly due to the presence of foreign bodies in contact with the implant (polyethylene terephthalate sock and tip), which are required to house the cylinders and anchor them to the pubic bone.

Penile prosthesis infection can be subdivided into acute and chronic. The former is characterized by sepsis, purulent collection around the implant, swelling and erythema, while in the latter the symptoms are generally mild and usually patients complain of dull ache at the level of the phallus and pain while cycling the device.

In case of penile prosthesis infection, all the components of the device have to be removed, including the polyethylene terephthalate tip and sock, and the cavity irrigated with antiseptic and antibiotic solutions. Salvage procedures have not been described in these patients, and a new attempt of penile prosthesis implantation should be deferred for at least 4–6 months to allow for a complete healing process to occur.

Rates of mechanical failure of the device can be as high as 50 % at 4 years, which is significantly higher than in virgin male patients [13]. This is because of the lack of the tunica albuginea, which naturally protects the cylinders, and of a lax, loose scrotum, which guarantees an adequate shelter for the tubing and the pump. This is why the most common locations of device failure are the cylinders, due to the continuous friction with the polyethylene terephthalate tip and sock, and at the level where the tubings exit from the pump, as they are forcibly bent to be accommodated in a stiff, small neo-scrotum.

In case of mechanical failure, the faulty component of the device needs to be identified and replaced. If the prosthesis has been implanted more than 3 years before, all the components of the device should be replaced, as they have almost reached their full life expectancy [13].

Malposition of the device has been described in up to 15 % of cases and can cause pain when cycling the implant or having sexual intercourse. Revision surgery, which involves repositioning the device in the correct location, should not be postponed as malposition of the device can lead to premature wearing of the device or erosion.

36.7 Surgical Outcome

As penile prosthesis implantation in a phallus is a very uncommon procedure, no standardized validated questionnaires are available in the literature to evaluate surgical outcome and patient's satisfaction. Surgical outcome is assessed subjectively by the surgeon, and patients are directly questioned to investigate satisfaction rates. In particular, a straight phallus with enough rigidity to allow successful penetrative intercourse and a pump that is easy to access and cycle are considered a satisfactory surgical outcome.

Clearly complication rates tend to be high, and therefore adequate preoperative counselling of the patient is mandatory to make sure they have realistic expectations from surgery and therefore are more likely to be satisfied with the surgical outcome.

Despite of a high overall complication rate, in the largest series published so far, after a median follow-up of 30 months, after revision surgery, 108 out of 129 patients (84 %) have a functional erectile device, are potentially able to have penetrative sexual intercourse and are satisfied with the surgical outcome [13].

Conclusions

Two- and three-piece inflatable penile prosthesis implantation represent the only solution in female-to-male patients who have undergone total phallic reconstruction and wish to achieve the rigidity necessary for penetrative sexual intercourse.

The procedure is complex, and complication rates are still significantly higher than penile prosthesis implantation in ED patients and therefore should be carried out only by experienced surgeons in large volume dedicated centres.

References

1. Garaffa G, Christopher AN, Ralph DJ (2010) Total phallic reconstruction in female-to-male transsexuals. Eur Urol 57(4):715–722
2. Doornaert M, Hoebeke P, Ceulemans P, T'sjoen G, Heylens G, Monstrey S (2011) Penile reconstruction with the radial forearm flap: an update. Handchir Mikrochir Plast Chir 43(4):208–214
3. Bogoras N (1936) Über die volle plastische Wiederherstellung eines zum Koitus fähigen Penis (Peniplastica totalis). Zentralbl Chir 22:1271–1276
4. Hage JJ, Bloem JJA, Bouman FG (1993) Obtaining rigidity in the neophallus of female-to-male transsexuals: a review of the literature. Ann Plast Surg 30:327–333
5. Puckett CL, Montie JE (1978) Construction of male genitalia in the transsexual, using a tubed groin flap for the penis and a hydraulic inflation device. Plast Reconstr Surg 61:523–530
6. Garaffa G, Ralph DJ, Christopher AN (2010) Total urethral reconstruction with the use of the forearm free flap in the transsexual. BJU Int 106(8):1206–1210
7. Bettocchi C, Ralph DJ, Pryor JP (2004) Pedicled pubic phalloplasty in females with gender dysphoria. BJU Int 95:120–124
8. Carson CC, Mulcahy JJ, Govier FE (1997) Efficacy, safety and patient satisfaction outcomes of the AMS 700CX inflatable penile prosthesis. J Urol 158: 456–459
9. Levine LA, Estrada CR, Morgentaler A (2001) Mechanical reliability and safety of, and patient satisfaction with the Ambicor inflatable penile prosthesis: results of a 2 center study. J Urol 166:932–937
10. Henry GD, Donatucci CF, Conners W, Greenfield JM, Carson CC, Wilson SK et al (2012) An outcomes analysis of over 200 revision surgeries for penile prosthesis implantation: a multicenter study. J Sex Med 9(1):309–315
11. Levine LA, Zachary LS, Gottlieb LJ (1993) Prosthesis placement after total phallic reconstruction. J Urol 149:593–598
12. Hoebeke P, Cuypere G, Ceulemans P, Monstrey S (2003) Obtaining rigidity in total phalloplasty: experience with 35 patients. J Urol 169:221–223
13. Hoebeke P, Decaestecker K, Beysens M, Opdenakker Y, Lumen N, Monstrey S (2009) Erectile implants in female-to-male transsexuals: our experience in 129 patients. Eur Urol 57:334–341
14. Boyd SD, Martins FE (1995) Simultaneous Ultrex penile prosthesis reimplantation and Gore-Tex grafting corporoplasty. J Urol 153:359

15. Sansalone S, Garaffa G, Djinovic R, Egydio P, Vespasiani G, Miano R, Loreto C, Ralph DJ (2012) Simultaneous penile lengthening and penile prosthesis implantation in patients with Peyronie's Disease, refractory erectile dysfunction and severe penile shortening. J Sex Med 9(1):316–321
16. Ralph DJ, Garaffa G, Christopher AN (2010) Editorial comment on: erectile implants in female-to-male transsexuals: our experience in 129 patients. Eur Urol 57:340–341

37 Imaging

Michele Bertolotto, Francesca Cacciato, Cristina Cercato, Vincenzo Savoca, and Carlo Trombetta

37.1 Introduction

The goal of female-to-male sex reassignment surgery (FtM SRS) is to provide an aesthetically attractive and functional result, which permits for the new male voiding while standing and ability to penetrate preserving an orgasmic potential. In the standard clinical practice, imaging is not routinely performed. However, different imaging modalities can be considered in selected cases both before and after sex reassignment surgery to evaluate the integrity of the donor and the acceptor site for the neopenis, to investigate breast tissues and pelvic organs before hysteroannessiectomy and mastectomy, to identify postoperative complications, and to investigate the integrity of the neopenis before prosthesis implantation.

M. Bertolotto, MD (✉)
Department of Radiology, University of Trieste, Cattinara Hospital, Strada di Fiume 447, Trieste 34149, Italy
e-mail: bertolot@units.it

F. Cacciato • C. Cercato • V. Savoca
Department of Radiology, University of Trieste, Ospedale di Cattinara, Strada di Fiume 447, Trieste 34149, Italy
e-mail: francescacacciato@gmail.com; s129198@stud.units.it; enzosavoca@gmail.com

C. Trombetta
Department of Urology, University of Trieste, Cattinara Hospital, Strada di Fiume 447, Trieste 34149, Italy
e-mail: trombcar@units.it; trombcar@univ.trieste.it

37.2 MR Anatomy after FtM SRS

The superior soft tissue contrast resolution afforded by MR imaging provides an opportunity to advance the imaging evaluation of the postoperative anatomy in FtM SRS.

The new male anatomy is best estimated on T2-weighted images which show hysterectomy and oophorectomy, lengthening of the urethra, and creation of a scrotum containing testicular implants (Fig. 37.1). The vagina is usually closed or has been removed, but in some patients, it may be patent.

If the patient underwent phalloplasty, a hypertrophied clitoris is identified. The morphology and attachment of the neophallus vary depending on the surgical technique. In metoidioplasty, the clitoris is changed into a small neopenis.

37.3 Imaging of the Donor and Acceptor Site

If a free flap phalloplasty is chosen, the feeding vessels must be confirmed to be intact by a vascular Doppler ultrasound examination. With the radial forearm flap, this is particularly important in patients who have had fractures of the upper limb or have scarring from previous suicide

C. Trombetta et al. (eds.), *Management of Gender Dysphoria: A Multidisciplinary Approach*, DOI 10.1007/978-88-470-5696-1_37, © Springer-Verlag Italia 2015

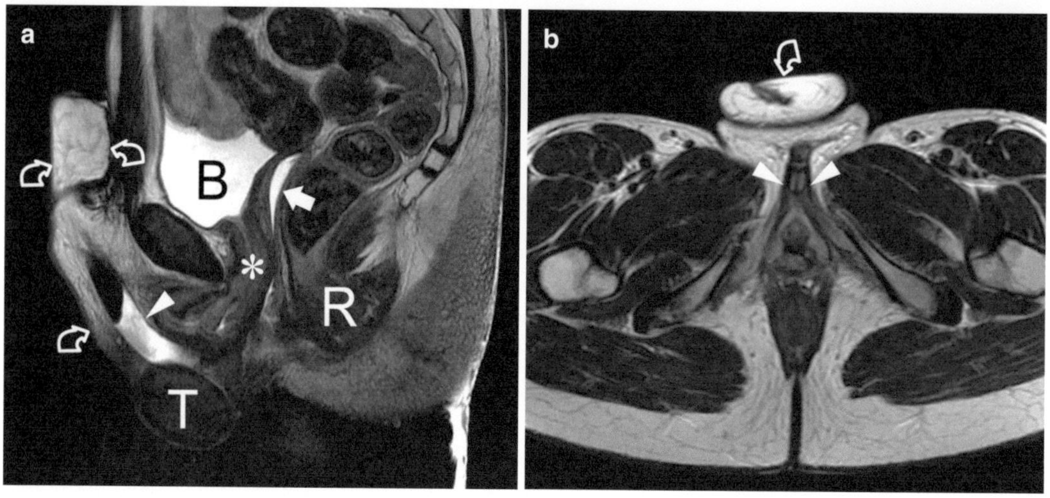

Fig. 37.1 Postoperative anatomy of the new male after FtM SRS. The patient had a urethral stenosis. (**a**) Sagittal T2-weighted image showing hysterectomy and patent vagina (*arrow*) which is distended by a small amount of fluid. In the neopenis (*curved arrows*), the urethra is dilated (*arrowhead*) and filled with saline. The native urethra (*) is not distended. *B* bladder, *T* testicular prosthesis, *R* rectum. (**b**) Axial T2-weighted image showing the neopenis (*curved arrow*) and the hypertrophied clitoris (*arrowheads*)

attempts. Doppler investigation of the vessels of the acceptor site is indicated to assess their patency and caliber in patients with previous abdominal surgery. In patients undergoing anterolateral thigh (ALT) flap phalloplasty, CT angiography is the state-of-the-art imaging modality for preoperative vascular mapping of the donor site [1]. The entire vascular tree supplying the flap is fully investigated from the femoral artery to the perforators. If the need arises, the acceptor site can also be studied with the same CT procedure (Fig. 37.2).

Perforators are then marked by using Doppler interrogation in the neighborhood of the points identified by CT [2]. Preoperative color Doppler sonography is valuable in identifying the location of the penetrating points and the suprafascial courses of skin perforators. It facilitates prefabrication of the urethra, assists in the design of the flap, prevents injury to skin perforators during elevation of the flap, and decreases the risk of flap necrosis.

Besides the evaluation of the perforators, preoperative MDCT provides also an accurate preoperative measurement of the subcutaneous fat tissue in the donor site which is necessary in order to allow an adequate patient and perforator selection and to determine the exact size of the flap [1].

37.4 Breast Imaging

Before sex reassignment surgery, preoperative breast imaging, either ultrasonography and/or mammography, is indicated according to age, if the patient meets the usual natal female requirements [3]. We routinely investigate the breast also during the workup for the subcutaneous mastectomy. Early after the mastectomy, imaging has a role in the assessment of postoperative complications, including hematoma, seroma, and abscess formation [3]. Imaging-guided drainage may be performed if clinically indicated. FtM transsexuals who have undergone bilateral subcutaneous mastectomy as part of sex reassignment surgery have dramatically decreased risk of breast cancer by nearly 90 % compared to women [4]. Although there remains a small possibility that breast cancer may develop in residual breast tissue, screening mammography is therefore not indicated.

37.5 Postoperative Evaluation of the Neourethra

For FtM transsexuals undergoing phalloplasty, the ability to void while standing is a high priority [5]. Unfortunately, the reported incidence

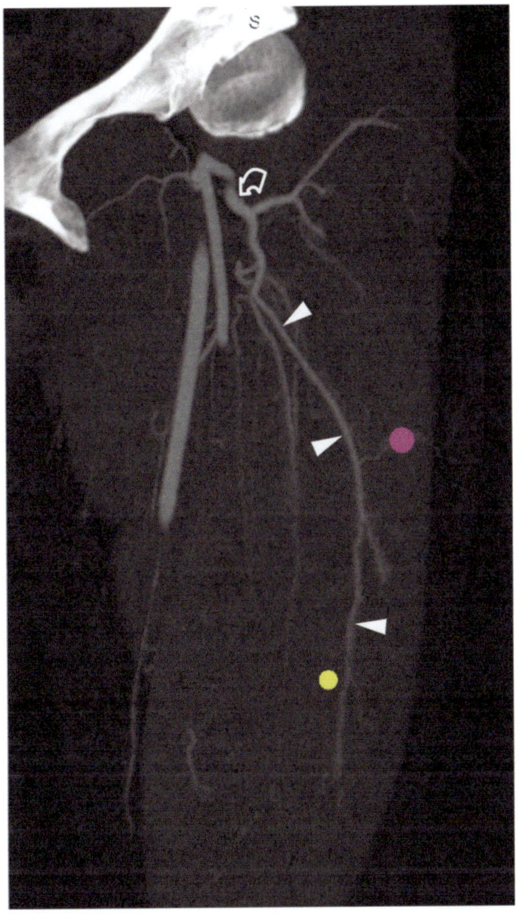

Fig. 37.2 Preoperative vascular mapping of the left thigh in a 30-year-old FtM transsexual patient undergoing anterolateral thigh (ALT) flap phalloplasty. CT angiography shows the descending branch (*arrowheads*) of the lateral femoral circumflex artery (*curved arrow*) and two dominant perforators supplying the ALT flap (*purple and yellow dots*)

of urological complications following urethral reconstruction is high in all series [1, 6]. For this reason, certain surgeons have even stopped reconstructing a complete neourethra [7, 8]. The most serious complications of urethral reconstruction are urethrocutaneous fistulas, stenoses, and strictures. Hair growth is a relatively common cause of germ proliferation in the neourethra and chronic inflammation. Urethrography is the imaging modality of choice to evaluate urethral abnormalities and is routinely performed before removal of the suprapubic catheter inserted during the operation to divert the urine (Fig. 37.3).

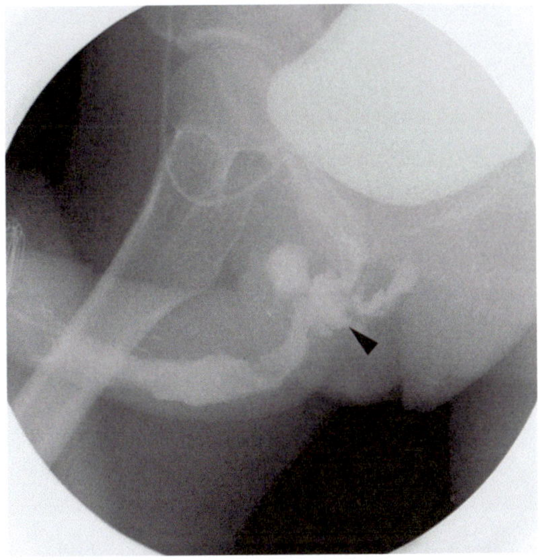

Fig. 37.3 Urethral fistula in a 31-year-old FtM transsexual with radial forearm flap phalloplasty. Voiding urethrogram shows contrast material extravasation at the anastomosis (*arrowhead*) between the native urethra and the neourethra

Ultrasonography allows also evaluation of hair growth in the neourethra [9].

37.6 Prosthesis Implantation

Most FtM patients want to use the neophallus for sexual experience. Care must be paid during prosthesis insertion to avoid injury to the neourethra and to the vascular pedicle of the neopenis.

Color Doppler ultrasound is able to identify the neourethra and the vascular pedicle of the neopenis in order to avoid incidental injury during prosthesis insertion (Fig. 37.4). Compared to color Doppler ultrasound, MR imaging provides a more panoramic view of the penoid and allows assessment of fibrotic changes resulting from inflammatory and ischemic complications (Fig. 37.5).

A major concern is as regards the long-term follow-up of prosthesis in FtM transsexuals. A recent study showed an explantation rate of 44 % in 130 patients, mainly due to malpositioning, technical failure, or infection [10]. MR imaging is the investigation of choice to evaluate the integrity and morphology of the prosthesis and to identify inflammatory complications.

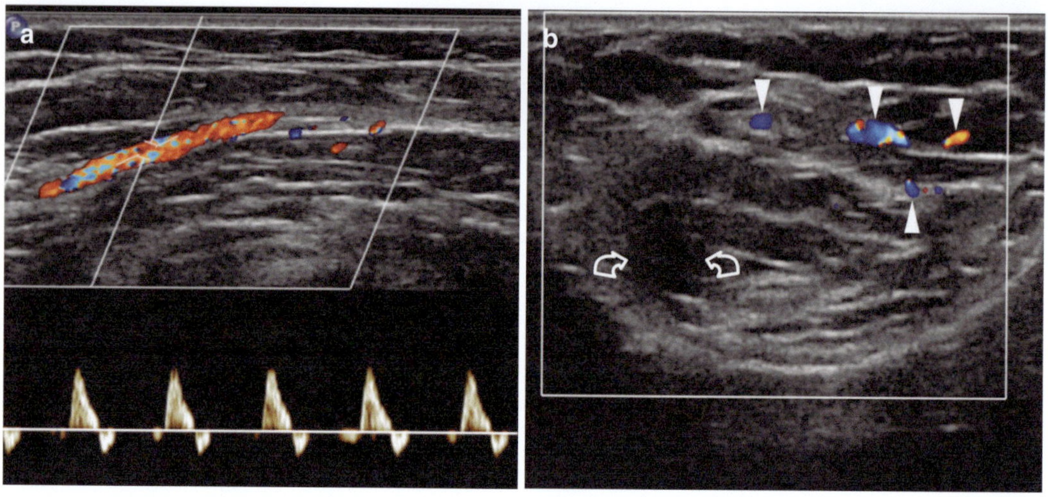

Fig. 37.4 Evaluation of the vascular pedicle of the neophallus before prosthesis insertion in a 46-year-old FtM transsexual with radial forearm flap phalloplasty. (**a**) Color Doppler image obtained along the course of the vascular pedicle of the penoid. (**b**) Transverse color Doppler ultrasound image of the neophallus showing the position of the vessels (*arrowheads*) and of the neourethra (*curved arrows*)

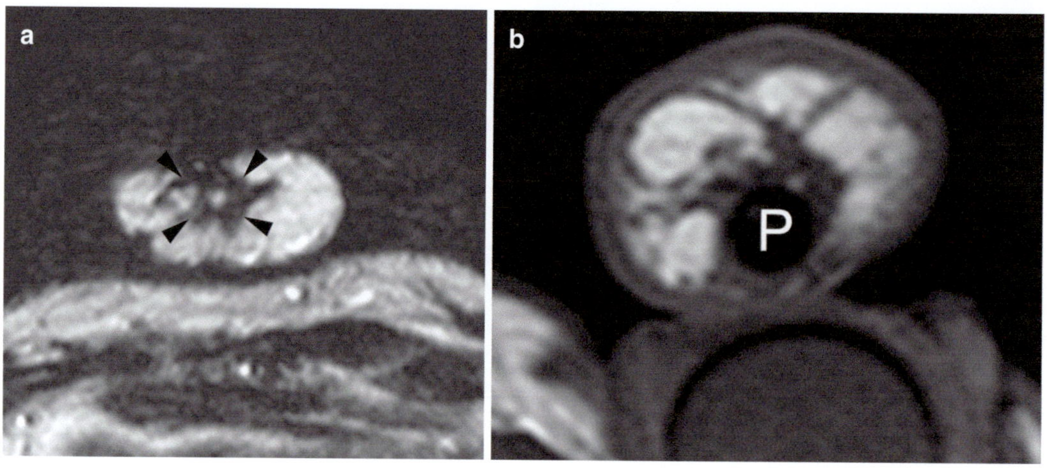

Fig. 37.5 Evaluation of the neophallus before prosthesis insertion in a 49-year-old FtM transsexual with radial forearm flap phalloplasty. The intervention was complicated by ischemia which resulted in severe fibrotic changes and required defunctionalization of the urethra. (**a**) Axial T2-weighted image obtained before prosthesis insertion shows the extension of the fibrotic changes (*arrowheads*). (**b**) Axial T2-weighted image obtained after a semirigid prosthesis was inserted within the scarring tissue to minimize the risk of vascular damage confirms the absence of postoperative complications. *P* prosthesis

Conclusions

The ideal flap for phalloplasty, besides the versatility of the flap and the low donor site morbidity, combines the shaping, the consistency and sensitivity of the neophallus, and the urethral reconstruction in the same operation stage for optimal patient satisfaction. A good patient selection is critical when considering the technique for phalloplasty. In particular, MDCT examination allows the preoperative evaluation of anatomic variations. It is valuable in identifying the course of skin perforators and assists in the design of the flap. Preoperative color Doppler sonography is valuable especially in the evaluation of the integrity of the vascularity of the acceptor site. Urethrography is the imaging modality of choice for the evaluation of the neourethra, while MR imaging has a role when planning prosthesis insertion.

References

1. Sinove Y, Kyriopoulos E, Ceulemans P, Houtmeyers P, Hoebeke P, Monstrey S (2013) Praoperative Planung der gestielten anterolateralen Oberschenkel-Lappenplastik fur Penis-Rekonstruktionen mittels Multidetektor-CT. Handchir Mikrochir Plast Chir. doi :10.1055/s-0032-1333271
2. Onoda S, Azumi S, Hasegawa K, Kimata Y (2013) Preoperative identification of perforator vessels by combining MDCT, doppler flowmetry, and ICG fluorescent angiography. Microsurgery 33:265–269. doi:10.1002/micr.22079
3. Phillips J, Fein-Zachary VJ, Mehta TS, Littlehale N, Venkataraman S, Slanetz PJ (2014) Breast imaging in the transgender patient. AJR Am J Roentgenol 202:1149–1156
4. Rebbeck TR, Friebel T, Lynch HT et al (2004) Bilateral prophylactic mastectomy reduces breast cancer risk in BRCA1 and BRCA2 mutation carriers: the PROSE Study Group. J Clin Oncol 22:1055–1062
5. Hage JJ, Bout CA, Bloem JJ, Megens JA (1993) Phalloplasty in female-to-male transsexuals: what do our patients ask for? Ann Plast Surg 30:323–326
6. Babaei A, Safarinejad MR, Farrokhi F, Iran-Pour E (2010) Penile reconstruction: evaluation of the most accepted techniques. Urol J 7:71–78
7. Felici N, Felici A (2006) A new phalloplasty technique: the free anterolateral thigh flap phalloplasty. J Plast Reconstr Aesthet Surg 59:153–157
8. Matti BA, Matthews RN, Davies DM (1988) Phalloplasty using the free radial forearm flap. Br J Plast Surg 41:160–164
9. Bertolotto M, Serafini G, Savoca G et al (2005) Color Doppler US of the postoperative penis: anatomy and surgical complications. Radiographics 25:731–748
10. Hoebeke P, Selvaggi G, Ceulemans P et al (2005) Impact of sex reassignment surgery on lower urinary tract function. Eur Urol 47:398–402

Part IV

Legislative, Ethical and Health Policy Aspects

Ethical Issues for the Practitioner Work in the Transgender Care

38

Cristoforo Pomara, Andrea Brincat, Daniel Cassar, Massimo Martelloni, Emanuela Turillazzi, and Stefano D'Errico

38.1 Introduction

All treatment decisions involve the tacit decision to treat or to withhold treatment. Although often not expressed, the "not to treat" side of the analysis of risks versus benefits is quite important and should be explored in patients with gender identity dysphoria (GID) and its variants [1]. The availability of somatic treatments as accepted interventions for the overall management of GID raises a number of bioethical issues. The medical literature rarely is as rife with affect as when this issue is discussed by those who oppose the application of surgical treatments as part of the treatment plan for gender transmutation.

This passing fad for what is miscalled "transsexualism" has led to the most tragic betrayal of human expectation in which medicine and modern endocrinology and surgery have been engaged [2].

Psychiatrists' responses to requests for treatment from those with GID range from the nearly cavalier referral for hormones and sex reassignment surgery to an inflexible reticence to entertain any such referrals, erecting the defensive facades of "do no harm" and "never deliberately remove a healthy organ."

In spite of the fact that somatic treatments have been used for over 30 years, clinical decisions must be made in the absence of well-controlled trials that compare multimodal treatment (which includes hormones and sex reassignment surgery – SRS) to purely psychiatric interventions [3–6]. Although there is far more evidence in favor of utilizing somatic treatments as part of the treatment plan for carefully evaluated persons with GID [7, 8], decisions must be made with the awareness that the psychiatrist shares the "moral responsibility for that decision (i.e., whether or not to refer for SRS) with the surgeon who accepts that recommendation" [9].

The decision to withhold somatic treatments carries with it a significant risk that must also be taken into consideration [10]. For example, the incidence of suicidal behavior and genital self-mutilatory behavior appears to be greater in those denied SRS than in those referred for this procedure [11–13]. Along with psychotic decompensation [14], postoperative suicide due to regrets over having had SRS is often cited as the most

C. Pomara (✉)
Department of Forensic Medicine, University of Foggia, Foggia, Italy

Department of Anatomy, University of Malta, Msida, Malta
e-mail: cristoforopomara@hotmail.com

A. Brincat • D. Cassar
Department of Anatomy, University of Malta, Msida, Malta

M. Martelloni • S. D'Errico
Department of Legal Medicine, USL2 Lucca, Lucca, Italy

E. Turillazzi
Department of Forensic Medicine, University of Foggia, Foggia, Italy

C. Trombetta et al. (eds.), *Management of Gender Dysphoria: A Multidisciplinary Approach*,
DOI 10.1007/978-88-470-5696-1_38, © Springer-Verlag Italia 2015

compelling reason to withhold this intervention [10, 15, 16].

Both of these negative outcomes are actually quite unusual, however, as noted by follow-up studies in countries that have the ability to monitor outcomes in fairly homogeneous societies with centralized health-care registries [12]. Given the very low rate of requests for reversal in many recent studies from around the world, it appears that some of the earlier concerns about somatic treatments have not been borne out.

In spite of a preponderance of clinical reports supportive of providing somatic treatments in carefully selected patients, clinicians faced with the evaluation and treatment of gender-dysphoric persons must address both countertransference issues and bioethical concerns in the absence of well-controlled, prospective studies of large numbers of patients over lengthy follow-up periods. While the medical community seems to have few qualms about genital surgery on minors (with substituted consent) for inborn biological errors such as ambiguous genitalia conditions and pseudohermaphroditism [17, 18], the same detached approach has not been applied to altering the anatomy of adults and adolescents with bona fide GID.

Patients with severe GID often have pervasive disturbances in their sense of self and are willing to seek out mental health-care professionals who are able to confront their own ethical, moral, and spiritual standards in an attempt to provide compassionate care or competent referrals.

An additional bioethical issue that is still actively debated is whether to provide SRS for applicants who are HIV infected. Some persons with GID engage in commercial sex work or are otherwise at increased risk for acquiring blood-borne infections [19, 20]. Indeed, an HIV test is usually part of the required preoperative testing. Speaking to this issue, the Harry Benjamin International Gender Dysphoria Association (HBIGDA) adopted a resolution in September 1997 that states, "The availability of sex reassignment surgery should not be denied solely on the basis of blood seropositivity for blood borne infections (such as HIV, hepatitis B or C, etc.)." This resolution has not been embraced by all health-care providers, however, and it is often difficult for otherwise qualified, appropriate candidates for SRS to receive this treatment due to reticence on the part of some surgeons who perform this procedure [21]. Many state medical licensing boards also make it illegal to discriminate on the basis of HIV seropositivity in the delivery of health-care services. However, there remains controversy in surgical circles over the ethical issue of balancing risks to surgeons and the rights of patients referred for this procedure [22].

38.2 Ethical Issues for Practitioners

38.2.1 Background

Zandvliet defined gender "as the sum of a person's non-physical and non-biological characteristics that determine their sense of being male, female or neither or any combination" [23]. More recently, Nagoshi and Burzuzy defined gender as "an identity that exists separate from the constraints of physical sex characteristics and the dictates of a binary that our society has imposed" [24].

Transsexual is a medical term. Transgender is frequently indicated as an "umbrella term" that is used to describe individuals whose gender self-identification or expression transgresses established gender norms [25, 26]. Specifically, it is the state of one's gender identity (self-identification as male, female, both, or neither) not matching one's assigned gender (identification by others as male or female based on natal sex) [27].

In 1980, the American Psychiatric Association included transsexualism and gender identity disorder of childhood in DSM-III-R [28, 29]. It was not until publication of the DSM-IV that the diagnosis GID as applied to adults was codified [30].

According to the DSM-IV, gender identity disorder, or transsexuality, involves "a strong and persistent cross-gender identification (not merely a desire for any perceived cultural advantages of being the other sex), persistent discomfort with his or her sex or sense of inappropriateness in the gender role of that sex, clinically significant distress or impairment in social, occupational, or other important areas of functioning, all without having a physical intersex condition" [30–32].

In contrast to the American Psychological Association, it has been argued that transsexuality is *not* a mental disorder, but rather a physical problem which can be alleviated by means of a combination of physical therapies designed to change the body ("application of these diagnostic labels unnecessarily pathologizes transgender and gender-variant people"). Whether transsexuality is viewed as a mental disorder or whether it is viewed as simply another category of gender that should be accepted by society as legitimate, *the moral tension on the issue of GRS remains strong since GRS is an invasive surgery or group of surgeries which requires lots of medical resources that may, at times, be scarce.*

The availability of sex reassignment surgery as an intervention in the overall management of transsexualism raises a number of bioethical issues for physicians.

For those who accept the idea that transsexuality is a psychiatric disorder, there is moral tension regarding whether it is the duty of surgery to solve problems that could possibly be dealt with by means of a psychosocial approach or whether surgery is ever a morally acceptable, medically appropriate solution to the mind-body incongruity that exists in transsexual individuals.

People who maintain that all psychiatric disorders should be treated solely by psychologists and psychiatrists hold that GRS is not an acceptable solution to transsexualism. Additionally, it could be argued that surgeries which limit the function of healthy organs or produce significant health risk, as GRS does, should not be performed since surgery should only be done if it benefits a patient medically.

Those who believe that transsexualism is a physical problem, on the other hand, maintain that for some transsexuals, surgery is a medically appropriate treatment that has the potential to emotionally heal and provide a source of inner peace for those who feel their biological gender is incompatible with their inner gender identity [33, 34].

38.2.2 The Ethical Dilemma and Bioethical Principles

Considerations regarding the status of GID as a disorder and its relation to access to GRS are important since many people who identify as transsexual strongly desire body modification as the last step of their identity achievement. Serious incongruity between body and soul can, understandably, be very disquieting for an individual. Some transsexuals can achieve an adequate sense of body-soul congruency through hormonal therapies and cross-dressing, but for some, body modification is perceived as an integral part of achieving an identity as a member of the opposite gender. In order to achieve full body modification, surgery is often required for patient satisfaction. Hormone therapies can only do so much for patients; they can give male-to-female transsexuals breasts, but they can never give them a vagina. Cross-dressing and hormone therapies can give a female-to-male transsexual some sense of being male, but when he looks in the mirror, it is still a woman's soft face which looks back at him [35].

Since the inner struggle that goes with transsexuality is something that can be fixed by changing the body through surgery, *is surgery a viable treatment option?* If someone wants to achieve a desired image that he or she feels "matches what's on the inside" along with enough competence to fully understand the risks and benefits of undergoing surgery, then he or she *has the right to do so? All gender-dysphoric patients should be* approved for surgery?

It has been said for the moral permissibility of GRS that in cases in which "adult patients have been suffering from a severe gender-related mind-body imbalance which interferes with their everyday life functions, gender reassignment surgery is a morally permissible treatment option, provided that the patients requesting it are competent and are able to pay for the surgery out of pocket as an elective surgery without any serious financial detriment to their dependent family members" [36].

Patient autonomy. Competent adults who have identified themselves as transsexuals have the right to self-determination. Those who have the right to self-determination have the right to decide what to do with their bodies. Therefore, competent, adult individuals have the right to request and receive GRS [37].

Competence is the key when it comes to who should be able to obtain access to GRS. In this sense, the decision to undergo GRS has to represent the final step toward completion of a long, arduous journey of identity realization as a member of the opposite sex.

Most gender-variant people, in fact, go through stages in achieving their desired gender identity; some people stop at cross-dressing and hormone therapy, while others continue on to request GRS. Autonomy should be highly respected, but it should be especially respected for those making decisions which have such profound social risks.

Though it is true that the goals of medicine are diametrically opposed to the intentional, nonprophylactic removal of healthy organs, it is also true that in some cases, organs are not needed for certain goals of patients. Here, the role of patient autonomy is important. If a competent patient has determined that an organ is unnecessary to his or her goals for personal well-being and that, furthermore, said organ is causing him or her some type of discomfort, it can be considered morally permissible for a doctor to remove the said organ so long as removing the said organ will not profoundly and negatively affect other people.

Primum non nocere – do not harm. Physician response may be to ally with the patient in his all-encompassing quest for somatic treatment, leading to prescription of hormones and referral for SRS. Alternatively, physicians may be extremely reticent to entertain such treatment requests, erecting the defensive facades of "do no harm" and "never deliberately remove a healthy organ" [1]. The replacement of biological sex organs with nonfunctional sex organs can have a significant impact on the psychological well-being of the patient and should, therefore, be considered as having positive moral weight when one is evaluating the moral permissibility of removing healthy organs such as the mammary glands. It has been argued that men and women who are certain that they do not want to bear anymore children ask to undergo vasectomies and tubal ligations that will almost guarantee no more offspring will result from sexual intercourse. These procedures essentially incapacitate the sexual reproductive organs in males and females.

So, one cannot make the claim that there is a qualitative moral difference between such procedures and the procedures that remove sex organs in transsexuals during GRS.

The determination by some physicians to consider SRS an ethical therapeutic adjunct is largely a matter of personally witnessing individuals as they undergo the painful process of gender reorientation, which may include SRS and hormonal treatments. Numerous authors have reached the conclusion that SRS can contribute to the relief of suffering, enable better psychosocial adjustment, and impart a sense of well-being to these distressed individuals.

Physicians are faced with a complex dilemma that revolves around two central questions: What constitutes suffering in the gender-dysphoric patient? What are the ethically and morally viable interventions available to relieve suffering in these patients? The *Oath of Hippocrates* reminds us that the relief of suffering is the quintessential task of all of medicine.

The gender-dysphoric patient relates his or her subjective experience of suffering very clearly, but *what the physician may do to relieve it is unclear*; it is still unknown whether SRS is the most effective form of treatment for transsexualism. Clinical decisions must be made in the absence of definitive, prospective, long-term studies of the effectiveness of SRS compared to nonsurgical treatment modalities [1]. Others have disputed these claims, noting that positive outcome studies are seriously flawed by researcher bias and the lack of control groups.

Standards of care. Just as resourceful patients are able to obtain hormones illicitly, they can also obtain some forms of SRS from surgeons unaffiliated with established gender clinics. Many of these individuals have been subjected, in the past, to "inferior surgical techniques and preoperative selection procedures" with outcomes anecdotally reported as "horrifying" [37, 38].

Civil liability could be incurred by a surgeon in cases where the patient is dissatisfied with cosmetic and/or functional outcomes on the grounds that negligence occurred in preoperative evaluation. The case against the surgeon would be strengthened if the evaluation was brief and/or inconsistent with the standards of care, which clearly state that a minimum of two qualified mental health professionals must thoroughly evaluate the patient longitudinally, prior to recommendations for SRS [39]. Criminal charges could be filed as well, with prosecution based on the premeditated "act of intentionally mutilating a person's body or injuring it so as to deprive him of a limb or any organ of the body. The probability of a poor outcome, including postoperative suicide, is believed to be increased in patients who receive SRS without proper evaluation and lengthy preoperative preparation" [1].

Surgery alone is not curative or rehabilitative. SRS is only one component of a multidisciplinary approach to the rehabilitation process and should be viewed as confirmation of what the patient has already achieved with medical assistance.

38.3 Transsexualism in Children and Adolescents

Estimating the prevalence of GID for adolescents and adults is very difficult due to the lack of population-based studies. Estimates of adults with GID have generally been based on the numbers of individuals who have had sexual reassignment operations or those seeking services at specialized clinics. The prevalence of childhood GID is not known with any certainty, and estimates come principally from small studies and clinical experience [40]. Researchers assume that it is more common in children than in adults, based on the observation that the childhood diagnosis does not usually persist until adulthood. In both adults and children, GID occurs more frequently in males than females; the effect of social and cultural factors to explain the differences is not clear. There is some support for the view that boys are identified more often because parents, teachers, and peers are less tolerant of cross-gender behavior in boys, and girls may need to display more cross-gender behavior than boys before a referral is initiated.

Gender identity begins to develop early in childhood. Traditional views of gender identity have been categorical, asserting that one is either male or female and that this is fixed over time.

Cross-gender identification often emerges in childhood. A more developed psychologic sense of gender identity usually emerges in adolescence; although as transgender persons become more visible in everyday life and in the media, youth may examine and label their gender identities at earlier ages than in the past.

Most children aged 5–12 years diagnosed as having GID do not persist in having GID as adolescents; rather, most become homosexual or bisexual adolescents and adults [41–43].

Studies suggest that gender identity is fluid in childhood and even, although less so, into adolescence. GID in childhood very often does not persist into adulthood, and adolescent manifestations of GID sometimes do not continue into adulthood. In many instances, the adult outcome of childhood and adolescent GID manifests as homosexuality without the gender dysphoria; thus, for the adolescent, even allowing reversible treatment and allowing the adolescent to present in the opposite sex has future consequences if it solidifies a gender presentation that might have otherwise been later abandoned.

The issues surrounding treatment of children prior to puberty is even more difficult than that posed by treatment in adolescence. In children the issue is not whether to facilitate change, since hormonal treatment is not recommended prior to the onset of puberty, but instead whether GID can or should be suppressed. Currently there is insufficient data to know whether psychiatric treatment can reduce gender dysphoria and change the adult outcome. Moreover, as for psychiatric treatment to alleviate GID, one has to question *whether the motivation is to prevent GID or the more common resulting homosexuality given that either outcome may occur.*

Although once considered so, homosexuality is no longer considered a psychiatric condition, and therefore treatment to prevent it would be inappropriate. On the other hand, GID remains a disputable psychiatric disorder.

Thus, *if parents desire such treatment, ethical issues arise concerning the objective* of treatment and whether parents have authority to consent to such treatment.

Unless there is disagreement among parents, physicians, and the child, in the United States, generally, parties need not seek judicial approval to provide care to minors. Courts in the United States exercise a circumspect role in medical decision-making generally. Under Australia's Family Law Act of 1975, the Family Court of Australia has jurisdiction over matters concerning the welfare of children. Family law is largely decided at the federal level; thus, the standards announced by the court are, except for the state of Western Australia, precedential throughout the country.

There is no single answer as to how to treat children and adolescents with GID. Instead, professionals must exercise clinical judgment in developing and proposing a care plan. Even when sound clinical judgment is exercised, there are substantial risks in treating and in not treating these minors.

38.3.1 Treatment in Childhood: Ethical Issues

Treatment of childhood GID has evoked considerable controversy. First, the diagnosis can be elusive because gender nonconformity does not always constitute GID, and for some children, it appears self-limiting. In preadolescent children, the issue is whether to offer therapy aimed directly at reducing gender nonconformity, in hopes of preventing adult GID. The various treatment options have not been tested, lacking data supporting the efficacy of such treatment, so there is the concern of subjecting children to financially costly treatment that might be pointless or, worse, harmful.

In childhood, empirical studies demonstrate gender identity is not static, and children diagnosed with GID may not be so as adults. In fact, in the majority of children, GID remits by adolescence, if not earlier. Follow-up studies of boys who have GID indicate that a desistance of GID with a co-occurring homosexual orientation is the most common outcome, while GID may persist into adulthood for others, and for still others may desist "with a co-occurring heterosexual sexual orientation" [44, 45]. Less is known about the outcome in girls because insufficient numbers of girls with GID have been followed prospectively to draw conclusions about long-term outcome [46].

There is some professional thought that intervention with young children can alleviate GID, although this treatment option is not without critics [36].

Finally, depending on what outcome is desired, the treatment goal may itself raise ethical issues:

1. *The inappropriateness of preventing homosexuality as an end goal of treatment*
2. *Fundamental skepticism that gender identity dysphoria should be classified as a disorder at all*

Perhaps the most acute ethical issue concerns the relations between GID and a later homosexual orientation. Follow-up studies of boys with GID, largely untreated, indicate that homosexuality is the most common long-term psychosexual outcome. *Is ethically admissible parents' request of treatment for their child with GID to divert the probability of a later homosexual orientation*?

Zucker points out that it "has not been shown that any form of treatment for GID during childhood affects later sexual orientation and from an ethical standpoint… the clinician has an obligation to inform parents about the state of the empiric database." Zucker also cautions that "… the clinician must explain the distinctness of sexual orientation and gender identity in their psychoeducational work with parents. Yet, because it is beneficial to assist children with GID to resolve the conflicts that are associated with the disorder, regardless of the child's eventual sexual orientation, treatment is appropriate."

Therapy can include such things as helping parents create opportunities for the child to experience successful gender conforming experiences, develop same sex friendships, and develop a closer relationship with the same sex parent. It might also include behavior modification that results in reinforcement of gender-typical behavior during therapy sessions and extinction of cross-gender behavior, gradual shaping of gender-typical behavior, and desensitizing fear of failure. Despite the many treatment approaches, controlled studies do not exist.

Other therapists consider treating the children to prevent homosexuality unethical, because homosexuality is not a psychiatric disorder [47].

Cohen-Kettenis and Pfäfflin write: "Even therapists of opposing backgrounds will agree that certain forms of suffering should be alleviated under all circumstances. Such distress may come from social ostracism, non-GID psychiatric or family problems, or intense unhappiness about one's sex characteristics and being a boy or a girl."

38.3.2 Treatment in Adolescents: Ethical Issues

In adolescents, the ethical problems involve whether to treat certain youth with persistent GID with reversible and partially reversible hormonal treatment before adulthood when psychosocial treatment alone does not alleviate their distress. As with children, the ethical issues of whether and how to treat adolescents is made difficult by the lack of solid research. But in adolescents, *the issue is not how to "prevent GID" but how much to facilitate the gender transition.* The problems here again are threefold:

1. The lack of solid data concerning who should be treated
2. Whether such treatment is appropriate before adulthood
3. Whether the treatment might eventually prove disadvantageous

Zucker describes the difficulties of deciding when to treat adolescents: "Although early hormonal treatment is controversial, it may be the treatment of choice after the clinician is confident that other options have been exhausted." Importantly, clinicians must explore sexual orientation with their adolescent patients and help them to determine whether GID treatment is truly desirable.

The HBIGDA Standards of Care caution: "Before any physical intervention is considered, extensive exploration of psychological, family and social issues should be undertaken." Furthermore, "…identity beliefs in adolescents may become firmly held and strongly expressed, giving a false impression of irreversibility; more fluidity may return at a later stage" [48].

Treatment in adolescents is divided into three stages: reversible, puberty-delaying treatment, irreversible hormonal treatment, and surgical interventions. As to surgery, HBIGDA states that this should be delayed until the age of maturity.

Reversible treatment, according to HBIGDA, is designed to delay puberty. The standard of care permits "puberty-delaying hormones as soon as pubertal changes have begun." HBIGDA explains the justification for reversible treatment.

Two goals justify this intervention: (a) to gain time to further explore the gender identity and other developmental issues in psychotherapy and (b) to make passing easier if the adolescent continues to pursue sex and gender change. For some adolescents who are trying to make a transition, early treatment may help facilitate their psychological and social adjustment. Offering reversible puberty-delaying treatment may help to alleviate the adolescent's discomfort at the prospect of developing unwanted sex characteristics. It makes it easier to socially pass in the identified gender.

It delays pubertal changes and so makes a later transition surgically and psychologically easier. Moreover, it can help to confirm the diagnosis; delaying puberty "gains time to further explore the gender identity and other developmental issues" while keeping the maturing adolescent's options open.[1]

[1] The SOC criteria for eligibility for reversible treatment state the following. In order to provide puberty-delaying hormones to an adolescent, the following criteria must be met: (1) throughout childhood the adolescent has demonstrated an intense pattern of cross-sex and cross-gender identity and aversion to expected gender role behaviors; (2) sex and gender discomfort has significantly increased

HBIGDA Standards of Care also accept that "partially reversible interventions" may be instituted in 16-year olds with certain safeguards. HBIGDA does not recommend surgical (irreversible) interventions until adulthood, and then only after the 2-year real-life experience has been completed.[2] Irreversible interventions should not be carried out prior to adulthood or prior to a real-life experience of at least 2 years in the gender role of the sex with which the adolescent identifies.

Conclusions

Clinicians faced with the evaluation and treatment of gender-dysphoric individuals are plagued with difficult bioethical issues. While we, as a medical community, have no qualms about genital surgery for inborn biological errors, e.g., ambiguous genitalia conditions and pseudohermaphroditism, the same detached approach has not been applied to altering the anatomy of transsexuals.

"Above all, do no harm" is to be heeded with special care by mental health professionals facing both a lack of knowledge and an abundance of ethical dilemmas. This could, and should, lead to the restriction of SRS to centers involved in a multiuniversity research project aimed at addressing the relevant extant clinical questions.

In spite of proclamations that nothing else holds promise for the treatment of transsexualism other than SRS, less invasive interventions have been shown to be useful for some patients, e.g., expressive group psychotherapy, hormonal treatment in conjunction with psychotherapy, and behavior therapy.

Ethical dilemmas related to *denial* of SRS continue, such as the reported increased rate of suicide attempts and withholding treatment considered by some experts to be life saving. Controlled, prospective studies comparing treatment modalities are needed.

Is SRS then an elective cosmetic procedure as most insurance carriers claim? Is it the treatment of choice for selected gender-dysphoric patients or a well-intentioned mutilation tantamount to mayhem? There are no generalizations to adhere to and no convenient "rules of thumb." But there are patients with severe, pervasive disturbances in their sense of self who seek out those health-care professionals who are willing to confront their own ethical and moral standards in an attempt to provide appropriate care.

Unaddressed negative countertransference responses to gender-dysphoric patients, who are often manipulative and driven, may interfere with clinical decision-making and contribute to the suffering these patients endure.

Appendix: Jurisprudence [49]

Gender identity is receiving increasing recognition as a prohibited ground of discrimination at international and national levels. The UN system and the Council of Europe have highlighted its pertinence in the implementation of international and European human rights standards. Explicit references to gender identity can also be found in recent national equal treatment legislation in a growing number of countries.

One focal point for these developments was the publication, by a group of international human rights experts in 2007, of *Principles on*

with the onset of puberty; and (3) the family consents and participates in the therapy.

[2] The Standards of Care state: *Partially Reversible Interventions.* Adolescents may be eligible to begin masculinizing or feminizing hormone therapy, as early as age 16, preferably with parental consent. In many countries 16-year olds are legal adults for medical decision-making and do not require parental consent. Mental health professional involvement is an eligibility requirement for triadic therapy during adolescence. For the implementation of the real-life experience or hormone therapy, the mental health professional should be involved with the patient and family for a minimum of 6 months. While the number of sessions during this 6-month period rests upon the clinician's judgment, the intent is that hormones and the real-life experience be thoughtfully and recurrently considered over time. In those patients who have already begun the real-life experience prior to being seen, the professional should work closely with them and their families with the thoughtful recurrent consideration of what is happening over time.

the application of international human rights law in relation to sexual orientation and gender identity, usually referred to as the Yogyakarta Principles.

In February 2010, the US Tax Court in *O'Donnabhain v. Commissioner* ruled that sex-transitioning treatments were tax deductible.

Anti-discrimination legislation protecting jobs and housing is becoming increasingly popular, and the Affordable Care Act removed some barriers to better health care. These changes demonstrate greater legal recognition and social acceptance of transgender people in the United States.

From Biologic to Functionality

The so-called *transgender jurisprudence* in the common law world was inaugurated with the English decision of Corbett v. Corbett; Mr Corbett sought to have his marriage to A. A., a male-to-female transgender person who had undergone sex reassignment procedures, declared a nullity [49]. While the practical effect of such a finding related to questions of maintenance, the key legal question required a determination as to the sex of A. A. for marriage purposes. In answering this question, Ormrod J. held that "*sex is determined at birth*" and by a congruence of chromosomal, gonadal, and genital factors. According to this A. A. was determined to be a male person.

The decision has been subject to sustained and almost universal criticism within academic and law reform circles. Despite this, the Corbett decision has been followed consistently by the English courts and has been influential throughout the common law world.

The first superior court decision to depart from the biologic that is given expression in Corbett was the New York case of Re Anonymous. In this case which involved an application by a male-to-female transgender person to have her birth certificate changed to reflect surgical intervention, Pecora J. held the applicant to be female because her anatomy had been brought into conformity with her psychological sex. Unlike the Corbett analysis, *the decision created a legal space for the postoperative transgender body while it simultaneously drew a clear distinction between that body and pre- or nonsurgical transgender bodies*. The judgment appears to understand "harmony" as dependent on postoperative vaginal capacity for (hetero) sexual intercourse.

The "psychological and anatomical harmony" test formulated by Pecora J. in Re Anonymous was consolidated in MT v. JT; in this case the New Jersey Supreme Court considered valid a 2 years marriage between a biological man and a postoperative male-to-female transgender person. Recognition for the purposes of marriage proves to be dependent on the additional requirement of heterosexual desire. Law desires to know her desire, to know that it is heterosexual, and to be assured through that knowledge as to the "authenticity" of MT's transsexuality. The court explored in some detail her genital topography and finally noted that MT had "a vagina and labia which were adequate for sexual intercourse and could function as any female vagina, that is, for traditional penile/vaginal intercourse." Functionality of MT's vagina in this regard finds further expression in the evidence of Dr Ihlenfeld, who pointed out that MT's vagina had been "lined initially by the skin of [her] penis" that it would, in all likelihood, later take on "the characteristics of normal vaginal mucosa", and that though at "a somewhat different angle was not really different from a natural vagina in size, capacity, and the feeling of the walls around it".

From Functionality to Aesthetics

The judgment of the Federal Court of Australia in Secretary, Department of Social Security v SRA represents the shift from function to aesthetics within transgender jurisprudence. After expressing satisfaction with regard to postoperative male-to-female heterosexual capacity, Lockhart J. contended that "the female-to-male transsexual is probably in a rather different situation because even successful surgery cannot cause him to be a fully functional male, although he can be given the appearance of male genitals."

The significance of Lockhart J.'s statement lies in the fact that this in no way precludes legal recognition for the purposes of social security provisions. Lockhart J. makes it quite clear that the postsurgical female-to-male transgender body is to be regarded as male irrespective of a capacity for heterosexual intercourse.

The case is concerned with marriage, an area of law traditionally most resistant to transgender sex claims. Moreover, it is clear that the decision applies to both male-to-female and female-to-male transgender persons. The attorney general made an application on behalf of the Registrar of Marriages for "a declaration as to whether two persons of the same genetic sex may by the law of New Zealand enter into a valid marriage where one of the parties to the proposed marriage has adopted the sex opposite to that of the proposed marriage partner through sexual reassignment by means of surgery or hormone administration or both or by any other medical means."

The uncoupling of sex reassignment surgery from the capacity for heterosexual intercourse is significant as it serves to highlight law's concern over bodily aesthetics.

References

1. Brown GR (1988) Bioethical issues in the management of gender dysphoria. Jefferson J Psychiatry 6:23–34
2. Kubie L (1974) The drive to become both sexes. Psychoanal Q 43:349–426
3. Eldh J, Berg A, Gustafsson M (1997) Long-term follow up after sex reassignment surgery. Scand J Plast Reconstr Surg Hand Surg 31:39–45
4. Green R (1985) Gender identity in childhood and later sexual orientation: follow-up of 78 males. Am J Psychiatry 142:339–341
5. Mate-Kole C, Freschi M, Robin A (1990) A controlled study of psychological and social change after surgical gender reassignment in selected male transsexuals. Br J Psychiatry 157:261–264
6. Strapko N, Seil D, Buck T et al (1999) Physiological and psychological outcome of sex reassignment surgery in patients seen by members of New England Gender Specialists. Paper presented at the 16th Biennial Symposium of the Harry Benjamin International Gender Dysphoria Association, London, Aug 1999
7. Huang TT (1995) Twenty years of experience in managing gender dysphoric patients, I: surgical management of male transsexuals. Plast Reconstr Surg 96: 931–934
8. van Kesteren P, Lips P, Gooren LJ et al (1998) Long-term follow-up of bone mineral density and bone metabolism in transsexuals treated with cross-sex hormones. Clin Endocrinol (Oxf) 48:347–354
9. Walker P (1987) Transsexualism: character disorders and results of MMPI profiles. Paper presented at the 10th Biennial Symposium of the Harry Benjamin International Gender Dysphoria Association, Amsterdam, June 1987
10. Abramowitz S (1986) Psychosocial outcomes of sex reassignment surgery. J Consult Clin Psychol 54:183–189
11. Gallarda T, Amado I, Coussinoux S et al (1997) The transsexualism syndrome: clinical aspects and therapeutic prospects [in French]. Encéphale 23: 321–326
12. Lundstrom B, Pauly I, Walinder J (1984) Outcome of sex reassignment surgery. Acta Psychiatr Scand 70:289–294
13. Pauly IB (1992) Terminology and classification of gender identity disorders. In: Bockting WO, Coleman E (eds) Gender dysphoria: interdisciplinary approaches to clinical management. Haworth, New York
14. Van Putten T, Fawzy FI (1976) Sex conversion surgery in a man with severe gender dysphoria. A tragic outcome. Arch Gen Psychiatry 33:751–753
15. Sorensen T (1981) A follow-up study of operated transsexual females. Acta Psychiatr Scand 64:50–64
16. Sorensen T (1981) A follow-up study of operated transsexual males. Acta Psychiatr Scand 63:486–503
17. Money J (1994) The concept of gender identity disorder in childhood and adolescence after 39 years. J Sex Marital Ther 20:163–177
18. Money J (1994) Sex errors of the body and related syndromes: a guide to counseling children, adolescents, and their families. Paul H Brookes, Baltimore
19. Bockting WO, Coleman E (1992) A comprehensive approach to the treatment of gender dysphoria. In: Bockting WO, Coleman E (eds) Gender dysphoria: interdisciplinary approaches in clinical management. Haworth, New York, pp 131–155
20. Reback CJ, Lombardi E (1999) HIV risk behaviors of male-to-female transgenders in a community-based harm reduction program. Int J Transgenderism 3(1–2). http://www.symposion.com/ijt/hiv_risk/reback.htm
21. Meyer WJ (1999) HBIGDA HIV committee report. Newsletter of the Harry Benjamin International Gender Dysphoria Association, Inc. 9(2):2–3
22. Pang H, Pugh K, Catalan J (1994) Gender identity disorder and HIV disease. Int J STD AIDS 5(2): 130–132
23. Zandvliet T (2000) Transgender issues in therapy. In: Neal C, Davies D (eds) Issues in therapy with lesbian, gay, bisexual and transgender clients. Open University Press, Buckingham, UK, pp 176–190
24. Nagoshi JL, Burzuzy S (2010) Transgender theory: embodying research and practice. Affilia 25(4): 431–443

25. Markman ER (2011) Gender identity disorder, the gender binary, and transgender oppression: implications for ethical social work. Smith Coll Stud Soc Work 81:314–327
26. Stein E (2012) Commentary on the treatment of gender variant and gender dysphoric children and adolescents: common themes and ethical reflections. J Homosex 59:480e500
27. Grossman AH, D'Augell AR (2007) Transgender youth and life-threatening behaviours. Suicide Life Threat Behav 37(5):527–537
28. American Psychiatric Association (1980) Diagnostic and statistical manual of mental disorders, 3rd edn. American Psychiatric Association, Washington, DC
29. Meyerowitz J (2002) How sex changed: a history of transsexuality in the United States. Harvard University Press, Cambridge
30. American Psychiatric Association (1994) Diagnostic and statistical manual of mental disorders, 4th edn. Author, Washington, DC
31. American Psychological Association Task Force on Gender Identity and Gender Variance (2009) Report of the APA task force on gender identity and gender variance. American Psychological Association, Washington, DC
32. American Psychiatric Association (2000) Diagnostic and statistical manual of mental disorders, vol Text Revision, 4th edn. American Psychiatric Association, Washington, DC
33. Cohen-Ketenis PT, Plaffin F (2010) The DSM diagnostic criteria for gender identity disorder in adolescents and adults. Arch Sex Behav 39(2): 499–513
34. Girshick LB (2008) Transgender voices. University Press of New England, Lebanon
35. Kelley W (2010) Gender identity disorder reform. GID Reform Advocates. Web. 8 Nov 2010. http://www.gidreform.org/
36. Lev AI (2004) Transgender emergence: therapeutic guidelines for working with gender-variant people and their families. The Haworth Press, Binghamton, New York
37. Hume MC (2011) Sex, lies, and surgery: the ethics of gender reassignment surgery. Res Cogitans 2:37–48
38. Gottlieb A (1978) Three atypical results. Arch Sex Behav 7:371–375
39. Fisk N (1978) Five spectacular results. Arch Sex Behav 7:351–369
40. Terryann CC et al (2014) The Health and well being of transgender high school students: results from the new Zealand adolescent health survey (youth'12). J Adolesc Health 55:93–99
41. Drummond KD, Bradley SJ, Peterson-Badali M, Zucker KJ (2008) A follow up study of girls with gender identity disorder. Dev Psychol 44(1):34–35
42. Wallien MSC, Cohen-Keltens PT (2008) Psychosexual outcome of gender-dysphoric children. J Am Acad Child Adolesc Psychiatry 47(12):1413–1423
43. Olson J, Forbes C, Belzer M (2011) Management of the transgender adolescent. Arch Pediatr Adolesc Med 165(2):171–176
44. Beh H, Diamond M (2005) Ethical concerns related to treating gender nonconformity in childhood and adolescence: lessons from the family court of Australia. Health Matrix 15(2):239–283
45. Zucker KJ (2004) Gender identity development and issues. Child Adolesc Psychiatr Clin N Am 13:551, 554
46. Cohen-Kettenis PT, Pfäfflin F (2003) Transgenderism intersexuality childhood adolescence, SAGE Publications, Inc., UK. pp 64–66, 83
47. Arriola ER (1998) The penalties for puppy love: institutionalized violence against lesbian, gay, bisexual, and transgendered youth. J Gend Race Just 1:429, 469–470
48. The Harry Benjamin Int'l Gender Dysphoria Ass'n, Standards of Care for Gender Identity Disorders, Sixth version (2001). At: www.hbigda.org/socv6.html
49. Sharpe A (2006) From functionality to aesthetics: the architecture of transgender jurisprudence. 621–631. In The Transgender Studies Reader. Stryker S and Whittle S (eds). New York: Routledge

Transgender Identity and Sexually Transmitted Diseases Including HIV

39

Roberto Luzzati and Cristina Maurel

39.1 Current State of Art

The term sexually transmitted diseases (STDs) is used to refer to a variety of clinical syndromes caused by pathogens that can be acquired and transmitted through sexual activity. STDs are among the most common infectious diseases in all social contests and comprise over 30 infections with prevalent or frequent sexual transmission. In Table 39.1 are listed the most important of these.

Despite diagnostic and therapeutic advances, STD incidence rates remain high in most of the world, particularly in the younger age groups and in developing countries. Some of these infections, such as syphilis, gonorrhea, HIV infection, and hepatitis B virus (HBV), are more commonly found in key populations characterized by multiple sex partners and very frequent sexual activity. These high-risk populations include some male homosexual groups and sex workers and their clients. Other STDs are distributed more evenly among all populations. For example, chlamydial genital infections, human papillomavirus (HPV) infections, and genital herpes simplex virus (HSV) are efficiently transmitted also in low-risk populations [1]. Transmission of hepatitis A virus (HAV) during sexual activity occurs due to fecal-oral contact or contamination. Although not common, hepatitis C virus (HCV) can be transmitted through sexual activity.

HIV infection is of major public health importance worldwide and in Europe. At the end of 2011, about 34 million people were living with HIV infection, according to estimates by WHO and the Joint United Nations Programme on HIV/AIDS (UNAIDS). Only about half of them knew their HIV status, 2.5 million became newly infected, and 1.7 million died of AIDS [2]. The surveillance results suggest that HIV transmission continues to represent an important challenge in most countries worldwide. Although HIV incidence has declined in some countries, it is stable or increasing in others. In the WHO European Region, it is estimated an overall rate of 7.8 diagnoses per 100,000 population. The rates are highest in the east of the region.

The main transmission mode varies by geographical area; worldwide the heterosexual-acquired HIV infections are the most reported. In

Table 39.1 Main sexually transmitted agents

Neisseria gonorrhoeae
Chlamydia trachomatis
Treponema pallidum
Trichomonas vaginalis
Herpes simplex virus type 2 (HSV-2)
Human papillomavirus (HPV)
Hepatitis B virus (HBV)
Hepatitis A virus (HAV)
Human immunodeficiency virus (HIV)

R. Luzzati (✉) • C. Maurel
Infectious Diseases Unit, University Hospital of Trieste, Piazza dell'Ospitale 1, Trieste 34100, Italy
e-mail: roberto.luzzati@aots.sanita.fvg.it; cristina.maurel@hotmail.it

C. Trombetta et al. (eds.), *Management of Gender Dysphoria: A Multidisciplinary Approach*, DOI 10.1007/978-88-470-5696-1_39, © Springer-Verlag Italia 2015

Eastern Europe and Central Asia, there is still a high percentage of new diagnoses in people who inject drugs, while, in the western part of the European Region and the United States, the epidemic remains concentrated among men who have sex with men (MSM) and migrants from countries with generalized epidemics. Overall groups at greater risk of infection are the socially marginalized and people whose behavior is socially stigmatized or illegal, including sex workers, MSM, transgender people, and people who inject drugs [3].

HIV prevalence is continuously rising as a result of antiretroviral treatment and efficient health-care assistance that ensure an improved and prolonged life for infected patients. Fewer people living with HIV are dying from AIDS-related causes in many countries while new infections continue to occur [4].

39.2 Epidemiology of HIV in Transgender People

Transgender communities are among the groups at highest risk for HIV and other STD infections. It has been estimated that HIV prevalence for transgender women is nearly 50 times as high as for other adults of reproductive age [5]. The average prevalence in this population is about 27.7 %.

Reliable information on how many transgender people are infected with HIV is lacking because it is very difficult to collect data uniformly. Gender expression may fluctuate for some transgender people, and there is great diversity in orientation and behavior in this population. In addition some transgender people may not identify as transgender due to fear of discrimination or previous negative experiences [6].

Data collected by local health departments and scientists studying these communities in the United States show high levels of HIV infection and racial disparities. In 2010, the Centers for Disease Control and Prevention (CDC) reported that the highest percentage of newly identified HIV-positive test results was among transgender people. Among transgender people, the highest percentages of newly identified HIV-positive test results were among ethnic minorities above all African Americans, followed by Latinos. Most studies confirm that black transgender women are more likely to become infected with HIV than nonblack transgender women [7]. Over half of newly diagnosed transgender women were in their twenties. Also, among newly diagnosed, it is very likely to report documentation in medical records of substance use, commercial sex work, homelessness, incarceration, and sexual abuse as compared with other people who were not transgender [8, 9].

Although there remains globally a poor understanding of the burden of HIV among transgender women, it is evident that they are a higher-risk population and in urgent need of prevention, treatment, and care services [10].

Transgender men's sexual health has been understudied. Compared to transgender women, little is known about HIV risk and sexual health needs among transgender men. This is because they have not traditionally been considered at risk for HIV due to different sexual exposure. Prevalence of HIV infection among female-to-male (FTM) is considerably lower than among male-to-female (MTF) transgender people [11].

39.3 Risk Assessment for STD Including HIV

The high burden of HIV infection among transgender people is not attributable only to individual behaviors such as unprotected sexual intercourse and promiscuity. Also many cultural, socioeconomic, and health-related factors contribute to the HIV epidemic spread in transgender communities. Behaviors and factors that contribute to high risk of HIV infection among transgender people include higher rates of drug and alcohol abuse, sex work, incarceration, homelessness, attempted suicide, unemployment, lack of familial support, violence, stigma and discrimination, limited health-care access, and negative health-care encounters. In addition to biological and network-level factors, the structural risks for HIV infection, such as social exclusion, economic marginalization, and unmet health-care needs, transcend the level of the individual and might also help explain why HIV rates are so high in transgender women compared with other adults [12].

Discrimination and social stigma can hinder access to education, employment, and housing opportunities. And this statement may help explain why transgender people who experience significant economic difficulties often pursue high-risk activities, including sex work, to meet their basic survival needs. In general, sex workers have been shown to experience risk for various adverse health conditions, including HIV and other sexually transmitted infections [13, 14].

Health-care provider insensitivity to transgender identity or sexuality can be a barrier for HIV-infected transgender people seeking health care. Although research shows a similar proportion of HIV-positive transgender women have health insurance coverage as compared with other infected people who are not transgender, HIV-infected transgender women are less likely to be on antiretroviral therapy. Indicator of this situation is unawareness of one's serostatus. As a matter of fact, CDC has reported that most of the transgender women who were tested HIV positive were unaware of their status and potential unknowing transmitters of infection.

A primary driver of HIV infection in transgender women, similar to MSM, is the very high transmission probability of unprotected receptive anal intercourse [12, 15]. Since transgender women have been consistently identified as engaging in receptive anal sex with men, this biological vulnerability to HIV acquisition is undoubtedly an important factor in the high acquisition risk identified. Anal intercourse is a much more efficient mode of HIV transmission than penile-vaginal intercourse. However, there is still little research on HIV acquisition risks from neovaginal intercourse after vaginoplasty as well as from sex between transgender women and female partners. As a matter of fact, consistent condom use with appropriate lubricants is an essential prevention method for anyone engaging in anal sex.

Other individual-level risks for HIV include high rates of depression that may drive to drug abuse as well as risk of parenteral acquisition through illicit hormone and silicone injections [16, 17].

Additional research is needed to identify factors that prevent HIV in this population. Several behavioral HIV prevention interventions developed for transgender people have been reported in studies, such as encouraging frequent HIV testing for identifying transgender people with undiagnosed HIV infection and safe sex practices. Most have shown at least modest reductions in HIV risk behaviors among transgender women, such as fewer sex partners and/or unprotected anal sex acts. Behavioral HIV prevention interventions developed for other at-risk groups with similar behaviors have been adapted for use with transgender people; however, their effectiveness is still unknown.

39.4 Prevention Strategies of HIV Infection

In the absence of a vaccine, HIV prevention involves combinations of strategies including behavioral interventions, widespread condom use with appropriate lubricants, male circumcision, STD treatment, early initiation of antiretroviral therapy (ART) after infection, and preexposure and postexposure antiretroviral prophylaxis (Table 39.2) [18].

In a recent study, ART in combination with condom use and counseling was found to reduce

Table 39.2 Prevention strategies of sexually transmitted HIV infection

Preexposed individuals	Exposed individuals	Infected individuals
HIV vaccine	Antiretroviral nPEP	Treatment of HIV infection
Behavioral interventions		
Male circumcision		
Condoms		
Treatment of STDs		
Antiretroviral PrEP		

STDs sexual transmitted diseases, *PrEP* preexposure prophylaxis, *nPEP* nonoccupational postexposure prophylaxis

HIV transmission by 96 % among 1,763 serodiscordant couples (97 % heterosexual) in which the HIV-infected partner had a CD4 count of 350–550 cells/mm^3 [19]. The outstanding results of this study also showed that earlier ART can provide significant benefit even to HIV-infected individuals with reduction of clinical events including extrapulmonary tuberculosis and others. According to these results, the World Health Organization (WHO) and the US Department of Health and Human Services (DHHS) recommend immediate ART for people in HIV discordant relationships, irrespective of CD4 cell count [20, 21]. Earlier epidemiological studies as well as mathematical models support the theory that promoting treatment of HIV will decrease HIV incidence. However, the effectiveness of HIV treatment as prevention among other individuals (i.e., homosexuals, transgender, intravenous drug users, sex workers) and settings (i.e., resource-limited countries) is still debatable. Furthermore, the treatment as prevention strategy also seems to be undermined by lack of universal agreement about when to start ART, whether for individual health, to prevent HIV transmission, or for both benefits combined [18]. To address these and other concerns, several studies are being planned or ongoing to evaluate the effectiveness of ART as part of combined prevention strategies [22].

Administration of antiretroviral drugs to uninfected persons at high risk of infection to protect against HIV acquisition is known as preexposure prophylaxis (PrEP). Over the last 3 years, several trials have shown that PrEP (including oral and topical tenofovir-based compounds) can decrease the incidence of HIV infection in various high-risk patient populations. However, other studies were discontinued early because of lack of efficacy of such strategy due to suboptimal adherence or different risk behaviors among participants. Thus, other trials including oral tenofovir-emtricitabine and pericoitally administered tenofovir gel are ongoing [22]. The first study demonstrating that PrEP can protect against HIV acquisition in humans showed that the pericoital use of tenofovir vaginal gel was associated with 39 % decrease in the risk for HIV acquisition among at-risk South African women after 2.5 years compared with placebo [23]. Several months later, a study in 2,499 MSM or transgender women receiving daily oral emtricitabine-tenofovir reported a 44 % reduction in new HIV infection. In addition, the result in participants with detectable antiretroviral drug levels in plasma was a 92 % reduction. All subjects received risk-reduction counseling, condoms, HIV testing, and treatment of sexually transmitted diseases. Elevation of serum creatinine levels was more frequent in the tenofovir group than in the placebo group. However, the two groups had similar rates of serious adverse events. In summary, although more information is needed about possible side effects regarding bone mineral density and drug resistance, the findings of such trial showed that a dual oral antiretroviral regimen provided protection against the acquisition of HIV infection among MSM or transgender women [24]. More recently, two studies demonstrated that daily oral PrEP with tenofovir-emtricitabine, given also in the context of other prevention services, reduced the risk of HIV acquisition by the HIV-uninfected partner in serodiscordant, heterosexual couples. The first trial showed a 75 % reduction in new infections with daily oral tenofovir-emtricitabine, and 67 % with tenofovir, again with results in patients with detectable drug levels [25]. In the second trial, daily oral tenofovir-emtricitabine decreased HIV incidence by 62 % [26]. Both trials showed that the efficacy of preexposure prophylaxis depends largely on adherence to the medication, and rates of serious adverse events were similar across the study groups. However, the active study medications were associated with increased reports of gastrointestinal side effects and, in the latter trial [26], significant decline in bone mineral density as compared with placebo. After data of these studies were available, the US Food and Drug Administration (FDA) approved tenofovir-emtricitabine for PrEP for HIV-uninfected MSM, HIV-uninfected partners in serodiscordant couples, and other individuals at risk of acquiring HIV through sexual activity. The CDC published guidance for the prescription of daily oral tenofovir-emtricitabine as PrEP to at-risk males who have sex with men [27]. The CDC recommended that providers document negative HIV antibody test results immediately before starting PrEP, test for acute HIV infection if symptoms consistent with this syndrome are present, and undergo serial, regular HIV testing during PrEP use. Persons who acquire HIV infection should immediately discontinue PrEP use to reduce the risk of drug resistance. The CDC also advised screening for other STDs, including hepatitis B virus. In summary, daily ingestion of oral PrEP may result to be desirable when potential exposure to HIV is frequent (i.e., serodiscordant couples, MSM with multiple partners, sex workers). On the other hand, pericoital topical PrEP allows high local drug exposure with lower systemic drug levels, probably leading to a decreased likelihood of drug toxicity and increased adherence. However, topical PrEP will result to be difficult to use without partner knowledge [28]. A study assessed the acceptability of oral PrEP and rectal PrEP during unprotected receptive anal intercourse among MSM and transgender women in Peru. Among 532 individuals, high acceptance of either oral daily (96 %) or rectal (92 %) PrEP products were reported. If both products were efficacious and available, 29 % would prefer a pill, 57 % a rectal lubricant, and 14 % either products. Therefore, the development of an effective antiretroviral-based rectal gel is likely to have high acceptability among subjects practicing receptive anal sex because of rates of rectal lubricant use that are high in such populations. In conclusion, the findings of this study suggest that efficacious oral or rectally formulated HIV PrEP interventions would be highly acceptable among MSM and transgender women practicing receptive anal sex and with concomitant high-risk sexual behavior [29]. The efficacy of administering PrEP to the HIV-uninfected partner of a monogamous couple, whose HIV-infected partner is receiving ART, is actually unknown. Integrating these two strategies into current behavioral interventions could allow to reduce considerably the incidence of new HIV infections among serodiscordant couples.

Nonoccupational postexposure antiretroviral prophylaxis (nPEP) is the provision of antiretroviral drugs to prevent HIV infection after unanticipated sexual exposure. nPEP cannot replace behaviors that help to avoid HIV exposure (e.g., sexual abstinence, sex only in a mutually monogamous relationship with a noninfected partner, consistent and correct condom use). Once HIV crosses a mucosal barrier, it may take up to 48–72 h before HIV can be detected within regional lymph nodes and up to 5 days before HIV can be detected in blood [30]. Data from animal transmission models, perinatal clinical trials, and studies of health-care workers undergoing occupational exposures indicate that nPEP might sometimes reduce the risk for HIV infection after nonoccupational exposures [31]. The most direct evidence supporting the efficacy of PEP is a case-control study of needlestick injuries among health-care workers (HCW) showing that the prompt initiation of zidovudine prophylaxis was associated with an 81 % decrease in the risk for acquiring HIV [32]. In another study, in a high-risk HIV incidence cohort in Brazil, HIV seroincidence was 0.7 per 100 person-years among MSM who began taking nPEP after a self-identified high-risk exposure and 4.1 per 100 person-years among MSM who did not take nPEP [33]. Although studies do not provide definitive evidence of the efficacy of nPEP following sexual and other nonoccupational HIV exposure, recommendations from both the DHHS [31] and from the British Association for Sexual Health and HIV [34] support that nPEP initiated soon after exposure and continued for 28 days might reduce the risk for acquiring HIV infection. In a recent study, an antiretroviral regimen including tenofovir, emtricitabine, and raltegravir was found to be well tolerated as nPEP and resulted in levels of adherence almost 90 % with no participant becoming infected among 120 MSM [35]. All individuals seeking care after HIV exposure should be tested for the presence of HIV antibodies at baseline and at 4–6 weeks, 3 months, and 6 months after exposure to determine whether HIV infection has occurred. In addition, testing for STD, HBV, and HCV and pregnancy should be offered. The risk of an individual acquiring HIV following an exposure is dependent upon the risk that the source is HIV positive and the specific exposure from an

Table 39.3 Estimated risk for HIV acquisition following an unprotected exposure from an HIV-positive subject

Exposure route	Median (range) risk of HIV transmission per exposure (%)
Receptive anal intercourse	1.11 (0.042–3.0 %)
Insertive anal intercourse	0.06 (0.06–0.065 %)
Receptive vaginal intercourse	0.1 (0.004–0.32 %)
Insertive vaginal intercourse	0.082 (0.011–0.38 %)
Receptive oral sex	0.02 (0–0.04 %)
Insertive oral sex	0

HIV-positive individual [34] (Table 39.3). Indeed, the probability of HIV transmission depends not only upon the exposure characteristics but also upon the infectivity of the source (high plasma and genital tract HIV viral load, concomitant STDs, non-circumcision, occurring ejaculation) and the host susceptibility (breaches in the mucosal barrier, concomitant STDs, menstruation). Circumcision has been shown to significantly reduce HIV acquisition among heterosexual men in high-prevalence countries [36]. On the other hand, a meta-analysis of observational studies among MSM suggests circumcision has little impact upon HIV acquisition in these individuals [36]. Several factors influence the efficacy of PEP including delayed initiation of PEP, presence of resistant virus in the source patient, different penetration of drugs into tissue compartments, poor adherence, and further high-risk sexual exposures. PEP may be less or ineffective if initiated later than 72 h after exposure and is not recommended according to both the DHHS and the British Association for Sexual Health and HIV [31, 34]. However, clinicians should evaluate risks and benefits of nPEP on a case-by-case basis. The potential risks from nPEP include possible decrease in risk-reduction behaviors, the occurrence of adverse effects from antiretroviral therapy, and potential selection of resistant viruses, particularly if adherence is poor during the nPEP course. Although serious side effects (e.g., hepatitis) have been reported in literature, evidence indicates that these risks due to nPEP might not be a major problem. In the US nPEP surveillance registry, among 107 exposure for which nPEP was taken, the antiretroviral regimen initially prescribed was stopped or modified in 22 % of cases; in half of them, this occurred because of side effects [37]. Similarly, a 10-year retrospective analysis of nPEP administration showed that 396 (56 %) of 710 individuals who started nPEP reported side effects, especially gastrointestinal intolerance and fatigue. However, only 39 (3.7 %) individuals had to interrupt antiretroviral treatment for serious side effects [38]. Because nPEP is not 100 % effective in preventing HIV transmission and because antiretroviral agents carry a possible risk of adverse effects, nPEP should be used only for infrequent use (e.g., condom failure). Even if nPEP is cost-effective for the highest-risk exposures, behavioral interventions including risk-reduction interventions are most cost-effective and should be implemented to reduce the occurrence of future HIV exposure [31, 34].

The use of antiretroviral agents as postexposure prophylaxis (PEP) is the most important strategy for preventing occupationally acquired HIV infection since 1990 [39]. A recent report of the CDC updates previous recommendations for the management of HCW who experience occupational exposure to blood and/or other body fluids that might contain HIV [40]. An exposure that might place HCW at risk for HIV infection is defined as a percutaneous injury (e.g., a needlestick or cut with a sharp object) or contact of mucous membrane or non-intact skin (e.g., exposed skin that is chapped, abraded, or afflicted with dermatitis) with blood, tissue, or other body fluids that are potentially infectious. In addition to blood and visibly bloody body fluids, semen and vaginal secretions are also considered potentially infectious. Other fluids also considered potentially infectious are cerebrospinal fluid, synovial fluid, pleural fluid, peritoneal fluid, pericardial fluid, and amniotic fluid. The average risk for HIV transmission after a percutaneous exposure to HIV-infected blood has been estimated to be approximately 0.3 % [41] and that after a mucous membrane exposure to be approximately 0.09 % [42]. The risk for transmission after exposure to fluids or tissue other than HIV-infected blood also has not been quantified but is probably considerably lower than for blood exposures. The recent CDC recommendations emphasize the importance of a primary prevention strategy, the prompt reporting and management of occupational exposures, adherence to recommended HIV PEP regimens when indicated, expert consultation in management of exposures, follow-up of exposed HCW to improve adherence to PEP, and careful monitoring for adverse events related to treatment, as well as for virologic, immunologic, and serologic signs of infection. The CDC guidelines recommend three antiretroviral agents (preferred regimen: tenofovir, emtricitabine, and raltegravir), which should be selected to optimize side effect and toxicity profiles. PEP should be initiated as soon as possible, preferably within hours from exposure. HCW receiving PEP should complete a full 4-week regimen, if tolerated. The recommendations apply to situations in which a HCW has been exposed to a source person who has HIV infection or for whom there is reasonable suspicion of HIV infection. If PEP is offered and taken and the source is later determined to be HIV negative, PEP should be discontinued, and no further HIV follow-up testing is indicated for the exposed HCW. Otherwise, postexposure HIV testing should be performed at 6 weeks, 12 weeks, and 6 months after exposure. Finally, exposed personnel should be advised to use precautions (e.g., use of barrier contraception, avoidance of blood or tissue donations, pregnancy and, if possible, breast-feeding) to prevent secondary transmission, especially during the first 6–12 weeks after exposures.

References

1. Kasper DL, Braunwald E (2005) Harrison's principles of internal medicine, 16th edn. McGraw-Hill, New York
2. Hankins C (2013) Overview of the current state of the epidemic. Curr HIV/AIDS Rep 10:113–123
3. HIV/AIDS surveillance in Europe 2012. http://www.euro.who.int/en/health-topics/communicable-diseases/hivaids/publications/2012/hivaids-surveillance-in-europe-2011
4. UNAIDS (2012) Global report 2012 UNAIDS report on the global AIDS epidemic. United Nations Publications, Geneve
5. HIV among transgender people. http://www.cdc.gov/hiv/transgender/
6. Institute of Medicine (2011) The health of lesbian, gay, bisexual and transgender people: building a foundation for better understanding. The National Academies Press, Washington, DC
7. New York City Department of Health and Mental Hygiene (2011) Surveillance slide sets: HIV among transgender persons in New York City, 2005–2009. Accessed Oct 2013
8. Herbst JH, Jacobs ED, Finlayson TJ, McKleroy VS, Neumann MS, Crepaz N (2008) Estimating HIV prevalence and risk behaviors of transgender persons in the United States: a systematic review. AIDS Behav 12(1):1–17
9. Operario D, Soma T, Underhill K (2008) Sex work and HIV status among transgender women: systematic review and meta-analysis. J Acquir Immune Defic Syndr 48:97–103
10. Baral SD, Poteat T, Strömdahl S, Wirtz AL, Guadamuz TE, Beyrer C (2013) Worldwide burden of HIV in transgender women: a systematic review and meta-analysis. Lancet Infect Dis 13:214–222
11. Clements-Nolle K, Marx R, Guzman R, Katz M (2001) HIV prevalence, risk behaviors, health care use, and mental health status of transgender persons: implications for public health intervention. Am J Public Health 91:915–921
12. Baggaley RF, White RG, Boily MC (2010) HIV transmission risk through anal intercourse: systematic review, meta-analysis and implications for HIV prevention. Int J Epidemiol 39:1048–1063
13. Coan DL, Schrager W, Packer T (2005) The role of male sexual partners in HIV infection among male-to-female transgendered individuals. Int J Transgenderism 8:21–30
14. Vandepitte J, Lyerla R, Dallabetta G et al (2006) Estimates of the number of female sex workers in different regions of the world. Sex Transm Infect 82(Suppl 3):S18–S25
15. Beyrer C, Baral SD, van Griensven F et al (2012) Global epidemiology of HIV infection in men who have sex with men. Lancet 380:367–377
16. Grant JM, Mottet LA, Tanis J, Harrison J, Herman JL, Keisling M (2011) Injustice at every turn: a report of the national transgender discrimination survey. The National Gay and Lesbian Task Force and the National Center for Transgender Equality, Washington, DC
17. Melendez RM, Pinto R (2007) 'It's really a hard life': love, gender and HIV risk among male-to-female transgender persons. Cult Health Sex 9:233–245
18. Cohen MS, Smith MK, Muessig KE, Hallett TB, Powers KA, Kashuba AD (2013) Antiretroviral treatment of HIV-1 prevents transmission of HIV-1: where do we go from here? Lancet 382:1515–1524
19. Cohen MS, Chen YQ, McCauley M et al; the HPTN 059 Study Team (2011) Prevention of HIV-1 infection

with early antiretroviral therapy N Engl J Med 365:493–505
20. World Health Organization. Consolidated guidelines on the use of antiretroviral drugs for treating and preventing HIV infection (2013) http://www.who.int/hiv/pub/guidelines/arv2013/download/en/index.html. Accessed 19 Aug 2013
21. US Department of Health and Human Services. Panel on antiretroviral guidelines for adults and adolescents (2012): guidelines for the use of antiretroviral agents in HIV-1 infected adults and adolescents (2012) http://aidsinfo.nih.gov/contentfiles/lvguidelines/adultandadoloscentgl.pdf. Accessed 3 Aug 2013
22. Mayer K, Gazzard B, Zuniga JM et al (2013) Controlling the HIV epidemic with antiretrovirals: IAPAC consensus statement on treatment as prevention and preexposure prophylaxis. J Int Assoc Provid AIDS Care 12:208–216
23. Abdool Karim Q, Abdool Karim SS, Frohlich JA et al (2010) Effectiveness and safety of tenofovir gel, an antiretroviral microbicide, for the prevention of HIV infection in women. Science 329:1168–1174
24. Grant RM, Larna JM, Anderson PL et al (2010) Preexposure chemoprophylaxis for HIV prevention in men who have sex with men. N Engl J Med 363:2587–2599
25. Baeten JM, Donnell D, Ndase P et al (2012) Antiretroviral prophylaxis for HIV prevention in heterosexual men and women. N Engl J Med 367:399–410
26. Thigpen MC, Kebaabetswe PM, Paxton LA et al (2012) Antiretroviral preexposure prophylaxis for heterosexual HIV transmission in Botswana. N Engl J Med 367:423–434
27. Centers for Disease Control and Prevention (CDC) (2011) Interim guidance: preexposure prophylaxis for prevention of HIV infection in men who have sex with men. Morb Mortal Wkly Rep 60:65–68
28. Krakower D, Mayer KH (2012) What primary care providers need to know about preexposure prophylaxis for HIV prevention. Ann Intern Med 157:490–497
29. Peinado J, Lama JR, Galea JT et al (2013) Acceptability of oral versus rectal HIV preexposure prophylaxis among men who have sex with men and transgender women in Peru. J Int Assoc Provid AIDS Care 12:278–283
30. Spira AI, Marx PA, Patterson BK et al (1996) Cellular targets of infection and route of viral dissemination after an intravaginal inoculation of simian immunodeficiency virus into rhesus macaques. J Exp Med 183:215–225
31. Smith DK, Grohskopf LA, Black RJ et al (2005) US Department of Health and Human Services. Antiretroviral postexposure prophylaxis after sexual, injection-drug use, or other nonoccupational exposure to HIV in the United States: recommendations from the U.S. Department of Health and Human Services. MMWR Recomm Rep 54:1–20
32. Cardo DM, Culver DH, Ciesielski CA et al (1997) A case-control study of HIV seroconversion in health care workers after percutaneous exposure to HIV-infected blood: clinical and public health implications. N Engl J Med 337:1485–1490
33. Harrison LH, Lago RF, Moreira RI, Schechter M (2000) Demand for post-sexual-exposure chemoprophylaxis for the prevention of HIV infection in Brazil. 7th Conference on retroviruses and opportunistic infections, San Francisco, Jan 30–Feb 2 2000 (Abstract 492)
34. Benn P, Fisher M, Kulasegaram R (2011) UK guideline for the use of post-exposure prophylaxis for HIV following sexual exposure. Int J STD AIDS 22:695–708
35. McAllister J, Read P, McNulty A, Tong W, Ingersoll A, Carr A (2014) Raltegravir-emtricitabine-tenofovir as HIV nonoccupational post-exposure prophylaxis in men who have sex with men: safety, tolerability and adherence. HIV Med 15:13–22
36. Millett GA, Flores SA, Marks G et al (2008) Circumcision status and risk of HIV and sexually transmitted infections among men who have sex with man: a meta-analysis. JAMA 300:1674–1684
37. Grohskopf LA, Smith DK, Kunches LK et al (2002) Surveillance of post-exposure prophylaxis for non-occupational HIV exposures through the U.S. national registry. Presented at the XIV international conference on AIDS, Barcelona, July 7–12 2002 (Abstract MoOrD1107)
38. Tissot F, Erard V, Dang T, Cavassini M (2010) Nonoccupational HIV post-exposure prophylaxis: a ten year retrospective analysis. HIV Med 11:584–592
39. Centers for Disease Control and Prevention (1990) Public Health Service statement on management of occupational exposure to human immunodeficiency virus, including considerations regarding zidovudine postexposure use. MMWR Recomm Rep 39:1–14
40. Kuhar DT, Henderson DK, Struble KA et al (2013) Updated US Public Health Service guidelines for the management of occupational exposures to human immunodeficiency virus and recommendations for postexposure prophylaxis. Infect Control Hosp Epidemiol 34:875–892
41. Bell DM (1997) Occupational risk of human immunodeficiency virus infection in healthcare workers: an overview. Am J Med 102:9–15
42. Ippolito G, Puro V, De Carli G, Italian Study Group on Occupational Risk of HIV infection (1993) The risk of occupational human immunodeficiency virus infection in health care workers: Italian multicenter study. Arch Intern Med 153:1451–1458

Answers to Fertility Request

40

Elisabetta Feliciani, Anna Pia Ferraretti, Maria Cristina Magli, Irene L.F. Terracina, and Luca Gianaroli

As in all living beings, human reproduction has the fundamental role of allowing survival and evolution of the species. However, contrary to what happens for other species, for human beings alongside biological pushes, there are also unique emotional factors related to the fulfilment of the wish for parenthood. For this reason, reproduction is an issue that should interest everyone, even those who apparently do not have reproductive problems or reproductive desires.

Reproduction in the human species is a very complex process and the functioning of many of its aspects has not been completely understood and described yet. It implies several steps, each of which must occur perfectly and in perfect timing with the other ones.

The different steps of the reproductive process in human beings are outlined in Fig. 40.1:

- Regular ovulation cycle.
- Production of viable gametes. Female: production of oocytes suitable for fertilisation and generation of a vital embryo. Male: production of sperms suitable for fertilisation and activation of embryo development.
- Contact between viable gametes and their subsequent fusion (fertilisation). These phases take place inside the Fallopian tubes.
- Regular development of the embryo.
- After 3 or 4 days of development inside the tubes, the embryo reaches the uterine cavity.
- Nesting of the embryo in the uterus (implantation).
- Development of a regular pregnancy inside the uterus.

The condition of infertility is defined as the inability to conceive a child within 2 years of regular unprotected sexual intercourse. It is estimated that infertility affects about 12–15 % of the total of couples in reproductive age throughout the world, and it can be therefore considered a social issue.

Every year in Italy about 50,000–70,000 among newly formed couples are destined to suffer from reproductive problems in their future relational experiences. All these couples represent the so-called infertile population. Alongside its medical significance – because inability to procreate is considered a "disease" to all intents and purposes by WHO (World Health Organization) – infertility involves other psychological, familiar and relational aspects.

Heterosexual, homosexual or transsexual, fertile or sterile, the couple remains a symbol of the matching of the two gametes: an archetype that is present in everybody [1]. For this reason, once the transsexual person has completed the transitioning process from both the psychological

E. Feliciani • A.P. Ferraretti • M.C. Magli
I.L.F. Terracina • L. Gianaroli (✉)
S.I.S.Me.R. Reproductive Medicine Unit,
Via Mazzini 12, Bologna 40138, Italy
e-mail: elisabetta.feliciani@sismer.it;
annapia.ferraretti@sismer.it; cristina.magli@sismer.it;
congress@sismer.it; luca.gianaroli@sismer.it

C. Trombetta et al. (eds.), *Management of Gender Dysphoria: A Multidisciplinary Approach*,
DOI 10.1007/978-88-470-5696-1_40, © Springer-Verlag Italia 2015

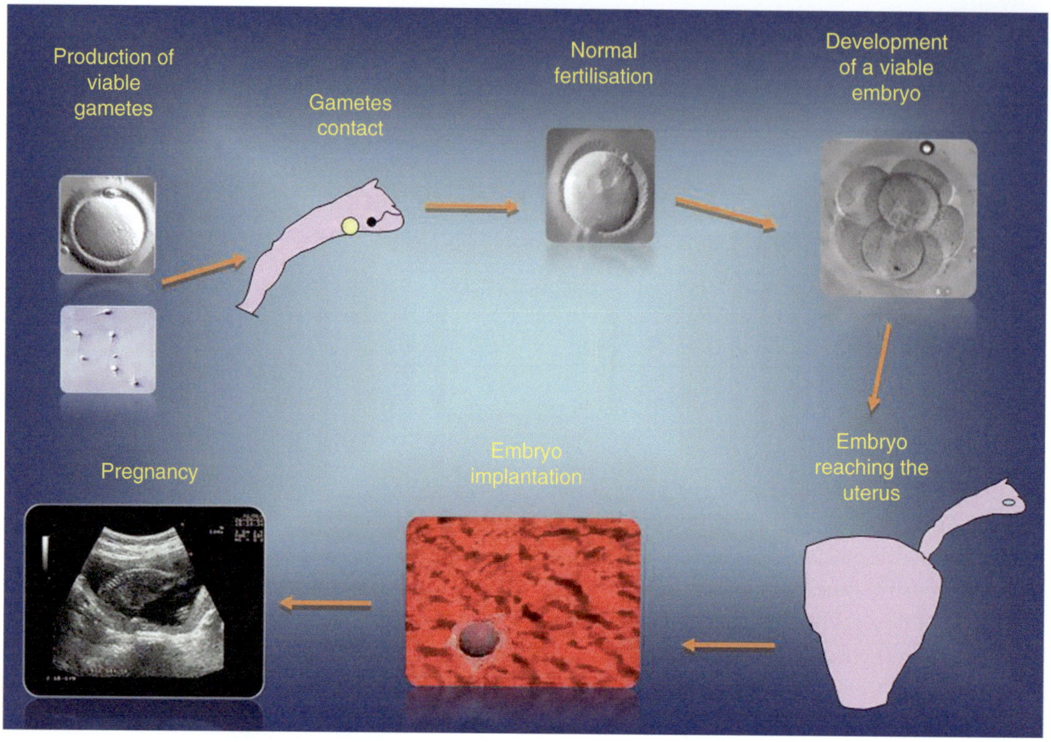

Fig. 40.1 Physiological reproductive process in human beings

and the physical point of view[1] she/he may also feel the desire to form a couple that might permit a complete fulfilment of her/his life.

In a context of sexual uncertainty like that of transition, the condition of "couple" may be felt as a strong instrument for the individual existential fulfilment, often superior even to family, work and sexual power.

While in the general population infertility or sterility is usually secondary to a pathology or other physiological factors (e.g. age, genetic factors, etc.), in a transsexual couple they are the direct consequence of the medical surgical procedures that transsexual people undertake to complete their transition.

Nowadays, ARTs (assisted reproductive technologies) include a variety of medical treatments that can provide a solution for many different kinds of infertility factors.

Assisted reproduction techniques are divided in:

- Techniques that imply an "in vivo" conception
  - Ovarian stimulations
  - IUI (intrauterine inseminations)
- Techniques that require surgical oocyte retrieval
  - IVF (in vitro fertilisation)
  - ICSI (intracytoplasmic sperm injection)
  - Cryopreservation of oocytes and embryos or percutaneous retrieval of sperms from testicles
- Techniques that require laparoscopy or surgical retrieval of sperms from testicles
- Gamete (sperm or oocytes) or embryo donation
- Surrogacy ("womb for rent")

The different ART techniques that can apply to transsexual couples depend on several factors, including the kind of modification of one's sexual traits and, consequently, the type of couple that is formed in the end [7, 8]. These techniques are summarised in Table 40.1.

1 Physical aspects include medical therapy as well as the surgical approach that has been elaborated and perfected during the last 50 years [2, 3].

Among the first group of techniques, intrauterine insemination with heterologous sperm (also known as AID – artificial insemination by donor) is suitable for couples formed by a trans man (FtM) and a cissexual woman [9]. Artificial insemination cannot be considered an assisted reproductive technique proper because the whole fertilisation process happens "in vivo". It is recommended in those cases when the tubal patency of the female partner has been medically ascertained. It entails the introduction of seminal fluid provided by a donor into the uterine cavity, using an atraumatic catheter which allows a painless passage through the cervical canal. This procedure requires that cryopreserved sperm is thawed and conveniently prepared for insemination.

Several studies stress that success rates of intrauterine insemination (either with heterologous or with homologous sperm) increase when this technique is combined to an ovarian hyperstimulation, which allows the maturation of a higher number of ovulatory follicles.

However, it has to be considered that hyperstimulation can lead to complications such as multiple pregnancies and OHSS (ovarian hyperstimulation syndrome). Therefore, the use of mild stimulation protocols and a regular monitoring of the ovarian response by ultrasound and (if necessary) hormonal tests are recommended.

Furthermore, it is advisable to perform intrauterine insemination only when the number of follicles is less than or equal to 3 and their dimension is greater than or equal to 16 mm.

Among the second group of techniques, in vitro fertilisation with heterologous sperm is applicable to the same kind of couple (trans man and cissexual woman) in case the female partner suffers from a tubal factor of infertility which makes it impossible to perform intrauterine insemination.

The fundamental stages of IVF (in vitro fertilisation) include surgical oocyte retrieval, their extracorporeal (in vitro) fertilisation of oocytes collected and the subsequent transfer into the maternal uterus of the embryos generated.

As for IVF, insemination is performed putting each of the retrieved oocytes into contact with a certain number of motile and morphologically normal sperms, in a set quantity of culture medium. The different stages of fertilisation (i.e. crossing of the oocyte barrier, fusion with the plasma membrane and penetration of the sperm into the oocyte) happen spontaneously, although in "in vitro" conditions.

The use of cryopreserved semen may require the technique known as ICSI (intracytoplasmic sperm injection) whenever at the moment of thawing the total motility of the semen sample makes it unsuitable for IVF. This is due to the fact that, in some cases, cryopreservation can compromise the total motility compared to the one observed at the moment of ejaculation.

ICSI entails the injection of one selected sperm directly into the oocyte cytoplasm using a micromanipulator.

In the case of a man that has completed the transition to woman (MtF), the couple (trans woman and cissexual man) can resort to egg donation with surrogate mother (see Table 40.1).

Egg donation is a technique that implies the donation of oocytes by a female donor that accepts undergoing hyperstimulation and retrieval of her oocytes. These oocytes are fertilised in vitro using the seminal fluid of the male partner, and the embryos obtained are subsequently transferred in the uterus of a third woman,

Table 40.1 Possible ARTs techniques in different transitioning processes

Transitioning process		Formed couple	Requested technique
♀ → ♂t		♂t – ♀	Sperm donation with IUI/IVF/ICSI
♂ → ♀t		♂ – ♀t	Egg donation with surrogate mother
♀ → ♂t	♂ → ♀t	♂t – ♀t	Embryo donation with surrogate mother
♀ → ♂t in absence of hysterectomy and annexectomy	♂ → ♀t with prior sperm cryopreservation	♂t – ♀t	In vitro fertilisation with the partner's cryopreserved semen

the so-called surrogate mother. Surrogacy, or gestational surrogacy, takes place when a woman takes the responsibility of carrying to term a pregnancy and giving birth on behalf of another couple. The surrogate mother gives up all parental rights and obligations towards the newborn. Before performing embryo transfer, the treatment implies the preparation of the uterine mucosa by means of a specific hormone therapy. Surplus embryos can be cryopreserved for potential use in future cycles.

Even though it is possible to cryopreserve human oocytes, the best results are obtained when a "fresh" egg donation is performed. In this case, the menstrual cycle of the surrogate mother is synchronised with that of the egg donor so that her endometrium is ready to receive embryos just when the donor's oocytes are fertilised [10].

Such synchronisation is obtained through a specific hormone replacement therapy (estrogens to be taken orally or transdermally and progesterone).

Initially, all the donors remained anonymous – which meant that the born child could not trace down who the oocyte donor was nor vice versa. Recently, some countries have made traceability compulsory, entitling the child born following gamete donation to have the legal right of gaining information about the identity of the person who donated the gametes that led to her/his birth.

When a couple is formed by two partners who have both transitioned to the other sex, the only possibility is embryo donation with surrogate mother. Notwithstanding this, whereas a biological female has undertaken a transitioning process without undergoing hysterectomy and annexectomy (in the countries where this is possible), conception can be achieved through sperm donation. In this case, the woman that has started a transition to become a man (FtM) will carry the baby to term, implying a suspension of the medical treatment for transition which will be resumed once the baby is born. After delivery, when the personal detail about sex in the civil registry is changed, the biological mother will be listed on the vital records as father.

Another possible option is a man transitioned to woman (MtF) who pre-emptively cryopreserved his seminal fluid and is therefore able to conceive through egg donation and surrogate mother. Also in this case, in presence of a change of the personal detail about sex in the civil registry, the biological father will be listed on the vital records as mother. Such therapeutic options are available thanks to the technology that permits cryopreservation of sperms, oocytes, zygotes and embryos and to the enhancement of these same techniques.

Until few years ago performing cryopreservation meant using a so-called "slow" process, during which embryos were gradually exposed to temperatures below zero degrees Celsius making use of cryoprotectants, substances used to protect biological tissues from freezing damage due to the formation of ice crystals within the cells.

Nevertheless, ice crystal formation at the moment of thawing could not be avoided, hence the pregnancy rates recorded were inferior compared to those obtained transferring fresh embryos.

In order to solve these problems, also and especially for what regards oocytes – which are more delicate – a new methodology called "vitrification" has been developed [5].

As it takes only a few minutes to vitrify a sample, by all means this technique prevents the formation of ice crystals by impeding the freezing of water molecules. Besides, the use of sucrose on the sample before it is vitrified causes the expulsion of all the water (and its replacement by cryoprotectant substances) before performing cryopreservation. Embryos can be vitrificated at any stage of their development [11].

While they can be applied to solve a wide range of infertility cases, gamete and embryo donation and surrogacy are ethically controversial techniques, and for these reasons they are prohibited in several countries. This generated a great legislative disparity among the various countries in the world and also within the same continent. This discrepancy has originated the phenomenon of "cross-border reproductive care". Cross-border reproductive care, also known as "reproductive tourism", refers to the travelling of citizens from their country of residence to another country in order to receive fertility treatment through assisted reproductive technology [4].

In conclusion, it is important to stress that cross-sex identification per se does not make transsexual people unsuitable to parenthood. In fact, their sexual identities do not impair their ability to understand the nature and consequences of pregnancy nor predictably interfere with the ability to raise children. Moreover, no evidence suggests that being born to and raised by transgender parents can affect negatively the psychosocial development of the newborn in a way that would justify exclusion of trans-identified men and women from ARTs as a class [6].

References

1. Cociglio G, Fontana D, Massobrio M, Rovera GG (eds) (1999) La coppia. Nuove realtà, nuovi valori, nuovi problemi. Franco Angeli, Milano
2. Trombetta C, Liguori G, Pascone M, Bucci S, Guaschino S, Papa G, Belgrano E (2002) Total sex-reassignment surgery in female-to-male transsexuals: a one-stage technique. BJU Int. doi:10.1046/j.1464-410X.2002.03009.x
3. Trombetta C, Liguori G, Buttazzi L, Bucci S, Ciciliato S, Belgrano E (2002b) La femminilizzazione dei genitali esterni e la creazione della neovagina. In: Nadalin DA, Stella P (eds) Transiti: percorsi e significati dell'identità di genere: convegno scientifico internazionale: Aula Absidale di S. Lucia, Via De' Chiari 25/a, 28-29-20 giugno 2002. Regione Emilia-Romagna, Bologna, pp 111–118
4. Ferraretti AP, Pennings G, Gianaroli L, Natali F, Magli MC (2009) Cross border reproductive care: a phenomenon focusing the controversial aspects of reproductive technologies. Reprod Biomed Online. doi:10.1016/j.rbmo.2009.11.009
5. Kuleshova L, Gianaroli L, Magli MC, Ferraretti AP, Trounson AO (1999) Birth following vitrification of a small number of human oocytes. Hum Reprod. doi:10.1093/humrep/14.12.3077
6. Murphy TF (2010) The ethics of helping transgender men and women have children. Perspect Biol Med. doi:10.1353/pbm.0.0138
7. T'sjoen G, Van Caenegem E, Wierckx K (2013) Transgenderism and reproduction. Curr Opin Endocrinol Diabetes Obes. doi:10.1097/01.med.0000436184.42554.b7
8. Wierckx K, Van Caenegem E, Pennings G, Elaut E, Dedecker D, Van de Peer F, Weyers S, De Sutter P, T'Sjoen G (2012) Reproductive wish in transsexual men. Hum Reprod. doi:10.1093/humrep/der406
9. Faccio E, Bordin E, Cipolletta S (2013) Transsexual parenthood and new role assumptions. Cult Health Sex. doi:10.1080/13691058.2013.806676
10. Ferraretti AP, Pennings G, Gianaroli L, Magli MC (2006) Semen donor recruitment in an oocyte donation programme. Hum Reprod. doi:10.1093/humrep/del204
11. Gianaroli L, Resta S, Magli MC, Ferraretti AP (2009) Vitrification of the human oocyte: a practical approach. In: Rao KA (ed) The infertility manual, 3rd edn. Jitendar P Vij. Location: New Delhi. pp 588–594

MIX
Papier aus verantwortungsvollen Quellen
Paper from responsible sources
FSC® C105338

If you have any concerns about our products,
you can contact us on
ProductSafety@springernature.com

In case Publisher is established outside the EU,
the EU authorized representative is:
Springer Nature Customer Service Center GmbH
Europaplatz 3, 69115 Heidelberg, Germany

Printed by Libri Plureos GmbH
in Hamburg, Germany